Current Research in Brain Cancer

Current Research in Brain Cancer

Editor: Carmen Ferguson

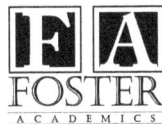

FA
FOSTER
ACADEMICS

www.fosteracademics.com

www.fosteracademics.com

FA
FOSTER
A C A D E M I C S

Cataloging-in-Publication Data

Current research in brain cancer / edited by Carmen Ferguson.
      p. cm.
Includes bibliographical references and index.
ISBN 978-1-63242-743-4
1. Brain--Cancer. 2. Brain--Cancer--Research. 3. Brain--Tumors. I. Ferguson, Carmen.
RC280.B7 C87 2019
616.994 81--dc23

Foster Academics,
118-35 Queens Blvd., Suite 400,
Forest Hills, NY 11375, USA

ISBN 978-1-63242-743-4 (Hardback)

Contents

Preface

Over the recent decade, advancements and applications have progressed exponentially. This has led to the increased interest in this field and projects are being conducted to enhance knowledge. The main objective of this book is to present some of the critical challenges and provide insights into possible solutions. This book will answer the varied questions that arise in the field and also provide an increased scope for furthering studies.

Brain cancers occur when an abnormal growth of cells occurs in the brain. Some types of brain cancer are medulloblastoma, astrocytoma, meningiomas, etc. A form of astrocytoma called glioblastoma is the most aggressive form of brain cancer. Symptoms of brain cancer include headaches, vomiting, seizures, altered vision and mental changes. It is diagnosed using computed tomography (CT) or magnetic resonance imaging (MRI) scans and the result is confirmed usually through a biopsy. The treatment of brain cancer may involve a combination of chemotherapy, radiation therapy and surgery. No therapy has yet shown any progress in increasing life expectancy in people with malignant gliomas. However, cancer immunotherapy is being actively studied. Research is also being pursued in the use of vesicular stomatitis virus and retroviral replicating vectors as management strategies for brain cancer. The objective of this book is to give a modern perspective on brain cancer. Different approaches, evaluations, methodologies and advanced studies on brain cancer have been included in this book. Students, researchers, experts and all associated with neurology, neuroscience, surgical oncology, clinical oncology and radiation oncology will benefit alike from this book.

I hope that this book, with its visionary approach, will be a valuable addition and will promote interest among readers. Each of the authors has provided their extraordinary competence in their specific fields by providing different perspectives as they come from diverse nations and regions. I thank them for their contributions.

Editor

Analysis of cellular and molecular antitumor effects upon inhibition of SATB1 in glioblastoma cells

Anja Frömberg[1], Michael Rabe[2], Henry Oppermann[3], Frank Gaunitz[3] and Achim Aigner[1*]

Abstract

Background: The Special AT-rich Sequence Binding Protein 1 (SATB1) regulates the expression of many genes by acting as a global chromatin organizer. While in many tumor entities SATB1 overexpression has been observed and connected to pro-tumorigenic processes, somewhat contradictory evidence exists in brain tumors with regard to SATB1 overexpression in glioblastoma and its association with poorer prognosis and tumor progression. On the functional side, initial data indicate that SATB1 may be involved in several tumor cell-relevant processes.

Methods: For the detailed analysis of the functional relevance and possible therapeutic potential of SATB1 inhibition, we employ transient siRNA-mediated knockdown and comprehensively analyze the cellular and molecular role of SATB1 in glioblastoma.

Results: In various cell lines with different SATB1 expression levels, a SATB1 gene dose-dependent inhibition of anchorage-dependent and –independent proliferation is observed. This is due to cell cycle-inhibitory and pro-apoptotic effects of SATB1 knockdown. Molecular analyses reveal SATB1 knockdown effects on multiple important (proto-) oncogenes, including Myc, Bcl-2, Pim-1, EGFR, β-catenin and Survivin. Molecules involved in cell cycle, EMT and cell adhesion are affected as well. The putative therapeutic relevance of SATB1 inhibition is further supported in an in vivo tumor xenograft mouse model, where the treatment with polymeric nanoparticles containing SATB1-specific siRNAs exerts antitumor effects.

Conclusion: Our results demonstrate that SATB1 may represent a promising target molecule in glioblastoma therapy whose inhibition or knockdown affects multiple crucial pathways.

Keywords: SATB1, Glioblastoma, RNAi, siRNA, PEI nanoparticles

Background

Malignant glioblastoma is the most common primary adult brain tumor in Western nations [1]. Despite aggressive treatment regimens including surgery, chemo- and radiotherapy, the prognosis for patients with the highest grade tumor, glioblastoma multiforme (GBM), has remained very poor. In fact, the overall survival rate is 12–15 months and the 5-years survival rate is only 5%. Limitations in complete resection and resistance towards adjunct radio- and chemotherapy account for this failure of treatment strategies and demonstrate the need for other therapeutic approaches based on novel targets. An optimal candidate should be overexpressed in the tumor tissue, with less expression and relevance in normal tissue, and its inhibition should ideally lead to multiple cellular and molecular effects harmful to the tumor cell.

The Special AT-rich Sequence Binding Protein 1 (SATB1) has been shown to regulate the expression of a large number of genes by acting as a global chromatin organizer [2]. More specifically, SATB1 interacts with the altered sugar-phosphate backbone of the DNA, that is specific for double-stranded base-unpairing regions (BURs) often found in matrix attachment regions (MARs) at the base of chromatin loops [3]. In the nuclei of thymocytes, SATB1 has a cage-like network distribution

* Correspondence: achim.aigner@medizin.uni-leipzig.de
[1]Rudolf-Boehm-Institute for Pharmacology and Toxicology, Clinical Pharmacology, University of Leipzig, Haertelstrasse 16 – 18, D-04107 Leipzig, Germany
Full list of author information is available at the end of the article

and tethers specialized DNA sequences onto its network [4]. Additionally, SATB1 binds and connects so-called "chromatin-remodeling complexes" to DNA and thus functions as a "landing platform" for chromatin remodeling enzymes [5]. In this way, SATB1 folds chromatin into loops and allows SATB1 to control the expression of a multitude of genes in a manner that is dependent on cell type and cell function [4, 6–9]. SATB1 is required in some physiological processes including the development of thymocytes [7] and the activation of Th2 cells [6]; it furthermore participates in the development of epidermis and epidermal differentiation [10], in X-chromosome inactivation [11], cortical development [12] and in the differentiation of mouse embryonic stem cells [13].

More importantly, SATB1 has been found to be overexpressed in various tumors and associated with prognosis and clinicopathological features. Examples include aggressive breast cancer [2], gastric cancer [14, 15], prostate cancer [16], liver cancer [17], laryngeal squamous cell carcinoma [18], ovarian carcinoma [19, 20], cervical carcinoma [21], pancreatic carcinoma [22], colorectal cancer [23–27] and malignant melanoma [28]. In different tumor entities including breast cancer, small cell lung cancer, liver cancer, osteosarcoma, prostate cancer and colorectal cancer, the stable RNAi-mediated knockdown of SATB1 has revealed multiple effects on the cellular level, including cell cycle [17, 22, 26], cell proliferation [2, 17, 22, 25, 26, 29], apoptosis [17, 25, 29], epithelial-mesenchymal transition (EMT) [17], invasiveness [2, 16, 22, 25, 26, 29] and/or tumor growth [2, 16, 17, 26, 27, 29].

In brain tumors, the situation appears so far to be more complex. A significant association of SATB1 levels with histological grade and poor survival has been described in low and high grade astrocytoma including glioblastoma [29, 30]. According to the recent WHO classification, glioblastoma is defined as grade IV astrocytoma. Chu et al. demonstrated that SATB1 mRNA and protein expression was low in normal brain and in grade I-II astrocytoma specimens but highly upregulated in grade III-IV astrocytoma patients [31]. SATB1 expression was positively correlated with astrocytoma pathological grade, while a negative correlation with patients' overall survival was found [31]. In contrast, another study found an inverse correlation between SATB1 expression and tumor grade/patient survival, and identified only phospho-SATB1 as relevant [32]. Likewise, a Rembrandt/TCGA database analysis (http://www.betastasis.com/glioma/rembrandt/gene_expression_in_glioma_subtypes/) did not support the notion of SATB1 overexpression in brain tumors. In another study, initial results in one cell line indicated a possible role of SATB1 in some cellular and molecular processes [29]. Despite opposite findings with regard to SATB1 expression in glioblastoma and tumor grade/

prognosis, another study found inhibitory effects of a SATB1 decoy on cell proliferation and invasion [32].

Taken together, this clearly warrants a more detailed analysis of the molecular and cellular consequences of SATB1 inhibition in glioblastoma, in order to establish the functional relevance of different levels of SATB1 expression in this tumor and to evaluate the putative therapeutic value of SATB1 inhibition, beyond a therapeutically less relevant stable knockdown. In fact, in order to avoid possible adaptive processes upon constitutive knockdown or overexpression, we employed a transient siRNA-mediated knockdown strategy in this paper. We comprehensively analyze the cellular and molecular role of SATB1 in various glioblastoma cell lines with different SATB1 expression levels, establishing in vitro and in vivo the functional relevance of SATB1 in glioblastoma, and the possible therapeutic potential of SATB1 inhibition.

Methods

Cell lines, primary cultures and cell culture conditions

Glioblastoma cell lines T98G, U-87 MG, U373 and LN-229 were obtained from the American type culture collection (ATCC). MZ-54 and MZ-18 cell lines were kindly provided by Dr. Donat Kögel (Experimental Neurosurgery, Frankfurt University Clinic, Frankfurt, Germany) [33], and the G55T2 cell line was a kind gift from Dr. Katrin Lamszus (Dept. of Neurosurgery, University Medical Center Hamburg-Eppendorf, Hamburg, Germany) [34]. U343 cells were established by B. Westermark [35]. All cell lines were cultivated under standard conditions (37 °C, 5% CO_2) in Iscove's Modified Dulbecco's Medium (IMDM; Sigma-Aldrich, St. Louis, MO), supplemented with 10% fetal calf serum (FCS) and 2 mM stable L-Alanyl-L-Glutamine (Biochrom GmbH, Berlin, Germany) unless stated otherwise. Depending on the cell lines and the experimental setup, appropriate plate sizes and cell densities were chosen to reach 80 to 90% cell confluency at the end of the experiment. Cell lines were regularly tested for (absence of) mycoplasma, using the Venor GeM kit (Biostep, Berlin, Germany) based on very sensitive PCR detection.

Primary cell cultures from surgically removed glioblastoma tissues were established as described [36]. Briefly, freshly removed tumor tissue was washed with PBS (phosphate buffered saline) and minced with a scalpel blade. After mincing, small tissue pieces were transferred to a 25 cm^2 culture flask (TPP, Trasadingen, Switzerland) sprinkled with AmnioMax complete medium (Thermo Fisher Scientific, Darmstadt, Germany). Cells were incubated for 30 min at room temperature and finally, 1 ml AmnioMax complete medium was added. Incubation was then performed at 37 °C, 5% CO_2 and humidified air in an incubator. Medium was changed after

72 h. As soon as a confluent layer was obtained, cells were removed from culture flasks by use of accutase (PAA, Pasching, Austria) and transferred to 75 cm^2 culture flasks (TPP). AmnioMax Medium with AmnioMax Supplement was used for the first 2–3 weeks of cultivation. Thereafter, and in the experiments described, DMEM Medium supplemented with 2 mM Glutamax, streptomycin and penicillin and 10% fetal calf serum (Biochrome, Berlin, Germany) was used for cultivation.

Analysis of SATB1 expression in primary glioblastoma and normal brain tissue

For the RNA isolation from primary tissue, fresh surgically obtained tumor tissue was transferred into RNAlater (Qiagen, Hilden; Germany) immediately after removal in order to stabilize RNA. Then, total RNA from 40 to 80 mg of stabilized tissue was extracted using the miRNeasy kit (Qiagen) and the RNA was stored at –80 °C until further use. For the isolation of mRNA from cultured cells and cell lines 0.5×10^6 cells were used and also prepared using the miRNeasy kit according to manufacturer's instructions. All patients provided written informed consent according to the German laws, as confirmed by the local ethics committee. Surgery was performed between 2010 and 2013 at the University of Leipzig, Medical Faculty, Department of Neurosurgery. The samples were histopathologically confirmed as glioblastoma multiforme. For cDNA synthesis the ImProm-II™ Reverse Transcription System (Promega, Mannheim, Germany) was employed according to manufacturer's protocol, using 500 ng of total RNA. qRT-PCR was performed on a Rotor-Gene 3000 system (Qiagen) with SYBR Green (Maxima SYBR Green/ROX qPCR Master Mix, Thermo Scientific, Germany). Data analysis was performed using the Rotor-Gene 6 software (Version 6.1/Build 93; Corbett Research) and relative mRNA expression was calculated by the $2^{-\Delta Ct}$ method using TBP (TATA box binding protein) as housekeeping gene. cDNA from normal brain tissue was obtained from BioCat (Heidelberg, Germany).

Transient transfection

SiRNAs were purchased from Sigma-Aldrich (Taufkirchen, Germany) or Eurofins MWG Operon (Ebersberg, Germany); see Additional file 1: Table S1 for sequence information. SiRNAs targeting luciferase (pGL3) were used as negative control. Prior to transfection, cells were seeded in appropriate cell culture plates and maintained overnight under standard conditions. 2.5 nM siRNA were transfected using INTERFERin™ (Polyplus, Illkirch, France), at 1 µl INTERFERin™/pmol siRNA (U-87 MG) or 0.5 µl INTERFERin™/pmol siRNA (G55T2, U343, MZ-18) according to the manufacturer's protocol.

RNA preparation and qRT-PCR in cell lines

Total RNA was isolated using TRI Reagent® (Sigma-Aldrich) according to manufacturer's instructions. The RevertAid™ H Minus First Strand cDNA Synthesis Kit (Fermentas, St. Leon-Roth, Germany) was used to reversely transcribe 1 µg of total RNA with random hexamer primers. For quantitative PCR, a LightCycler® 2.0 (Roche, Mannheim, Germany) and the Absolute™ QPCR SYBR® Green Capillary Mix (Thermo Scientific) were used as described previously [37]. Quantification of gene expression was performed based on the $\Delta\Delta C_t$ method, with β-actin as reference housekeeping gene. Control experiments revealed that very similar results were obtained for β-actin vs. TBP as housekeeping genes, indicating the usefulness of both primer sets for normalization. Primers were purchased from Eurofins MWG Operon (for sequences, see Additional file 2: Table S2).

Western blotting

5×10^4 G55T2 or U-87 MG cells were seeded in 6-well plates and transfected as described above. 72 h (G55T2) or 96 h (U-87 MG) after transfection, cells were washed with PBS and lysed as described previously [37]. 50 µg (U-87MG) or 10–20 µg (G55T2) total protein was separated by SDS-PAGE, prior to transfer onto a 0.2 µM or 0.45 µM PROTRAN® nitrocellulose membrane (Whatman, Dassel, Germany). Membranes were blocked with 5% (w/v) non-fat dry milk in TBST (10 mM Tris/HCl, pH 7.6, 150 mM NaCl, 0.1% Tween 20), washed with TBST and incubated overnight with primary antibodies at 4 °C as detailed in Additional file 3: Table S3. After washing with TBST, membranes were incubated with horseradish peroxidase-coupled secondary antibodies (Additional file 3: Table S3) for 1 h at room temperature. Bound antibodies were visualized using the chemiluminescence ECL kit from Thermo Scientific. For parallel detection of phosphorylated proteins and their corresponding unphosphorylated counterpart, membranes were incubated in stripping buffer (0.2 M glycin, 3.5 mM sodium dodecyl sulfate, 1% (v/v) Tween-20, pH 2.2) for 30 min at room temperature, washed with TBST and blocked again with 5% (w/v) non-fat dry milk in TBST, prior to further processing as described above.

Anchorage-dependent and -independent proliferation

Anchorage-dependent proliferation was analyzed using a WST-1 colorimetric assay (Roche). 200 cells/well were seeded in 96-well plates and transfected as described above. At the time points indicated in the Figures, viable cells were quantified in triplicate wells using WST-1 colorimetric assay according to manufacturer's protocol. To measure anchorage-independent proliferation, U-87 MG cells were seeded in 6-well plates and transfected as described above. 48 h after transfection, soft agar assays were performed as described previously [37]. Soft agars were run in triplicate wells and incubated under standard conditions. At the time points indicated, colonies > 50 μm were counted by at least two blinded investigators.

Cell cycle analysis

For cell cycle analysis, 1×10^4 U-87 MG or G55T2 cells were seeded into 24-well plates and transfected as described above. 72 h after transfection, cells were treated with 100 ng/ml nocodazole (Merck-Calbiochem®, Darmstadt, Germany) in IMDM/10% FCS for 8 h to induce a G2/M arrest. The cells were harvested by trypsinization, washed with PBS and fixed with 70% ethanol at 4 °C overnight. Prior to addition of 50 μg/ml propidium iodide (Sigma-Aldrich), cells were incubated with 50 μg/ml RNase A for 30 min at 37 °C and subsequently analyzed by flow cytometry using an Attune® Acoustic Focusing Cytometer (Life Technologies, Darmstadt, Germany).

Apoptosis assays

To quantify the activity of caspases 3 and 7, the bioluminescent Caspase-Glo® 3/7 assay (Promega, Mannheim, Germany) was used. 300 cells (U-87 MG) or 750 cells (G55T2) were seeded per well in 96-well plates, transfected as described above and maintained under standard conditions for 96 h. The Caspase-Glo® assay was performed according to the manufacturer's protocol. Luminescence was measured using a POLARstar Omega reader (BMG Labtec, Jena, Germany) after 1 h of incubation at room temperature in the dark. A WST-1 assay was performed in parallel on the same plate as described above, to normalize for slight variations in cell densities.

Mouse xenograft model

To investigate the effects of RNAi-mediated SATB1-knockdown on tumor growth in vivo, 3×10^6 U-87 MG cells in 150 μl PBS were injected into both flanks of 6–8 weeks old athymic nude mice (Crl:CD1-Foxn1nu, Charles River Laboratories, Sulzfeld, Germany). When solid tumors were established, mice were randomized into treatment and control groups. The tumors were treated with intratumoral injections of 2 μg siRNA complexed with 10 μg PEI F25-LMW [38] in a total volume of 30 μl. The tumors were treated every 2 to 3 days and tumor growth was monitored as indicated in Fig. 4a. Animal studies were conducted according to the national regulations of animal welfare and approved by the local authorities (Regierungspräsidium Giessen, Germany).

Statistics

Statistical analysis was performed by Student's t-test and significance levels are $* = p < 0.05$, $** = p < 0.01$, $*** = p < 0.001$, $\# =$ not significant as compared to siCtrl, unless indicated otherwise. Values are shown as means +/− s.e.m.

Results

Determination of SATB1 expression in primary glioblastoma tissue and cells, compared to normal brain tissue

In contrast to other tumor entities where SATB1 upregulation as compared to normal tissue has been well established, the situation in glioblastoma appears less clear (see Background). Therefore, we first analyzed SATB1 mRNA levels of ten different primary tumor samples. While all tumors showed SATB1 expression, levels varied considerably between different samples, with a maximum ~10-fold difference (Additional file 4: Figure S1, center). The same was true for primary tumor cells derived from these tumors, with values often, but not in all cases being comparable between a primary tumor and its corresponding primary cell line (Additional file 4: Figure S1, center). Notably, in comparison to normal brain tissue no SATB1 upregulation was observed in tumors, with tumor levels rather being even lower (Additional file 4: Figure S1, left). From these data, we conclude that SATB1 expression levels may only poorly predict its functional relevance, thus requiring more detailed analyses in a panel of cell lines with different SATB1 expression levels.

Expression of SATB1 in various glioblastoma cell lines and comparison to SATB2

Based on the heterogeneous situation with regard to SATB1 expression levels in glioblastoma, we screened a set of eight commercially available and well-established glioblastoma cell lines for SATB1 levels. qRT-PCR results demonstrated substantial expression of SATB1 in 7/8 cell lines, with the only exception being T98G cells that showed almost no SATB1 (Additional file 4: Figure S1, right). Some variations between positive cell lines were observed with a maximum ~9-fold difference in SATB1. SATB2, which is considered as a functional counterpart of SATB1, was analyzed as well. Here, expression was observed in all 8 cell lines (Additional file 5: Figure S2). The comparison between SATB1 and SATB2 levels revealed no correlation in expression levels.

The expression of SATB1 in almost all glioblastoma cell lines provided the basis for subsequent functional studies. To this end, four glioblastoma cell lines (U-87 MG, MZ-18, G55T2 and U343) with high or low SATB1 levels, thus covering the broad range of SATB1 expression, were selected for transient RNAi-mediated knockdown. To exclude false-positive results due to off-target effects and to allow the establishment of gene-dose effects, two siRNAs validated previously for specific

SATB1 knockdown to different degrees were employed and compared to untreated as well as to negative control transfected cells (siRNA targeting the luciferase gene which is not expressed in glioblastoma cells). In all cell lines, qRT-PCR after single transfection with the less potent SATB1-specific siRNA (si989) revealed a ~ 50% SATB1 knockdown in comparison to negative controls (wt and siCtrl). A > 60% knockdown was observed with the more potent si467 (Fig. 1a and Additional file 6: Figure S3A), with only minor differences between the four selected cell lines. Knockdown results were confirmed on the protein level by Western blots, showing a concomitant reduction of SATB1 with bands upon si467 transfection being close to the limit of detection (Fig. 1b). This was also true at later time points (e.g., 120 h, 144 h after transfection; data not shown). We thus concluded that the transient siRNA

transfection provides an efficient tool for specific SATB1 downregulation.

Inhibitory effects of SATB1 knockdown on cell proliferation

To initially explore the effects of SATB1 knockdown on overall cell proliferation and viability, WST-1 proliferation assays were performed. Growth curves revealed a marked reduction of cell proliferation upon transfection with si989 in all cell lines (Fig. 1c and Additional file 6: Figure S3B). Except for G55T2 cells, no nonspecific transfection effects were observed. Using the more potent si467, cell proliferation was reduced by > 80%, indicating very profound effects of the SATB1 knockdown on the number of viable cells. These results were confirmed in a soft agar assay, which resembles more closely the in vivo situation. Upon siRNA transfection of U87

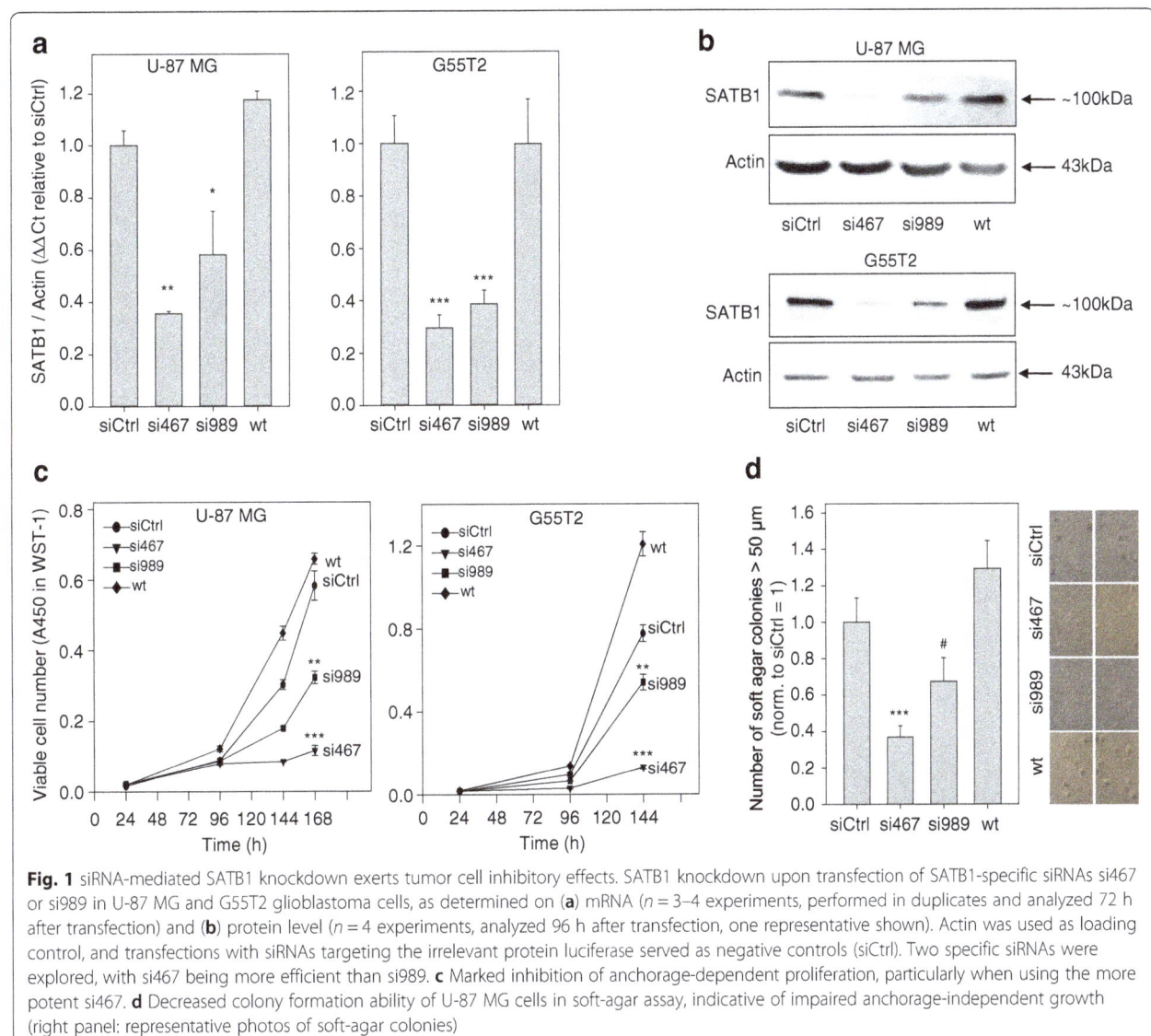

Fig. 1 siRNA-mediated SATB1 knockdown exerts tumor cell inhibitory effects. SATB1 knockdown upon transfection of SATB1-specific siRNAs si467 or si989 in U-87 MG and G55T2 glioblastoma cells, as determined on (a) mRNA (n = 3–4 experiments, performed in duplicates and analyzed 72 h after transfection) and (b) protein level (n = 4 experiments, analyzed 96 h after transfection, one representative shown). Actin was used as loading control, and transfections with siRNAs targeting the irrelevant protein luciferase served as negative controls (siCtrl). Two specific siRNAs were explored, with si467 being more efficient than si989. c Marked inhibition of anchorage-dependent proliferation, particularly when using the more potent si467. d Decreased colony formation ability of U-87 MG cells in soft-agar assay, indicative of impaired anchorage-independent growth (right panel: representative photos of soft-agar colonies)

MG cells, a reduction in the anchorage-independent colony formation was observed, which was again dependent on the siRNA efficacy and reached a > 60% decrease in colonies in the case of si467 (Fig. 1d).

Cell cycle inhibition and induction of apoptosis upon SATB1 knockdown

To further explore the underlying cellular mechanisms of the reduction of the number of viable cells upon SATB1 knockdown, we next analyzed effects on cell cycle. Here and in subsequent experiments, we selected the two cell lines, U-87 MG and G55T2. Cells were transfected with the respective siRNAs and 72 h later nocodazole treatment was started in order to implement a G2/M block. When cells were propidium iodide-stained and analyzed by flow cytometry upon 8 h

nocodazole treatment, 40% (U87 MG) or 70% (G55T2) of the cells were in G2/M (Fig. 2a). In contrast, upon transfection with SATB1-specific siRNAs si989 and especially si467 this percentage was reduced, indicative of cell cycle deceleration/arrest in G_0/G_1 with a smaller number of cells reaching the block within the selected time frame. Consequently, a larger fraction of cells was determined in the G_0/G_1 phase (Fig. 2a, right panels). In both cell lines, the degree of cell cycle inhibition was dependent on the siRNA efficacy and thus the residual SATB1 levels, with si467 showing more profound effects.

In addition to cell cycle deceleration, SATB1 knockdown led to the induction of apoptosis as indicated by increasing caspase-3/-7 activity. More specifically, while the transfection with si989 led to little or no effects

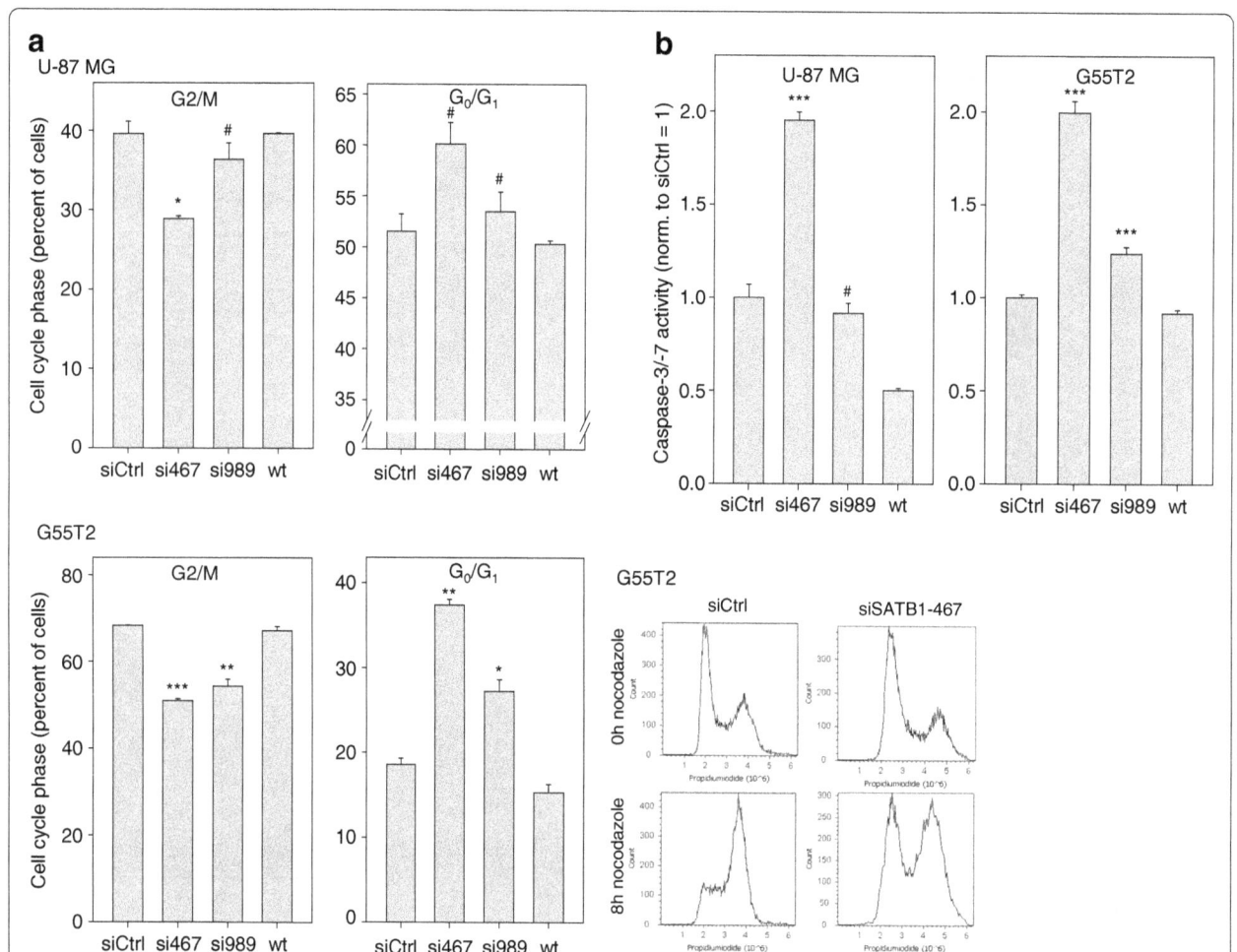

Fig. 2 Effects of SATB1 knockdown on cell cycle and apoptosis. **a** Transient SATB1 knockdown leads to a decreased percentage of cells in G2/M and an increase of cells in G_0/G_1, as determined in U-87 MG (upper panel) and G55T2 glioblastoma cells (lower panel). Cell cycle inhibition is more pronounced when using the more efficient si467, indicating a SATB1 gene-dose effect. Measurements were performed 8 h after addition of nocodazole (see text for details; $n = 2$ experiments per cell line). Lower right: representative flow cytometry histograms. **b** Induction of apoptosis upon transient SATB1 knockdown, as determined by increased caspase-3/-7 activity. Effects are seen in both U-87 MG (left) and G55T2 glioblastoma cells (right) and are dependent on the degree of SATB1 reduction

depending on the cell line, the more potent si467 resulted in a profound up to 2-fold increase in caspase activity.

Molecular consequences of SATB1 knockdown

The siRNA-mediated knockdown of SATB1 revealed effects on the expression levels of a broad spectrum of (proto-) oncogenes and various molecules involved in cell cycle, EMT, signal transduction and cell adhesion, as detected on the mRNA level by quantitative RT-PCR and on the protein level by Western blotting in G55T2 cells. Although the other family member, SATB2, is considered as a potential functional counterpart with opposite roles, qRT-PCR revealed it was downregulated by siRNAs 467 and 989 in parallel with SATB1 (Fig. 3a). By analyzing the siRNA sequences with regard to sequence

homologies, it was firmly excluded that this observation was due to unwanted off-target effects of SATB1-specific siRNAs on SATB2 based on any partial sequence homology [39]. Additionally, the observed absence of decreased SATB2 levels upon SATB1 knockdown in cells from another tumor entity further substantiates the notion of SATB2 reduction as a specific effect downstream of SATB1. In line with the observed cell cycle deceleration, cell cycle proteins Cyclin B1 and D1 that are often overexpressed in tumor cells were downregulated upon SATB1 knockdown. Again, the transfection with the more potent si467 led to a more profound reduction of Cyclin mRNAs with a > 50% decrease in the case of Cyclin B1. Rather mild effects were observed on TGFβ or the transcription factors Slug and Twist, with slightly increased mRNA levels upon SATB1 knockdown. In

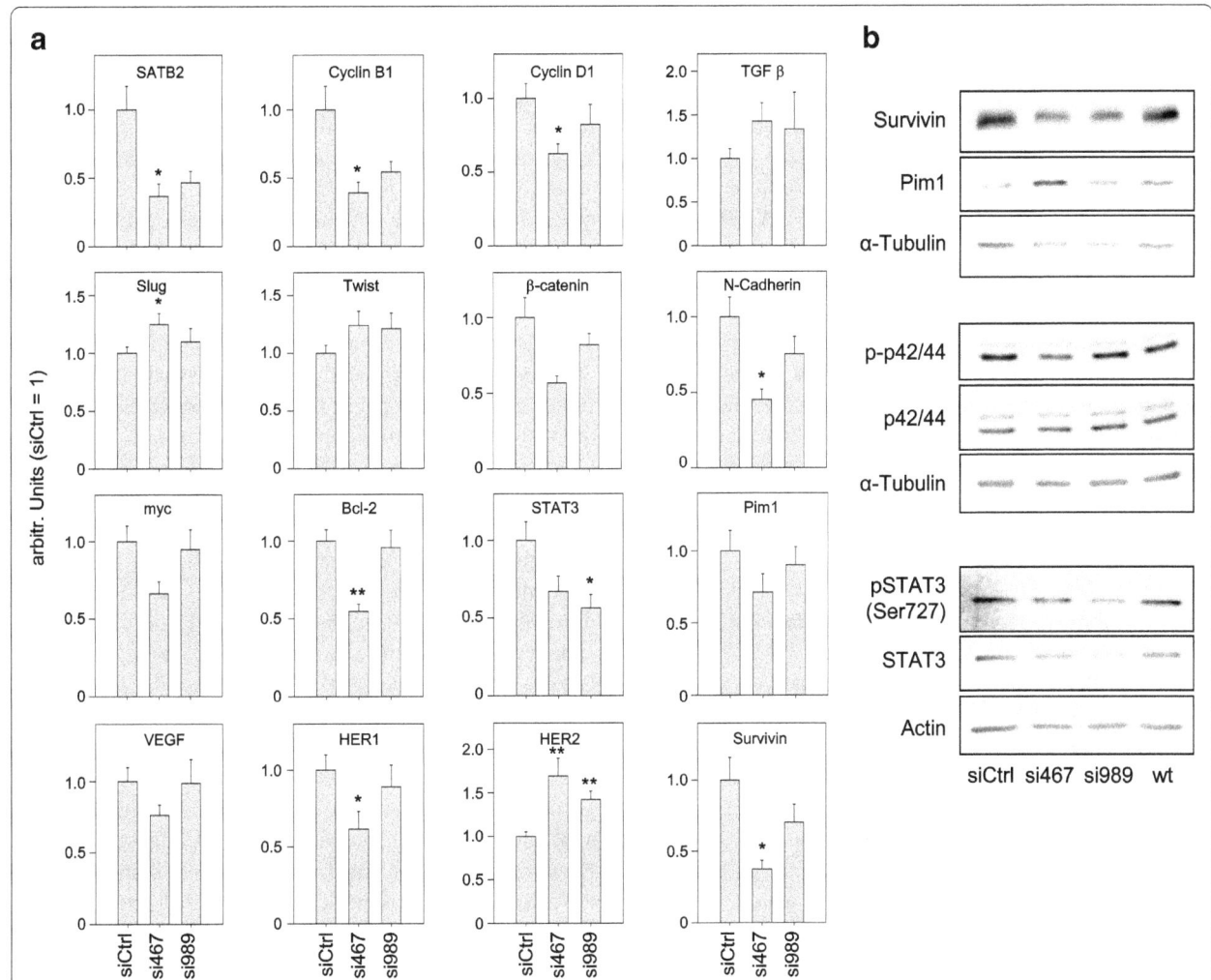

Fig. 3 Analysis of molecular consequences of SATB1 knockdown in G55T2 cells. The siRNA-mediated knockdown of SATB1 affects the expression levels of a broad spectrum of (proto-) oncogenes and various molecules involved in cell cycle, EMT, signal transduction and cell adhesion, as determined on the mRNA level by quantitative RT-PCR at 48 – 72 h after transfection (**a**) and on the protein level by Western blotting (**b**). For details, see text. In (**a**), differences that reached significance are indicated (n = 5–6 experiments determined at 72 h after transfection; Slug and Twist: n = 9 experiments determined at 48 – 72 h after transfection)

contrast, profound inhibitory effects were detected on the cell adhesion and gene transcription regulating proto-oncogene β-catenin and on N-Cadherin which were again dependent on the siRNA efficacy and led to ~50% reduced levels in the case of si467. While si989 exerted effects as well, albeit to a lesser degree, in the case of Myc and Bcl-2 downregulated mRNA levels were only observed with si467, indicative of a threshold of minimally required SATB1 knockdown. The same was true for the (rather mild) reduction in mRNA levels of the pro-angiogenic VEGF, while in the case of the proto-oncogenes Pim1 and HER1 si989 slightly reduced mRNA expression while si467 led again to a more profound decrease up to 60–70% residual level. Opposite to HER1, the SATB1 knockdown led to an increase in HER2 expression which was again gene-dose dependent and thus most profound upon si467 transfection. Finally, profound inhibitory effects on the mRNA level were also observed on STAT3 and Survivin (Fig. 3a). The latter finding correlated well with decreased protein levels of the anti-apoptotic protein Survivin as determined in Western blot experiments, with si467 showing the most profound effects (Fig. 3b, upper panel). Interestingly, the same siRNA led to an increase, rather than decrease, in Pim1 protein levels. Consequences of SATB1 knockdown were also explored with regard to downstream signaling. While the total expression of p42/44 (ERK1/2) remained unchanged, ERK phosphorylation was reduced (Fig. 3b, center panel). Again, this effect was only observed upon si467 transfection indicative of the requirement of sufficiently profound SATB1 knockdown. Quite in contrast, effects of SATB1 knockdown on STAT3 were already observed on the level of protein expression (Fig. 3b, lower panel), thus being in line with the qRT-PCR data, with a concomitant and parallel decrease of phospho-STAT3.

Tumor inhibitory effects of SATB1 knockdown in vivo

The consequence of siRNA-mediated SATB1 knockdown was finally tested in a more relevant in vivo situation by exploring tumor-inhibitory effects in an s.c. xenograft model. Rather than using stably transfected cells, which may well interfere with tumor xenograft formation, the SATB1 knockdown was performed in already established tumors. To this end, mice were treated with siRNAs formulated in polymeric, polyethylenimine (PEI)-based nanoparticles, which mediate siRNA protection, cellular delivery and intracellular release. As shown previously by our group, PEI/siRNA nanoparticles allow for the knockdown of the respective target gene (see e.g. [40, 41]). Indeed, a ~ 40% inhibition of the growth of established tumors was observed as compared to untreated or PEI/negative control siRNA-treated mice (Fig. 4a). Results from

tumor size measurements were paralleled and confirmed by a reduction of tumor mass, as detected upon termination of the experiment by excision of the tumor xenografts for weight determination (Fig. 4b).

Discussion

In the light of conflicting results regarding a positive [29–31] or negative [32] correlation between SATB1 expression and clinicopathological features of glioblastoma, and thus the relevance of SATB1 in these tumors, a deeper understanding of the cellular and molecular roles of SATB1 in glioblastoma cells is required. Indeed, our qRT-PCR screening data presented here do not support the notion of SATB1 overexpression in glioblastoma. While a recent analysis in colorectal cancer [42] has identified divergent expression patterns of SATB1 on the mRNA and protein level versus normal tissues, which may offer an explanation for rather low mRNA levels in tumors, only in-depth functional studies allows for evaluating the relevance of SATB1 in glioblastoma.

Here, the approach of transient RNAi, avoiding issues related to stable cell transfection with constitutive knockdown or overexpression, offers an excellent avenue. Notably, we found proliferation inhibitory effects of SATB1 knockdown in *all* glioblastoma cell lines tested, thus being independent of initial SATB1 expression levels. This emphasizes the general relevance of SATB1 beyond differences in mRNA levels and suggests SATB1 inhibition as a promising therapeutic avenue. Subsequent cellular analyses also revealed that this tumor cell inhibition upon SATB1 knockdown is based on the induction of apoptosis, as indicated previously [29], but also on cell cycle deceleration. This supports the notion that SATB1 acts on several pathways and its inhibition thus exerts multiple effects in parallel. In line with this, various key players are affected by SATB1 knockdown on the molecular level. This includes the downregulation of Cyclins B1 and D1 (deceleration of cell cycle in the transition from G2 to M and from G1 to S, respectively), the activation of caspase-3/-7 (induction of apoptosis) and the decrease in the pro-survival protein Survivin. The latter finding supports our previous studies in colon carcinoma [39, 43] suggesting a SATB1 – Pim1 – Survivin axis that leads to a parallel Survivin decrease upon SATB1 knockdown. However, we found Pim1 protein levels being even elevated instead. This indicates that Pim1 expression is not merely determined on the level of transcription, but that the Pim1 protein is also post-transcriptionally regulated and subject to degradation/stabilization as described previously ([44] and references therein).

Our results furthermore support the previous hypothesis [29] that SATB1 knockdown may also affect the anti-apoptotic proto-oncogene Bcl-2. Here like in the

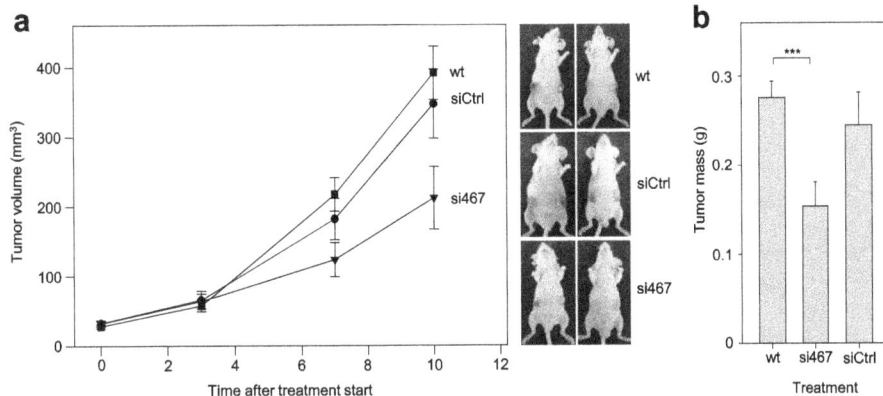

Fig. 4 Inhibition of tumor growth *in vivo* upon SATB1 knockdown. **a** Subcutaneous U-87 MG tumor xenografts were established in athymic nude mice. Upon randomization, mice were treated by i.t. injection of 2 μg siRNAs specific for SATB1 (si467) vs. negative control siRNAs (siCtrl). For siRNA delivery, siRNAs were formulated in polymeric nanoparticles based on a low-molecular weight polyethylenimine (PEI F25-LMW). Untreated mice ('wt') served as additional negative control for the absence of non-specific treatment effects. Right: representative pictures of mice (*n* = at least 13 tumor xenografts per group). **b** The determination of masses of the tumor xenografts explanted upon termination of the experiment confirmed the tumor growth inhibition

case of another important proto-oncogene, Myc, it should be noted that, when comparing siRNAs with different SATB1 knockdown efficacies, a knockdown below a certain threshold is required for altering on Myc or Bcl-2 mRNA levels. Thus, while our knockdown studies reveal a 'SATB1 gene dose effect' on the expression of many genes (e.g., Cyclin B1, Cyclin D1, N-Cadherin, β-catenin, Survivin, HER2), other mRNAs (Myc, Bcl-2, VEGF, HER1) are only affected by very profound SATB1 inhibition (si467). Alterations are also seen in the transcription factor STAT3. At first glance, the observed differences in STAT3 phosphorylation could be attributed to HER1 (EGFR) downregulation with subsequently decreased EGFR-STAT3 signaling (as previously shown to be relevant for example in peripheral nerve sheath tumors [45]). It should be noted, however, that here differences in band intensities actually reflect differences in STAT3 expression, as shown on mRNA and protein level. To the contrary, the observed decrease in phospho-p42/44 (p-ERK 1/2) rests on reduced phosphorylation rather than differences in expression. The downregulation of HER1 (EGFR) upon SATB1 knockdown is in line with previous studies in other tumor entities [2, 39]. Interestingly, however, this is not true for another member of the EGFR family, HER2, where upregulation rather than downregulation is observed, thus suggesting activation rather than inactivation of an oncogene upon SATB1 knockdown. Since previously direct effects of SATB1 on HER2 have been shown [2], one explanation for this discrepancy may be mutual effects of one HER receptor (here: EGFR) on the expression of other family members (here: HER2), as found in other tumor entities (Gutsch and Aigner, unpublished). This also demonstrates that the functional relevance and molecular effects of a given target gene (in this case SATB1) need to be evaluated in the precise tumor context.

The EGFR pathway is one of the most significant signaling pathways in glioblastoma, and EGFR is among the major genetic factors affecting the pathogenesis and prognosis of GBM. This emphasizes the relevance of SATB1 knockdown on reducing EGFR expression. Another central player in glioblastoma is β-catenin which has been found overexpressed for example in astrocytic tumors and correlated with poor prognosis and short patient survival [46, 47]. Here we describe β-catenin downregulation upon SATB1 knockdown. While activating mutations are not prevalent in glioblastoma, it was shown previously that proliferation of several glioblastoma cells could be significantly inhibited by siRNA-mediated targeting of β-catenin [48]. Thus, β-catenin downregulation may well contribute to the observed inhibitory effects of SATB1 inhibition. Our findings are also in line with a recent study in colorectal cancer, where SATB1 was found to be a target of Wnt/β-catenin signaling while in turn simultaneously regulating β-catenin expression [27]. Taken together, this establishes a SATB1 knockdown effect on two central factors in glioblastoma, EGFR and β-catenin.

Finally, inhibitory effects of SATB1 knockdown were also observed on two molecules relevant in other important processes. While the very profound effect on in N-Cadherin expression connects SATB1 expression with tumor cell motility and invasiveness, it should be noted that in high grade glioblastomas N-Cadherin has been found to be inversely correlated with invasive behavior [49]. This suggests that the N-Cadherin decrease observed here upon SATB1 knockdown may rather enhance invasive properties. On the other hand, albeit downregulated to a lesser extent, the reduction of VEGF provides a molecular explanation for the previous finding that SATB1 inhibition leads to anti-angiogenesis [29].

Conclusion

The transient knockdown approach chosen here reflects a therapeutic situation and, by using an siRNA delivery system based on polymeric nanoparticles developed in our lab, can also be employed in vivo. This allowed to study SATB1 knockdown in established tumors, thus clearly distinguishing inhibitory effects of SATB1 knockdown on tumor growth from just reducing tumor cell grafting. In light of this, and considering the multiple effects of targeting SATB1, the observed tumor-inhibitory effects are very promising with regard to future therapeutic implications. Our findings, also in the context of previous studies, provide a basis for the explanation of the observed antitumor effects on the cellular and molecular level.

Additional files

Additional file 1: Table S1. Sequences of siRNAs used in this study.

Additional file 2: Table S2. Primers used in this study.

Additional file 3: Table S3. Primary and secondary antibodies used for Western blotting in this study, and the specifications of the buffers used for dilution.

Additional file 4: Figure S1. SATB1 mRNA levels in normal brain tissue versus primary glioblastoma tissue and primary cell lines derived thereof, and established cell lines. Expression levels were determined by qRT-PCR. Denominations of the primary material on the x-axis refer to patients' IDs.

Additional file 5: Figure S2. Expression of SATB2 in various glioblastoma cell lines, as determined on the mRNA level by qRT-PCR.

Additional file 6: Figure S3. siRNA-mediated SATB1 knockdown and tumor cell inhibition. (A) SATB1 knockdown upon transfection of SATB1-specific siRNAs si467 or si989 in U343 and MZ-18 glioblastoma cells, as determined on mRNA level ($n = 2$–3 experiments performed in duplicates and analyzed 72 after transfection). Actin was used as loading control. (B) Marked inhibition of anchorage-dependent proliferation, particularly when using the more potent si467.

Abbreviations

GBM: Glioblastoma multiforme; IMDM: Iscove's Modified Dulbecco's Medium; PBS: Phosphate-buffered saline; qRT-PCR: Quantitative real-time polymerase chain reaction; SATB1: Special AT-rich sequence binding protein 1; SDS: Sodium dodecyl sulfate; siRNA: Small interfering RNA

Acknowledgments

We are grateful to Bärbel Obst and Andrea Wüstenhagen for expert technical assistance.

Funding

The authors declare no funding for this study.

Authors' contributions

AF, MR and AA designed the functional study experiments, AF and MR performed the functional study experiments, HO and FG performed the experiments on SATB1 levels in primary tissues and cells, AA drafted and wrote the manuscript, with text contributions from AF and FG. All authors have read and approved the final manuscript. All the contributors listed meet the ICMJE guidelines for authorship and have approved publication.

Competing interests

The authors declare that they have no competing interests.

Author details

[1]Rudolf-Boehm-Institute for Pharmacology and Toxicology, Clinical Pharmacology, University of Leipzig, Haertelstrasse 16 – 18, D-04107 Leipzig, Germany. [2]Present address: Deptartment of Pediatrics, University Clinic Heidelberg, Heidelberg, Germany. [3]Department of Neurosurgery, University Hospital Leipzig, Leipzig, Germany.

References

1. Louis DN, Ohgaki H, Wiestler OD, Cavenee WK, Burger PC, Jouvet A, Scheithauer BW, Kleihues P. The 2007 WHO classification of tumours of the central nervous system. Acta Neuropathol. 2007;114(2):97–109.
2. Han HJ, Russo J, Kohwi Y, Kohwi-Shigematsu T. SATB1 reprogrammes gene expression to promote breast tumour growth and metastasis. Nature. 2008;452(7184):187–93.
3. Dickinson LA, Joh T, Kohwi Y, Kohwi-Shigematsu T. A tissue-specific MAR/SAR DNA-binding protein with unusual binding site recognition. Cell. 1992;70(4):631–45.
4. Cai S, Han HJ, Kohwi-Shigematsu T. Tissue-specific nuclear architecture and gene expression regulated by SATB1. Nat Genet. 2003;34(1):42–51.
5. Yasui D, Miyano M, Cai S, Varga-Weisz P, Kohwi-Shigematsu T. SATB1 targets chromatin remodelling to regulate genes over long distances. Nature. 2002;419(6907):641–5.
6. Cai S, Lee CC, Kohwi-Shigematsu T. SATB1 packages densely looped, transcriptionally active chromatin for coordinated expression of cytokine genes. Nat Genet. 2006;38(11):1278–88.
7. Alvarez JD, Yasui DH, Niida H, Joh T, Loh DY, Kohwi-Shigematsu T. The MAR-binding protein SATB1 orchestrates temporal and spatial expression of multiple genes during T-cell development. Genes Dev. 2000;14(5):521–35.
8. Kumar PP, Bischof O, Purbey PK, Notani D, Urlaub H, Dejean A, Galande S. Functional interaction between PML and SATB1 regulates chromatin-loop architecture and transcription of the MHC class I locus. Nat Cell Biol. 2007;9(1):45–56.
9. Wang L, Di LJ, Lv X, Zheng W, Xue Z, Guo ZC, Liu DP, Liang CC. Inter-MAR association contributes to transcriptionally active looping events in human beta-globin gene cluster. PLoS One. 2009;4(2):e4629.
10. Fessing MY, Mardaryev AN, Gdula MR, Sharov AA, Sharova TY, Rapisarda V, Gordon KB, Smorodchenko AD, Poterlowicz K, Ferone G, et al. p63 regulates Satb1 to control tissue-specific chromatin remodeling during development of the epidermis. J Cell Biol. 2011;194(6):825–39.
11. Agrelo R, Souabni A, Novatchkova M, Haslinger C, Leeb M, Komnenovic V, Kishimoto H, Gresh L, Kohwi-Shigematsu T, Kenner L, et al. SATB1 defines the developmental context for gene silencing by Xist in lymphoma and embryonic cells. Dev Cell. 2009;16(4):507–16.
12. Balamotis MA, Tamberg N, Woo YJ, Li J, Davy B, Kohwi-Shigematsu T, Kohwi Y. Satb1 ablation alters temporal expression of immediate early genes and reduces dendritic spine density during postnatal brain development. Mol Cell Biol. 2012;32(2):333–47.
13. Savarese F, Davila A, Nechanitzky R, De La Rosa-Velazquez I, Pereira CF, Engelke R, Takahashi K, Jenuwein T, Kohwi-Shigematsu T, Fisher AG, et al. Satb1 and Satb2 regulate embryonic stem cell differentiation and nanog expression. Genes Dev. 2009;23(22):2625–38.
14. Cheng C, Lu X, Wang G, Zheng L, Shu X, Zhu S, Liu K, Wu K, Tong Q. Expression of SATB1 and heparanase in gastric cancer and its relationship to clinicopathologic features. APMIS. 2010;118(11):855–63.
15. Lu X, Cheng C, Zhu S, Yang Y, Zheng L, Wang G, Shu X, Wu K, Liu K, Tong Q. SATB1 is an independent prognostic marker for gastric cancer in a Chinese population. Oncol Rep. 2010;24(4):981–7.

16. Shukla S, Sharma H, Abbas A, MacLennan GT, Fu P, Danielpour D, Gupta S. Upregulation of SATB1 is associated with prostate cancer aggressiveness and disease progression. PLoS One. 2013;8(1):e53527.

17. Tu W, Luo M, Wang Z, Yan W, Xia Y, Deng H, He J, Han P, Tian D. Upregulation of SATB1 promotes tumor growth and metastasis in liver cancer. Liver Int. 2012;32(7):1064–78.

18. Zhao XD, Ji WY, Zhang W, He LX, Yang J, Liang HJ, Wang LL. Overexpression of SATB1 in laryngeal squamous cell carcinoma. ORL. 2010;72(1):1–5.

19. Xiang J, Zhou L, Li S, Xi X, Zhang J, Wang Y, Yang Y, Liu X, Wan X. AT-rich sequence binding protein 1: contribution to tumor progression and metastasis of human ovarian carcinoma. Oncol Lett. 2012;3(4):865–70.

20. Nodin B, Hedner C, Uhlen M, Jirstrom K. Expression of the global regulator SATB1 is an independent factor of poor prognosis in high grade epithelial ovarian cancer. J Ovarian Res. 2012;5(1):24.

21. Wang S, Wang L, Zhang Y, Liu Y, Meng F, Ma J, Shang P, Gao Y, Huang Q, Chen X. Special AT-rich sequence-binding protein 1: a novel biomarker predicting cervical squamous cell carcinoma prognosis and lymph node metastasis. Jpn J Clin Oncol. 2015;45(9):812–8.

22. Chen Z, Li Z, Li W, Zong Y, Zhu Y, Miao Y, Xu Z. SATB1 promotes pancreatic cancer growth and invasion depending on MYC activation. Dig Dis Sci. 2015;60(11):3304–17.

23. Meng WJ, Yan H, Zhou B, Zhang W, Kong XH, Wang R, Zhan L, Li Y, Zhou ZG, Sun XF. Correlation of SATB1 overexpression with the progression of human rectal cancer. Int J Color Dis. 2012;27(2):143–50.

24. Nodin B, Johannesson H, Wangefjord S, O'Connor DP, Lindquist KE, Uhlen M, Jirstrom K, Eberhard J. Molecular correlates and prognostic significance of SATB1 expression in colorectal cancer. Diagn Pathol. 2012;7:115.

25. Zhang J, Zhang B, Zhang X, Sun Y, Wei X, McNutt MA, Lu S, Liu Y, Zhang D, Wang M, et al. SATB1 expression is associated with biologic behavior in colorectal carcinoma in vitro and in vivo. PLoS One. 2013;8(1):e47902.

26. Fang XF, Hou ZB, Dai XZ, Chen C, Ge J, Shen H, Li XF, Yu LK, Yuan Y. Special AT-rich sequence-binding protein 1 promotes cell growth and metastasis in colorectal cancer. World J Gastroenterol. 2013;19(15):2331–9.

27. Mir R, Pradhan SJ, Patil P, Mulherkar R, Galande S. Wnt/beta-catenin signaling regulated SATB1 promotes colorectal cancer tumorigenesis and progression. Oncogene. 2016;35(13):1679-91.

28. Chen H, Takahara M, Oba J, Xie L, Chiba T, Takeuchi S, Tu Y, Nakahara T, Uchi H, Moroi Y, et al. Clinicopathologic and prognostic significance of SATB1 in cutaneous malignant melanoma. J Dermatol Sci. 2011;64(1):39–44.

29. Chu SH, Ma YB, Feng DF, Zhang H, Zhu ZA, Li ZQ, Jiang PC. Upregulation of SATB1 is associated with the development and progression of glioma. J Transl Med. 2012;10:149.

30. Chu SH, Ma YB, Feng DF, Li ZQ, Jiang PC. Correlation between SATB1 and Bcl-2 expression in human glioblastoma multiforme. Mol Med Rep. Mol Med Rep. 2013;7(1):139-43.

31. Chu SH, Ma YB, Feng DF, Zhang H, Qiu JH, Zhu ZA, Li ZQ, Jiang PC. Relationship between SATB1 expression and prognosis in astrocytoma. J Clin Neurosci. 2013;20(4):543–7.

32. Han S, Xia J, Qin X, Han S, Wu A. Phosphorylated SATB1 is associated with the progression and prognosis of glioma. Cell Death Dis. 2013;4:e901.

33. Hetschko H, Voss V, Horn S, Seifert V, Prehn JH, Kögel D. Pharmacological inhibition of Bcl-2 family members reactivates TRAIL-induced apoptosis in malignant glioma. J Neuro-Oncol. 2008;86(3):265–72.

34. Kunkel P, Ulbricht U, Bohlen P, Brockmann MA, Fillbrandt R, Stavrou D, Westphal M, Lamszus K. Inhibition of glioma angiogenesis and growth in vivo by systemic treatment with a monoclonal antibody against vascular endothelial growth factor receptor-2. Cancer Res. 2001;61(18):6624–8.

35. Libermann TA, Friesel R, Jaye M, Lyall RM, Westermark B, Drohan W, Schmidt A, Maciag T, Schlessinger J. An angiogenic growth factor is expressed in human glioma cells. EMBO J. 1987;6(6):1627–32.

36. Renner C, Seyffarth A, de Arriba SG, Meixensberger J, Gebhardt R, Gaunitz F. Carnosine inhibits growth of cells isolated from human glioblastoma multiforme. Int J Pept Res Ther. 2008;14(2):127–35.

37. Schulze D, Plohmann P, Hobel S, Aigner A. Anti-tumor effects of fibroblast growth factor-binding protein (FGF-BP) knockdown in colon carcinoma. Mol Cancer. 2011;10:144.

38. Werth S, Urban-Klein B, Dai L, Hobel S, Grzelinski M, Bakowsky U, Czubayko F, Aigner A. A low molecular weight fraction of polyethylenimine (PEI) displays increased transfection efficiency of DNA and siRNA in fresh or lyophilized complexes. J Control Release. 2006;112(2):257–70.

39. Fromberg A, Rabe M, Aigner A. Multiple effects of the special AT-rich binding protein 1 (SATB1) in colon carcinoma. Int J Cancer. 2014;135(11):2537–46.

40. Hobel S, Koburger I, John M, Czubayko F, Hadwiger P, Vornlocher HP, Aigner A. Polyethylenimine/small interfering RNA-mediated knockdown of vascular endothelial growth factor in vivo exerts anti-tumor effects synergistically with Bevacizumab. J Gene Med. 2010;12(3):287–300.

41. Hendruschk S, Wiedemuth R, Aigner A, Topfer K, Cartellieri M, Martin D, Kirsch M, Ikonomidou C, Schackert G, Temme A. RNA interference targeting survivin exerts antitumoral effects in vitro and in established glioma xenografts in vivo. Neuro-Oncology. 2011;13(10):1074–89.

42. Kowalczyk AE, Godlewski J, Krazinski BE, Kiewisz J, Sliwinska-Jewsiewicka A, Kwiatkowski P, Pula B, Dziegiel P, Janiszewski J, Wierzbicki PM, et al. Divergent expression patterns of SATB1 mRNA and SATB1 protein in colorectal cancer and normal tissues. Tumour Biol. 2015;36(6):4441–52.

43. Weirauch U, Beckmann N, Thomas M, Grunweller A, Huber K, Bracher F, Hartmann RK, Aigner A. Functional role and therapeutic potential of the pim-1 kinase in colon carcinoma. Neoplasia. 2013;15(7):783–94.

44. Bachmann M, Moroy T. The serine/threonine kinase Pim-1. Int J Biochem Cell Biol. 2005;37(4):726–30.

45. Wu J, Patmore DM, Jousma E, Eaves DW, Breving K, Patel AV, Schwartz EB, Fuchs JR, Cripe TP, Stemmer-Rachamimov AO, et al. EGFR-STAT3 signaling promotes formation of malignant peripheral nerve sheath tumors. Oncogene. 2014;33(2):173–80.

46. Liu X, Wang L, Zhao S, Ji X, Luo Y, Ling F. beta-Catenin overexpression in malignant glioma and its role in proliferation and apoptosis in glioblastma cells. Med Oncol. 2011;28(2):608–14.

47. Rossi M, Magnoni L, Miracco C, Mori E, Tosi P, Pirtoli L, Tini P, Oliveri G, Cosci E, Bakker A. beta-catenin and Gli1 are prognostic markers in glioblastoma. Cancer Biol Ther. 2011;11(8):753–61.

48. Pu P, Zhang Z, Kang C, Jiang R, Jia Z, Wang G, Jiang H. Downregulation of Wnt2 and beta-catenin by siRNA suppresses malignant glioma cell growth. Cancer Gene Ther. 2009;16(4):351–61.

49. Asano K, Duntsch CD, Zhou Q, Weimar JD, Bordelon D, Robertson JH, Pourmotabbed T. Correlation of N-cadherin expression in high grade gliomas with tissue invasion. J Neuro-Oncol. 2004;70(1):3–15.

2

An advanced glioma cell invasion assay based on organotypic brain slice cultures

Tanja Eisemann[1], Barbara Costa[1], Jens Strelau[2], Michel Mittelbronn[3,4,5,6,7], Peter Angel[1]* and Heike Peterziel[1,8,9,10]

Abstract

Background: The poor prognosis for glioblastoma patients is caused by the diffuse infiltrative growth pattern of the tumor. Therefore, the molecular and cellular processes underlying cell migration continue to be a major focus of glioblastoma research. Emerging evidence supports the concept that the tumor microenvironment has a profound influence on the functional properties of tumor cells. Accordingly, substantial effort must be devoted to move from traditional two-dimensional migration assays to three-dimensional systems that more faithfully recapitulate the complex in vivo tumor microenvironment.

Methods: In order to mimic the tumor microenvironment of adult gliomas, we used adult organotypic brain slices as an invasion matrix for implanted, fluorescently labeled tumor spheroids. Cell invasion was imaged by confocal or epi-fluorescence microscopy and quantified by determining the average cumulative sprout length per spheroid. The tumor microenvironment was manipulated by treatment of the slice with small molecule inhibitors or using different genetically engineered mouse models as donors.

Results: Both epi-fluorescence and confocal microscopy were applied to precisely quantify cell invasion in this ex vivo approach. Usage of a red-emitting membrane dye in addition to tissue clearing drastically improved epi-fluorescence imaging. Preparation of brain slices from of a genetically engineered mouse with a loss of a specific cell surface protein resulted in significantly impaired tumor cell invasion. Furthermore, jasplakinolide treatment of either tumor cells or brain slice significantly reduced tumor cell invasion.

Conclusion: We present an optimized invasion assay that closely reflects in vivo invasion by the implantation of glioma cells into organotypic adult brain slice cultures with a preserved cytoarchitecture. The diversity of applications including manipulation of the tumor cells as well as the microenvironment, permits the investigation of rate limiting factors of cell migration in a reliable context. This model will be a valuable tool for the discovery of the molecular mechanisms underlying glioma cell invasion and, ultimately, the development of novel therapeutic strategies.

Keywords: migration, organotypic brain slices, tumor microenvironment, glioblastoma, three-dimensional invasion assay

Background

Glioblastoma is the most frequent and malignant primary brain tumor, with a median survival of 12–15 months after diagnosis. Despite extensive surgical resection, chemo-, and radiotherapy, glioblastoma is still considered incurable [1–3]. The diffuse infiltration of tumor cells into adjacent healthy brain tissue is a major cause of treatment failure, and so the characterization of signaling pathways and effector molecules that drive glioblastoma invasion is a major aim in glioblastoma research (for reviews see [4, 5]).

Most studies of tumor cell migration involve simple and inexpensive two-dimensional methods like the in vitro scratch and Boyden chamber/transwell assays. However, recent studies have shown striking differences in protein functions in two- and three-dimensional contexts [6–8]. Furthermore, in vivo tumor cells are embedded in a three-dimensional matrix consisting of the extracellular matrix (ECM) and multiple cell types, which can all interact with tumor cells. Emerging evidence highlights the substantial impact of these reciprocal interactions within the tumor microenvironment on tumor cell invasion [9], and therefore the requirement for an invasion assay that closely mimics the environmental milieu

* Correspondence: p.angel@dkfz.de
[1]Division of Signal Transduction and Growth Control, DKFZ/ZMBH Alliance, Heidelberg, Germany
Full list of author information is available at the end of the article

that glioma cells encounter in vivo. Invading glioblastoma cells follow distinct anatomical features called Scherer's structures. These include meninges and the subjacent subarachnoid space, blood vessels, myelinated nerve fibers and the extracellular space between neuronal or glial processes in the brain parenchyma [10]. Taking into account that glioblastoma cells migrate along these pre-existing multicellular structures - that cannot simply be mimicked by co-cultivation of the relevant cell types - we used organotypic murine brain slice cultures as a three-dimensional invasion matrix. Preserving essential features of the host tissue such as neuronal connectivity, glial-neuronal interactions and an authentic ECM, organotypic brain slice cultures have mainly been used to study developmental, structural and electrophysiological aspects of neuronal circuits (for reviews see [11, 12]). Previously, these organotypic cultures have also been presented as a novel tool to examine the migratory behavior of ex vivo implanted tumor cells [13–16]. However, the reported methods were based on human brain slices, or the extent of invasion observed was rather low and did not reflect the high infiltration capacity of glioblastoma cells in vivo. Here, we present an optimized and reproducible protocol to assess highly infiltrating glioma cells in an adult murine brain slice. In particular, we show that the usage of a membrane dye with red-shifted fluorescence spectra and tissue clearing results in greatly increased image quality. Finally, we present a selection of application examples, including the treatment of tumor cells or the manipulation of the tumor cell environment by pharmacological inhibitors and the use of genetically modified mice as brain slice donors. Knowledge gained from in vitro and high-throughput approaches can be functionally validated by this method, accentuating its value as link between in vitro and animal studies.

Methods
Preparation of brain slices
6–8 week old C57Bl/6 wild-type or knockout mice were euthanized, the brain was isolated and the cerebellum removed with a scalpel. Using insect forceps the brain was transferred to the vibratome (Leica VT1200 S) platform and immediately fixed to this device by applying a drop of superglue. The lateral short side of the brain was placed facing the blade, in order to reduce mechanical stress. 350 μm thick coronal slices were cut with a maximal speed of 0.2 mm/s. Up to three slices were gathered per filter (Millipore #PICM03050). The transfer of the slices was facilitated by a brush and addition of brain slice medium on top of the filter. The brain slice medium is composed of MEM (Sigma # M2279), 25% heat-inactivated horse serum (Life Technologies # 26050070), 25 mM HEPES (Sigma # H0887-100 mL), 1 mM L-glutamine (Sigma, # G7513), 5 mg/ml glucose (Sigma #

G8769), 100 U/ml penicillin/streptomycin (Sigma # P4333). For cultivation at 37 °C and 5% CO_2 the medium was removed from the filter and 1 ml of fresh brain slice medium was added below. The medium was refreshed after 18-24 h and then every other day. Brain slices were cultivated air-exposed. To prevent dehydration the tissue was moistened with a drop of medium every day, and remaining excess medium removed. Although the brain slices can be cultivated for at least one week, experiments were performed at d2 and, due to the high migratory capacity of glioma cells, terminated on d4.

Preparation of fluorescently labeled spheroids
Murine (SMA560) and human (LN319; U87MG; U251MG) glioma cell lines cultivated in serum-containing medium (DMEM, Sigma # D5671; 10% FBS, Sigma # F7524; 2 mM L-glutamine) were trypsinized and counted. 1×10^6 cells/ml PBS were incubated with 5 μl lipophilic dye DiD (1 mg/ml in DMSO, Biotium #60014) or 5 μl DiI (Biotium # 30022) for 30 min at 37 °C. After two washing steps 500 cells/well were seeded in a flat-bottom 96-well plate coated with 50 μl low melt agarose (Genaxxon # M3049.0010; 1% in PBS). SMA560 and U87MG spheroids were cultivated in serum-containing DMEM medium, whereas the spheroid formation of LN319 and U251MG required cultivation in serum-free neurobasal medium (Thermo Fisher Scientific # 10888022) containing B27 supplement (Thermo Fisher Scientific # 17504044), 20 ng/ml of both EGF (Promokine # C-60170) and FGFb (Promokine # C-60240), 2 μg/ml heparin sodium salt (Sigma # H3149), 2 mM L-glutamine and 1% penicillin/streptomycin (p/s; 100 U/ml).

Human and murine primary cells were cultivated as spheroids in serum-free medium. Primary human cells were kept in neurobasal medium, and primary murine cells were cultivated in DMEM/F12 (Thermo Fisher Scientific # 21331020) medium containing N 2 supplement (Life Technologies # 17502048), 20 ng/ml of both EGF and FGFb, 2 mM L-glutamine and 1% penicillin/streptomycin (100 U/ml). To generate spheroids for subsequent implantations, cells were labeled as described above and seeded in agarose-free U-bottom 96-well plates (500 cells/well; Greiner # 650185).

Most glioma cell lines and primary cells we tested formed spheroids under the described conditions. However, in some cases the protocol might have to be adjusted to cultivation in neurobasal medium, or to the hanging drop culture protocol. The last cultivation technique requires medium supplementation with 20% methyl cellulose. The single cell suspension is pipetted in drops of 20 μl on the inside of a dish which is then slowly inverted.

For generation of heterotypic spheroids, astrocytes were isolated from 3 day old neonatal mice. Briefly, brains were isolated and the meninges removed. Cortical tissue was ground on a 70 µm cell strainer with a glass pestle. After three washes, cells were cultured in DMEM (10% FBS, 2 mM L-glutamine and 1% p/s) on poly-lysine-coated culture vessels. After a cultivation period of at least 10 days astrocytes were used for co-implantation experiments. Astrocytes were labeled with DiI and co-cultivated as heterotypic multicellular spheroids with DiD labeled murine SMA560 glioma cells line in a ratio of 3:2 in agarose coated 96-well plates for two days.

Due to the different growth rates of the tumor cells used in the experiments and the difficulty of precisely measuring the number of cells in an established spheroid, we seeded a fixed number of 500 cells and implanted the tumor cell spheroids when they reached a diameter of approximately 150 µm.

The murine cell line SMA560 was provided by Prof. Michael Platten (Department of Neurology, University Heidelberg). The human cell lines LN319 and U251 were provided by Prof. Wolfgang Wick (University Hospital Heidelberg), and Prof. Michael Weller (Department of Neurology, University Zurich) provided the human cell line U87MG. Human and murine primary glioblastoma cultures were generated in our laboratory.

Tumor cell and brain slice treatment with jasplakinolide

500 DiD labeled SMA560 glioma cells were seeded in spheroid-forming conditions per well of a 96-well plate. 18 h prior to implantation, spheroids or brain slices were treated with 1 µM jasplakinolide (Cayman #11705) or DMSO (Sigma # 41639-100ML). 24 h after implantation, brain slices were fixed and imaged by confocal microscopy.

Cell viability in vitro was measured with trypan blue staining (Sigma # 93595-50ML).

Spheroid implantation

8–10 spheroids per brain slice were manually implanted using a blunt Hamilton syringe (701 N; 10 µl; 26 s/51/3) and a binocular microscope. For this purpose, a single spheroid was aspirated in a maximum volume of 0.5 µl and implanted by release of the total volume into the tissue. This procedure was repeated until 8–10 spheroids were implanted along the cortex (see Fig. 1 for implantation sites). There are several factors that are essential for maximum invasion. Most important in this context is proper implantation of the spheroids. It might help to completely penetrate through the tissue to the filter to estimate its depth; however, it is crucial to not release the spheroid onto the filter. The spheroid must be implanted within the tissue, as release of the spheroid below or on top of the brain tissue will not result in tumor cell invasion but in proliferation or in some cases in collective migration along the tissue surface. Furthermore, tissue integrity is an essential factor for correct implantation. Dehydration of brain slices impedes penetration of the tissue with the needle tip, as the tissue surface becomes too rigid. Conversely, excessive immersion of the brain slice in medium results in tissue degeneration and disintegration upon penetration with the needle tip. Thus, we recommend moistening the brain slices every other day, followed by removal of excessive medium. If these instructions are carefully followed, a successful implantation rate of at least 80% can be achieved.

Following implantation, medium was refreshed and the slices cultivated at 37 °C and 5% CO_2. Experiments were terminated 2d after implantation unless otherwise stated. For fixation brain slice medium was removed and 1 - 2 ml 4% PFA added on top of the filter for 2 h at RT

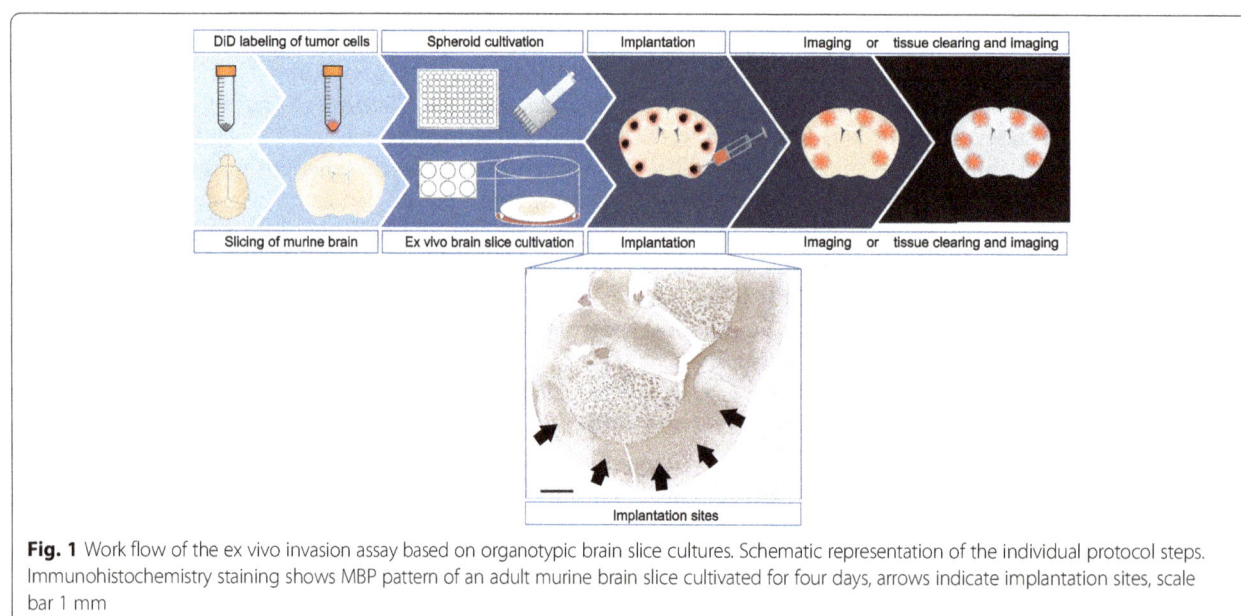

Fig. 1 Work flow of the ex vivo invasion assay based on organotypic brain slice cultures. Schematic representation of the individual protocol steps. Immunohistochemistry staining shows MBP pattern of an adult murine brain slice cultivated for four days, arrows indicate implantation sites, scale bar 1 mm

or o/n at 4 °C. Fixed slices were transferred with a spatula from the filter into a new 6-well plate containing 2 ml PBS/well. Although the slices can be stored in the parafilm-sealed plate for at least three months in the dark at 4 °C, slices were imaged by epi-fluorescence or confocal microscopy as soon as possible.

Tissue clearing

To obtain high quality epi-fluorescence microscopy images, autofluorescent brain slices were cleared according to the SeeDB protocol [17]. After incubation in 20% clearing solution for 4-8 h in the dark with gentle shaking, the clearing solution was changed to 40% and subsequently 60% clearing solution each for 4-8 h. Slices were sequentially incubated in 80%, 100% and 115% clearing solution o/n. As clearing solutions of 100% and 115% tend to crystalize, incubation steps were performed in a humid chamber. Cleared slices were stored in the 115% clearing solution in a dark humid chamber at RT. All clearing solutions contain 0,5% α-thioglycerol (Sigma # M1753) and the above given wt/vol percentage of (D-) fructose (Sigma # F0127).

Imaging and quantification of invasion

For epi-fluorescence imaging the slices were kept in 6-well plates containing PBS or, if the slices had been cleared, 115% clearing solution. For confocal imaging slices were transferred with a spatula onto an object slide and loosely covered with a coverslip.

Z-stack images were transformed to a maximum projection image by using ImageJ [18]. Image quality was optimized by adjusting brightness, contrast and gamma. Migratory cells were visible as spikes emerging from the bulk of the spheroids that had been formed by cells establishing an infiltration path. These invasion sprouts were traced from the center of the mass to the tip using the freehand tool. The radius of the spheroid body (if not determinable spheroid body radius from d0) was subtracted from the measured sprout length. Subsequently, we calculated the average cumulative sprout length by adding up the length of all sprouts of a spheroid and dividing this sum by the number of analyzed spheroids. This statistic integrates sprout length and the number of sprouts to estimate the migratory capacity of the cells. Calculation of the cumulative sprout length is a common tool in angiogenesis research, where it is used as reliable quantification of cell movement and proliferation in a three-dimensional environment [19–22].

Statistical analysis

Welch's t-test was performed to evaluate the difference between the cumulative sprout lengths of experimental groups. Differences in the grade of invasion were considered significant if $p < 0.05$. Bonferroni correction of p-values was applied for multiple comparisons (in particular, comparison of jasplakinolide treated cells, cells implanted in jasplakinolide treated slices and control cells).

Immunohistochemistry

4d after brain slice preparation the tissue was fixed and pre-embedded in 2% agar (Carl Roth # 5210.3)- 2.5% gelatin (Merck Millipore # 1040700500; in PBS) without sponge pads and subsequently processed for paraffin embedding. 4-6 μm thick sections were stained according to standard immunohistochemistry protocols. The antibodies used were specific for: glial fibrillary acidic protein (GFAP) (Biolegend # 644701; diluted 1:500), laminin (Progen Biotech # 10765; diluted 1:200), myelin basic protein (MBP) (Abcam # 7349; diluted 1:200) and ionized calcium-binding adapter molecule 1 (Iba1) (Wako # 019–19,741; diluted 1:500).

Results

Adult slice cultures retain cytoarchitecture of the brain

The majority of previous publications utilized brain slices from perinatal donors that show a high degree of resistance to mechanical trauma during slice preparation [23]. However, as high grade gliomas are most common among adult patients, we used adult mice with a fully developed brain, including completed myelination, as donors for the preparation of brain slices. To determine whether the cytoarchitecture is preserved, we performed immunohistochemical staining on adult brain slices embedded 4 days after slicing. We observed that blood vessels and myelinated fiber tracts were present and morphologically intact; astrocytes (GFAP) and microglia (Iba1) were slightly activated within the brain slice, presumably induced by the mechanical trauma of cutting (Fig. 2). In contrast to the survival of astrocytes, microglia and endothelial cells, neuronal survival in brain slices has been reported as a major challenge, especially for slices prepared from adult donors [24]. This is partly attributed to the fact that neuronal cell death is induced by axotomy during the process of tissue slicing. However, the structure of myelinated nerve tracts remains intact and provides the same structural surfaces glioma cells encounter in vivo. Taken together, we confirm that the cytoarchitecture of the adult murine brain is retained in the slices which, thus, represent a suitable three-dimensional matrix to study glioma cell invasion.

Assessment of invasive capacity

To demonstrate that our ex vivo invasion assay protocol allows a high degree of glioma cell invasion, we manually implanted a panel of DiD labeled human and murine glioma spheroids into adult brain slices that had been adapted to in vitro conditions for 2 days. 48 h after implantation we fixed the slices and performed confocal

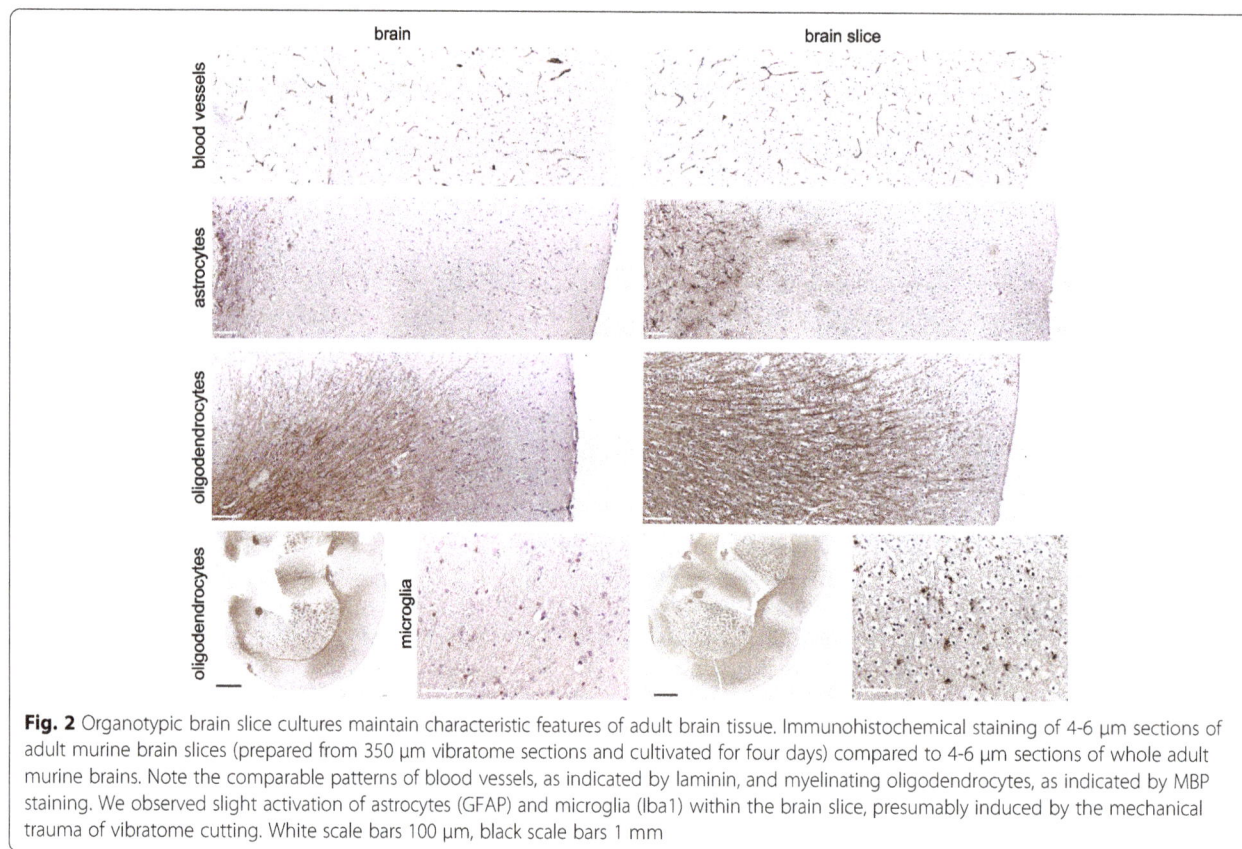

Fig. 2 Organotypic brain slice cultures maintain characteristic features of adult brain tissue. Immunohistochemical staining of 4-6 μm sections of adult murine brain slices (prepared from 350 μm vibratome sections and cultivated for four days) compared to 4-6 μm sections of whole adult murine brains. Note the comparable patterns of blood vessels, as indicated by laminin, and myelinating oligodendrocytes, as indicated by MBP staining. We observed slight activation of astrocytes (GFAP) and microglia (Iba1) within the brain slice, presumably induced by the mechanical trauma of vibratome cutting. White scale bars 100 μm, black scale bars 1 mm

imaging. As depicted in Fig. 3 all types of implanted glioma cells invaded strongly into the surrounding tissue. These observations suggest that the invasive capacity of different tumor cells can be reliably assessed and compared using this ex vivo invasion assay protocol.

DiD labeling of tumor cells and optional tissue clearing enables high-contrast imaging

Although previous studies have used ectopic GFP expression or the carbocyanine dye DiI for membrane labeling and tracing of cell invasion [13, 14, 16], we experienced high autofluorescence of the brain slice and a poor contrast between tissue and tumor cells when imaged with short excitation/emission wavelengths. To reduce this autofluorescent background we used the lipophilic carbocyanine dye DiD, an analog of DiI with markedly red-shifted fluorescence excitation and emission spectra. As autofluoresence decreases dramatically at longer wavelengths, DiD labeling resulted in strikingly sharper images compared to DiI (Fig. 4) and is moreover preferable for live cell imaging applications due to reduced photodamaging effects. To further improve epi-fluorescence imaging we cleared the brain tissue according to the SeeDB protocol [17]. As shown in Fig. 5 the quality of epifluorescence images of cleared brain slices was dramatically improved

when compared to uncleared tissue. Taken together, our results show that tumor cell labeling with the carbocyanine dye DiD and brain slice clearing produce high-contrast epi-fluorescence images, representing a comparable alternative to confocal microscopy.

Brain slices prepared from genetically engineered mice are suitable to study the stromal impact on tumor cell invasion

The influence of the microenvironment on the invasive behavior of tumor cells has been increasingly recognized. To illustrate that the ex vivo invasion assay enables the study of tumor cell/microenvironment interactions, we used brain slices prepared from a genetically engineered mouse with a global loss of a cell surface protein. We observed a substantial reduction in tumor cell invasion upon spheroid implantation in knockout compared to control wild-type brain slices (Fig. 6a-c). Thus, our results demonstrate the suitability of this assay to study the impact of stromal components on tumor cell invasion by using brain slices from genetically engineered mice.

Heterotypic spheroids allow direct comparison of different cell types and their mutual influence on invasion

To examine the mutual influence of different cell types on their invasive properties, we performed implantations

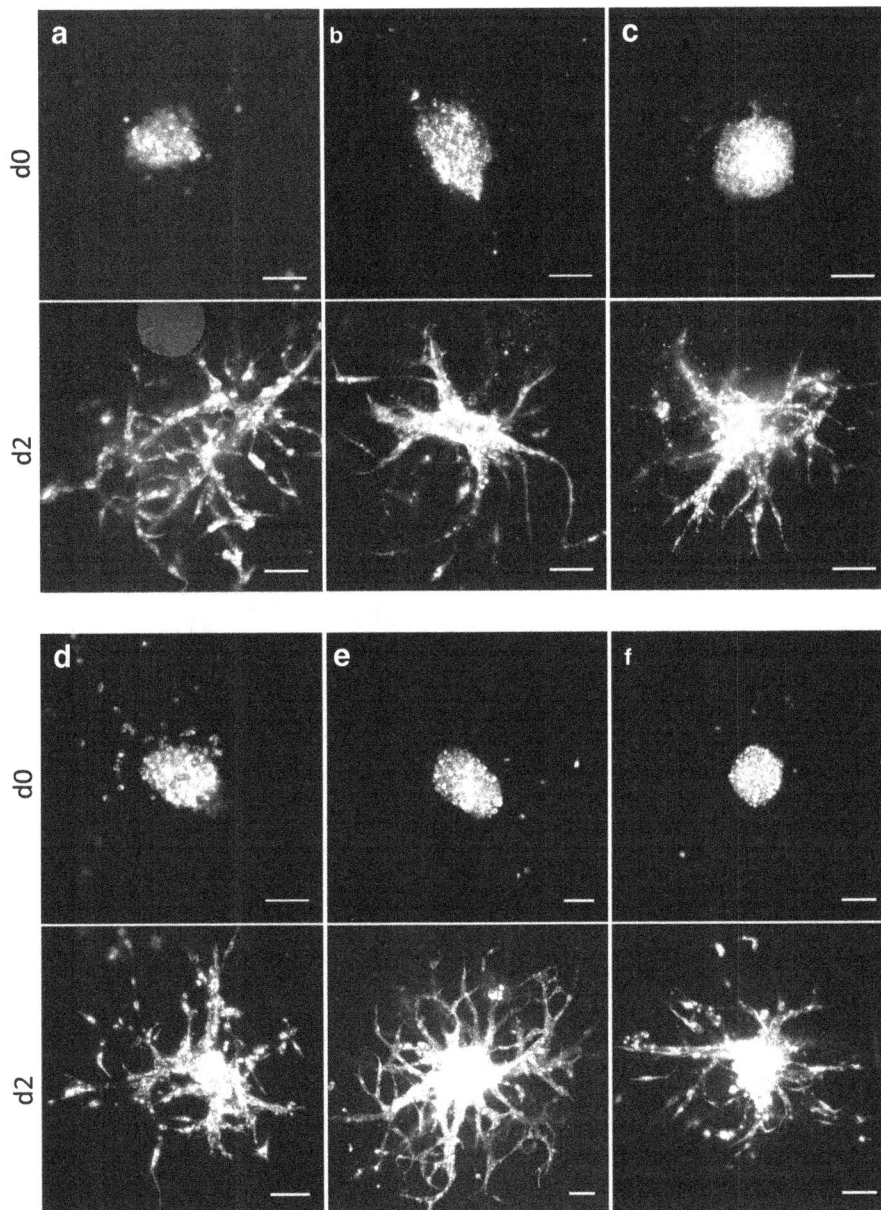

Fig. 3 Improved ex vivo cell invasion assay. Representative confocal images of DiD labeled primary glioma cells (human (**a**), murine (**b**)) and established glioma cell lines (murine SMA560 (**c**) and human LN319 (**d**), U87MG (**e**) and U251MG (**f**)) implanted in adult brain slice cultures. Images were acquired at d0 (top) and d2 (bottom). Scale bars 100 μm, image quality was optimized by adjustment of brightness, contrast and gamma

of heterotypic spheroids composed of tumor cells and other cell types differentially labeled with fluorescent dyes. In heterotypic spheroids generated from tumor cells and reactive astrocytes, we observed migration of both cell types (Fig. 6d) without identifying one cell type as the leading cell. Similarly, this method allows for the co-cultivation of control and genetically modified tumor cells, i.e. harboring gain or loss of specific proteins, and direct comparison of their invasive behavior.

The ex vivo invasion assay as a tool to identify small molecules affecting invasion

Finally, we evaluated whether the system is suitable for small molecule treatment for the testing of cell invasion modulating compounds. In our experimental setting the drug can be applied either directly to the tumor cells or to the environment. As a proof of principle, we treated tumor spheroids before implantation with jasplakinolide, a known inhibitor of migration [25, 26]. Previously, an inhibitory effect of 1 μM jasplakinolide on actin

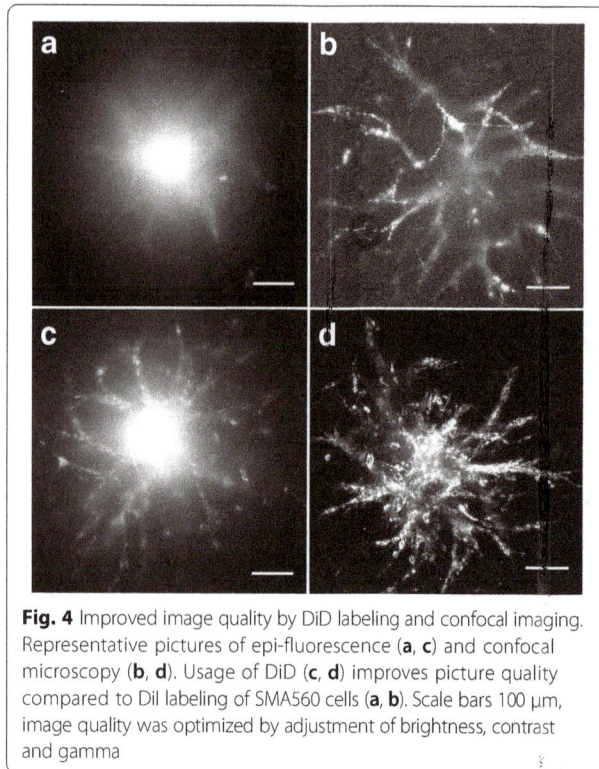

Fig. 4 Improved image quality by DiD labeling and confocal imaging. Representative pictures of epi-fluorescence (**a**, **c**) and confocal microscopy (**b**, **d**). Usage of DiD (**c**, **d**) improves picture quality compared to DiI labeling of SMA560 cells (**a**, **b**). Scale bars 100 μm, image quality was optimized by adjustment of brightness, contrast and gamma

depolymerization and thus cell migration had been described [26, 27]. Consistent with this, we observed significantly less tumor cell invasion upon tumor cell treatment with 1 μM jasplakinolide for 18 h (Fig. 6e, f, h). Importantly, cell death was not induced under these conditions (Fig. 6i). We obtained similar results when treating the brain slice with 1 μM jasplakinolide 18 h prior to implantation (Fig. 6g). This result highlights the application of our method to drug discovery and preclinical evaluation, by permitting the selection of compounds affecting tumor cell invasion prior to in vivo testing.

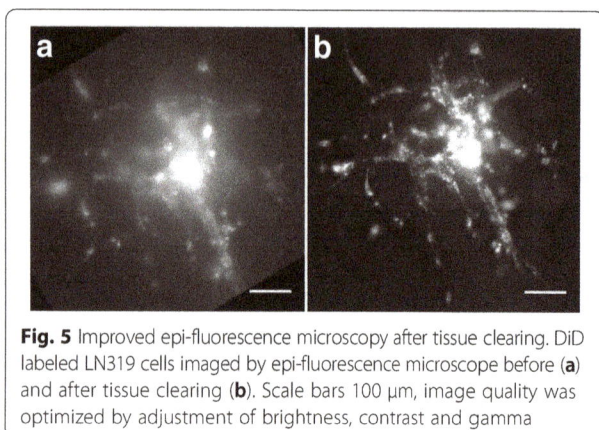

Fig. 5 Improved epi-fluorescence microscopy after tissue clearing. DiD labeled LN319 cells imaged by epi-fluorescence microscope before (**a**) and after tissue clearing (**b**). Scale bars 100 μm, image quality was optimized by adjustment of brightness, contrast and gamma

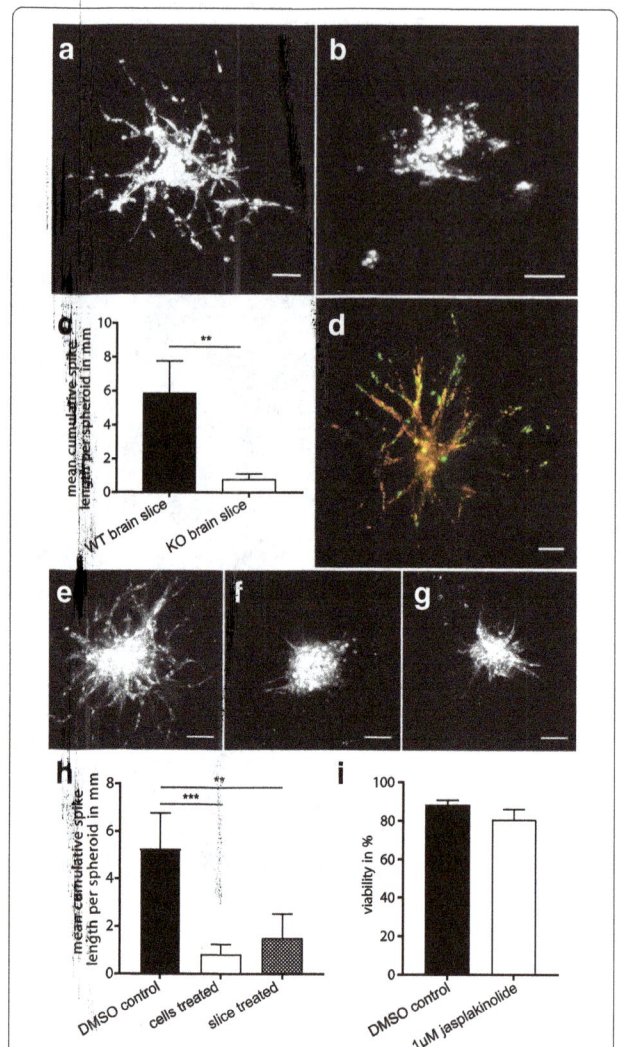

Fig. 6 Multiple applications of the ex vivo invasion assay. Representative confocal images, scale bars 100 μm, image quality was optimized by adjustment of brightness, contrast and gamma. **a-c** Brain slices of genetically modified mice as a tool to modulate the microenvironment. Human glioma cell line LN319 implanted in **a** wild-type and **b** knockout brain slices. The deletion of a specific cell surface protein in the microenvironment significantly inhibits tumor cell invasion as quantified in (**c**). Error bars represent 95% confidence interval, (A) $n = 7$; (B) $n = 5$; **$p < 0.001$, Welch's t-test. **d** Co-implantation of different cell types. Reactive astrocytes (pseudocolored in green, DiI labeled) and the murine glioma cell line SMA560 (red, DiD labeled) were co-cultured in a ratio of 3:2 as heterotypic multicellular spheroids and implanted in a wild-type brain slice. **e-i** The ex vivo invasion assay as a tool to identify invasion modulating compounds. 500 SMA560 glioblastoma cells were seeded per well to induce spheroid growth. 18 h prior to implantation, spheroids or brain slices were treated with 1 μM jasplakinolide. 24 h after implantation, brain slices were fixed and imaged by confocal microscopy. In contrast to **e** the highly invasive control-treated SMA560, **f** the treatment of the tumor cells or **g** brain slices with jasplakinolide significantly reduced their ability to invade without inducing cell death as examined by trypan blue staining (**i**). **h** Quantification of invasion. Error bars show 95% confidence interval, **e** $n = 12$; **f**, **g** $n = 7$; **i** $n = 3$; **$p < 0.001$; ***$p \leq 0.0001$; Welch's t-test, p-values Bonferroni corrected

Discussion

In the past decades tumor cell invasion has primarily been assessed by inexpensive and rapid two-dimensional assays. However, these cell culture models are very limited in their power to accurately predict the effect of proteins or small molecules on cell invasion in vivo, probably due to functional differences of proteins between two- and three-dimensional migration and the absence of environmental influences [28]. Although animal models are thought to represent the most reliable method of investigating cell invasion, they involve not only high cost but also ethical and technical concerns. The laborious and time inefficient application of mouse models is especially disadvantageous for co-clinical and personalized treatment studies that rely on a rapid read out and the exclusion of false-positive candidate compounds identified by conventional two-dimensional assays [29]. This has resulted in attempts to bridge the gap between over-simplified cell culture approaches and the more meaningful, but inefficient, in vivo models with reproducible ex vivo techniques. The current state of the art to mimic the natural environment of glioma cells are organotypic brain slice cultures that can be cultivated ex vivo for several days to weeks without considerable loss of their cytoarchitecture. Retaining their physiological structure, brain slices provide an optimal three-dimensional matrix for ex vivo invasion assays. To our knowledge, mostly perinatal donors have been used for the preparation of organotypic brain slices due to their high mechanical and ischemic resistance. However, in rodents the ECM is substantially remodeled starting from 2 weeks after birth. This remodeled and thus significantly firmer ECM is subsequently maintained throughout adulthood [30]. Similarly, myelination of nerve fibers occurs predominantly postnatally and can be extended to adulthood [31]. Hence, absent or incomplete myelination and the immature and loose extracellular matrix are profound differences between neonatal and mature adult brain tissue. In order to reflect the age related disease of adult glioma, we decided to use adult brain slices that exhibit a mature myelination pattern and ECM composition.

While there are previous reports that use organotypic brain slices for tumor cell invasion assessment, we still lack a simple, standardized, and reproducible protocol that allows its application in basic and preclinical research. Various approaches for the co-cultivation of tumor cells and slices and the measurement of cell invasion have been published. For brain metastasis research, tumor cells have been seeded in a matrigel plug adjacent to the brain slice in order to investigate interactions between cancer and glial cells by fluorescence microscopy [32]. However, this model is unsatisfactory when used to examine the invasion of primary brain tumor cells, as they arise and migrate within the brain tissue and moreover do not encounter an environment comparable to matrigel. Other publications have developed this approach by seeding single cells on top of the slices [33]. However, we see disadvantages in this technique, as it is disturbed by the diffusion of single cells after seeding and requires life cell imaging, preferably by an upright confocal microscope, which is not universally available. Moreover, we have observed reduced invasion when the tumor cells were seeded on top instead of within the tissue, as the cells migrate on the slice surface instead of efficiently penetrating the tissue. In contrast, we implant tumor cells as spheroids within the tissue in order to position them at a specific location of the brain slice and to provide a comparable starting point for the assay. Indeed, other publications have reported this approach; however, they show a low grade of invasion that does not reflect the aggressive infiltration observed in patients [13, 15, 16]. Following our protocol, we could observe strong invasion in a panel of human and murine glioma cell lines as well as primary cells. Moreover, we could improve the imaging quality of implanted tumor cells using DiD, which drastically reduces autofluorescence compared to the commonly applied DiI. Epi-fluorescence microscopy was further optimized by tissue clearing according to the SeeDB protocol [17]. Thus, we have generated an optimized and standardized protocol that acts as the basis of a set of functional applications, some of which we describe here. The possibility of specifically manipulating either one or both compartments involved in tumor cell migration, the microenvironment and the tumor cells themselves, and to monitor the consequences of the manipulation on tumor cell invasion is a major advantage of this improved protocol. Here, we demonstrate the flexibility of the protocol by manipulating the microenvironment with exogenous small molecule treatment or using genetically modified mice as donors for the organotypic brain slice cultures. This allows the investigation of the effects of global inactivation of a gene or gene product of interest, as well as cell type-specific deletion or overexpression, depending on the mouse model used. In addition, this assay is suitable for direct manipulation of the tumor cells themselves by gain- or loss-of-function approaches. Consequently, the combination of both strategies is a powerful tool i) to identify critical factors in tumor cells and their putative interaction partners in the tumor microenvironment and ii) to dissect their mode of action in tumor cell invasion, ultimately yielding potential novel targets for brain tumor therapy.

Conclusion

As growing evidence suggests the tumor microenvironment as a key factor in tumor cell invasion, we optimized an ex vivo invasion assay that can reliably and quantitatively measure glioma cell movement in an environment that more accurately recapitulates the physiological state in vivo. The functional applications described demonstrate the power and versatility of this method as an advance over previous work, and will encourage the use of more relevant models than traditional two-dimensional migration assays.

Abbreviations
DiD: 1,1'-dioctadecyl-3,3,3',3'- tetramethylindodicarbocyanine, 4-chlorobenzenesulfonate salt; DiI: 1,1'-dioctadecyl-3,3,3',3'-tetramethylindocarbocyanine; DMEM: Dulbecco's Modified Eagle Medium; DMSO: Dimethyl sulfoxide; ECM: extracellular matrix; EGF: Epidermal growth factor; FGFb: Basic fibroblast growth factor; GFAP: glial fibrillary acidic protein; GFP: Green fluorescent protein; HEPES: 4-(2-hydroxyethyl)-1-piperazineethanesulfonic acid buffer; Iba1: ionized calcium-binding adapter molecule 1; MBP: myelin basic protein; MEM: Minimum Essential Medium; PBS: Phosphate Buffered Saline

Acknowledgements
We thank Dr. Annette Kopp-Schneider for advice on statistical analysis, Dr. Michael Fletcher for proofreading the manuscript, Sabrina Lohr for technical support and Tobias Schmidt for helpful discussions. MM would like to thank the Luxembourg National Research Fond (FNR) for the support (FNR PEARL P16/BM/11192868 grant).

Funding
This work was supported by the Helmholtz Alliance Preclinical Comprehensive Cancer Center (to PA).

Authors' contributions
TE and HP designed the study; TE and BC conducted the experiments; JS helped with brain slice preparation; MM provided primary human brain tumor material; data was interpreted and discussed by TE, BC, JS, MM, PA, HP; the manuscript was written by TE, PA and HP. All authors have read and approved the final version of this manuscript.

Competing interests
The authors declare that they have no competing interests.

Author details
[1]Division of Signal Transduction and Growth Control, DKFZ/ZMBH Alliance, Heidelberg, Germany. [2]Functional Neuroanatomy, University of Heidelberg, Heidelberg, Germany. [3]Institute of Neurology (Edinger-Institute), University Hospital Frankfurt, Goethe University, Frankfurt, Germany. [4]Luxembourg Centre of Neuropathology (LCNP), Dudelange, Luxembourg. [5]Laboratoire National de Santé, Dudelange, Luxembourg. [6]Luxembourg Centre for Systems Biomedicine (LCSB), University of Luxembourg, Esch-sur-Alzette, Luxembourg. [7]Department of Oncology, NORLUX Neuro-Oncology Laboratory, Luxembourg Institute of Health (L.I.H.), Strassen, Luxembourg. [8]Present address: Translational Program, Hopp Children's Cancer Center at NCT Heidelberg (KiTZ), University Hospital and DKFZ Heidelberg, Heidelberg, Germany. [9]Present address: Clinical Cooperation Unit Pediatric Oncology, DKFZ, Heidelberg, Germany. [10]German Consortium for Translational Cancer Research (DKTK), Heidelberg, Germany.

References
1. Chaudhry NS, Shah AH, Ferraro N, Snelling BM, Bregy A, Madhavan K, Komotar RJ. Predictors of long-term survival in patients with glioblastoma multiforme: advancements from the last quarter century. Cancer Investig. 2013;31(5):287–308. https://doi.org/10.3109/07357907.2013.789899

2. Johnson DR, O'Neill BP. Glioblastoma survival in the United States before and during the temozolomide era. J Neuro-Oncol. 2012;107(2):359–64. https://doi.org/10.1007/s11060-011-0749-4.

3. Krex D, Klink B, Hartmann C, von Deimling A, Pietsch T, Simon M, Sabel M, Steinbach JP, Heese O, Reifenberger G, et al. long-term survival with glioblastoma multiforme. Brain. 2007;130(Pt 10):2596–606. https://doi.org/10.1093/brain/awm204.

4. Paw I, Carpenter RC, Watabe K, Debinski W, Lo HW. Mechanisms regulating glioma invasion. Cancer Lett. 2015;362(1):1–7. https://doi.org/10.1016/j.canlet.2015.03.015.

5. Xie Q, Mittal S, Berens ME: Targeting adaptive glioblastoma: an overview of proliferation and invasion. Neuro-Oncology 2014, 16(12):1575–1584.

6. Khatau SB, Bloom RJ, Bajpai S, Razafsky D, Zang S, Giri A, Wu PH, Marchand J, Celedon A, Hale CM, et al. The distinct roles of the nucleus and nucleus-cytoskeleton connections in three-dimensional cell migration. Sci Rep. 2012;2:488.

7. Madsen CD, Hooper S, Tozluoglu M, Bruckbauer A, Fletcher G, Erler JT, bates PA, Thompson B, Sahai E. STRIPAK components determine mode of cancer cell migration and metastasis. Nat Cell Biol. 2015;17(1):68–80. https://doi.org/10.1038/ncb3083.

8. Skau CT, Fischer RS, Gurel P, Thiam HR, Tubbs A, Baird MA, Davidson MW, Piel M, Alushin GM, Nussenzweig A, et al. FMN2 makes perinuclear actin to protect nuclei during confined migration and promote metastasis. Cell. 2016;167(6):1571–85 e1518. https://doi.org/10.1016/j.cell.2016.10.023.

9. Joyce JA, Pollard JW. Microenvironmental regulation of metastasis. Nat Rev Cancer. 2009;9(4):239–52. https://doi.org/10.1038/nrc2618.

10. Cuddapah VA, Robel S, Watkins S, Sontheimer H. A neurocentric perspective on glioma invasion. Nat Rev Neurosci. 2014;15(7):455–65. https://doi.org/10.1038/nrn3765.

11. Huang Y, Williams JC, Johnson SM. Brain slice on a chip: opportunities and challenges of applying microfluidic technology to intact tissues. Lab Chip. 2012;12(12):2103–17. https://doi.org/10.1039/c2lc21142d.

12. Lossi L, Alasia S, Salio C, Merighi A. Cell death and proliferation in acute slices and organotypic cultures of mammalian CNS. Prog Neurobiol. 2009;88(4):221–45. https://doi.org/10.1016/j.pneurobio.2009.01.002.

13. Aaberg-Jessen C, Norregaard A, Christensen K, Pedersen CB, Andersen C, Kristensen BW. Invasion of primary glioma- and cell line-derived spheroids implanted into corticostriatal slice cultures. Int J Clin Exp Patho. 2013;6(4):546–60.

14. Jung S, Kim HW, Lee JH, Kang SS, Rhu HH, Jeong YI, Yang SY, Chung HY, Bae CS, Choi C, et al. Brain tumor invasion model system using organotypic brain-slice culture as an alternative to in vivo model. J Cancer Res Clin Oncol. 2002;128(9):469–76. https://doi.org/10.1007/s00432-002-0366-x.

15. Petterson SA, Jakobsen IP, Jensen SS, Aaberg-Jessen C, Nielsen M, Johansen J, Kristensen BW. Implantation of glioblastoma spheroids into organotypic brain slice cultures as a model for investigating effects of irradiation: a proof of concept. Int J Clin Exp Patho. 2016;9(4):4816–23.

16. Xu WL, Wang Y, Wu J, Li GY. Quantitative analysis of U251MG human glioma cells invasion in organotypic brain slice co-cultures. Eur Rev Med Pharmaco. 2016;20(11):2221–9.

17. Ke MT, Fujimoto S, Imai T. SeeDB: a simple and morphology-preserving optical clearing agent for neuronal circuit reconstruction. Nat Neurosci. 2013;16(8):1154–U1246. https://doi.org/10.1038/nn.3447.

18. Schneider CA, Rasband WS, Eliceiri KW. NIH image to ImageJ: 25 years of image analysis. Nat Methods. 2012;9(7):671–5. https://doi.org/10.1038/nmeth.2089.

19. Heiss M, Hellstrom M, Kalen M, May T, Weber H, Hecker M, Augustin HG, Korff T. Endothelial cell spheroids as a versatile tool to study angiogenesis in vitro. FASEB J. 2015;29(7):3076–84. https://doi.org/10.1096/fj.14-267633.

20. Korff T, Augustin HG. tensional forces in fibrillar extracellular matrices control directional capillary sprouting. J Cell Sci. 1999;112(Pt 19):3249–58.

21. Stahl A, Wu X, Wenger A, Klagsbrun M, Kurschat P. Endothelial progenitor cell sprouting in spheroid cultures is resistant to inhibition by osteoblasts: a model for bone replacement grafts. FEBS Lett. 2005;579(24):5338–42. https://doi.org/10.1016/j.febslet.2005.09.005.

22. Weber H, Claffey J, Hogan M, Pampillon C, Tacke M. Analyses of Titanocenes in the spheroid-based cellular angiogenesis assay. Toxicol in Vitro. 2008;22(2):531–4. https://doi.org/10.1016/j.tiv.2007.09.014.

23. Cho S, Wood A, Bowby MR. Brain slices as models for neurodegenerative disease and screening platforms to identify novel therapeutics. Curr Neuropharmacol. 2007;5(1):19–33. https://doi.org/10.2174/157015907780077105

24. Humpel C. Organotypic brain slice cultures: a review. Neuroscience. 2015;305:86–98. https://doi.org/10.1016/j.neuroscience.2015.07.086.

25. Ivkovic S, Beadle C, Noticewala S, Massey SC, Swanson KR, Toro LN, Bresnick AR, Canoll P, Rosenfeld SS. Direct inhibition of myosin II effectively blocks glioma invasion in the presence of multiple motogens. Mol Biol Cell. 2012;23(4):533–42.

26. Ponti A, Machacek M, Gupton SL, Waterman-Storer CM, Danuser G. Two distinct actin networks drive the protrusion of migrating cells. Science. 2004;305(5691):1782–6. https://doi.org/10.1126/science.1100533.

27. Mseka T, Cramer LP. Actin depolymerization-based force retracts the cell rear in polarizing and migrating cells. Curr Biol. 2011;21(24):2085–91. https://doi.org/10.1016/j.cub.2011.11.006.

28. Pampaloni F, Reynaud EG, Stelzer EH. The third dimension bridges the gap between cell culture and live tissue. Nat Rev Mol Cell Biol. 2007;8(10):839–45. https://doi.org/10.1038/nrm2236.

29. Jensen SS, Petterson SA, Halle B, Aaberg-Jessen C, Kristensen BW. effects of the lysosomal destabilizing drug siramesine on glioblastoma in vitro and in vivo. BMC Cancer. 2017;17(1):178.

30. Zimmermann DR, Dours-Zimmermann MT. Extracellular matrix of the central nervous system: from neglect to challenge. Histochem Cell Biol. 2008;130(4):635–53. https://doi.org/10.1007/s00418-008-0485-9.

31. Semple BD, Blomgren K, Gimlin K, Ferriero DM, Noble-Haeusslein LJ. Brain development in rodents and humans: identifying benchmarks of maturation and vulnerability to injury across species. Prog Neurobiol. 2013;106-107:1–16. https://doi.org/10.1016/j.pneurobio.2013.04.001.

32. Chuang HN, Lohaus R, Hanisch UK, Binder C, Dehghani F, Pukrop T. Coculture system with an organotypic brain slice and 3D spheroid of carcinoma cells. J Vis Exp. 2013;(80) https://doi.org/10.3791/50881.

33. Chadwick EJ, Yang DP, Filbin MG, Mazzola E, Sun Y, Behar O, Pazyra-Murphy MF, Goumnerova L, Ligon KL, Stiles CD, et al. A brain tumor/Organotypic slice co-culture system for studying tumor microenvironment and targeted drug therapies. J Vis Exp. 2015;105:e53304.

3

The allosteric AKT inhibitor MK2206 shows a synergistic interaction with chemotherapy and radiotherapy in glioblastoma spheroid cultures

Ravi S. Narayan[1], Carlos A. Fedrigo[1], Eelke Brands[1], Rogier Dik[1], Lukas J.A. Stalpers[2], Brigitta G. Baumert[3,4], Ben J. Slotman[1], Bart A. Westerman[5], Godefridus J. Peters[6] and Peter Sminia[1*]

Abstract

Background: Glioblastoma multiforme (GBM) is the most common, invasive and deadly primary type of malignant brain tumor. The Phosphatidylinositol-3-Kinase/AKT (PI3K/AKT) pathway is highly active in GBM and has been associated with increased survival and resistance to therapy. The aim of this study is to investigate the effects of AKT inhibition in combination with the current standard of care which consists of irradiation and temozolomide (TMZ) on human malignant glioma cells growing adherent and as multicellular spheroids in vitro.

Methods: The effects of the allosteric inhibitor MK2206 combined with irradiation and TMZ were assessed on glioma cells growing adherent and as multicellular 3D spheroids. The interaction was studied on proliferation, clonogenic cell survival, cell invasion, −migration and on expression of key proteins in the PI3K-AKT pathway by western blot.

Results: A differential effect was found at low- (1 μM) and high dose (10 μM) MK2206. At 1 μM, the inhibitor reduced phosphorylation of Thr308 and Ser473 residues of AKT in both adherent cells and spheroids. Low dose MK2206 delayed spheroid growth and sensitized spheroids to both irradiation and TMZ in a synergistic way (Combination index <0.35). In contrast, neither low nor high dose MK2206 did enhance therapy sensitivity in adherent growing cells. Effective inhibition of invasion and migration was observed only at higher doses of MK2206 (>5 μM).

Conclusions: The data show that a 3D spheroid model show different sensitivity to irradiation when combined with AKT inhibition. Thereby we show that MK2206 has potential synergistic efficacy to the current standard of care for glioma patients.

Keywords: Glioma, Radiosensitization, Akt, Spheroid cultures, MK2206, Synergy

Background

Glioblastoma multiforme (GBM) is the most common and aggressive primary brain tumor in adults, with an overall incidence rate of approximately 3 per 100,000 persons per year [1]. The unique characteristics of GBM, such as high mitotic capacity, microvascular proliferation, pseudopallisading necrosis and infiltrative growth, confer a poor prognosis, with a median overall survival of approximately 15 months after diagnosis [2]. Postoperative radiotherapy (RT) with concomitant temozolomide (TMZ) has become the standard procedure in the treatment of patients with newly diagnosed GBM, based on the results of a large European-Canadian phase III trial [3]. Despite these encouraging results, the majority of patients still succumb from locally recurrent disease, which is due to the diffuse infiltrative growth characteristics of this tumor type and high level of resistance to radiotherapy and chemotherapy [4]. The treatment

* Correspondence: p.sminia@vumc.nl
[1]Department of Radiation Oncology, VU University Medical Center/Cancer Center Amsterdam, P.O. Box 7057, Amsterdam 1007, MB, The Netherlands
Full list of author information is available at the end of the article

response and prognosis are related to several (epi)genetic characteristics of glioma like methylation status of O6-methylguanine–DNA methyltransferase (MGMT) and genetic events in GBM core pathways including the phosphatidylinositide 3-kinase (PI3K) pathway [5]. PI3K is a central upstream node related to cell survival and cell proliferation [6]. Its primary downstream effector protein AKT plays a pivotal role in the pathway activation via phosphorylation of AKT on two critical residues, Thr308 (through PI3K) and Ser473 (mediated predominantly via mTORC2) [6, 7]. AKT exists in three isoforms, AKT1, −2 and −3, of which AKT2 and −3 are found to be important in glioma cells [7, 8]. Experimental data has indicated that phosphorylated AKT is required for proper DNA-damage response (DDR) during Non-Homologous end-joining (NHEJ) by binding to DNA-PKcs and promoting its auto-phosphorylation [9, 10]. Pharmacological inhibition of AKT has therefore also been found to sensitize cancer cells to DNA damaging agents and radiotherapy [11, 12]. In recent years many specific PI3K/AKT/mTOR pathway targeted agents have become available for preclinical studies and clinical evaluation [13]. MK2206 is an oral allosteric AKT inhibitor which can inhibit all isoforms of AKT [14]. Early clinical feasibility studies already demonstrated that MK2206 monotherapy is well tolerated in patients [15]. Emerging data show MK2206 to enhance the activity of chemotherapeutic agents in various types of cancers both pre-clinical [14, 16–21] and in patients [15, 22]. Data on MK2206 additional to the current standard GBM therapy are however not available. In the present study, we investigated the effect of MK2206 alone and its ability to synergize with radiation and TMZ to inhibit glioma growth, invasion and migration using monolayer human glioma cells and multicellular glioma spheroids.

Methods

Monolayer and spheroid/organoid cell culture

Experiments were performed using the established glioma cell lines U87MG (ATCC-HTB-14) and U251 (cell line was kindly provided by Dr. C.H. Langevel, Dept. Neurology, VU University Medical Center, Amsterdam, The Netherlands) and on two primary cell lines VU28 and VU122 (derived directly from surgical specimens from the VU University Medical Center). Cells were cultured at 37 °C in Dulbecco's modified Eagle's medium (D-MEM; Gibco BRL, UK) containing 10% fetal calf serum, 100 IU ml − 1 penicillin and 100 IU ml − 1 streptomycin, in at 5% CO2-humidified atmosphere. The AKT-inhibitor MK-2206 (Selleck Chemicals®, Houston, Texas, USA) was dissolved to a 10 mM stock solution in DMSO and stored at −20 °C. The alkylating agent temozolomide (Schering-Plough®, Utrecht, The Netherlands) was freshly dissolved at 100 mM in DMSO before each treatment.

Cells and spheroids were irradiated at room temperature radiation from a Cobalt-60 source at a dose rate of 516 Gy/h (Gammacell 220®; Atomic Energy of Canada, Mississauga, Ontario, Canada).

Cell proliferation

U87MG Cells were plated at a density of 2000 cells/well in a 96-well plate 24 h prior to drug treatment. Subsequently, cells were exposed to a serial dilution of MK2206 for 72 h in sextuple. Cell viability was determined using Cell-titer Glo 3D (Promega), which dissociates the spheroids. Relative light units (RLU) were measured using the BioTek Synergy HT Microplate Reader RLUs were normalized against the untreated controls.

Western blot

Expression of total AKT (Cell Signaling #9272, Boston, USA, 60 kDa), phospho-AKT Ser473 (Cell Signaling #9271, 60 kDa), phospho-AKT Thr308 (Cell Signaling #9275, 60 kDa), phospho-H2A.X (#9718) with loading control total-S6 (#2217) proteins were evaluated by western blot. Cells were either treated with 1 μM MK-2206 1 h before being irradiated, and collected at indicated time points for analysis.

Migration assay

Cells were plated at high density of 30.000 cells/well in 96-wells plates. A day later wells were uniformly scratched using a guided 96-well pin tool (Peira, Turnhout, Belgium) to create wounds of approximately 300 μm wide. Wells were washed with PBS and growth medium was added with MK2206. Images were automatically captured on a Leica DMI3000 microscope (Leica, Rijswijk, The Netherlands) using Universal Grab 6.3 software (DCILabs, Keerbergen, Belgium). Scratch sizes were determined using Scratch Assay 6.2 (DCILabs), and absolute wound closure (μm²) was expressed as a percentage of control wells.

Invasion assay

Cellular invasion was evaluated using Boyden chamber assay. In short, 2×10^5 cells were seeded into each insert of a 24-well plate (Falcon #353504, Fisher Scientific, USA) containing serum-free medium in the upper compartment and complete medium in the lower compartment, separated by a matrigel (10%) membrane in D-MEM. MK-2206 (1–10 μM) was added to both compartments. After 16 h of cell seeding the invasive capacity was assessed using a fluorescent microscope to count the number of cells that crossed the membrane. Fluorescence was achieved with addition of 5 μM Calcein-AM to the lower compartment in the last half hour of the experiment. For the combination with irradiation, exponential growing cells were exposed to 1 μM of MK-2206 for 1 h or 24 h, followed by 4 Gy irradiation and incubation at 37 °C for one hour and then transferred to inserts.

Spheroid growth and migration

U87MG tumor spheroids were prepared from monolayer cells which were trypsinised and seeded at a density of 5×10^6 cells/well in 6-well ultra-low attachment plate (Corning #3471, Boston, USA) containing complete DMEM. After 2 days, round spheroids were formed and those with 150–250 µm diameter were collected with a micropipette in an inverted microscope, transferred and cultured individually again with complete DMEM in 24-well ultra-low attachment plates (Corning #3473) for analysis for spheroid growth. For migration analysis these spheroids were transferred to regular adhesive 24-well culture plates. The size of the spheroids was measured every 3-days over a 15-day period. A SONY DSC-HX1 camera was attached to the microscope and the pictures were always taken with the same resolution and configuration: 2048x1536px, horizontal and vertical resolution of 72 dpi, Bit depth 24, Exposure time 1/30 s, Focal length 5 mm. The software IMAGE-J was used for the measurement of the diameters used for the calculations of area and volume.

Synergy calculation and statistics

Statistical analysis was done using one-way ANOVA to compare different groups. Two-way repeated measures ANOVA was used for the experiments with several time points. Bonferroni post hoc test was utilized to compare differences between groups. The value of p was adjusted to the number of groups. Differences between two sets of data were considered statistically significant at $p < 0.05$ (95% CI). The combination index (CI) for n amount of treatments that were combined, was calculated using a adapted formula from Chou and Talalay [23, 24] which was used on normalized growth data, where v is cell viability in %.

$$CI[ndrugs] = \frac{\sum \left[\frac{1}{Vn}\right] - \left[\frac{n-1}{100}\right]}{\frac{1}{V1..n}}$$

Results

MK2206 does not lead to temozolomide/radiation sensitization in glioma monolayer cultures.

We investigated the efficacy of MK2206 at attenuating U87 glioma cell proliferation and found it to be effective at 1 µM and higher (Fig. 1a). Protein analysis showed complete AKT dephosphorylation at 1 µM (Fig. 1c). In the combination of MK2206 with 4 Gy irradiation or 5 µM TMZ no synergistic interaction was found. Synergy calculations show a combination index (CI) > 1.2, indicating a slight antagonism (Fig. 1a). Next we tested the combination with irradiation on clonogenic cell survival using U251 glioma cells. None of the different MK2206 treatment schedules showed a reduction in clonogenic survival (Fig. 1b). In line with these findings, the expression of γH2A.X phosphorylation was not increased at 24 h after 4 Gy irradiation in cells treated with MK2206 (Fig. 1c). The data show that in monolayer growing cell cultures MK2206 was not able to induce sensitization to DNA damaging therapies and actually showed antagonistic tendencies.

Low dose MK2206 sensitizes long-term U87 multicellular spheroid cultures to irradiation and temozolomide

To further study the ability of MK2206 to sensitize glioma cells, we used the capability of U87 to easily form spheroids in low-attachment plates [25]. The growth of spheroids was inhibited after single exposure to 1 µM MK2206 and their growth was completely abrogated at 10 µM (Fig. 2a). Next, we treated the spheroids with fractionated irradiation in the presence of 5 µM TMZ and/or 1 µM MK2206. Spheroids were irradiated 3 days after start of MK2206 treatment, and TMZ was given 1 h prior to irradiation (Fig. 2b). MK2206 sensitized U87 spheroids to radiation with the lowest CI at 0.33 and 0.42 for TMZ. Furthermore, combining all three treatment modalities resulted in a strong synergy (CI > 0.33, Fig. 2c & d) which is dependent on MK, since TMZ and RT do not show any synergy (Fig. 2c). Spheroids showed complete pAKT inhibition and increased γH2A.X expression after irradiation combined with MK2206 (Fig. 2e). The data show that low-dose MK2206 can sensitize glioma spheroids to both irradiation and TMZ.

High dose MK2206 inhibits glioma migration and invasion.

An important aspect of glioma therapy resistance is the ability for the cells to invade and migrate throughout the brain. Therefore, we investigated the effect of AKT inhibition on the mobility of glioma cells on the established cell lines U87 and U251 and on the primary cell lines VU28 and VU122. In Fig. 3a the invasive capabilities of each cell line were quantified in the presence of increasing doses of MK2206. U251 and VU122 showed a decrease in invasion at a relatively high dose of 5 µM with a further decrease at 10 µM ($p < 0.01$). The invasion of VU28 was modestly attenuated at the low dose of 1 µM. Higher doses did not decrease the invasion further. Interestingly no inhibition of invasion was observed in U87 cells. Combining MK2206 (1 µM & 10 µM) with irradiation yielded an additive interaction for invasion inhibition for all cell lines (CI > 0.8) (Additional file 1: Figure S1A). Wound healing experiments were performed to assess migration inhibition, using 1 µM and 10 µM MK2206 at multiple time-points up to 8 h after start treatment (Additional file 1: Figure S1B). All cells showed a modest yet significant

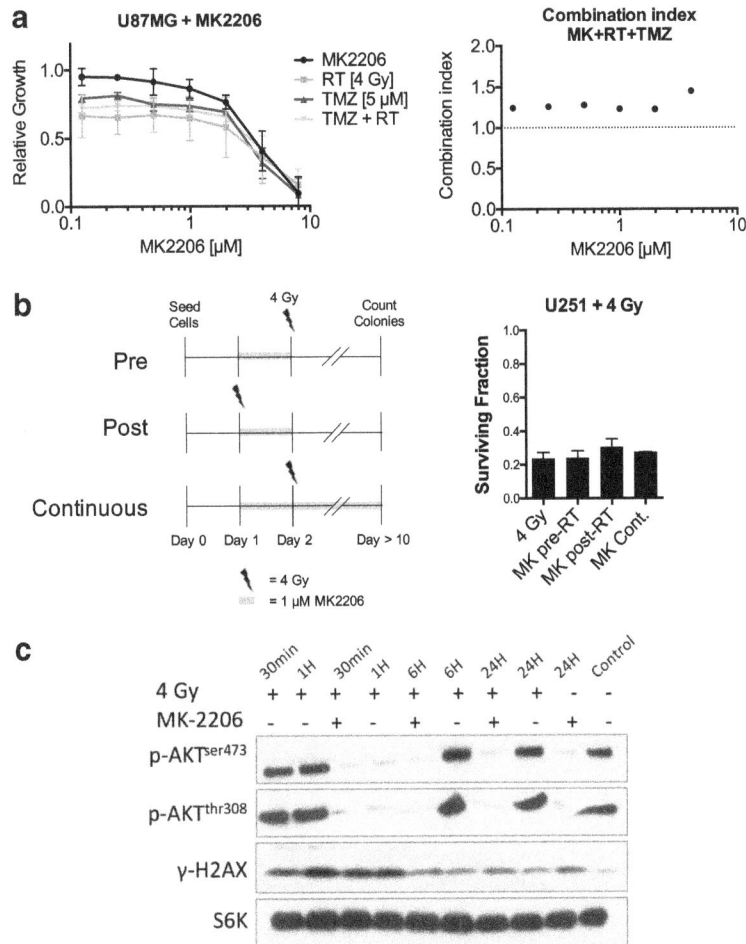

Fig. 1 MK2206 does not lead to temozolomide/radiation sensitization in glioma monolayer cultures. **a** U87MG cells were treated for 72 h with MK2206 at indicated concentrations and treated with 5 μM TMZ or 4 Gy irradiation or the combination of both. The combination index of the triple combination was calculated at each time point. A CI < 0.8 indicates synergy, 0.8 < > 1.2 additive, > 1.2 antagonism. Data points represent means, ±SD (n = 3). **b** U251 cells were treated with 1uM MK2206 and or 4 Gy irradiation in different schedules. *Top*: MK was given 24 h before (Pre-RT) irradiation and plated for colony formation; *Middle*: cells were treated with MK and immediately irradiated (Post-RT), cells were plated 24 h later for colony formation; *Bottom*: cells were treated with MK 24 h before irradiation and cells were plated for colony formation in the presence of 1 μM MK2206. Columns represent means, ±SD (n = 2). **c** U87MG cells were treated with 1 μM MK and/or with 4 Gy irradiation and lysed at indicated time points

inhibition of migration at 10 μM (Fig. 3b). VU28 was the only cell line to have inhibition of migration at a low dose of 1 μM. Furthermore, we set up a spheroid outgrowth assay to study the effect of (low dose) AKT inhibition combined with irradiation on a longer time-scale of 4 days (Additional file 1: Figure S1B). Figure 3c shows that the VU28 cell line is the only cell line in which both radiation and MK alone significantly reduced migration and when combined leads to a mild synergistic interaction (CI = 0.79). These results show that AKT inhibition and irradiation do not preferentially synergize in glioma mobility inhibition. However, strong attenuation of the AKT pathway does lead to a decrease in invasion and a mild decrease in migration.

Discussion

In the present study, we investigated the effect of AKT inhibition by MK2206 on adherent growing human glioma cells and on multicellular spheroids. The most important finding is that low dose MK2206 is able to synergistically sensitize glioma spheroids to the current standard treatment modalities in GBM therapy, i.e. irradiation and TMZ. This is in contrast to adherent growing which showed at best modest additivity for the combinatorial treatments. This has not described earlier in the context of radiosensitization since the golden standard for radiosensitization has always been monolayer clonogenic assays. Hence, studies for evaluation of radiosensitizing agents should take in to account the biological and physiological limitations of

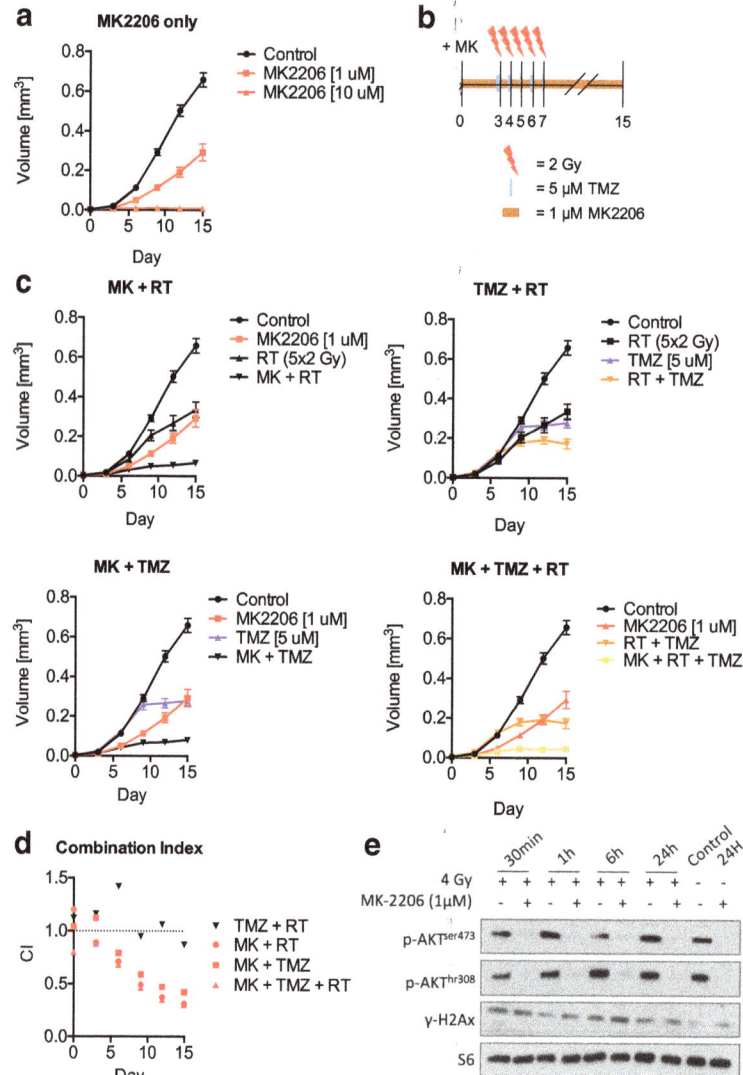

Fig. 2 Low dose MK2206 sensitizes long-term U87MG multi-cellular spheroid cultures to irradiation and temozolomide. **a** U87 multicellular spheroids were treated for 15 days with 1 μM or 10 μM MK2206. Data points represent means, ±SD (n = 8 spheroids). **b-c** U87 spheroids were treated for 15 days with 1 μM MK2206 together with fractions of 5 μM TMZ or 2 Gy irradiation. Points are means, ±SD (n = 8 spheroids). **d** Combination index for all combinations of MK/TMZ/RT for each time point. CI < 1 indicates synergy, CI > 1 indicates antagonism. **e** U87 spheroids were treated with 1 μM MK and/or with 4 Gy irradiation and lysed at indicated time points

monolayer cultures. Cells growing in multicellular structures more faithfully resemble the context of real life tumors. Cells in this context deal with complex interactions due to heterotypic cell-to-cell contact, signaling, extracellular matrix deposition and intracellular structure. This micro milieu results in gradients of oxygen, nutrients and biomolecules can result in hypoxia/oxidative stress [26, 27], which has been shown to culminate to an increase of the autophagic flux near the core of spheroids [28]. Cheng and colleagues have previously shown that the treatment of glioma cells with MK2206 preferentially leads to an increased autophagic flux and that this could be increased synergistically with gefitinib leading to autophagic cell death [29, 30].

In our study RT and TMZ were used to induce genotoxic stress (DNA-damage) which is a well-known inducer of autophagy [31, 32]. We therefore hypothesize that AKT inhibition together with RT/TMZ in spheroids tips the autophagic equilibrium towards autophagic cell death which cannot be achieved in adherent cells. The presence of these mechanisms and the concomitant different phenotype makes spheroids a preferred model over adherent monolayer growing cells for studying radiosensitizing potential of targeted agents [33]. Recently, a study has shown similar results where the authors show that AKT inhibition does not radiosensitize U87 monolayer cells but does sensitize primary glioma stem-like cell cultures to irradiation [34]. U87

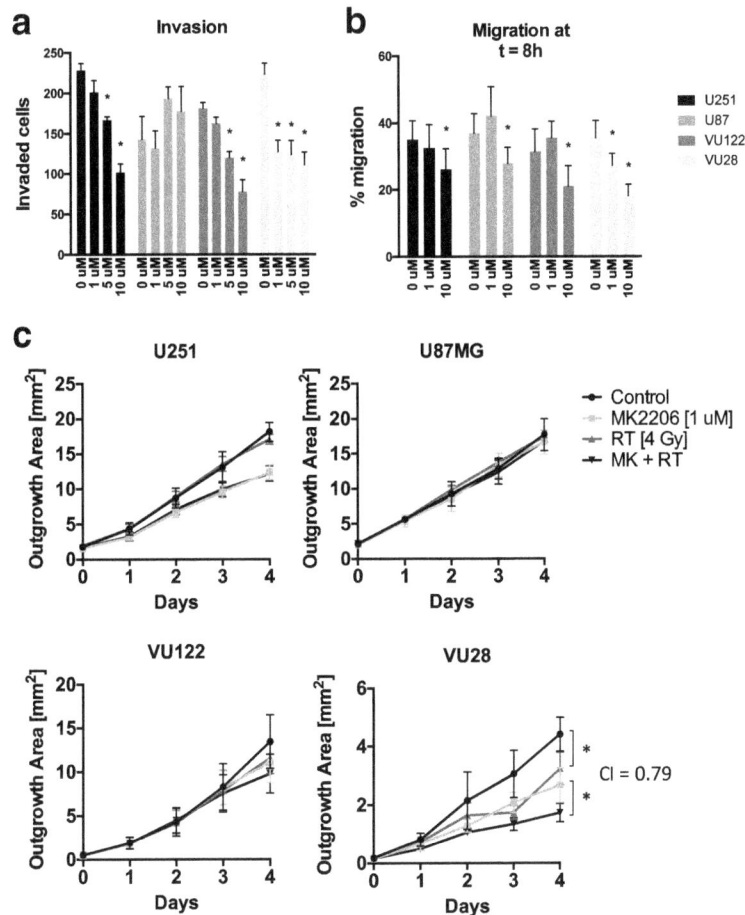

Fig. 3 High dose MK2206 inhibits glioma migration and invasion. **a** Number of cells invaded through matrigel after 16 h in the presence of 1 μM, 5 μM, or 10 μM MK2206. Columns represent means, ±SD ($n = 3$), * = $p < 0.05$. **b** Percentage of scratch area remaining compared to 0 h. Columns represent means, ±SD ($n = 10$ replicates), * = $p < 0.05$. **c** Area of spheroid outgrowth. Spheroids were treated with 1 μM MK and 4 Gy irradiation and plated in regular culture plates. Data points represent means, ±SD, ($n = 8$ replicates), * = $p < 0.05$

cells grown as spheroids have been shown to have elevated levels of the stem cell marker CD133 [35], indicating another mechanism of how the structural organization of cells influence internal signaling and drug response.

The ability of glioma cells to invade into the brain and migrate to different regions of the brain is one of the most important physical means of therapy resistance. AKT is thought to stimulate cell migration through signaling routes [36]. Cellular invasiveness can be inhibited by irradiation, which has been reported before [37]. However, our data shows a modest attenuation of glioma cell mobility through AKT inhibition and shows synergy in only one of the four cell lines tested (Figure 3). Nevertheless, this modest inhibition together with the synergistic effect the combination therapy shows on growth inhibition warrant further investigation in an orthotopic in vivo glioma model. Cheng and colleagues have shown MK2206 alone to have inhibitory effects on in vivo glioma growth [30].

Conclusions

Taken together, low dose MK2206 enhanced the effect of radiotherapy and TMZ on brain tumor spheroids in vitro which was not seen in adherent growing cell lines. Furthermore, High dose MK2206 inhibited migration and invasion of glioma cells and also synergized with irradiation in a primary GBM line. Our findings indicate the AKT pathway to be a promising target to be combined with the current standard of care for GBM therapy.

Author details

[1]Department of Radiation Oncology, VU University Medical Center/Cancer Center Amsterdam, P.O. Box 7057, Amsterdam 1007, MB, The Netherlands. [2]Department of Radiation Oncology, Academic Medical Center, Amsterdam, The Netherlands. [3]Clinical Cooperation Unit Neurooncology, MediClin Robert Janker Klinik & University of Bonn Medical Center, Bonn, Germany. [4]Department of Radiation Oncology, Maastro Clinic, Maastricht, The Netherlands. [5]Department of Neurosurgery, Neuro Oncology Research

Group, VU University Medical Center, Amsterdam, The Netherlands.
[6]Department of Medical Oncology, VU University Medical Center, Amsterdam, The Netherlands.

Abbreviations

GBM: Glioblastoma; RT: Radiotherapy; TMZ: Temozolomide; MGMT: O6-methylguanine–DNA methyltransferase; PI3K: phosphatidylinositide 3-kinase; DDR: DNA-damage response; NHEJ: Non-Homologous end-joining; CI: Combination Index

Acknowledgements

None.

Funding

This project was funded by the Dutch Cancer Foundation (KWF), Grant No. VU2010–4874. Funding was granted after a review process of the design of the study. The funding body had no further involvement thereafter.

Authors' contributions

RSN, CAF, EB, RD: conducted all laboratory experiments, RSN: performed the data analysis and wrote the manuscript. BGB, LJS, PS, BJS: conceptualized, initiated and supervised the project. GJP, BAW: experimental design, figure design, constructive discussions. PS, GJP, BAW: Manuscript review. All authors read and approved the final manuscript.

Competing interests

The authors declare that they have no competing interests.

References

1. Ostrom QT, Gittleman H, Liao P, Rouse C, Chen Y, Dowling J, et al. CBTRUS statistical report: primary brain and central nervous system tumors diagnosed in the United States in 2007-2011. Neuro-Oncology. 2014; 16(Suppl 4):iv1–63.
2. Louis DN, Perry A, Reifenberger G, von Deimling A, Figarella-Branger D, Cavenee WK, et al. The 2016 World Health Organization classification of tumors of the central nervous system: a summary. Acta Neuropathol. Springer. Berlin Heidelberg. 2016;131:1–18.
3. Stupp R, Hegi ME, Mason WP, van den Bent MJ, Taphoorn MJ, Janzer RC, et al. Effects of radiotherapy with concomitant and adjuvant temozolomide versus radiotherapy alone on survival in glioblastoma in a randomised phase III study: 5-year analysis of the EORTC-NCIC trial. Lancet Oncol Elsevier Ltd. 2009;10:459–66.
4. Campos B, Olsen LR, Urup T, Poulsen HS. A comprehensive profile of recurrent glioblastoma. Oncogene Nature Publishing Group. 2016;1–7
5. Brennan CW, Verhaak RGW, McKenna A, Campos B, Noushmehr H, Salama SR, et al. The somatic genomic landscape of glioblastoma. Cell. 2013;155: 462–77.
6. Fan Q-W, Weiss WA. Targeting the RTK-PI3K-mTOR axis in malignant glioma: overcoming resistance. Curr Top Microbiol Immunol. 2010;347:279–96.
7. Mure H, Matsuzaki K, Kitazato KT, Mizobuchi Y, Kuwayama K, Kageji T, et al. Akt2 and Akt3 play a pivotal role in malignant gliomas. Neuro-Oncology. 2010;12:221–32.
8. Joy A, Kapoor M, Georges J, Butler L, Chang Y, Li C, et al. The role of AKT isoforms in glioblastoma: AKT3 delays tumor progression. J Neuro-Oncol. Springer US. 2016;130(1):43-52.
9. Toulany M, Lee K-J, Fattah KR, Lin Y-F, Fehrenbacher B, Schaller M, et al. Akt promotes post-irradiation survival of human tumor cells through initiation, progression, and termination of DNA-PKcs-dependent DNA double-strand break repair. Mol Cancer Res. 2012;10(7):945-57.
10. Fraser M, Harding SM, Zhao H, Coackley C, Durocher D, Bristow RG. MRE11 promotes AKT phosphorylation in direct response to DNA double-strand breaks. Cell Cycle. 2011;10:2218–32.
11. Narayan RS, Fedrigo CA. Stalpers LJ a, Baumert BG, Sminia P. Targeting the Akt-pathway to improve radiosensitivity in glioblastoma. Curr. Pharm. Des. 2013;19:951–7.
12. Toulany M, Rodemann HP. Potential of Akt mediated DNA repair in radioresistance of solid tumors overexpressing erbB-PI3K-Akt pathway. Transl Cancer Res. 2013;2(3):190–202.
13. Rodon J, Dienstmann R, Serra V, Tabernero J. Development of PI3K inhibitors: lessons learned from early clinical trials. Nat. Rev. Clin. Oncol. Nat Publ Group. 2013;10:143–53.
14. Hirai H, Sootome H, Nakatsuru Y, Miyama K, Taguchi S, Tsujioka K, et al. MK-2206, an allosteric Akt inhibitor, enhances antitumor efficacy by standard chemotherapeutic agents or molecular targeted drugs in vitro and in vivo. Mol Cancer Ther. 2010;9:1956–67.
15. Yap TA, Yan L, Patnaik A, Fearen I, Olmos D, Papadopoulos K, et al. First-in-man clinical trial of the oral pan-AKT inhibitor MK-2206 in patients with advanced solid tumors. J Clin Oncol. 2011;29:4688–95.
16. Duan L, Perez RE, Hansen M, Gitelis S, Maki CG. Increasing cisplatin sensitivity by schedule-dependent inhibition of AKT and Chk1. Cancer Biol. Ther. 2014;15:1600–12.
17. Rebecca VW, Massaro RR, Fedorenko IV, Sondak VK, Anderson ARA, Kim E, et al. Inhibition of autophagy enhances the effects of the AKT inhibitor MK-2206 when combined with paclitaxel and carboplatin in BRAF wild-type melanoma. Pigment Cell Melanoma Res. 2014;27:465–78.
18. Almhanna K, Cubitt CL, Zhang S, Kazim S, Husain K, Sullivan D, et al. MK-2206, an Akt inhibitor, enhances carboplatinum/paclitaxel efficacy in gastric cancer cell lines. Cancer Biol Ther. 2013;14:932–6.
19. Sangai T, Akcakanat A, Chen H, Tarco E, Wu Y, Do K-A, et al. Biomarkers of response to Akt inhibitor MK-2206 in breast cancer. Clin Cancer Res. 2012; 18:5816–28.
20. Tao K, Yin Y, Shen Q, Chen Y, Li R, Chang W, et al. Akt inhibitor MK-2206 enhances the effect of cisplatin in gastric cancer cells. Biomed reports. 2016; 4:365–8.
21. Lin Y-H, Chen BY-H, Lai W-T, Wu S-F, Guh J-H, Cheng A-L, et al. The Akt inhibitor MK-2206 enhances the cytotoxicity of paclitaxel (Taxol) and cisplatin in ovarian cancer cells. Naunyn Schmiedeberg's Arch Pharmacol. 2015;388:19–31.
22. Molife LR, Yan L, Vitfell-Rasmussen J, Zernhelt AM, Sullivan DM, Cassier PA, et al. Phase 1 trial of the oral AKT inhibitor MK-2206 plus carboplatin/paclitaxel, docetaxel, or erlotinib in patients with advanced solid tumors. J Hematol Oncol. 2014;7:1.
23. Chou TC, Talalay P. Generalized equations for the analysis of inhibitions of Michaelis-Menten and higher-order kinetic systems with two or more mutually exclusive and nonexclusive inhibitors. Eur J Biochem. 1981;115:207–16.
24. Chou TC, Talaly P. A simple generalized equation for the analysis of multiple inhibitions of Michaelis-Menten kinetic systems. J Biol Chem. 1977;252:6438–42.
25. Vinci M, Gowan S, Boxall F, Patterson L, Zimmermann M, Court W, et al. Advances in establishment and analysis of three-dimensional tumor spheroid-based functional assays for target validation and drug evaluation. BMC Biol. BioMed Central Ltd2012;10:29.
26. Hubert CG, Rivera M, Spangler LC, Wu Q, Mack SC, Prager BC, et al. A three-dimensional organoid culture system derived from human glioblastomas recapitulates the hypoxic gradients and cancer stem cell heterogeneity of tumors found in vivo. Cancer Res. 2016;1–14
27. Boonstra J, Post JA. Molecular events associated with reactive oxygen species and cell cycle progression in mammalian cells. Gene. 2004;337:1–13.
28. Lin HH, Li X, Chen J-L, Sun X, Cooper FN, Chen Y-R, et al. Identification of an AAA ATPase VPS4B-dependent pathway that modulates epidermal growth factor receptor abundance and signaling during hypoxia. Mol Cell Biol. 2012;32:1124–38.
29. Cheng Y, Ren X, Zhang Y, Patel R, Sharma A, Wu H, et al. eEF-2 kinase dictates cross-talk between autophagy and apoptosis induced by Akt inhibition, thereby modulating cytotoxicity of novel Akt inhibitor MK-2206. Cancer Res. 2011;71:2654–63.
30. Cheng Y, Zhang Y, Zhang L, Ren X, Huber-Keener KJ, Liu X, et al. MK-2206, a novel allosteric inhibitor of Akt, synergizes with gefitinib against malignant glioma via modulating both autophagy and apoptosis. Mol Cancer Ther. 2012;11:154–64.
31. Rodriguez-Rocha H, Garcia-Garcia A, Panayiotidis MI, Franco R. DNA damage and autophagy. Mutat Res. Fundam. Mol. Mech. Mutagen. Elsevier B.V2011; 711:158 66.

The allosteric AKT inhibitor MK2206 shows a synergistic interaction with chemotherapy and radiotherapy...

29

32. Sharma K, Goehe R, Beckta JM, Valerie K, Gewirtz DA. Autophagy and radiosensitization in cancer. EXCLI J. 2014;13:178–91.

33. Eke I, Cordes N. Radiobiology goes 3D: how ECM and cell morphology impact on cell survival after irradiation. Radiother Oncol Elsevier Ireland Ltd. 2011;99:271–8.

34. Mehta M. Khan a., Danish S, Haffty BG, Sabaawy HE. Radiosensitization of primary human glioblastoma stem-like cells with low-dose AKT inhibition. Mol Cancer Ther. 2015;1171–81

35. Hermansen SK, Christensen KG, Jensen SS, Kristensen BW. Inconsistent immunohistochemical expression patterns of four different CD133 antibody clones in glioblastoma. J Histochem Cytochem. 2011;59:391–407.

36. Joy AM, Beaudry CE, Tran NL, Ponce FA, Holz DR, Demuth T, et al. Migrating glioma cells activate the PI3-K pathway and display decreased susceptibility to apoptosis. J Cell Sci. 2003;116:4409–17.

37. Pei J, Park I-H, Ryu H-H, Li S-Y, Li C-H, Lim S-H, et al. Sublethal dose of irradiation enhances invasion of malignant glioma cells through p53-MMP 2 pathway in U87MG mouse brain tumor model. Radiat Oncol. 2015;10:164.

4

Survival time following resection of intracranial metastases from NSCLC-development and validation of a novel nomogram

Xiaoyu Ji[1], Yingjie Zhuang[2], Xiangye Yin[2], Qiong Zhan[1], Xinli Zhou[1] and Xiaohua Liang[1]*

Abstract

Background: Brain metastases (BM) from non-small cell lung cancer (NSCLC) are the most frequent intracranial tumors. To identify patients who might benefit from intracranial surgery, we compared the six existing prognostic indexes(PIs) and built a nomogram to predict the survival for NSCLC with BM before they intended to receive total intracranial resection in China.

Methods: First, clinical data of NSCLC presenting with BM were retrospectively reviewed. All of the patients had received total intracranial resection and were randomly distributed to developing cohort and validation cohort by 2:1. Second, we stratified the cohort using a recursive partitioning analysis(RPA), a score index for radiosurgery (SIR), a basic score for BM (BS-BM), a Golden Grading System (GGS), a disease-specific graded prognostic assessment (DS-GPA) and by NSCLC-RADES. The predictive power of the six PIs was assessed using the Kaplan–Meier method and the log-rank test. Third, univariate and multivariate analysis were explored, and the nomogram predicting survival of BMs from NSCLC was constructed using R 3.2.3 software. The concordance index (C-index) was calculated to evaluate the discriminatory power of the nomogram in the developing cohort and validation cohort.

Results: BS-BM could better predict survival of patients before intracranial surgery compared with other PIs. In the final multivariate analysis, KPS at diagnosis of BM, metachronous or synchronous BM and the histology of lung cancer appeared to be the independent prognostic predictors for survival. The C-index in the developing cohort and validation cohort were 0.75 and 0.71 respectively, which was better than the C-index of the other six PIs.

Conclusions: The new nomogram is a promising tool in further choosing the candidates for intracranial surgery among NSCLC with BM and in helping physicians tailor suitable treatment options before operation in clinical practice.

Keywords: Non-small-cell lung cancer, Brain metastases, Prognostic indexes, Intracranial surgery, Nomogram

Background

Brain metastases (BM) are the most frequent intracranial tumors, resulting in significant morbidity and mortality. Among these patients, non-small cell lung cancer (NSCLC) ranks as a leading cause. As a result of prolonged overall survival(OS) in NSCLC patients and better detection of subclinical lesions, incidences of BM are increasing [1]. The risk of developing BM in advanced NSCLC (stage III-IV) is approximately 30%–50%. Even in resected early stage patients (stage I-II), the risk of developing BM at 5 years is 10% [2].

Until recently the median survival time (MST) for patients with BM was still not good [3]. BM is a highly heterogeneous disease, and prognosis and treatment options should be determined depending on the patient's performance status, the number, size and location of BM, the pathologic type, and the control of the primary tumor and extracranial disease. Some candidates decided to receive

* Correspondence: xhliang66@sina.com
[1]Department of oncology, Huashan Hospital Fudan University, Shanghai 200040, China
Full list of author information is available at the end of the article

surgery if intracranial lesions could be totally resected. In clinical practice, only a portion of those candidates could benefit from the intensive treatment. There have been few studies on how to further identify those candidates who might benefit from surgery, and the individuals should avoid overtreatment before they decided to receive intracranial surgery.

Many prognostic indexes (PIs) for predicting the prognosis of BM have been developed based on retrospective studies [4]. In 1997, the Radiation Therapy Oncology Group established the first prognostic score called the recursive partitioning analysis (RPA) [5]. Then, the Score Index for Radiosurgery (SIR) [6], the basic score for BM (BSBM) [7], the Golden Grading System (GGS) [8], the disease-specific graded prognostic assessment (DS-GPA) [9] and the NSCLC-RADES [10] emerged (the details of the six PIs are shown in Table 1). The published PIs have been used to help physicians tailor suitable treatment options based on the prognosis prediction. However, they were mostly designed for BM patients who were treated with radiotherapy. Whether patients who received intracranial surgery as first line treatment can be stratified by the PIs is not known.

A nomogram is a graphical prediction model widely used to predict cancer prognosis. It combines several prognostic factors on the basis of the Cox proportional hazards model and reduces statistical predictive models into a single numerical estimate of the probability of an event, such as death or recurrence [11]. As a result, an individual prediction of a specific outcome can be provided for each patient. In this study, we analyzed a cohort of patients retrospectively, compared the prediction ability of six PIs, and developed a new nomogram to identify the NSCLC patients presenting with BM who might benefit from intracranial surgery more precisely and help physicians tailor more suitable treatment options.

Methods

Patients

We collected the data of 335 NSCLC patients presenting with BM between 01/2003 and 12/2009. All of the patients were diagnosed and treated at Huashan Hospital, Fudan University, Shanghai, China. They were randomly distributed to developing cohort and validation cohort by 2:1. The inclusion criteria was histologically confirmed BM from NSCLC, and BM lesions not exceeding three to ensure that they received total intracranial resection. Exclusion criteria were patients with leptomeningeal metastases (meningeal enhancement on MRI or tumor cells found in cerebral spinal fluid), and either histological or clinical evidence of other malignant tumors except NSCLC.

Data collection and follow-up

The data from the medical records included: age, gender, the KPS at the time of BM diagnosis, the time of the primary and metastatic tumor diagnosis, the pathology type of the tumor, the presence of extracranial metastases, the control of primary tumor, and brain involvement characteristics. Synchronous BM was defined as lesions in the brain that were detected within three months of NSCLC diagnosis. Metachronous BM was defined as there have been no evidence of BM within three months of the NSCLC diagnosis.

The follow-up was by phone-call or letter. All patients were followed until death or up to May 1, 2015. The information included: 1) follow-up treatments; 2) survival data; and 3) the date of death.

Statistical analysis

The primary end-point was OS, defined as the interval from the date of BM diagnosis to the date of death or failure of follow-up. Patients alive without

Table 1 Six prognostic indexes for patients with non-small cell lung cancer with brain metastases

Prognostic factors	RPA	SIR	BS-BM	GGS	DS-GPA	NSCLC-RADES
Sample	1200	65	110	479	5067	514
Age(years)	<65/≥65	≤50(2'), 51–59(1'), ≥60(0')	–	≥65(1'), <65(0')	<50(1'), 50–60(0.5'), >60(0')	
gender						M (2'), F (5')
KPS (%)	≥70/<70	80–100(2'), 60–70(1'), ≤50(0')	80–100(1'), ≤70(0')	<70(1'), ≥70(0')	90–100(1'), 70–80(0.5'), <70(0')	<70(1'), ≥70(5')
CPT	Y/N		Y (1'), N (0')			
ECM	Y/N	CR (2'), PR/stable (1'), PD (0')	N (1'), Y (0')	Y (1'), N (0')	N (1'), Y (0')	Y (2'), N (5')
Vol. of BM(cm³)	–	<5(2'), 5–13(1'), >13(0')	–	–	–	–
Number of BM	–	1(2'), 2(1'), ≥3(0')	–	–	1(1'), 2–3(0.5'), >3(0')	–
Class I	All 4 favorable factors	8–10'	3'	0'	0–1'	5–9'
Class II	others	4–7'	2'	1'	1.5–2'	11–12'
Class III	KPS < 70	1–3'	1'	2'	2.5–3'	15'
Class IV			0'	3'	3.5–4'	

RPA recursive partitioning analysis, SIR Score Index for Radiosurgery, BS-BM basic score for BM, GGS Golden Grading System, DS-GPA disease-specific graded prognostic assessment, CPT control of primary tumor, ECM extracranial metastases, BM brain metastases, Y yes, N no, M male, F female, KPS Karnofsky performance status, CR complete response, PR partial response, PD progressive disease events were censored at the end of the follow-up. The diagnosis of BM needed to be confirmed by at least two experienced pathologists. Two hundred and twenty-three patients were distributed to the developing cohort randomly and the other one hundred and twelve patients were distributed to the validation cohort. The developing cohort was stratified by RPA, SIR, BS-BM, GGS, DS-GPA, and NSCLC-RADES. The OS curves were drawn by subgroups of the six PIs. OS was estimated by the Kaplan–Meier method, and the MST of each subgroup was compared among subgroups using the log-rank test. Harrell's concordance Index (C-index) was used to assess the discriminating ability of the six PIs. The value of C-index ranges between 0.5 and 1. 0.5 represents completely inconsistent with the practical situation, indicating that the nomogram has no predictive effect; 1 means the predictive result of the nomogram is exactly the same with the practical situation. Prognostic factors found to be $p < 0.1$ on univariate analysis were further explored in a multivariate analysis used with the Cox proportional hazards model. The significant variables ($p < 0.05$ in the multivariable Cox model) were seen as prognostic factors in the final nomogram. The new nomogram predicting the prognosis of NSCLC presenting with BM was also measured by C-index in the developing cohort and validation cohort. we used the bootstrap-corrected C-index to measure discriminative ability of the nomogram.

The statistical analyses were calculated with SPSS Statistics23.0 (IBM, SPSS Inc. Chicago, IL, US) and R 3.2.3 software (https://www.r-project.org/).

Results

The developing cohort patients' characteristics

In the developing cohort, a total of 223 patients were qualified for the retrospective study. By May 1, 2015, all enrolled patients arrived at the end point, apart from the 25 individuals lost during the follow-ups and the 7 patients still alive. One hundred and sixty patients received only a gross total resection, and the others were treated in combination with whole brain radiation therapy (WBRT) or stereotactic radiation (SRS). The differences of MST between the only operative group and the postoperative radiation therapy group showed no statistical significance ($p = 0.260$). Most patients were male and the median age was 58 years (range 22–85 years). In the metachronous entity, the intervals from NSCLC diagnosis to the confirmation of BM ranged from 3 to 68 months. Detailed characteristics of patients are listed in Table 2.

Survival analysis and PIs comparison

The MST of the developing cohort was 15 months (95% confidence interval, 13.01–16.99 months), and

Table 2 Characteristics of the developing cohort patients and the validation cohort patients with brain metastases from non-small cell lung cancer

Characteristics	Developing cohort (n = 223)		Validation cohort (n = 112)
	N (%)	p value	N (%)
Gender		0.013	
Male	144 (64.6%)		73 (65.2%)
Female	79 (35.4%)		39 (34.8%)
Age of BM diagnosis(years)		0.311	
< 60	134 (60.1%)		61 (54.5%)
≥ 60	89 (39.9%)		51 (45.5%)
KPS (%)		<0.001	
≥ 80	99 (44.4%)		45 (40.6%)
< 80	124 (55.6%)		67 (59.4%)
Interval from NSCLC diagnosis to BM diagnosis		0.044	
Synchronous	159 (71.3%)		86 (76.8%)
Metachronous	64 (28.7%)		26 (23.2%)
Time from neural symptom onset to BM diagnosis(months)		0.759	
≤ 1	159 (71.3%)		81 (72.3%)
1–3	45 (20.2%)		25 (22.3%)
> 3	19 (8.5%)		6 (5.4%)
ECM when BM diagnosis		0.009	
Yes	85 (38.1%)		35 (31.3%)
No	138 (61.9%)		77 (68.8%)
Number of BM		0.925	
1	148 (66.3%)		70 (62.5%)
2	11 (5.0%)		14 (12.5%)
3	64 (28.7%)		28 (25.0%)
Tumor size(cm)		0.348	
≤ 2	62 (27.8%)		26 (23.2%)
> 2	124 (55.6%)		67 (59.8%)
Unknown	37 (16.6%)		19 (17.0%)
Histology		0.006	
Adenocarcinoma	116 (52.2%)		75 (67.0%)
Squamous cell lung cancer	25 (11.2)		20 (17.9%)
Poorly differentiated carcinoma or histology can't be distinguished	82 (36.8%)		17 (15.1%)

BM brain metastases, KPS Karnofsky performance status, ECM extracranial metastases

survival rates at 6-months, 1-, 2-, 3- and 5-years were 80.2%, 61.0%, 30.0%, 11.7% and 4.5% respectively. Population repartition and the MST in each subgroup are listed in Table 3. Survival curves were demonstrated in Fig. 1. All classes were represented by at least 10% of the patients, with the exception of class

Table 3 Distribution of the population and MST for each PI

PI	Number of patients	%	MST (months)	p value
RPA			15	<0.001
I	79	35.4	27	<0.001
II	118	52.9	13	0.144
III	26	11.7	8	
SIR			15	<0.001
I	33	14.8	33	0.003
II	164	73.5	15	0.003
III	26	11.7	9	
BS-BM			15	<0.001
I	27	12.1	5	0.036
II	63	28.3	11	<0.001
III	74	33.2	18	0.001
IV	59	26.4	31	
GGS			15	0.001
I	106	47.5	21	0.058
II	87	39.0	14	0.631
III	25	11.2	12	0.054
IV	5	2.3	5	
DS-GPA			15	0.003
I	27	12.1	11	0.799
II	68	30.5	14	0.261
III	100	44.8	15	0.003
IV	28	12.6	37	
NSCLC-RADES			15	<0.001
I	66	29.6	11	0.025
II	103	46.2	16	0.002
III	54	24.2	27	

IV in the GGS. The results showed that the six PIs could discriminate with statistical significance ($p < 0.05$). However, differences of MST in some contiguous classes showed no statistical significance. MST of RPA class II and class III ($p = 0.144$), every adjacent classes of GGS ($p = 0.058$, 0.631, 0.054 respectively), DS-GPA class I and class II ($p = 0.799$), DS-GPA class II and class III ($p = 0.261$) could not be discriminated well. Only SIR, BS-BM and NSCLC-RADES had statistical significance between every adjacent subgroup.

To further evaluate the discriminatory power of the six PIs, we calculated the C-index using R software. The C-index value of BSBM was 0.69, higher than the other five PIs (RPA: 0.64, SIR: 0.59, GGS: 0.58, DS-GPA: 0.59, NSCLC-RADES: 0.62).

Univariate and multivariate analysis

In the univariate analysis of the possible prognostic factors, we considered the nine variables listed in Table 2, and the following five factors, female ($p = 0.013$), KPS ≥80 ($p < 0.001$), metachronous ($p = 0.044$), absence of ECM ($p = 0.009$), and histology of lung adenocarcinoma ($p < 0.001$) were associated with prolonged OS. The final multivariate analysis is shown in Table 4. Independent prognostic predictors for better survival were KPS ≥80 at diagnosis of BM, metachronous BM and the histology of lung adenocarcinoma.

Establishment and validation of the nomogram

Following the multivariable Cox model, the three independent variables, KPS at the diagnosis of BM, metachronous/synchronous BM, and the pathologic type of NSCLC were selected in the final nomogram to predict the survival time of NSCLC presenting with BM before they decided to receive complete surgical resection. The nomogram was shown in Fig. 2.

One hundred twelve patients were included in the validation cohort, whose characteristics were similar to the counterpart in the developing cohort. They were also followed until May 1, 2015. All enrolled patients arrived at the end point, apart from the 5 individuals lost during the follow-ups and the 2 patients still alive. The median OS of the validating cohort was 15 months (95% confidence interval, 9.70–16.30 months), and the survival rates at 6-months,1-, 2-, 3- and 5-years were 77.7%, 51.0%, 27.4%, 13.2% and 5.7% respectively. Most patients were male and the median age was 58 years (ranging 38–80 years). Table 2 shows the detailed characteristics of the validation patients. The C-index for the developing cohort and the validation cohort were 0.75 and 0.71 respectively.

Discussion

Brain metastases are becoming an increasingly common challenge for the clinician. The role of complete surgical resection in brain metastatic patients is still controversial [12]. Traditionally, the treatment for BM generally relied on radiotherapy and chemotherapy. Even if intracranial lesions could be totally resected, the survival time would not be extended [13]. Meanwhile, the operations themselves might result in higher mortality rates. However, with the advances in surgical techniques, patients with BM might benefit from intracranial operations, as confirmed by some studies.

Since the 1980s, more studies have emphasized the importance of surgery in treatment for BM. They compared intracranial operations with other treatments, like WBRT or SRS [14]. Although the results were not always consistent, it could be concluded that some patients benefit from intracranial operation [15–17]. Moreover, surgery allows a relief of intracranial hypertension, seizures and focal neurological deficits, and is the most useful way to get a clear pathologic diagnosis. Surgery has become an important

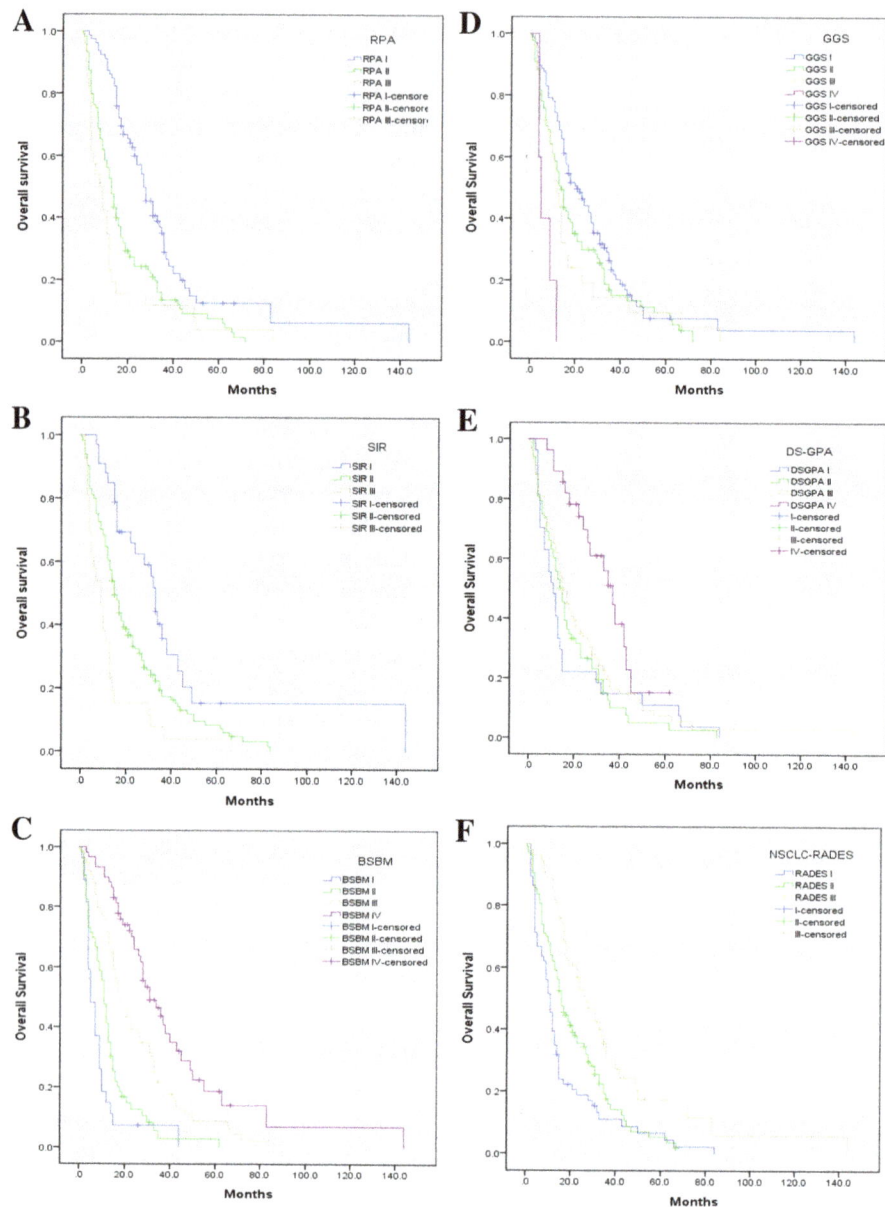

Fig. 1 Overall survival curves of the developing cohort subgrouped by six different prognostic indexes. The picture **a-f** represents overall survival curves of the developing cohort subgrouped by RPA、SIR、BS-BM、GGS、DS-GPA and NSCLC-RADES. The predictive abilities of the six PIs are different

Table 4 Multivariate analysis of prognostic factors

Prognostic factors	HR	95% CI	P value
Gender (male/female)	1.297	0.954–1.762	0.097
KPS (<80/≥80)	2.087	1.539–2.831	<0.001
Metachronous/Synchronous	0.685	0.489–0.961	0.028
ECM (N/Y)	0.749	0.054–1.012	0.060
Histology (non-adenocarcinoma/adenocarcinoma)	1.303	1.114–1.524	0.001

MST median survival time, *KPS* Karnofsky performance status, *ECM* extracranial metastases

therapeutic option for patients presenting with BM [16, 18]. As the NCCN guidelines recommend, for one to three brain metastatic lesions, and stable systemic diseases, surgical resection may be considered. However, clinical data show some eligible patients cannot benefit from intracranial operation whatsoever. Operative indications for BM are still ardently disputed. As such, identifying patients who might benefit from intracranial surgery more precisely and helping physicians tailor more suitable treatment options are crucial.

Currently, there is no research to compare the existing PIs in BM patients who were treated with intracranial

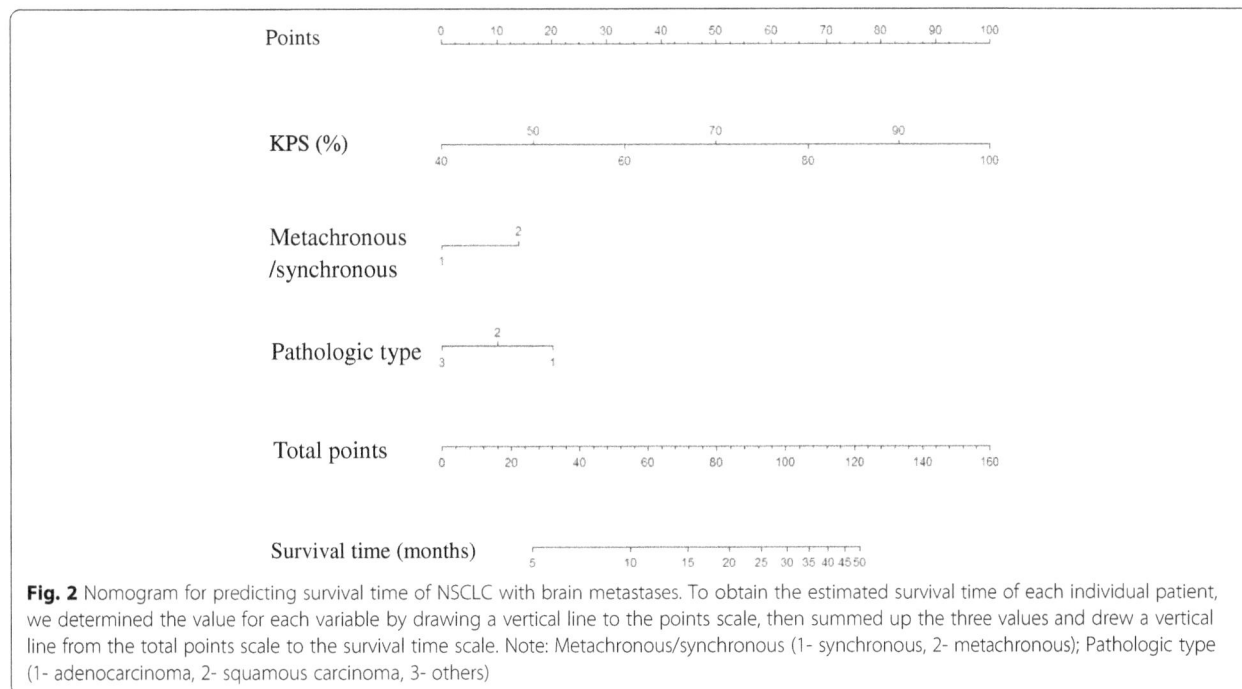

Fig. 2 Nomogram for predicting survival time of NSCLC with brain metastases. To obtain the estimated survival time of each individual patient, we determined the value for each variable by drawing a vertical line to the points scale, then summed up the three values and drew a vertical line from the total points scale to the survival time scale. Note: Metachronous/synchronous (1- synchronous, 2- metachronous); Pathologic type (1- adenocarcinoma, 2- squamous carcinoma, 3- others)

total resection [19]. We enrolled 335 eligible patients in this study. Completely surgical resection of intracranial lesions was used as the first line treatment option. We eliminated the possibilities that different treatments may affect the survival outcome, and explored the relationship between baseline situations and the prognosis.

RPA [5] is commonly used in the prognosis prediction. It was developed in patients who were treated with WBRT. Agboola [20], once applied in a cohort of surgical resected BM patients, showed the predictive value of RPA. However, the 1200 enrolled patients came from three different trials, and the criteria and the dose of WBRT were not same. SIR [6] resulted in BM-related variables: the numbers and sizes of BM. Some studies found that patients benefitted from surgical treatment for BM. BSBM [7] has been advocated as a convenient, easy to use PI, which was proposed on the basis of RPA and SIR. It was further evaluated in patients receiving WBRT with surgery and WBRT with or without SRS [21]. GGS [8] was constructed specifically for NSCLC patients. However, it failed to distinguish a good prognosis from a poor prognosis in our study. DS-GPA [9] was proposed in a large sample multi-center retrospective study. With the enrolled patients spanning from 1985 to 2007, it could not eliminate the influence of treatments, and different criteria, treatment measures, and selection bias were unavoidable. The newly proposed NSCLC-RADES [10] needs to be further validated in more studies.

With the six PIs targeting different populations, we could not demonstrate that one prognostic classification

was superior to the rest [22]. In our research, SIR, BSBM, NSCLC-RADES, especially BSBM better predicted the survival of BM from NSCLC who were treated with intracranial surgery in China. However, some patients were still misclassified to "good prognosis" and "poor prognosis" in BSBM. So the existing PIs are still not the ideal prognostic tool to help identify those patients who might benefit from intensive treatment like surgery, and the individuals should avoid overtreatments. The PIs need to be further optimized.

In our univariate and multivariate analyses, independent prognostic predictors for better survival were KPS at diagnosis of BM, metachronous BM and the histology of lung adenocarcinoma.

KPS at the BM diagnosis, which was also evaluated in the six studied PIs, was a significant prognostic factor in the study. Neurological symptoms, like headaches, motor impairment, dysphasia, seizures, and even coma, are always induced by intracranial lesions. Some discomfort, like coughing, sputum, and chest congestion are related to systematic cancer. All of these symptoms influence the KPS score and affect the prognosis. As a result, use of the KPS has been criticized because of its subjective nature, variability in scoring between observers, and the tendency for the score to be influenced by acute but self- limited events [23]. When we evaluate the variable, we should notice that and try to make KPS reliable. .

The pathological types of NSCLC were found to be a significant factor for prognosis, which was not involved in the six PIs. Lung adenocarcinoma (ADC) and squamous cell carcinoma (SCC) accounted for 80% of NSCLC. Our research showed significantly better OS for ADC. This result is in accordance with many other published studies [24]. There may be some reasons behind this phenomenon. First, the natural biological behaviors are not the same. The next-generation sequencing of the SCC subgroup identified entirely different genes [25]. Second, due to higher incidences of mutant genes (EGFR, ALK, ROS1, etc.) in ADC [26], the use of new targeted agents will enhance the response rates and prolong OS. We did not investigate the other rare types of NSCLC.

In 2012, our institution conducted a study to compare synchronous BM with metachronous BM. We found that the clinical characteristics, diagnoses, and treatment methods for synchronous BM and metachronous BM were different [24]. In our cohort, 73.1% of the patients were synchronous BM. As analyzed above, the MST in metachronous BM was longer than in the synchronous BM. The possible reasons for this are as follows: 1) control of primary tumor; 2) presence of ECM; 3) sizes of BMs; and 4) even dissimilitude driver genes of the two subgroups. Further research is needed to better understand these findings.

A nomogram is widely used for cancer prognosis, primarily because of its ability to integrate different variables on the basis of multivariate analysis to more accurately predict the survival of individuals. Kaizu [27] et al. established a nomogram to evaluate the risk of bone-metastasis in postoperative prostate cancer patients. Bevilacqua [28] developed a nomogram to predict the sentinel lymph node metastasis in early breast cancer and the survival of patients with breast cancer. Graesslin [29] even set up a nomogram to predict the incidence of brain metastasis in breast cancer. However, a nomogram for predicting the survival time of NSCLC patients with brain metastasis before they decided to receive complete surgical resection has not been previously investigated.

Our new nomogram is a predictive tool, which creates a simple graphical representation of a statistical predictive model to predict the survival time of individual NSCLC patient with brain metastasis for intracranial surgery. Through quantifying the risk of death with a variety of factors, the nomogram can help clinicians tailor treatment modalities and avoid good prognostic patients from giving up effective treatment and prevent the poor prognostic patients from receiving overtreatment. The C-index of the nomogram showed its superior ability to predict prognosis. In conclusion, before clinicians and NSCLC patients consider to have an intracranial resection surgery, our nomogram could be used as an effective tool to predict the survival of the patients and optimize treatment modalities in clinical practice.

Despite some findings of the present study, there are still several limitations. First, with the advent of targeted therapy, mutation testing has been standard practice with a NSCLC diagnosis. However, the gene expression patterns of our enrolled patients were unknown. As a result, we could not account for the molecular subtype. Although the efficacy of surgery may not be influenced by this factor, the patient's gene status should be as clear as possible in further studies. Second, as a single institution retrospective study, treatment protocols, patient selection, and follow-ups can bias the results. For all of the patients in our cohort who received intracranial surgery, the factors of KPS, age, ECM, and number of BMs were better than the average. Third, future multicenter studies are needed to confirm our developed nomogram.

Conclusions

In conclusion, we found that BS-BM could better predict survival of the BM patients after comparing the six existing PIs. In the final multivariate analysis, KPS ≥80 at diagnosis of BM, metachronous BM and the histology of lung adenocarcinoma appeared to be the independent prognostic predictors for better survival. Additionally, the new nomogram we built in the study is a predictive tool in further choosing the candidates for intracranial surgery among eligible NSCLC with BM. As a result, it helps to optimize NSCLC with BM patients' treatment modalities in clinical practice.

Abbreviations

ADC: Lung adenocarcinoma; BM: Brain metastases; BS-BM: Basic score for BM; C-index: Concordance index; CPT: Control of primary tumor; DS-GPA: Disease-specific graded prognostic assessment; ECM: Extracranial metastases; EGFR: Epidermal growth factor receptor; GGS: Golden Grading System; KPS: Karnofsky performance status; MST: Media survival time; NSCLC: Non-small cell lung cancer; OS: Overall survival; PIs: prognostic indexes; RPA: Recursive partitioning analysis; SCC: Squamous cell carcinoma; SIR: Score index for radiosurgery; SRS: Stereotactic radiation; WBRT: Whole brain radiation therapy

Acknowledgements

We thank Mr. Zhang for editing and the logistic support.

Funding

This work was financially supported by grants from the National Natural Science foundation of China (Nos. 81,302,010), Shanghai Health and Family planning Commission (Project Number: 201,440,584), the Science and Technology Development Program of Baoshan District, Shanghai, China (Project Number: 14-E-27). None of the funding bodies had any part in the design of the study and collection, analysis, and interpretation of data. The funding bodies supported the expense of the language editting of this manuscript.

Authors' contributions

Conception and design: XHL, XYJ, XLZ. Development of methodology: XYJ, YJZ, QZ. Acquisition of data (acquired and managed data, etc.): XYJ, YJZ, XYY. Analysis and interpretation of data (e.g., statistical, and computational analysis): QZ, YJZ, XYY. Writing, review the manuscript: XYJ, YJZ. All authors read and approved the final manuscript.

Competing interests

The authors declare that they have no competing interests.

Author details

[1]Department of oncology, Huashan Hospital Fudan University, Shanghai 200040, China. [2]Company 4, Battalion 1, Cadet Brigade 1, Fourth Military Medical University, Xi'an 710032, China.

References

1. Goldberg SB, Contessa JN, Omay SB, Chiang V. Lung Cancer Brain Metastases. Cancer journal (Sudbury, Mass) 2015;21(5):398–403. doi: 10.1097/ppo.0000000000000146.
2. Hubbs JL, Boyd JA, Hollis D, Chino JP, Saynak M, Kelsey CR. Factors associated with the development of brain metastases: analysis of 975 patients with early stage nonsmall cell lung cancer. Cancer. 2010;116(21):5038–46. doi:10.1002/cncr.25254.
3. Lin X, DeAngelis LM. Treatment of brain metastases. J Clinical Oncology : Official J American Soc Clin Oncology. 2015;33(30):3475–84. doi:10.1200/jco.2015.60.9503.
4. Venur VA, Ahluwalia MS. Prognostic scores for brain metastasis patients: use in clinical practice and trial design. Chin Clin Oncol. 2015;4(2):18. doi:10.3978/j.issn.2304-3865.2015.06.01.
5. Gaspar L, Scott C, Rotman M, Asbell S, Phillips T, Wasserman T, et al. Recursive partitioning analysis (RPA) of prognostic factors in three radiation therapy oncology group (RTOG) brain metastases trials. Int J Radiat Oncol Biol Phys. 1997;37(4):745–51.
6. Weltman E, Salvajoli JV, Brandt RA, de Morais Hanriot R, Prisco FE, Cruz JC, et al. Radiosurgery for brain metastases: a score index for predicting prognosis. Int J Radiat Oncol Biol Phys. 2000;46(5):1155–61.
7. Lorenzoni J, Devriendt D, Massager N, David P, Ruiz S, Vanderlinden B, et al. Radiosurgery for treatment of brain metastases: estimation of patient eligibility using three stratification systems. Int J Radiat Oncol Biol Phys. 2004;60(1):218–24. doi:10.1016/j.ijrobp.2004.02.017.
8. Golden DW, Lamborn KR, McDermott MW, Kunwar S, Wara WM, Nakamura JL, et al. Prognostic factors and grading systems for overall survival in patients treated with radiosurgery for brain metastases: variation by primary site. J Neurosurg. 2008;109(Suppl):77–86. doi:10.3171/jns/2008/109/12/s13.
9. Sperduto PW, Chao ST, Sneed PK, Luo X, Suh J, Roberge D, et al. Diagnosis-specific prognostic factors, indexes, and treatment outcomes for patients with newly diagnosed brain metastases: a multi-institutional analysis of 4,259 patients. Int J Radiat Oncol Biol Phys. 2010;77(3):655–61. doi:10.1016/j.ijrobp.2009.08.025.
10. Rades D, Dziggel L, Segedin B, Oblak I, Nagy V, Marita A, et al. A new survival score for patients with brain metastases from non-small cell lung cancer. Strahlentherapie und Onkologie : Organ der Deutschen Rontgengesellschaft [et al]. 2013;189(9):777–81. doi:10.1007/s00066-013-0362-x.
11. Iasonos A, Schrag D, Raj GV, Panageas KS. How to build and interpret a nomogram for cancer prognosis. J Clin Oncology : Official J American Soc Clin Oncology. 2008;26(8):1364–70. doi:10.1200/jco.2007.12.9791.
12. Ruda R, Franchino F, Soffietti R. Treatment of brain metastasis: current status and future directions. Curr Opin Oncol. 2016. doi:10.1097/cco.0000000000000326.
13. Patchell RA, Tibbs PA, Walsh JW, Dempsey RJ, Maruyama Y, Kryscio RJ, et al. A randomized trial of surgery in the treatment of single metastases to the brain. N Engl J Med. 1990;322(8):494–500. doi:10.1056/nejm199002223220802.
14. Muacevic A, Wowra B, Siefert A, Tonn JC, Steiger HJ, Kreth FW. Microsurgery plus whole brain irradiation versus gamma knife surgery alone for treatment of single metastases to the brain: a randomized controlled multicentre

phase III trial. J Neuro-Oncol. 2008;87(3):299–307. doi:10.1007/s11060-007-9510-4.
15. Metellus P, Reyns N, Voirin J, Menei P, Bauchet L, Faillot T, et al. Surgery of brain metastases. Cancer radiotherapie : J de la Societe Francaise de Radiotherapie Oncologique. 2015;19(1):20–4. doi:10.1016/j.canrad.2014.11.007.
16. Al-Shamy G, Sawaya R. Management of brain metastases: the indispensable role of surgery. J Neuro-Oncol. 2009;92(3):275–82. doi:10.1007/s11060-009-9839-y.
17. Rancoule C, Vallard A, Guy JB, Espenel S, Diao P, Chargari C, et al. Brain metastases from non-small cell lung carcinoma: changing concepts for improving patients' outcome. Crit Rev Oncol Hematol. 2017;116:32–7. doi:10.1016/j.critrevonc.2017.05.007.
18. Pessina F, Navarria P, Cozzi L, Ascolese AM, Maggi G, Rossi M, et al. The role of surgical resection in patients with single large brain metastases: feasibility, morbidity and local control evaluation. World neurosurgery. 2016. doi:10.1016/j.wneu.2016.06.098.
19. Kaul D, Angelidis A, Budach V, Ghadjar P, Kufeld M, Badakhshi H. Prognostic indices in stereotactic radiotherapy of brain metastases of non-small cell lung cancer. Radiation Oncology (London, England). 2015;10:244. doi:10.1186/s13014-015-0550-1.
20. Agboola O, Benoit B, Cross P, Da Silva V, Esche B, Lesiuk H, et al. Prognostic factors derived from recursive partition analysis (RPA) of radiation therapy oncology group (RTOG) brain metastases trials applied to surgically resected and irradiated brain metastatic cases. Int J Radiat Oncol Biol Phys. 1998;42(1):155–9.
21. Nieder C, Geinitz H, Molls M. Validation of the graded prognostic assessment index for surgically treated patients with brain metastases. Anticancer Res. 2008;28(5b):3015–7.
22. Nieder C, Mehta MP. Prognostic indices for brain metastases–usefulness and challenges. Radiation oncology (London, England). 2009;4:10. doi:10.1186/1748-717x-4-10.
23. Mor V, Laliberte L, Morris JN, Wiemann M. The Karnofsky performance status scale. An examination of its reliability and validity in a research setting. Cancer. 1984;53(9):2002–7.
24. Jin J, Zhou X, Liang X, Huang R, Chu Z, Jiang J, et al. Brain metastases as the first symptom of lung cancer: a clinical study from an Asian medical center. J Cancer Res Clin Oncol. 2013;139(3):403–8. doi:10.1007/s00432-012-1344-6.
25. Kuremsky JG, Urbanic JJ, Petty WJ, Lovato JF, Bourland JD, Tatter SB, et al. Tumor histology predicts patterns of failure and survival in patients with brain metastases from lung cancer treated with gamma knife radiosurgery. Neurosurgery 2013;73(4): 641–647; discussion 7 doi:10.1227/neu.0000000000000072.
26. Guo H, Xing Y, Mu A, Li X, Li T, Bian X, et al. Correlations between EGFR gene polymorphisms and pleural metastasis of lung adenocarcinoma. OncoTargets Therapy. 2016;9:5257–70. doi:10.2147/ott.s97907.
27. Hansen J, Becker A, Kluth LA, Rink M, Steuber T, Zacharias M, et al. Assessing the clinical benefit of a nomogram to predict specimen-confined disease at radical prostatectomy in patients with high-risk prostate cancer: an external validation. Urologic oncology 2015;33(9):384e1–384e8. doi:10.1016/jurolonc2015.02.017.
28. Bevilacqua JL, Kattan MW, Fey JV, Cody HS, 3rd, Borgen PI, Van Zee KJ. Doctor, what are my chances of having a positive sentinel node? A validated nomogram for risk estimation. Journal of clinical oncology : official journal of the American Society of Clinical Oncology 2007;25(24):3670–3679 doi:10.1200/jco.2006.08.8013.
29. Graesslin O, Abdulkarim BS, Coutant C, Huguet F, Gabos Z, Hsu L, et al. Nomogram to predict subsequent brain metastasis in patients with metastatic breast cancer. J Clin Oncology : Official J American Soc Clin Oncology. 2010;28(12):2032–7. doi:10.1200/jco.2009.24.6314.

5

Synergistic inhibition of tumor growth by combination treatment with drugs against different subpopulations of glioblastoma cells

Chia-Hsin Chang[1†], Wei-Ting Liu[1†], Hui-Chi Hung[1], Chia-Yu Gean[2], Hong-Ming Tsai[2], Chun-Lin Su[1] and Po-Wu Gean[1,3*]

Abstract

Background: Glioma stem cells (GSCs) contribute to tumor recurrence and drug resistance. This study characterizes the tumorigenesis of CD133[+] cells and their sensitivity to pharmacological inhibition.

Methods: GSCs from human U87 and rat C6 glioblastoma cell lines were isolated via magnetic cell sorting using CD133 as a cancer stem cell marker. Cell proliferation was determined using the WST-1 assay. An intracranial mouse model and bioluminescence imaging were used to assess the effects of drugs on tumor growth in vivo.

Results: CD133[+] cells expressed stem cell markers and exhibited self-renewal and enhanced tumor formation. Minocycline (Mino) was more effective in reducing the survival rate of CD133[+] cells, whereas CD133[−] cells were more sensitive to inhibition by the signal transducer and activator of transcription 3 (STAT3) inhibitor. Inhibition of STAT3 decreased the expression of CD133[+] stem cell markers. The combination of Mino and STAT3 inhibitor synergistically reduced the cell viability of glioma cells. Furthermore, this combination synergistically suppressed tumor growth in nude mice.

Conclusion: The results suggest that concurrent targeting of different subpopulations of glioblastoma cells may be an effective therapeutic strategy for patients with malignant glioma.

Keywords: Glioma, Cancer stem cells, Minocycline, STAT3, Combination therapy, Synergy

Background

Glioblastoma multiforme (GBM) is the most common type of primary brain tumor. Its infiltrative nature prevents complete resection [1]. In addition, GBM is highly resistant to radiation and chemotherapy. The median survival time is around 1–2 years [2]. Therefore, it is imperative to develop novel strategies and to identify more efficient therapeutic approaches for the treatment of GBM.

Accumulating evidence indicates that a small populaton of cells within the malignant neoplasm are capable of initiating and promoting tumor growth [3, 4]. These cells, termed cancer stem cells (CSCs) or tumor-initiating cells (TICs), can form neurospheres in vitro and initiate tumor growth in nude mice [3]. Thus, CSCs are thought to contribute to tumor recurrence and drug resistance after conventional treatment [5].

CSCs were first isolated from tumor tissues and later from tumor cell lines, including breast cancer, prostate cancer, epithelial ovarian carcinoma, melanoma, colon cancer, and brain tumors [6–9]. CD133 (prominin-1), a five-transmembrane glycoprotein, is commonly used as a surface marker for the identification of normal human stem cells. Previous studies showed that purified CD133[+] cells generated neurospheres in culture and promoted

* Correspondence: powu@mail.ncku.edu.tw
†Equal contributors
[1]Department of Pharmacology, College of Medicine, National Cheng Kung University, Tainan, Taiwan
[3]Department of Biotechnology and Bioindustry Sciences, College of Bioscience and Biotechnology, National Cheng Kung University, Tainan, Taiwan
Full list of author information is available at the end of the article

brain tumors in in vivo models [6, 10–12]. In the present study, we aimed at isolating and culturing CSCs from rat C6 and human U87 tumor cell lines. CSCs were purified via selection with CD133 magnetic microbeads. We found that STAT3 inhibitor increased the sensitivity of glioma cells to chemotherapeutic drugs. Thus, concurrent targeting of CD133$^+$ and CD133$^-$ cells may be an effective therapeutic strategy for patients with malignant glioma.

Methods

Animals

Mice were housed in animal rooms with controlled temperature (23 ± 2 °C) and humidity (55 ± 5%), exposed to a 12-h light-dark cycle, and allowed free access to water and food. All experimental procedures were in accordance with the National Institutes of Health guidelines and were approved by the National Cheng Kung University Medical Center Animal Care and Use Committee (project approval number #104064).

Cell culture

The human glioma cell line U87 was kindly provided by Dr. Michael Hsiao (Genomics Research Center, Academia Sinica, Taiwan) and rat glioma C6 cells was kindly provided by Dr. Shun-Fen Tzeng (National Cheng Kung University, Taiwan). The human glioma U87 cell line was cultured in Dulbecco's modified Eagle medium (DMEM, Caisson) supplemented with 10% fetal bovine serum (FBS, Sigma-Aldrich), 2 mM L-glutamine (Caisson), 100 U/ml penicillin, and 0.1 mg/ml streptomycin (Caisson). The rat glioma C6 cell line was cultured in DMEM/F12 (Caisson) supplemented with 10% FBS, 2 mM L-glutamine, 100 U/ml penicillin, and 0.1 mg/ml streptomycin. Cultured cells were maintained in a humidified incubator at 37 °C in 5% CO_2/95% air. The cells were labeled with 1 ml CD133/L micromagnetic beads per million cells using a CD133 cell isolation kit (Miltenyi Biotec, Bergisch Gladbach, Germany). CD133$^+$ and CD133$^-$ cells were plated onto 24-well culture dishes (5000 cells/well). CD133$^+$ cells were plated in serum-free medium containing 10 μg/ml fibroblast growth factor 2 (FGF-2) and 10 μg/ml epidermal growth factor (EGF) and gave rise to non-adherent spheres on Ultra Low Attachment Multiple Well Plates (CORNING). CD133$^+$ cells were allowed to form spheres/aggregates in a suspension culture, and were then dissociated and passaged using Accutase Cell Detachment Solution (BD Biosciences) at 37 °C for 30 min.

Magnetic cell sorting and flow cytometry

C6 and U87 glioblastoma parental cells were trypsinized and suspended with ice-cold phosphate-buffered saline (PBS), centrifuged at 800 g for 5 min, and then resuspended in 1 × PBS with 0.5% bovine serum albumin (BSA) and 2 mM EDTA. Magnetically labeled anti-CD133 antibody from the Miltenyi Biotec CD133 cell isolation kit was used to isolate glioma CD133$^+$ cells, as previously described [13]. CD133-PE conjugated antibody was applied for cell staining and evaluating the efficiency of magnetic separation via flow cytometry. The cell suspension was then placed within an autoMACS separator for magnetic separation. Labeled cells migrated toward the magnet; the unlabeled cells in suspension were drawn off. The remaining (labeled) cells were resuspended and then returned to the separator for further separation. The magnetic separation procedure was repeated twice to increase the efficiency of the magnetic separation. After the final elusion of the positive fraction of interest, the harvested cells suspended in culture medium were allowed for the downstream application. The separation purity was conducted via flow cytometry with a FACSCalibur machine (BD Biosciences).

Cell viability assay

Glioma cells (2×10^3 cells per well) were seeded in 96-well plates. Culture medium containing vehicle or drugs was added to the medium of each well, and cells were incubated at 37 °C for the indicated time. Cytotoxicity assayed via 2-(4-iodophenyl)-3-(4-nitrophenyl)-5-(2,4-disulfophenyl)-2H–tetrazolium monosodium salt (WST-1) reagent was used to measure cell viability. After aspirating drugs from wells, WST-1 was diluted in fresh culture medium (1:10) to a final volume of 100 μl and added into each well. The absorbance of soluble formazan was measured at 440 nm with a microplate reader. Cell viability is presented as the percentage of survivors relative to the vehicle-treated control culture. The absorbance of soluble formazan was measured at 440 nm with a microplate reader (Molecular Devices).

We used the response additivity approach [14]. In this approach, a positive drug combination effect occurs when the observed combination effect (E_{AB}) is greater than the expected additive effect given by the sum of the individual effects ($E_A + E_B$). The combination index (CI) was calculated as: $CI = (E_A + E_B)/E_{(A + B)}$.

Western blotting assay

Glioma cells were treated with medium containing minocycline (Mino), WP1066, or vehicle in a 10-cm dish at 37 °C. At the indicated time, cells were centrifuged at 4000 rpm and pellets were collected and stored at −80 °C. Cell pellets were lysed in a lysis buffer containing 50 mM Tris–HCl, pH 7.4, 150 mM NaCl, 1% Nonidet P-40, 0.25% sodium deoxycholate, 0.1% sodium dodecyl sulfate (SDS), and supplemented with protease (Roche) and phosphatase inhibitors (Roche). Lysates were shaken at 40 rpm on ice for 1 h and then centrifuged at 13,000 rpm for 30 min at 4 °C. Supernatants were collected and protein concentration was measured via the Bradford assay. The proteins were re-suspended in a 5X sample buffer (12.5 mM Tris, 25% glycerol, 4% SDS, 1.54% DTT, and 0.02% Bromophenol blue) and boiled in water for 10 min. Protein electrophoresis was conducted on 15%, 10%, or 9% SDS-polyacrylamide gel under 100 V. The separated proteins were transferred to a PVDF membrane (Immunobilon transfer membranes, Millipore) using a semi-dry transfer system (BIO-RAD) under 400 mA and 20 V for 2 h. The membrane was then immersed in 5% nonfat milk or 3% BSA) for 1 h at room temperature for non-specific blocking; it was reacted at 4 °C overnight with the following primary antibodies: CD133 (1:6000, Merck Millipore), NANOG (1:1000, ProSci Inc.), SOX-2 (1:1000, abcam), Caspase 3 (1:2000, Cell Signaling), Caspase 8 (1:2000, Cell Signaling), Caspase 9 (1:2000, Cell Signaling), and β-Actin (1:400,000, Millipore). HRP-conjugated secondary antibody (Jackson ImmunoResearch Lab., USA) was incubated at room temperature for 1 h. After three rinses with TBST for 10 min each, ECL-plus chemical reagents (PerkinElmer) were added to the membrane. The films were exposed and developed until an optimal image was obtained, but not saturated. The films were scanned and images were analyzed and quantified using ImageJ software (NIH) to evaluate the expression of proteins of interest. The protein levels in all groups are expressed as a percentage of those in controls.

Immunocytochemical staining of CD133⁺ cells

For immunostaining of non-adherent spheres, cells were seeded on Ultra Low Attachment Multiple Well Plates for 7 days. Cells were then fixed with 4% paraformaldehyde (PFA) in PBS and stained with primary antibodies against CD133 (mouse monoclonal; Merck Millipore), Nestin (rabbit polyclonal; Proteintech), SSEA-1 (rabbit polyclonal; Bioss), and SOX-2 (rabbit polyclonal; Abaca). The secondary antibodies used were Alexa Fluor®594-conjugated Goat-anti-rabbit IgG (Jackson ImmunoResearch) and Alexa Fluor®488-conjugated Sheep-anti-mouse IgG (Jackson ImmunoResearch). DAPI (4′,6-diamidino-2-phenylindole) (Sigma-Aldrich) dye was used to stain the nuclei.

Neurosphere formation assay

To count the total number of neurospheres, CD133⁺ and CD133⁻ cells were suspended and seeded at 2.5 × 10⁴ cells/well in Ultra Low Attachment Multiple Well Plates in stem cell medium. After incubation for 14–21 days at 37 °C, floating neutrospheres were counted using inverted fluorescence microscopy (Olympus IX71). A cluster of more than five single cells was counted as a neurosphere.

In vivo intracranial xenograft animal model and bioluminescence imaging

The lentiviral vector pAS2.EGFP construct was obtained from the National RNAi Core Facility at Academia Sinica, Taipei, Taiwan. Firefly luciferase cDNA was put into pAS2.EGFP and a bi-cistronic lentivirus expression vector was constructed. Lentiviruses were produced by co-transfecting the GFP-Luc-expressing lentiviral vector, the envelope plasmid (pMD2.G), and the packaging plasmid (pCMV-dR8.91) into 293 T cells using calcium phosphate. The culture medium was changed on day 2, and the viral supernatants were harvested and titrated.

For tumorigenesis, 10- to 12-week-old male nude mice (BALB/cAnN-Foxnlnu/CrlNarl mice, National Laboratory Animal Center) were subcutaneously injected with 1×10^4 CD133⁺ or CD133⁻ cells. For the intracranial tumor model, U87 and C6 glioma cells were transduced with a lentiviral vector expressing GFP and firefly Luc. Luciferase-expressing CD133⁺ cells (5×10^3 cells in Fig. 3b, 1×10^5 cells in Fig. 7) were injected intracranially into the 10- to 12-week-old male nude mice. The sorted cells were immediately implanted into the nude mice without further culture/amplification. Nude mice were anesthetized with chlorohydrate and placed on a stereotaxic device. Subsequently, a Hamilton syringe with a 30-gauge needle was mounted on the stereotaxic device. U87 luciferase-expressing glioma cells were injected 1.5 mm caudal and lateral to the bregma, and at a depth of 3.5–4 mm into the left side of the brain. Ten days after tumor implantation, Mino (50 mg/kg in saline with 10% DMSO), WP1066 (20 mg/kg in DMSO and polyethylene glycol), or their combination was injected intraperitoneally once per day for 10 days into the mice. Tumors were monitored via longitudinal bioluminescence imaging, for which mice were injected with 100 μg of luciferin (Caliper), simultaneously anesthetized with isoflurane, and subsequently imaged with a cooled charge-coupled device camera (IVIS-200, Xenogen). Tumor light output was quantitated using the Living Image 2.5 software package (Xenogen).

The method used to calculate combination drug interaction was based on previous reports [15, 16]. Fractional tumor volume (FTV) was calculated as tumor volume experimental/mean tumor volume control. Expected FTV was calculated as FTV of Minocycline × FTV of WP1066. A synergistic effect is suggested when the ratio of expected FTV/observed FTV is more than 1. A ratio of <1 indicates a less than additive effect.

Statistical analysis

Experiments were performed at least in triplicate. All results are presented as mean ± standard error of the mean (SEM). Independent experiments were analyzed using the unpaired t test. One-way analysis of variance

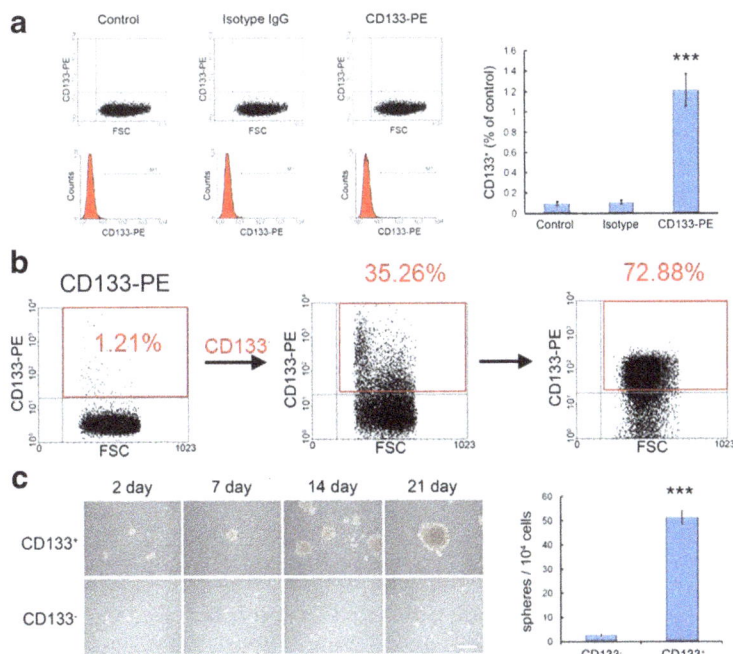

Fig. 1 Analysis, sorting, and characterization of CD133 positive cells via flow cytometry in C6 glioma cells. **a** Flow cytometry analysis of CD133 expression in C6 glioma cells. We detected 1.21% CD133 positive cells in C6 glioma cells. ***$p < 0.001$ vs. control. **b** C6 glioma cells were sorted for CD133 expression using magnetic bead cell sorting. CD133$^+$ cells were collected and cultured under the same conditions as those for unsorted parental cells. Purity of the CD133$^+$ populations was 35.26% at the second sorting and 72.88% after the third sorting. **c** Primary neurospheres derived from CD133$^+$ or CD133$^-$ cells of C6 glioma cells were dissociated and cultured. CD133$^+$ cells generated a greater number of secondary neurospheres than did CD133$^-$ cell. ***$p < 0.001$ vs. CD133$^-$. Scale bar: 100 μm

(ANOVA) was used to analyze differences in neurosphere numbers, various signaling inhibitors, and cell viability. Bonferroni multiple comparison tests were used as post hoc comparisons. Data were considered significant at the $p < 0.05$ level.

Results

CD133 has been demonstrated as a marker of brain normal and tumor stem cells [6, 17]. Analyzing CD133 expression via flow cytometry revealed that 1.21% of C6 glioma cells were CD133 positive (CD133$^+$) (Fig. 1a). Magnetic bead cell sorting was used to sort for CD133 expression in C6 glioma cells [18, 19]. Sorted CD133$^+$ and CD133$^-$ aliquots were checked with flow cytometry. The purity of the CD133$^+$ populations was 35.26% at the second sorting and 72.88% after the third sorting. Only 0.48% of the CD133$^-$ populations responded to CD133 antibody in the second sorting (Fig. 1b).

Primary neurospheres derived from CD133$^+$ or CD133$^-$ cells were dissociated and cultured. Over 3- to 21-day culture periods, CD133$^+$ cells generated a greater number of secondary neurospheres than did CD133$^-$ cells. CD133$^+$ cells were capable of growing as non-adherent spheres and continued to expand their population. Unpaired t tests showed that the self-renewal ability of CD133$^+$ cells at day 21 was significantly higher than that of CD133$^-$ cells ($t_{(6)} = 17.19$, $p < 0.001$) (Fig. 1c). Similar isolation of CD133$^+$ cells was performed from U87 glioma cells. A previous study revealed that the CD133$^+$ cell fraction accounted for 0.5% of the total population in U87 cells [20]. The number of neuroseres derived from CD133$^+$ cell at day 14 was significantly greater than that derived from CD133$^-$ cells ($t_{(4)} = 11.28$, $p < 0.001$).

Nestin, a cytoskeletal protein, is known to be a neural stem/progenitor cell marker [21]. NANOG is a transcription factor important for the self-renewal of embryonic stem cells [22, 23]. Stage-specific embryonic antigen 1 (SSEA-1) is a marker of murine normal and stem-like cells [24]. Western blotting analysis showed that nestin, NANOG, and SSEA-1 were present in the CD133$^+$ cells derived from C6 glioma cells (Fig. 2a). Furthermore, neurospheres derived from CD133$^+$ cells were positive for nestin and Musashi, an RNA-binding protein that is selectively expressed in neural progenitor cells [25] (Fig. 2b). These stem cell markers were also present in the CD133$^+$ cells derived from U87 glioma cells (data not shown).

To address whether CD133$^+$ and CD133$^-$ cells differed in their ability to form tumors in vivo, we inoculated CD133$^+$ or CD133$^-$ cells derived from C6 glioma cells (1×10^4) subcutaneously into the nude mice. Ten days after the inoculation, tumors were observed in 6 out of 6

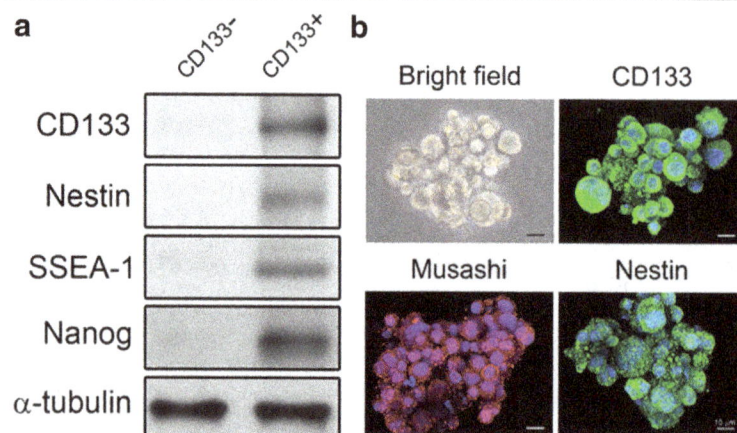

Fig. 2 Neurospheres derived from CD133 positive cells exhibit stem cell-like markers. Western blotting (**a**) and immunochemical staining (**b**) of neurospheres derived from CD133$^+$ cells. The neurospheres were positive for nestin, NANOG, and SSEA-1, markers for neural stem cells, embryonic stem cells, and pluripotent stem cells respectively. Scale bar: 10 μm

mice inoculated with CD133$^+$ cells. In nude mice inoculated with CD133$^-$ cells, in contrast, no tumors formed (0 out of 6 mice tested) (Fisher's exact test, $p < 0.01$) (Fig. 3a). We determined whether CD133$^+$ cells promoted tumor formation in an intracranial tumor model. To monitor intracranial tumor growth, Luc-expressing CD133$^+$ cells (5×10^3 cells) derived from U87 glioma cells were injected intracranially into athymic mice, and tumor growth was assessed using the IVIS-200 imaging system. Consistently,

tumors were observed in 4 out of 4 mice injected intracranially with CD133$^+$ cells. No tumors formed in nude mice injected with CD133$^-$ cells (0 out of 4 mice tested, Fisher's exact test, $p < 0.05$) (Fig. 3b).

We determined the signal pathways associated with neutrosphere formation activity by testing the effect of various signal pathway inhibitors on the self-renewal capacity of CD133$^+$ cells derived from C6 glioma cells. CD133$^+$ cells were treated with EGFR inhibitors

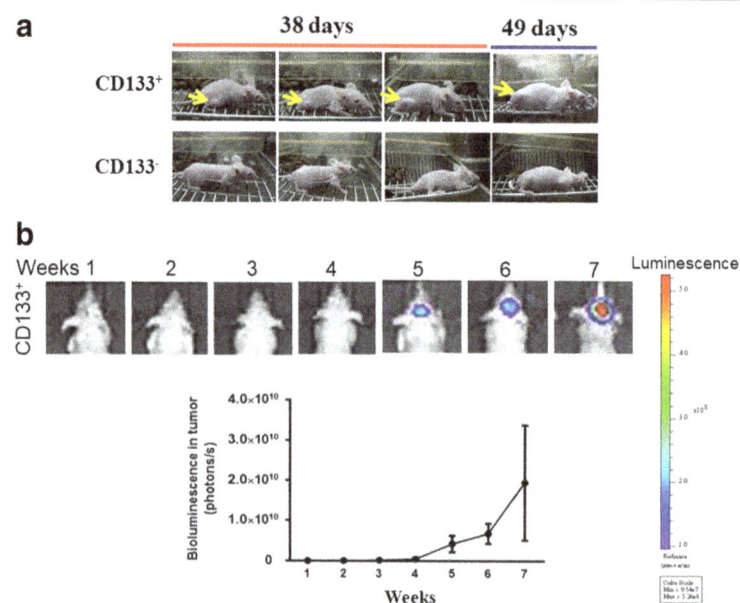

Fig. 3 CD133$^+$ but not CD133$^-$ cells are able to form tumors in vivo. **a** CD133$^+$ or CD133$^-$ cells (1×10^4) derived from C6 glioma cells were inoculated subcutaneously into the nude mice. Ten days after the inoculation, tumors were observed in 6 out of 6 mice inoculated. In contrast, no tumors formed in nude mice inoculated with CD133$^-$ cells (0 out of 6 mice tested) (Fisher's exact test, $p < 0.01$). **b** Luc-expressing CD133$^+$ cells derived from U87 glioma cells were injected intracranially into athymic mice, and tumor growth was assessed using the IVIS-200 imaging system. Tumors were observed in 4 out of 4 mice injected intracranially with CD133$^+$ cells. No tumors formed in 4 out of 4 mice injected with CD133$^-$ cells (Fisher's exact test, $p < 0.05$)

(PD153035 and PD168393) [26, 27], PI3K inhibitor (LY294002) [28], Akt inhibitor (Akt inhibitor VIII) [29], mTOR inhibitors (rapamycin, Pl103), JNK inhibitor (SP600125), MEK inhibitor (PD98059), cSrc inhibitor (PP2) [30], p38 MEK inhibitor (SB203580), JAK inhibitor (AG490) [31], STAT3 inhibitor (WP1006) [32], TGFβ inhibitor (SB431542) [33], or β-catenin inhibitor (FH535) [34] for 24 h and the number of neurospheres was measured. As shown in Fig. 4a, STAT3 inhibitor exhibited a potent effect on reducing the number of neutrospheres derived from CD133$^+$ cells. In parallel, CD133$^+$ cells were treated with various signal pathway inhibitors for 24 h and the survival rate was determined using the WST-1 assay. STAT3 inhibitor also had a potent effect on reducing the survival rate of CD133$^+$ cells (Fig. 4b).

Previously, we showed that Mino induced cell death in C6 glioma cells [35]. We compared the sensitivities of CD133$^+$ and CD133$^-$ cells to Mino treatment. CD133$^+$ and CD133$^-$ cells derived from U87 cells were treated with Mino (25 μM) for 48 h and cell viability was measured using the WST-1 assay. As shown in Fig. 5a,

CD133$^-$ cells were more sensitive to Mino than were CD133$^+$ cells. Mino at a concentration of 25 μM decreased the number of CD133$^-$ cells by 40% but only decreased the number of CD133$^+$ cells by 7% ($t_{(8)}$ = 4.271, $p < 0.01$). Conversely, STAT3 inhibitor WP1066 at a concentration of 5 μM reduced the number of CD133$^+$ cells by 92% but only reduced the number of CD133$^-$ cells by 27.5% ($t_{(18)}$ = 11.29, $p < 0.001$) (Fig. 5b).

We also compared the activated states of STAT3 among CD133$^+$, CD133$^-$, and their parental cells from C6 glioma cells and found that CD133$^+$ exhibited the highest phosphorylated state (Fig. 5c). CD133$^+$ C6 glioma cells were treated with STAT3 inhibitors WP1066 (5 μM) or S3 l-201 (50 μM) [36] for 24 h and p-STAT3, STAT3, CD133, Nestin, SSES-1, and NANOG were measured using Western blotting analysis. As expected, the phosphorylated states of STAT3 were markedly inhibited by WP1066 and S3 l-201 (Fig. 5d), so as the cancer stem cell markers Nestin, SSES-1, and NANOG (Fig. 5e).

We determined whether Mino (5 μM) alone or in combination with WP1006 induced synergistic

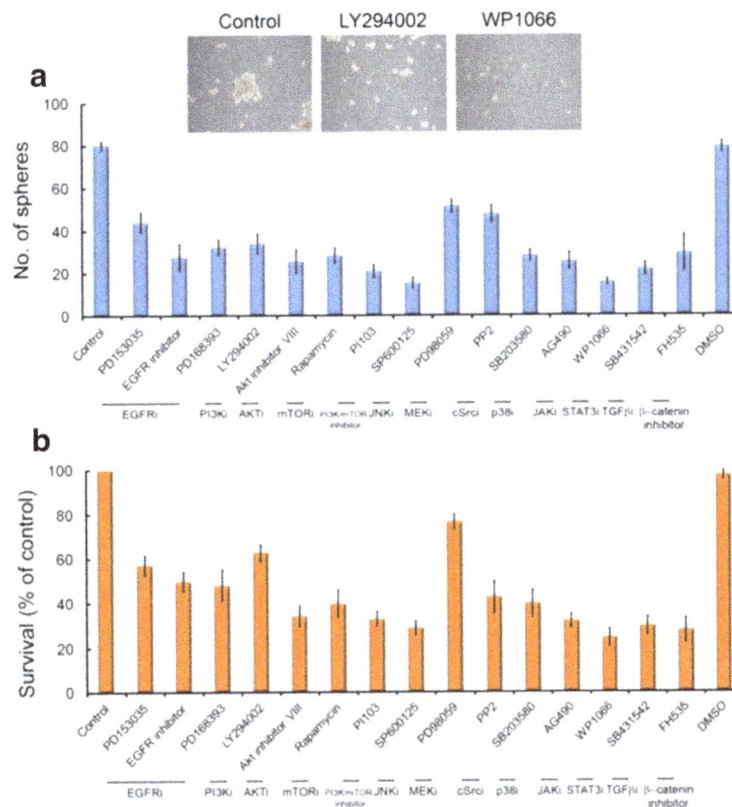

Fig. 4 Effects of various signal pathway inhibitors on the number of neurospheres derived from CD133$^+$ cells and the survival rate of C6 glioma cells. **a** Primary neurospheres derived from CD133$^+$ were dissociated and cultured. They were then treated with EGFR inhibitors (PD103035 and PD168393), PI3K inhibitor (LY294002), Akt inhibitor (Akt inhibitor VIII), mTOR inhibitors (rapamycin, Pl103), JNK inhibitor (SP600125), MEK inhibitor (PD98059), cSrc inhibitor (PP2), p38 MEK inhibitor (SB203580), JAK inhibitor (AG490), STAT3 inhibitor (WP1006), TGFβ inhibitor (SB431542), or β-catenin inhibitor (FH535) for 24 h and number of neurospheres were measured. **b** CD133$^+$ cells were treated with various signal pathway inhibitors for 48 h and the survival rate was measured using the WST-1 assay

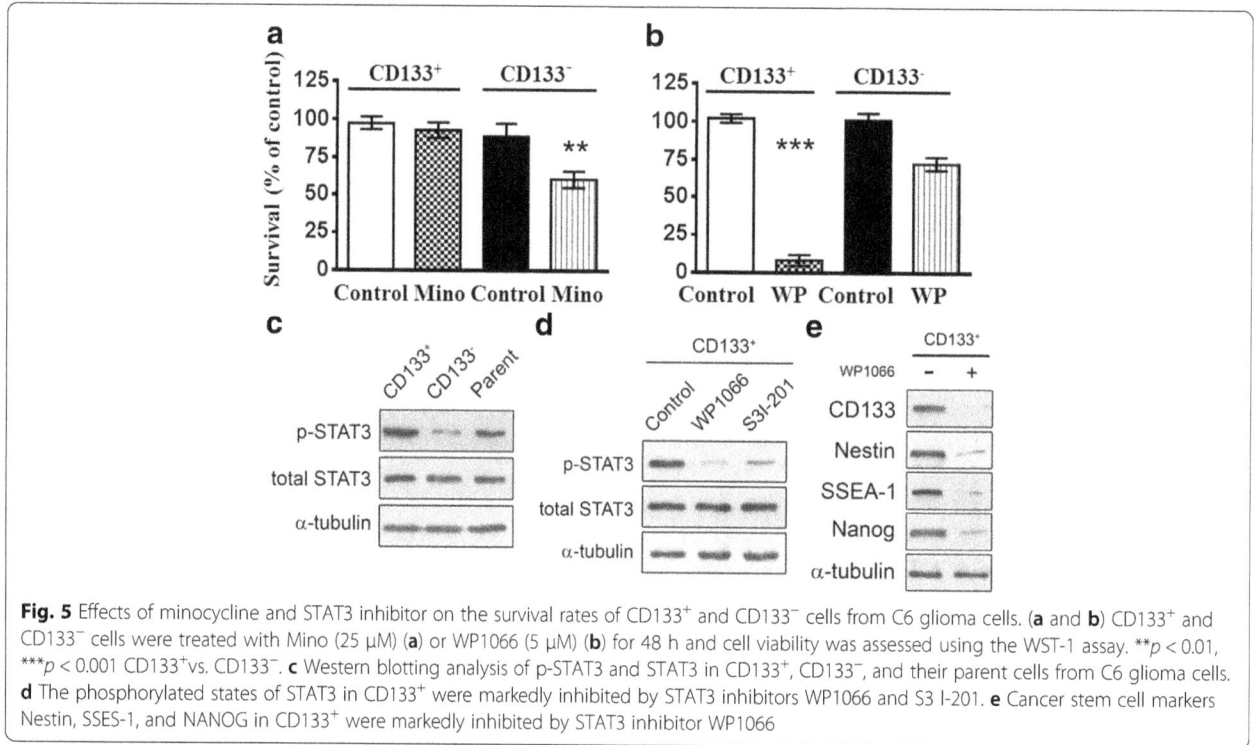

Fig. 5 Effects of minocycline and STAT3 inhibitor on the survival rates of CD133$^+$ and CD133$^-$ cells from C6 glioma cells. (**a** and **b**) CD133$^+$ and CD133$^-$ cells were treated with Mino (25 μM) (**a**) or WP1066 (5 μM) (**b**) for 48 h and cell viability was assessed using the WST-1 assay. **p < 0.01, ***p < 0.001 CD133$^+$vs. CD133$^-$. **c** Western blotting analysis of p-STAT3 and STAT3 in CD133$^+$, CD133$^-$, and their parent cells from C6 glioma cells. **d** The phosphorylated states of STAT3 in CD133$^+$ were markedly inhibited by STAT3 inhibitors WP1066 and S3 I-201. **e** Cancer stem cell markers Nestin, SSES-1, and NANOG in CD133$^+$ were markedly inhibited by STAT3 inhibitor WP1066

cytotoxicity toward glioma cells. U87 glioma cells were treated with Mino (5 μM), WP1006 (25 μM), or Mino (5 μM) plus WP1006 (25 μM) and cell viability was assessed using the WST-1 assay. Mino alone reduced survival rate by 2.6% whereas WP1006 reduced survival rate by 23.3%. Mino plus WP1006 inhibited cell growth by 64% (Fig. 6a). The combination drug index (CDI) for WP1006 (25 μM) and Mino (5 μM) was 0.481. Similarly, Mino (50 μM) alone reduced survival rate by 9% and Mino plus WP1006 inhibited cell growth by 67.7%. CDI for WP1006 (25 μM) and Mino (50 μM) was 0.462. The CDI values are less than 1, indicating a synergistic effect.

U87 glioma cells were treated with Mino (50 μM) plus WP1066 (5 μM) for different times, as indicated. We found that the cleaved fragment of caspase 3 was increased at 48 h after treatment (Fig. 6b). Furthermore, U87 glioma cells were treated with Mino (50 μM), WP1066 (5 μM), or their combination for 48 h. The expression of the cleaved fragment of caspase 3 was determined using Western blotting analysis. Figure 6c shows that the expression of the cleaved fragment of caspase 3 was higher after a combined application of Mino (50 μM) and WP1006 (5 μM) than those after the application of Mino or WP1006 alone.

We used the intracranial tumor model to determine whether Mino plus WP1006 could synergistically inhibit tumor growth. Transduced glioma cells were injected intracranially into athymic mice (Fig. 7a). At day 10 after injection, Mino (50 mg/kg), WP1006 (20 mg/kg), or

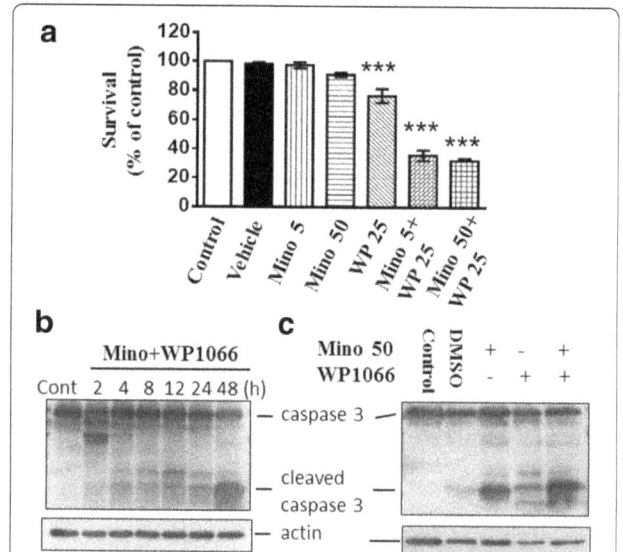

Fig. 6 Effects of Mino and WP1066 alone or in combination on the cell survival and caspase-3 activation in U87 glioma cells. **a** U87 glioma cells were treated with Mino (5 or 50 μM) and WP1066 (25 μM) alone or in combination and cell survival was assessed 48 h after the treatment using the WST-1 assay. Mino plus WP1066 synergistically inhibited cell growth. ***p < 0.001 vs. control. **b** Western blotting analysis of cleaved caspase-3. U87 glioma cells were treated with Mino (50 μM) and WP1066 (5 μM) for the indicated times. The expression of the cleaved fragment of caspase 3 was significantly increased. **c** U87 glioma cells were treated with Mino (50 μM), WP1066 (5 μM), or their combination for 48 h. The expression of the cleaved fragment of caspase 3 was determined using Western blotting analysis

their combination was injected intraperitoneally once per day into the mice for 10 days and tumor growth was observed for 15 more days (Fig. 7b). At day 35, Mino inhibited tumor growth by 63.3% and WP1006 inhibited tumor growth by 13%. Mino plus WP1006 in combination inhibited tumor growth by 98.9%. The expected fractional tumor volume (FTV) was 0.319 and the observed FTV was 0.011. The ratio of expected FTV/observed FTV was 29. A ratio of >1 indicates a synergistic effect and a ratio of <1 indicates a less than additive effect [15, 16]. These results suggest that a combination of Mino and WP1006 synergistically inhibits the intracranial growth of U87 glioma cells. The body weight of the mice was measured every 4 days. There were no differences among control, Mino, WP1006, and combination groups at day 35 (Fig. 7c).

Discussion

Although brain tumors are composed of a heterogeneous mass of cells, a subpopulation of cells called tumor stem cells is capable of self-renewal and initiating the formation of neurospheres [3–5]. Here, we established a method for the isolation, culture, and purification of tumor stem cells from rat C6 and human U87 glioblastoma cell lines using magnetic beads coupled to anti-CD133 antibody. These CD133$^+$ cells exhibited immunophenotypic characteristics of neural stem cells. First, CD133$^+$ cells were capable of initiating the formation of neurospheres, whereas CD133$^-$ cells were unable

to form tumors at the cell number tested. Second, neurospheres derived from CD133$^+$ cells were positive for nestin, NANOG, and SSEA-1, markers for neural stem cells, embryonic stem cells, and pluripotent stem cells, respectively. Third, when CD133$^+$ cells were inoculated into the nude mice, they were able to form tumors in vivo. In contrast, CD133$^-$ cells were unable to form tumors. These results indicate that we successfully established a process for the isolation and culture of glioblastoma stem cells.

In the present study, we demonstrated that the survival of CD133$^+$ stem-like cells in glioblastoma depends on STAT3 activity. We showed that the phosphorylated and activated level of STAT3 was higher in CD133$^+$ cells than in CD133$^-$ cells. STAT3 inhibitor WP1066 exhibited a potent effect on decreasing the number of neurospheres derived from CD133$^+$ cells. In addition, the survival rate of glioma cells and the expression of cancer stem cell markers Nestin, SSES-1, and NANOG were attenuated by WP1066. These results are consistent with previous reports showing that the STAT3 signaling pathway contributes to the progression of neurosphere-initiating tumor cells [32, 33].

We next examined the effect of WP1066 in combination with Mino, which was more effective in reducing the survival of CD133$^-$ cells than CD133$^+$ cells. Mino plus WP1006 synergistically inhibited the survival of glioma cells in vitro as well as the intracranial growth of U87 glioma cells in vivo. Furthermore, the expression of

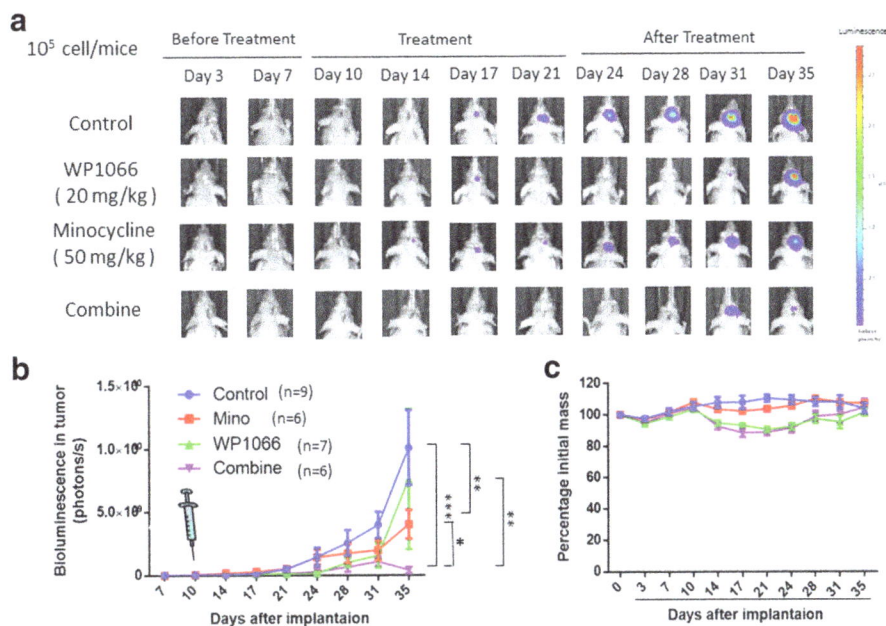

Fig. 7 Minocycline and WP1066 in combination synergistically inhibit intracranial tumor growth. **a** U87 glioma cells were injected intracranially into athymic mice and tumor growth was studied using the IVIS-200 imaging system. **b** At day 10 after intracranial injection of tumor cells, Mino (50 mg/kg), WP1006 (20 mg/kg), or their combination was administered intraperitoneally once per day for 10 days and tumor growth was observed for 15 days after the cessation of treatment. **c** Weight measurements were taken every 4 days. There were no differences among the four groups at day 35

the cleaved fragment of caspase 3 was increased, suggesting that the combination of Mino and WP1066 induced cell death through caspase-dependent apoptosis.

We found that inhibiting both CD133$^+$ and CD133$^-$ cells is more effective than inhibiting CD133$^+$ cells only. The results suggest that CD133$^-$ cells if untreated may undergo de-differentiation or reprogramming such that they can be converted to CD133$^+$ cells. Since STAT3 inhibitor reduced the viability of CD133$^+$ cells, STAT3 activation may promote reprogramming. Previous reports showing that STAT3 signaling is sufficient to promote somatic cell reprogramming [37–39] support this hypothesis.

Chemotherapy has not effectively increased the survival of patients with GBM because it usually targets the fast growing tumor mass, leaving cancer stem cells less affected. Combination therapy, on the other hand, is advantageous because it may not only lower the nonspecific toxicity produced by a high dose of single treatment but can also target different subpopulations of cancer cells. There may be adverse effects, as several inhibitors have been withdrawn from clinical trials due to serious side effects, including systemic STAT3 inhibition [40, 41].

Conclusion

We isolated cancer stem-like cells from human U87 and rat C6 glioblastoma cells via magnetic cell sorting using CD133 as a marker. We found that Mino was more effective in reducing the viability of CD133$^-$ cells, whereas STAT3 inhibitor was more effective in reducing the viability of CD133$^+$ cells. Mino and STAT3 inhibitor in combination produced a synergistic effect in reducing the cell viability of glioma cells in vitro and inhibited tumor growth in nude mice. This suggests that simultaneously targeting different subpopulations of glioblastoma cells may be an effective therapeutic strategy for patients with malignant glioma.

Abbreviations

CDI: Combination drug index; CSCs: Cancer stem cells; FTV: Fractional tumor volume; GBM: Glioblastoma Multiforme; GSCs: Glioma stem cells; Mino: Minocycline; STAT3: Signal transducer and activator of transcription 3; TICs: Tumor-initiating cells; WST-1: 2-(4-iodophenyl)-3-(4-nitrophenyl)-5-(2,4-disulfophenyl)-2H–tetrazolium

Acknowledgments

We would like to thank Dr. Michael Hsiao (Genomics Research Center, Academia Sinica, Taiwan) for providing human U87 glioma cell lines and Dr. Shun-Fen Tzeng (National Cheng Kung University, Taiwan) for providing rat glioma C6 cells.

Funding

This study was supported by the Ministry of Sciences and Technology of Taiwan (grant MOST 104–2320-B-006-007-MY3). The funding body had no role in the design of the study, collection, analysis, and interpretation of data, and in writing the manuscript.

Authors' contributions

CHC: collection and assembly of data, data analysis, and interpretation. WTL: conception and design, data analysis, and interpretation.CYG: data analysis and interpretation. HMT: conception and design. HCH: conception and design of experiments, manuscript writing. CLS: conception and design of experiments. PWG: conception and design of experiments, and manuscript writing. All authors approved the final manuscript.

Competing interest

The authors declare that they have no competing interest.

Author details

[1]Department of Pharmacology, College of Medicine, National Cheng Kung University, Tainan, Taiwan. [2]Department of Diagnostic Radiology, National Cheng Kung University Hospital, Tainan, Taiwan. [3]Department of Biotechnology and Bioindustry Sciences, College of Bioscience and Biotechnology, National Cheng Kung University, Tainan, Taiwan.

References

1. Bleau AM, Hambardzumyan D, Ozawa T, Fomchenko EI, Huse JT, Brennan CW, Holland EC. PTEN/PI3K/Akt pathway regulates the side population phenotype and ABCG2 activity in glioma tumor stem-like cells. Cell Stem Cell. 2009;4:226–35.
2. Wen PY, Kesari S. Malignant gliomas in adults. N Engl J Med. 2008;359: 492–507.
3. Vinogradov S, Wei X. Cancer stem cells and drug resistance: the potential of nanomedicine. Nanomedicine. 2012;7:597–615.
4. Medema JP. Cancer stem cells: the challenges ahead. Nat Cell Biol. 2013;15: 338–44.
5. Bao S, Wu Q, Sathornsumetee S, Hao Y, Li Z, Hjelmeland AB, Shi Q, McLendon RE, Bigner DD, Rich JN. Stem cell-like glioma cells promote tumor angiogenesis through vascular endothelial growth factor. Cancer Res. 2006;66:7843–8.
6. Singh SK, Clarke ID, Terasaki M, et al. Identification of a cancer stem cell in human brain tumors. Cancer Res. 2003;63:5821–8.
7. Li C, Heidt DG, Dalerba P, Burant CF, Zhang L, Adsay V, Wicha M, Clarke MF, Simeone DM. Identification of pancreatic cancer stem cells. Cancer Res. 2007;67:1030–7.
8. O'Brien CA, Pollett A, Gallinger S, Dick JE. A human colon cancer cell capable of initiating tumour growth in immunodeficient mice. Nature. 2007; 445:106–10.
9. Prince ME, Sivanandan R, Kaczorowski A, Wolf GT, Kaplan MJ, Dalerba P, Weissman IL, Clarke MF, Ailles LE. Identification of a subpopulation of cells with cancer stem cell properties in head and neck squamous cell carcinoma. Proc Natl Acad Sci U S A. 2007;104:973–8.
10. Galli R, Binda E, Orfanelli U, Cipelletti B, Gritti A, De Vitis S, Fiocco R, Foroni C, Dimeco F, Vescovi A. Isolation and characterization of tumorigenic, stem-like neural precursors from human glioblastoma. Cancer Res. 2004;64:7011–21.
11. Stupp R, Hegi ME. Targeting brain-tumor stem cells. Nat Biotech. 2007; 25:193–4.
12. Angelastro JM, Lame MW. Overexpression of CD133 promotes drug resistance in C6 glioma cells. Mol Cancer Res. 2010;8:1105–15.
13. Annabi B, Lachambre MP, Plouffe K, Sartelet H, Beliveau R. Modulation of Invasive Properties of CD133(+) Glioblastoma Stem Cells: A Role for MT1-MMP in Bioactive Lysophospholipid Signaling. Mol Carcinogenesis. 2009;48:910–9.
14. Slinker BK. The statistics of synergism. J Mol Cell Cardiol. 1998;30:723–31.
15. Yu DC, Chen Y, Dilley J, Li Y, Embry M, Zhang H, Nguyen N, Amin P, Oh J, Henderson DR. Antitumor synergy of CV787, a prostate cancer-specific adenovirus, and paclitaxel and docetaxel. Cancer Res. 2001;61(2):517–25.
16. Yokoyama Y, Dhanabal M, Griffioen AW, Sukhatme VP, Ramakrishnan S. (2000) Synergy between angiostatin and endostatin: inhibition of ovarian cancer growth. Cancer Res. 15;60(8):2190-2196.
17. Pallini R, Ricci-Vitiani L, Montano N, Mollinari C, Biffoni M, Cenci T, Pierconti F, Martini M, De Maria R, Larocca LM. Expression of the stem cell marker CD133 in recurrent glioblastoma and its value for prognosis. Cancer. 2011;117:162–74.

18. Chiou SH, Kao CL, Chen YW, Chien CS, Hung SC, Lo JF, Chen YJ, Ku HH, Hsu MT, Wong TT. Identification of CD133-positive radioresistant cells in atypical teratoid/rhabdoid tumor. PLoS One. 2008;3:e2090.

19. Yang YP, Chang YL, Huang PL, Chiou GY, Tseng LM, Chiou SH, Chen MH, Chen MT, Shih YH, Chang CH, Hsu CC, Ma HI, Wang CT, Tsai LL, Yu CC, Chang CJ. Resveratrol suppresses tumorigenicity and enhances radiosensitivity in primary glioblastoma tumor initiating cells by inhibiting the STAT3 axis. J Cell Physiol. 2012;227:976–93.

20. Wang Z, Wang B, Shi Y, Xu C, Xiao HL, Ma LN, Xu SL, Yang L, Wang QL, Dang WQ, Cui W, Yu SC, Ping YF, Cui YH, Kung HF, Qian C, Zhang X, Bian XW. Oncogenic miR-20a and miR-106a enhance the invasiveness of human glioma stem cells by directly targeting TIMP-2. Oncogene. 2015;34:1407–19.

21. Michalczyk K, Ziman M. Nestin structure and predicted function in cellular cytoskeletal organisation. Histol Histopathol. 2005;20:665–71.

22. Chambers I, Colby D, Robertson M, Nichols J, Lee S, Tweedie S, Smith A. Functional expression cloning of Nanog, a pluripotency sustaining factor in embryonic stem cells. Cell. 2003;113:643–55.

23. Mitsui K, Tokuzawa Y, Itoh H, Segawa K, Murakami M, Takahashi K, Maruyama M, Maeda M, Yamanaka S. The homeoprotein Nanog is required for maintenance of pluripotency in mouse epiblast and ES cells. Cell. 2003;113:631–42.

24. Liu S, Liu H, Tang S, Pan Y, Ji K, Ning H, Wang S, Qi Z, Li L. Characterization of stage-specific embryonic antigen-1 expression during early stages of human embryogenesis. Oncol Rep. 2004;12:1251–6.

25. Kaneko Y, Sakakibara S, Imai T, Suzuki A, Nakamura Y, Sawamoto K, Ogawa Y, Toyama Y, Miyata T, Okano H. Musashi 1: an evolutionarily conserved marker for CNS progenitor cells including neural stem cells. Dev Neurosci. 2000;22:139–53.

26. Bos M, Mendelsohn J, Kim YM, Albanell J, Fry DW, Baselga J. PD153035, a tyrosine kinase inhibitor, prevents epidermal growth factor receptor activation and inhibits growth of cancer cells in a receptor number-dependent manner. Clin Cancer Res. 1997;3:2099–106.

27. Fry DW, Bridges AJ, Denny WA, Doherty A, Greis KD, Hicks JL, Hook KE, Keller PR, Leopold WR, Loo JA, Mcnamara DJ, Nelson JM, Sherwood V, Smaill JB, Trumpp-Kallmeyer S, Dobrusin EM. Specific, irreversible inactivation of the epidermal growth factor receptor and erbB2, by a new class of tyrosine kinase inhibitor. Proc Natl Acad Sci U S A. 1998;95:12022–7.

28. Sauveur-Michel M, Stauffer F, Schnell C, Garcia-Echeverria C. PI3K inhibitors for cancer treatment: where do we stand? Biochem Soc Trans. 2009;37:265–72.

29. Zhong Z, Dang Y, Yuan X, Guo W, Li Y, Tan W, Cui J, Lu J, Zhang Q, Chen X, Wang Y. Furanodiene, a natural product, inhibits breast cancer growth both in vitro and in vivo. Cell Physiol Biochem. 2012;30:778–90.

30. Hanke JH, Gardner JP, Dow RL, Changelian PS, Brissette WH, Weringer EJ, Pollok BA, Connelly PA. Discovery of a novel, potent, and Src family-selective tyrosine kinase inhibitor. Study of Lck- and FynT-dependent T cell activation. J Biol Chem. 1996;271:695–701.

31. Miyamoto N, Sugita K, Goi K, Inukai T, Iijima K, Tezuka T, Kojika S, Nakamura M, Kagami K, Nakazawa S. The JAK2 inhibitor AG490 predominantly abrogates the growth of human B-precursor leukemic cells with 11q23 translocation or Philadelphia chromosome. Leukemia. 2001;15:1758–68.

32. Hussain SF, Kong LY, Jordan J, Conrad C, Madden T, Fokt I, Priebe W, Heimberger AB. A novel small molecule inhibitor of signal transducers and activators of transcription 3 reverses immune tolerance in malignant glioma patients. Cancer Res. 2007;67:9630–6.

33. Inman GJ, Nicolás FJ, Callahan JF, Harling JD, Gaster LM, Reith AD, Laping NJ, Hill CS. SB-431542 is a potent and specific inhibitor of transforming growth factor-beta superfamily type I activin receptor-like kinase (ALK) receptors ALK4, ALK5, and ALK7. Mol Pharmacol. 2002;62:65–74.

34. Handeli S, Simon JA. A small-molecule inhibitor of Tcf/beta-catenin signaling down-regulates PPARgamma and PPARdelta activities. Mol Cancer Ther. 2008;7:521–9.

35. W.T. Liu, C.H. Lin, M. Hsiao, P.W. Gean, Minocycline inhibits glioma growth by inducing autophagy. Autophagy 7 (2011) 166-175.

36. Siddiqueea K, Zhang S, Guida WC, Blaskovich MA, Greedy B, Lawrence HR, Yip MLR, Jove R, McLaughlin MM, Lawrence NJ, Sebtid SM, Turkson J. Selective chemical probe inhibitor of Stat3, identified through structure-based virtual screening, induces antitumor activity. Proc Natl Aca Sci. 2007;104:7391–6.

37. Sherry MM, Reeves A, Wu JK, Cochran BH. STAT3 is required for proliferation and maintenance of multipotency in glioblastoma stem cells. Stem Cells. 2009;27:2383–92.

38. Tang Y, Luo Y, Jiang Z, Ma Y, Lin CJ, Kim C, et al. Jak/ Stat3 signaling promotes somatic cell reprogramming by epigenetic regulation. Stem Cells. 2012;30:2645–56.

39. van Oosten AL, Costa Y, Smith A, Silva JC. JAK/ STAT3 signalling is sufficient and dominant over antagonistic cues for the establishment of naive pluripotency. Nat Commun. 2012;3:817.

40. Chiba T. STAT3 inhibitors for cancer therapy –the rationale and remained problems. EC Cancer. 2016;1(S1):S1–8.

41. Takeda K, Noguchi K, Shi W, Tanaka T, Matsumoto M, Yoshida N, Kishimoto T, Akira S. Targeted disruption of the mouse Stat3 gene leads to early embryonic lethality. Proc Natl Aca Sci. 1997;94:3801–4.

6

Inhibition of glioblastoma dispersal by the MEK inhibitor PD0325901

Stephen Shannon[1], Dongxuan Jia[1], Ildiko Entersz[1], Paul Beelen[1], Miao Yu[3], Christian Carcione[1], Jonathan Carcione[1], Aria Mahtabfar[1], Connan Vaca[1], Michael Weaver[1], David Shreiber[2], Jeffrey D. Zahn[2], Liping Liu[3,4], Hao Lin[3] and Ramsey A. Foty[1*]

Abstract

Background: Dispersal of glioblastoma (GBM) cells leads to recurrence and poor prognosis. Accordingly, molecular pathways involved in dispersal are potential therapeutic targets. The mitogen activated protein kinase/extracellular signal regulated kinase (MAPK/ERK) pathway is commonly dysregulated in GBM, and targeting this pathway with MEK inhibitors has proven effective in controlling tumor growth. Since this pathway also regulates ECM remodeling and actin organization – processes crucial to cell adhesion, substrate attachment, and cell motility – the aim of this study was to determine whether inhibiting this pathway could also impede dispersal.

Methods: A variety of methods were used to quantify the effects of the MEK inhibitor, PD0325901, on potential regulators of dispersal. Cohesion, stiffness and viscosity were quantified using a method based on ellipsoid relaxation after removal of a deforming external force. Attachment strength, cell motility, spheroid dispersal velocity, and 3D growth rate were quantified using previously described methods.

Results: We show that PD0325901 significantly increases aggregate cohesion, stiffness, and viscosity but only when tumor cells have access to high concentrations of fibronectin. Treatment also results in reorganization of actin from cortical into stress fibers, in both 2D and 3D culture. Moreover, drug treatment localized pFAK at sites of cell-substratum adhesion. Collectively, these changes resulted in increased strength of substrate attachment and decreased motility, a decrease in aggregate dispersal velocity, and in a marked decrease in growth rate of both 2D and 3D cultures.

Conclusions: Inhibition of the MAPK/ERK pathway by PD0325901 may be an effective therapy for reducing dispersal and growth of GBM cells.

Keywords: Glioblastoma, Dispersal velocity, MEK inhibitor, 3D spheroids, Fibronectin matrix

Background

Early and continuing dispersal of tumor cells from the primary mass renders GBM refractory to complete surgical excision or targeted chemotherapy and directly leads to recurrence and dismal prognosis. Strategies aimed at containing the primary or recurrent tumor could significantly improve targeted delivery of chemotherapeutic agents and increase the likelihood of total surgical resection. To disperse, cells must first detach from the primary mass, a process that likely involves mechanisms that decrease cohesion between tumor cells [1]. Cells must also attach to substrates at strengths that optimize their motility and secrete factors to facilitate their interaction with parenchyma [2, 3]. In addition, tumor cells must also become relatively compliant so as to deform and "squeeze" through pores in a meshwork of ECM components [4], and in the case of GBM, astrocytes within the normal brain parenchyma. Accordingly, strategies aimed at preventing tumor cell detachment, limiting motility, and inhibiting changes in compliance offer an effective approach to reduce dispersal. Ideally, such strategies should employ pharmacological agents that can cross the blood–brain barrier and that specifically target molecular pathways involved in mediating cohesion, adhesion, and compliance.

* Correspondence: fotyra@rwjms.rutgers.edu
[1]Department of Surgery-Rutgers Robert Wood Johnson Medical School, Clinical Academic Building, 125 Paterson Street, New Brunswick, NJ 08901, USA
Full list of author information is available at the end of the article

Cadherins, integrins and the extracellular matrix (ECM) are potential therapeutic targets, and various studies have identified drugs that can modulate their expression or function. For example, gamma-linolenic acid (GLA) up-regulates E-cadherin expression and inhibits invasion of lung, colon, breast, melanoma, and liver cancer [5]. Invasion suppression here was likely due to an increase in the strength of intercellular cohesion mediated by up-regulation of E-cadherin. 5-aza-deoxycitidine (5 AC) has also been shown to effectively inhibit invasion by up-regulating E-cadherin expression [6]. Because the down-regulation of E-cadherin is often associated with up-regulation of N-cadherin during epithelial-mesenchymal transition, drugs that can block N-cadherin expression have also been shown to be effective in blocking invasion. Biflorin, a novel o-naphtoquinone, has been shown to inhibit expression of N-cadherin and to block invasion of breast cancer cells [7]. Such drugs could be of potential benefit for glioblastoma given the correlation between increased N-cadherin expression in high-grade gliomas and tissue invasion [8]. Various integrins, including αvβ3 and αvβ5 have also been targets of anticancer therapy. Cilengitide, a cyclic pentapeptide, is a specific inhibitor of these integrins and has been shown to have anti-invasive activity in various glioma models [9]. Given the complexity and heterogeneity of the ECM, and the likelihood that glioma cells tune their integrin receptor fingerprint to match the local ECM microenvironment, drugs that modulate the ECM may prove effective in reducing dispersal. Many of these drugs, including various corticosteroids, target the ECM as a by-product of the drugs' principal actions. Consequently, this activity may in part be beneficial to the drugs' disease-modifying properties [10]. An example of such a drug is Dexamethasone (Dex). Dex is currently used to treat brain tumor-related edema associated with mass effect from Glioblastoma [11]. A by-product of the effects of Dex in glioblastoma is its ability to restore fibronectin matrix assembly (FNMA) and decrease detachment of tumor cells from cultured 3D spheroids [1]. However, due to the relatively high doses required, Dex has many side-effects, often limiting its long-term use. Identification of other drugs that can have similar effects but more specifically target pathways involved in modulating integrins and the ECM could be of therapeutic value.

The MAPK/ERK pathway has been identified as a commonly dysregulated pathway in several cancers, most notably in melanoma. Combined targeting of this pathway can have a synergistic effect in controlling tumor growth [12]. Clinical trials using various MEK inhibitors, such as trametinib [13, 14], cobimetinib [15] and CI 1040 (PD184352) [16] have been shown to shrink some melanomas, specifically those with BRAF mutations. The MEK inhibitor PD0325901 has also demonstrated efficacy in melanoma cell lines independent of BRAF status [17]. Experimental models have demonstrated in vitro and in vivo efficacy of PD0325901 in controlling tumor growth in animal models of GBM [18], although studies have identified possible issues with limited access through the blood–brain barrier [19]. To our knowledge, there is only one ongoing phase-2 trial testing the effects of PD0325901 on tumor growth in patients with neurofibromatosis type –1 (NF1) or plexiform neurofibromas [20] NCT02096471), and none testing efficacy in GBM. The majority of these studies have focused mainly on inhibition of growth and on activation of apoptosis. Inasmuch as MEK inhibitors target pathways that can also influence actin organization and remodeling of the ECM, we asked whether PD0325901 could also serve to impact mechanisms that regulate dispersal of primary human GBM cells.

We first determined whether primary human GBM cells used in this study are sensitive to PD0325901. We then assessed the effects of MEK inhibition on integrin activation *vis à vis* restoration of FNMA and actin organization in both 2D and 3D cultures. We also quantified the effects of PD0325901 on spheroid mechanical properties including cohesion, stiffness and viscosity. We evaluated effects of PD0325901 in regulating the strength of cell-substrate adhesion, cell motility, dispersal of tumor cells from spheroids, and in an ex vivo dispersal assay. Finally, we determined whether PD0325901 could also influence the growth rate of both 2D and 3D cultures of GBM.

Methods

Cell lines, maintenance, treatment, and generation of 3D spheroids

Four human primary glioblastoma cell lines (GBM-1, GBM-2, GBM-3 and GBM-4) were previously isolated and characterized [21]. Samples were examined by a neuropathologist and stained for several markers to confirm their designation as human GBM. Microscopically, all lines were described as astrocytic neoplasms with moderate to high pleiomorphism, vascular endothelial hyperplasia, with areas of abundant necrosis. Lines are all GFAP positive. GBM-1 and GBM-4 exhibit PTEN loss and all lines appear to express p-AKT. All lines express Nestin and BMI-1, both markers of undifferentiated cells. Collectively, pathologic and molecular analysis confirms highly undifferentiated grade IV glioma/glioblastoma. Cells were maintained in Eagles' Minimal Essential Medium (EMEM)/10% fetal calf serum (FCS) and antibiotics/antimycotics. They were sub-cultured using standard protocols and used at 3rd to 6th passage. Normal human astrocytes (NHA) were purchased from Lonza (Allendale, NJ) and maintained in AGM™

Astrocyte Growth Medium as recommended by the manufacturer. Where required, cells were treated with PD 0325901, a powerful inhibitor of ERK1/2 phosphorylation, at a final concentration of 1 μM w/v DMSO for 24 h prior to assay. Spheroids were generated as previously described [1].

Immunoblot and immunofluorescence assays

To confirm that PD0325901 inhibited ERK1/2 phosphorylation, cells were treated with either dimethyl sulfoxide (DMSO, vehicle control) or 1 μM PD0325901 overnight under standard tissue culture conditions. Twenty μg of protein was separated by SDS-PAGE under reducing conditions. Gels were blotted to PVDF and probed with anti-phospho P44/42 MAPK or P44/42 MAPK antibodies (Cell Signaling Technologies, Danvers, MA) and appropriate HRP-conjugated secondary antibodies. Blots were developed using Amersham ECL Prime Western Blotting Detection reagent (GE Healthcare Life Sciences, Pittsburgh, PA) and a C-Digit Blot Scanner (Li-COR, Lincoln, NE). Assessment of FNMA, phospho-FAK and actin expression by GBM cells in conventional 2D culture was performed as previously described [1]. For assessment of actin organization in 3D spheroids, aggregates of GBM cells were fixed and permeabilized with 4% paraformaldehyde/0.5% Triton X-100 and incubated in 6nM rhodamine-phalloidin for 30 min. Aggregates were washed 4x with PBS, mounted onto slides, and imaged using a Zeiss AxioImager Z1 spinning disc confocal microscope attached to a Photometrics Evolve 512 EMCCD camera with Metamorph Premier imaging software.

Measurement of aggregate cohesion and viscoelasticity

Aggregate cohesion was measured by tissue surface tensiometry (TST). TST employs a custom-built instrument to compress spherical cellular aggregates between poly-HEMA coated parallel plates to which they cannot adhere. Measurements of aggregate geometry and resistance to the applied force are then applied to the Young-Laplace equation to calculate aggregate surface tension. The method has been described in detail [1, 22–24]. TST measurements are only valid when tissues behave like liquid systems [22–24]. Accordingly, the calculated surface tension of a liquid aggregate, when subjected to two successive compressions (σ_1 and σ_2), the second greater than the first, will remain constant. In such aggregates the ratio of σ_2/σ_1 will approach 1 and will be less than the ratio of the force applied at each successive compression (F_2/F_1). The surface tension of liquid aggregates will also be independent of aggregate size. Only measurements in which surface tension is independent of the applied force and size were used to calculate average σ for each cell line.

For measurement of viscoelasticity, aggregates ranging in size from 200-400 μm were loaded into the tensiometer and subjected to a compressive force for 30 s, whereupon the force was removed and aggregates were allowed to relax for 2 min. A high-speed camera captured 12 frames/s and the shape of the relaxing aggregates was extracted and analyzed using an in-house edge detection and analysis algorithm. Mechanical parameters were extracted from the shape dynamics with a continuum-based model which includes a Kelvin-Voigt bulk enclosed in a stressed surface. This advanced model is different than the simple spring-dashpot or compartmental models previously described [25]. Analysis of the relaxation dynamics was greatly facilitated by a closed-form, analytical solution that we derived. Details of the theory and the data analysis method, as well as preliminary data validating our approach are presented in Additional file 1.

Measurement of shear-flow induced detachment

Cell-ECM attachment was measured by subjecting adhering cells to flow-induced shear stress as previously described [1]. Briefly, DMSO or PD0325901-treated GBM cells were plated at a concentration of 5x10⁴ cells/ml onto 6-well polyethylene terephthalate cell culture inserts (Franklin Lakes, NJ) for 2 h and were then inverted into complete medium and incubated overnight. Inserts were then loaded into custom-designed flow chambers and subjected to 30 dynes/cm of shear stress for 3 h, whereupon inserts were washed in PBS and immersed in SYTO 16 green fluorescent nucleic acid stain (Life Technologies, Carlsbad, CA). Cells seeded onto inserts but not subjected to flow were used as growth rate controls. A Nikon Eclipse epifluorescence microscope was used to capture nine low magnification fields/insert and nuclei were counted in ImageJ. The average number of attached cells was then expressed as a percentage of the no-flow controls.

Measurement of cell motility

GBM cell motility was measured using a fluorescence bead phagokinetic assay [26] as previously described [1]. Briefly, wells of a six-well dish were coated with poly-D-lysine, whereupon 1 μM diameter fluorescent polystyrene microspheres (ThermoFisher Scientific, Grand Island, NY), adjusted to a concentration of 0.018% v/v in PBS were added and allowed to adhere to the poly-lysine for 2 h. Cells were plated in complete tissue culture medium (TCM) at a cell/area density of 4 cells/mm². Experiments were performed either in DMSO or in 1 μm PD0325901. Experiments were also performed with PD0325901-treated cells incubated in hFn 7.1, a mouse monoclonal anti-human fibronectin antibody, or with non-specific mouse IgG. Motile cells phagocytose beads as they move leaving behind non-fluorescent tracks. Cleared area was quantified in ImageJ.

Measurement of aggregate dispersal velocity

50–100 μm diameter aggregates of DMSO or PD0325901-treated GBM-1-4 were deposited into 12-well tissue culture plates containing 2mls of pre-warmed TCM. Plates were incubated for eight h. Images were captured for each aggregate every hour and diameter at each time point was measured. Dispersal velocity (DV) was represented by the slope as determined by linear regression analysis for change of diameter as a function of time. Only regression lines with r^2 values of 0.95 and greater were used to calculate DV for each GBM line. Data were normalized with initial aggregate diameter. Twelve aggregates were used to generate an average DV for each GBM line.

Measurement of z-axis dispersal distance by confocal microscopy

Dispersal of GBM cells through a NHA-seeded porous filter was measured as previously described [1]. Two-hundred μm thick, cross-linked polystyrene scaffolds (Alvetex, Reinnervate, Durham, UK) with tunnel diameters of 8–13 μm were seeded with $1x10^6$ NHA cells in 100 μL of tissue culture medium. After 60 min to allow NHA cells to adhere, scaffolds were placed in 12-well plates and incubated in 4mls of TCM for 48 h to permit incorporation of NHA cells throughout the scaffold. After 48 h, GBM cells that had been transfected with BacMam 2.0 GFPT (Life Technologies, Long Island, NY) were deposited onto each scaffold in a small volume of medium. Scaffolds were incubated for 48 h to allow time for tumor cells to infiltrate and disperse. To image dispersed cells, a Yokogawa CSU-X1 spinning disk confocal microscope with MetaMorph software was used to generate z-stacks of images taken at 1 μm intervals. Differential interference contrast microscopy was used to identify the z = 0 starting point for each z-stack. The z-axis position of each cell within each tissue-scaffold was scored. Within any given scaffold the mean average z-axis cell position from 5– 6 z-stacks was measured and recorded.

Measurement of cell growth in conventional 2D culture and in 3D spheroids

For measurement of growth in conventional 2D cultures, cells were plated at a concentration of $5x10^4$ cells/ml in wells of a 6-well dish in complete medium. Total and live cell counts were performed once/day for 4 days using a BioRad TC10 automated cell counter. For measurement of growth rate by 3D spheroids, aggregates were generated using the hanging drop method [1]. Single aggregates were plated onto wells of an agarose-coated 6-well dish. Agarose prevented aggregates from adhering to the bottom of the dish. The area of each aggregate was measured once/day for nine days. Growth rate was determined by plotting aggregate area as a function of time. Regression analysis was performed to calculate growth rates of 3D spheroids [1].

Results

Effects of PD0325901 on FNMA, actin organization and pFAK localization in primary GBM cells

Studies have previously demonstrated a growth-inhibitory role for PD0325901 in GBM [20]. Here, we explore another potential role as a suppressor of GBM dispersal. We first confirmed that the primary lines used in this study are sensitive to drug treatment. Figure 1a shows that PD0325901 treatment down-regulates p-ERK, the downstream effector of MEK, in all 4 primary GBM cell lines. Unlike Dex, PD0325901 did not induce FNMA (Fig. 1c) relative to DMSO controls (Fig. 1b). Rather, treatment resulted in a remarkable change in cell shape, treated cells (Fig. 1e) becoming flatter and larger than those treated with DMSO (Fig. 1d). PD0325901 treatment also gave rise to the organization of actin into stress fibers when cells were grown as conventional 2D culture (Fig. 1d, e), and a shift in actin organization from cortical to stress fibers when cells were incubated as 3D hanging drops (Fig. 1h, i). Moreover, PD0325901 treatment resulted in the localization of p-FAK at sites of cell-ECM attachment (Fig. 1g). These results indicate that PD0325901 treatment activates mechanisms involved in regulating cell motility and mechanical properties of single cells or cellular aggregates.

The effects of PD0325901 on spheroid mechanical properties are fibronectin dependent

We first generated measurements of aggregate cohesion for GBM-1-4 treated in either DMSO or PD0325901, and confirmed that the cohesion measured was reflective of a true tissue surface tension (Table 1). We demonstrated that all GBM samples exhibited the defining characteristics of liquid-like behavior: (1) they display a constant surface tension when subjected to two different degrees of compression. Accordingly, the means of σ_1 and σ_2 when compared by a paired t-test are not significantly different, (2) the ratio of σ_2/σ_1 approaches 1 and is less than the ratio of the applied force at each successive compression (F_2/F_1). Table 1 shows that for all lines, a t-test comparing the ratios of σ_2/σ_1 to F_2/F_1 resulted in a $p < 0.0001$, indicating that the ratio of σ_2/σ_1 was significantly different than that of F_2/F_1, and 3) the surface tension of the aggregates is independent of aggregate volume. For the 4 GBM lines, combined aggregate volumes were plotted as a function of surface tension. Linear regression analysis yielded correlation coefficients,

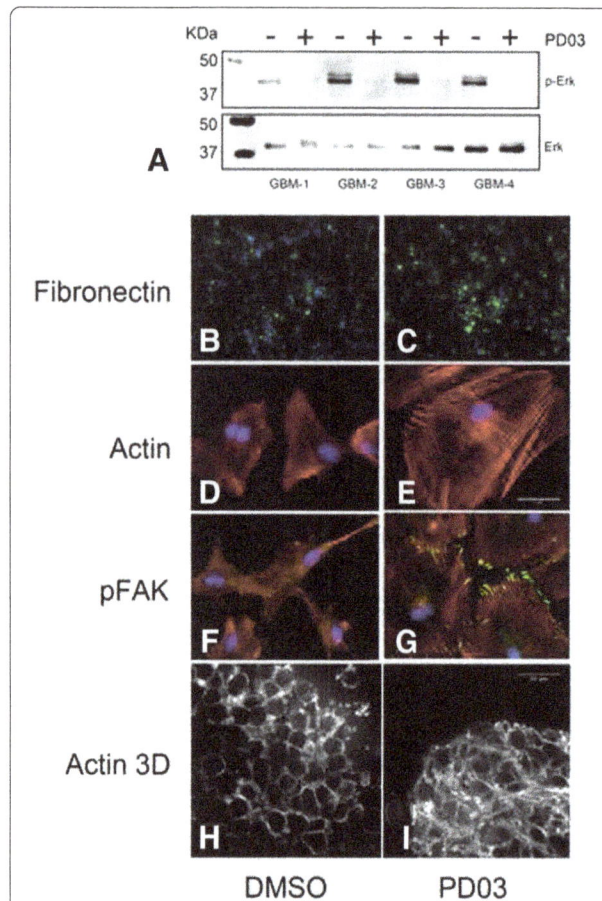

Fig. 1 Effects of PD0325901 on FNMA, actin organization and pFAK localization in primary GBM cells. Immunoblot analysis for phosho-ERK and ERK in response to overnight treatment with 1 μm PD0325901 or DMSO as vehicle control. PD0325901 significantly inhibited phosphorylation of ERK (**a**). Representative immunofluorescence images of FNMA by GBM-3 cells treated either with DMSO (**b**) or PD0325901 (**c**). Fibronectin is depicted in green and DAPI (blue) was used as counterstain. PD0325901 did not appear to induce FNMA by GBM-3 cells. Rhodamine-phalloidin staining of actin in DMSO-treated (**d**) or PD0325901-treated GBM-3 cells (**e**). Note significant cell shape change and actin fiber organization. Scale bar in (**e**) is 5 μm. Triple stain for actin (*red*), p-FAK (*green*) and DAPI (*blue*) in DMSO-treated (**f**) and PD0325901-treated (**g**) GBM-3 cells. PD0325901 appears to induce the localization of p-FAK at sites of cell-ECM attachment. Thirty-micron thick z-stack of DMSO (**h**) and PD0325901-treated (**i**) collected by confocal microscopy of multicellular aggregates of GBM-3. Note marked change in actin organization from cortical to stress fibers. Scale bar in (**i**) is 30 μm

r^2, of 0.031 and 0.071 for DMSO and PD0325901 treated aggregates, respectively, indicating that surface tension is independent of volume (Additional file 1: Figure S2). Figure 2a shows that PD0325901 treatment did not have an effect on aggregate surface tension. Surprisingly, however, generation of 3D spheroids in the presence of 300 μg/ml of serum fibronectin (sFn) resulted in a significant increase in aggregate cohesion (Fig. 2b),

suggesting that the effects of PD0325901 may be through enhancement of α5β1 integrin-fibronectin interaction. Since actin is a fundamental mediator of cell and tissue mechanics, we reasoned that PD0325901 mediated changes in actin reorganization should result in a change in aggregate stiffness and viscosity. Interestingly, for aggregates generated in 30 μg/ml sFn (30 sFn), PD0325901 treatment slightly increased stiffness (Fig. 2c) but had no effect on viscosity (Fig. 2d). However, when aggregates were generated in the presence of 300 μg/ml sFn, both stiffness (Fig. 2c) and viscosity (2D) markedly increased. This suggests that fibronectin is an absolute requirement for PD0325901 to alter mechanical properties.

PD0325901 increases resistance to shear-stress induced detachment, decreases cell motility and reduces dispersal velocity

The effects of PD0325901 on cell shape, actin reorganization and aggregate viscoelasticity translate to significant changes in tumor cell behavior. Notably, PD0325901 treatment rendered GBM cells more resistant to shear-induced detachment (Fig. 3a), suggesting a stabilization of cell-ECM adhesion and a decrease in area cleared by motile cells in a phagokinetic microbead assay. For all lines, cleared area was reduced approximately 3-fold in response to PD0325901 treatment, indicating a significant decrease in cell motility. When experiments were performed in TCM containing 5 μg/ml mouse monoclonal anti-human fibronectin antibody, the motility of PD0325901-treated cells was restored to levels comparable to those of DMSO controls (Fig. 3b). This effect was not observed when a non-specific mouse IgG was used (Additional file 1: Figure S4). These results indicate that the principal mechanism of PD0325901-mediated decrease in motility is α5β1 integrin-fibronectin dependent. Collectively, the observed increase in attachment strength to substrate and decreased motility gave rise to a significant overall decrease in aggregate dispersal velocity. Figure 3c shows that spheroids of GBM cells differ in baseline dispersal velocities and that PD0325901 treatment reduces DV relative to DMSO controls.

PD0325901 significantly alters pattern of dispersal and z-axis penetration

Treatment with the MEK inhibitor also resulted in a change in the pattern of dispersal. Whereas, the advancing edge of DMSO-treated aggregates dispersed as single cells (Fig. 4a, c), the leading edge of PD0325901-treated aggregates advanced as a sheet (Fig. 4b, d). Moreover, actin in advancing cells of DMSO-treated aggregates appeared to be cortical (Fig. 4b), whereas in treated aggregates, actin was arranged in stress fibers (Fig. 4d). This change in spreading behavior is likely associated with reduced cell motility, causing cells escaping the aggregate mass to

Table 1 Tissue surface tension measurements and confirmation of liquidity for DMSO-treated and PD0325901 treated aggregates of primary GBM cells

Line	σ_1 dynes/cm ± s.e.m	σ_2 dynes/cm ± s.e.m	$\sigma_{1,2}$ dynes/cm ± s.e.m	t-test σ_1 vs σ_2 p	σ_2/σ_1	F_2/F_1	t-test σ_2/σ_1 vs F_2/F_1 p
GBM-1 DMSO	16.9 ± 1.9	19.4 ± 2.3	18.2 ± 1.5	0.4082	1.14 ± 0.05	1.36 ± 0.01	0.0003
GBM-1 PD03	18.4 ± 1.3	17.9 ± 1.2	18.1 ± 0.9	0.7951	0.98 ± 0.04	1.36 ± 0.02	<0.0001
GBM-2 DMSO	15.5 ± 1.4	16.9 ± 2.0	16.2 ± 1.2	0.5638	1.07 ± 0.08	1.35 ± 0.03	0.0072
GBM-2 PD03	15.2 ± 1.4	15.1 ± 1.0	15.2 ± 0.8	0.9035	1.02 ± 0.07	1.37 ± 0.04	0.0003
GBM-3 DMSO	8.5 ± 0.6	8.6 ± 0.7	8.6 ± 0.4	0.9041	1.01 ± 0.04	1.36 ± 0.02	<0.0001
GBM-3 PD03	8.9 ± 0.7	10.1 ± 0.6	9.5 ± 0.5	0.2389	1.15 ± 0.03	1.42 ± 0.07	0.0017
GBM-3 DMSO 300 FN	7.5 ± 0.7	7.1 ± 0.7	7.3 ± 0.5	0.6725	0.95 ± 0.03	1.28 ± 0.03	<0.0001
GBM-3 PD03 300 FN	32.7 ± 5.8	37.9 ± 6.6	35.3 ± 4.3	0.5550	1.17 ± 0.03	1.32 ± 0.03	0.0047
GBM-4 DMSO	16.2 ± 1.8	15.8 ± 1.2	16.0 ± 1.1	0.8833	1.01 ± 0.05	1.34 ± 0.01	<0.0001
GBM-4 PD03	20.6 ± 1.2	20.2 ± 1.0	20.4 ± 1.8	0.8312	1.02 ± 0.04	1.35 ± 0.02	<0.0001

For all cell lines, PD0325901 treatment did not result in a change in surface tension (pair-wise comparison by Student t-test, $p > 0.05$). GBM-3 was used to determine effects of exogenous fibronectin on surface tension. Here, addition of 300 µg/ml of soluble fibronectin resulted in a significant increase in aggregate surface tension ($\sigma_{1,2}$) of 7.3 ± 0.5 to 35.3 ± 4.3 dynes/cm (pairwise Student t-test, $p < 0.0001$). Liquid behavior was confirmed by demonstrating that 1) surface tension measured at two different compressions, the second greater than the first, were not statistically different, and 2) that the ratio of σ_2/σ_1 approaches 1 and is less than the ratio of the applied force at each successive compression (F2/F1)

accumulate behind the advancing front. PD0325901 treatment also resulted in a significant reduction in z-axis dispersal for three of the four lines (Fig. 4e). The z-axis dispersal distance of PD0325901-treated GBM-1 and GBM-2 cells was approximately 2-fold less than that of the vehicle controls. GBM-3 cells responded more actively, their z-axis dispersal distance becoming reduced approximately 13-fold relative to controls.

PD0325901 reduces growth rates of conventional 2D cultures and 3D spheroids of GBM cells

Previous studies demonstrated that the growth rate of various immortalized GBM cell lines was markedly reduced by PD0325901 [20]. We tested our primary GBM lines to determine whether treatment had a similar effect when cells were grown as conventional 2D cultures and as spheroids. Figure 5 (a, b) shows that PD0325901

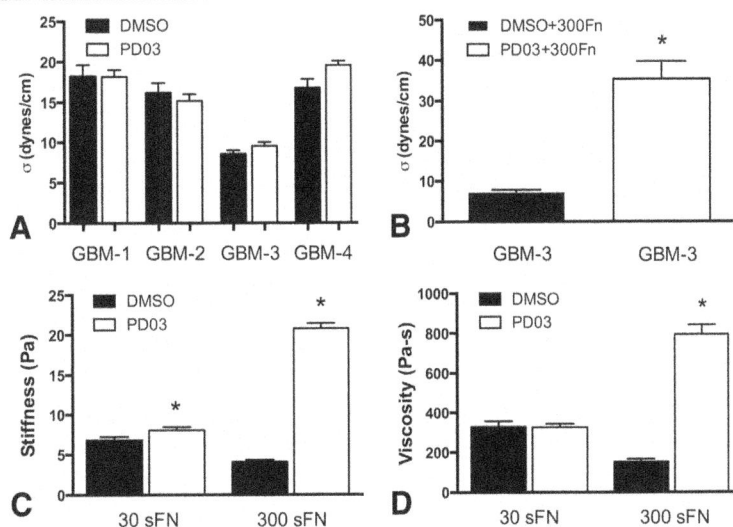

Fig. 2 Assessment of aggregate cohesion, stiffness, and viscosity in response to PD0325901 treatment. Surface tension measurements for GBM-1-4 aggregates generated using standard TCM and treated with either DMSO or PD0325901. $n = 20$, pair-wise comparison by Student t-test, $p > 0.05$ (**a**). Surface tension measurements of GBM-3 aggregates generated in fibronectin-depleted medium supplemented with 300 µg/ml of human fibronectin. $n = 20$, pair-wise comparison by Student t-test, $p < 0.0001$ (**b**). Stiffness (**c**) and viscosity (**d**) data for GBM-3 aggregates generated in fibronectin-depleted medium supplemented with either 30 µg/ml or 300 µg/ml human fibronectin. Asterisks represent statistical significance by pair-wise Student t-test, $p < 0.05$. Note significant increase in stiffness and viscosity in response to increased concentrations of fibronectin

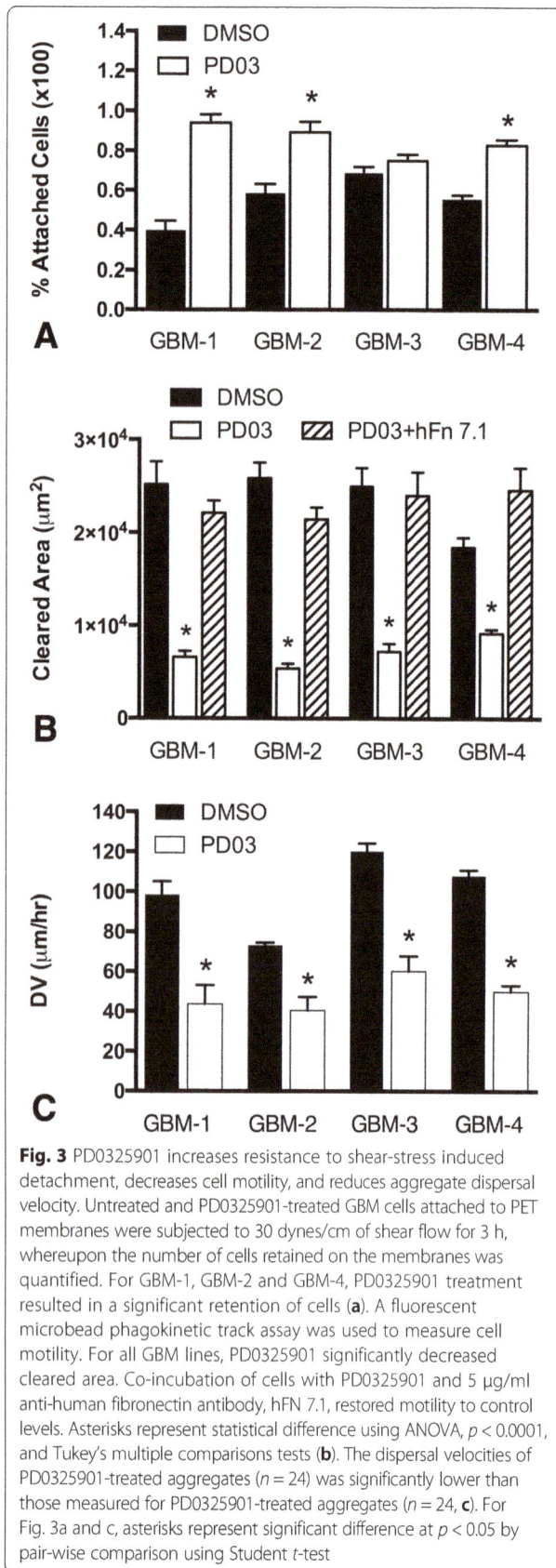

Fig. 3 PD0325901 increases resistance to shear-stress induced detachment, decreases cell motility, and reduces aggregate dispersal velocity. Untreated and PD0325901-treated GBM cells attached to PET membranes were subjected to 30 dynes/cm of shear flow for 3 h, whereupon the number of cells retained on the membranes was quantified. For GBM-1, GBM-2 and GBM-4, PD0325901 treatment resulted in a significant retention of cells (a). A fluorescent microbead phagokinetic track assay was used to measure cell motility. For all GBM lines, PD0325901 significantly decreased cleared area. Co-incubation of cells with PD0325901 and 5 μg/ml anti-human fibronectin antibody, hFN 7.1, restored motility to control levels. Asterisks represent statistical difference using ANOVA, $p < 0.0001$, and Tukey's multiple comparisons tests (b). The dispersal velocities of PD0325901-treated aggregates ($n = 24$) was significantly lower than those measured for PD0325901-treated aggregates ($n = 24$, c). For Fig. 3a and c, asterisks represent significant difference at $p < 0.05$ by pair-wise comparison using Student t-test

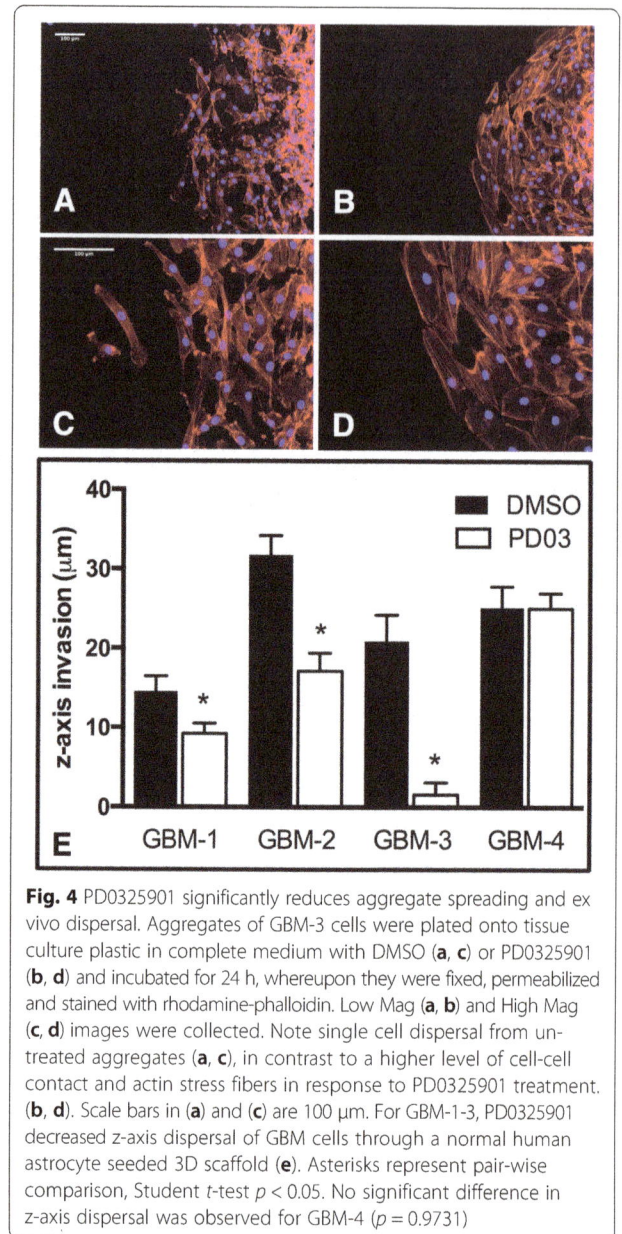

Fig. 4 PD0325901 significantly reduces aggregate spreading and ex vivo dispersal. Aggregates of GBM-3 cells were plated onto tissue culture plastic in complete medium with DMSO (**a**, **c**) or PD0325901 (**b**, **d**) and incubated for 24 h, whereupon they were fixed, permeabilized and stained with rhodamine-phalloidin. Low Mag (**a**, **b**) and High Mag (**c**, **d**) images were collected. Note single cell dispersal from untreated aggregates (**a**, **c**), in contrast to a higher level of cell-cell contact and actin stress fibers in response to PD0325901 treatment. (**b**, **d**). Scale bars in (**a**) and (**c**) are 100 μm. For GBM-1-3, PD0325901 decreased z-axis dispersal of GBM cells through a normal human astrocyte seeded 3D scaffold (**e**). Asterisks represent pair-wise comparison, Student t-test $p < 0.05$. No significant difference in z-axis dispersal was observed for GBM-4 ($p = 0.9731$)

significantly decreases the growth rate of conventional 2D cultures of GBM-1-4 as compared to DMSO controls. We then repeated the experiment using spheroids of GBM cells. Figure 5c-f shows that PD0325901 treatment significantly reduced the growth rate of GBM aggregates since the slope of the growth curves was significantly reduced by treatment relative to that of controls. Linear regression analysis of the 3D growth curves revealed a 2–11 fold reduction in growth rate when spheroids of GBM cells were treated with the drug. In fact, PD0325901 treated aggregates appeared to decrease in size over time. This suggests that cells are either dying and sloughing off the surface of the aggregate – this was not observed for aggregates incubated for

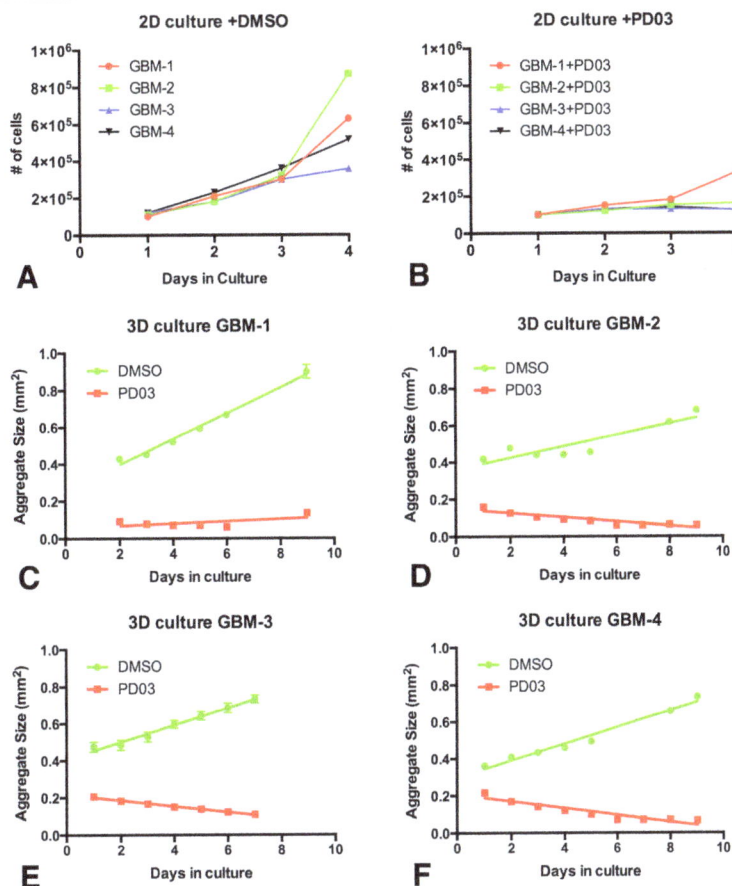

Fig. 5 PD0325901 reduces growth rates of conventional 2D cultures and 3D spheroids of GBM cells. Growth rate for conventional 2D cultures of the GBM lines was measured either in DMSO (**a**) or PD0325901 (**b**). Fifty-thousand cells were plated and proliferation was monitored over a 4-day period. PD0325901 treatment significantly reduced the growth rate of 2D cultures. Aggregates ($n = 6$ for each line and treatment) of GBM-1 (**c**), GBM-2 (**d**), GBM-3 (**e**) and GBM-4 (**f**) were cultured either in the absence or presence of PD0325901 and area was measured for each aggregate once/day for 9 days. Linear regression was used to analyze the data. Only regression lines with an r^2 of 0.95 or higher were used. Regression lines depicted are average area as a function of time. Growth rate was significantly reduced by PD0325901 for all GBM lines as demonstrated by a significant shallowing of the slope of the line (ANCOVA, $p < 0.0001$). For GBM-1-4, growth rate was reduced 11.6, 2.7, 2.9, and 2.5-fold, respectively

2 days (Additional file 1: Figure S3, panel a) or 4 days (Additional file 1: Figure S3, panel b) on agarose plates – or that aggregates became more compact over time. This appears to be the case inasmuch as PD0325901 treatment resulted in more compact aggregates (Additional file 1: Figure S3, Panel c). It is likely that the observed compaction was due to overall contraction of cell size.

Discussion

Therapies aimed at containing tumor cell dispersal could provide a powerful path towards extending the time of disease-free and overall survival of glioblastoma patients. Identifying drugs that can target molecular pathways involved in dispersal would provide valuable insight towards this goal. Our previous studies showed that Dexamethasone, an FDA approved drug to treat tumor-related edema in GBM, can also decrease in vitro and ex vivo dispersal of primary human GBM cells. It does so

by activating α5β1 integrin and subsequent restoration of FNMA and re-organization of cortical actin into stress fibers. In turn, these changes engender an increase in the strength of intercellular cohesion, increased attachment of tumor cells to substrate, and reduced cell motility. The net effect is an overall reduction in dispersal [1, 27]. The effects of Dex, however, are pleiotropic and the drug likely targets many pathways, which in part may explain the many side-effects associated with Dex treatment. Identifying drugs that are more specific in their targeting of dispersal-related pathways is therefore important.

In this study, we explore whether inhibition of the MAPK/ERK pathway, a critical regulator of processes underlying invasion and metastasis [28], could have similar effects on GBM dispersal. We tested the effects of the MEK inhibitor, PD0325901, on 4 primary GBM cell lines that were previously used to assess the effects of Dex on dispersal [1, 21]. Studies have shown that certain GBM lines do not respond to MEK inhibitors [20]. We therefore assessed whether our lines are responsive to PD0325901 by determining whether treatment results in a decrease in the levels of phospho-ERK. All 4 lines responded to the drug. We previously established that the cell lines were all deficient in their capacity for FNMA [1]. In contrast to Dex, treatment with PD0325901 did not result in a significant increase in FNMA. However, treatment with the MEK inhibitor resulted in a remarkable change in cell shape and in the reorganization of actin from cortical into stress fibers. This was particularly evident when actin was visualized in 3D spheroids. Given that the actin cytoskeleton is a fundamental mediator of cell and tissue stiffness [29], we posited that a shift in actin organization would correspond to a change in tissue stiffness.

Stiffening of the ECM is considered to be a hallmark of fibrotic lesions and has been demonstrated to modulate cell invasion and migration [30]. The current study focused on whether aggregate stiffness and viscosity could modulate dispersal. We quantified stiffness and viscosity using methods based on ellipsoid relaxation, specifically after the deforming external force is removed [31, 32]. The aggregate was modeled as a Kelvin-Voigt viscoelastic body [33, 34]. Unexpectedly, PD0325901 treatment only resulted in a modest increase in aggregate stiffness but not of viscosity. However, when aggregates were generated in higher concentrations of fibronectin, both stiffness and viscosity increased significantly. This is important for several reasons. First, the fibronectin gene has been shown to be up-regulated in GBM [35]. Accordingly, tumors able to respond to PD0325901 and in the presence of high concentrations of fibronectin, could, in principle, become stiffer and more viscous. Stiffer tumors have previously been shown to be less invasive and to grow more slowly [36]. Few studies have addressed the issue of tumor viscosity and those that have focus on applications of magnetic resonance elastography in liver tumors where fibrosis is a key parameter. In those studies, tumor viscosity appeared to be higher in malignant tumors [37]. In GBM, however, fibrosis is not typically observed. In GBM spheroids, the increase in viscosity in response to PD0325901 treatment was likely due to higher binding energy between the activated α5β1 integrin and fibronectin. This would effectively increase the friction between cells and the ECM. This increase in friction could significantly reduce the capacity for dispersal of tumor cells from the primary mass.

Treatment also resulted in the localization of p-FAK at sites of cell-substrate attachment. This is consistent with the observed resistance to flow-induced substrate detachment of GBM cells, and to decreased motility. Since cells require intermediate levels of cell-ECM adhesion to be optimally motile [38], an increase in the strength of cell-ECM adhesion past this point might stabilize adhesion to substrate to a point that significantly reduces cell movement, and consequently, dispersal. Decreased motility also appears to be associated with a significant decrease in dispersal velocity of GBM aggregates. Since PD0325901 treatment did not restore FNMA, it is likely that decreased motility rather than increased cohesion is the physical mechanism that restrains the detachment of tumor cells from the mass. Indeed, cells at the leading edge of treated aggregates appear to attach tightly to substrate causing cells behind them to pile up, again pointing to reduced motility as the primary restraint for detachment. For three of the four primary GBM lines, PD0325901 also significantly reduced the ability of single GBM cells to disperse through an astrocyte-seeded scaffold. It is not possible to differentiate between the effects of PD0325901 on decreased motility and ability to disperse through the scaffold, however, it is possible that on a single cell level, the re-organization of actin into stress fibers may have effectively rendered cells less compliant and inhibited their capacity to sufficiently deform and squeeze through pores established by the physical environment established by the scaffold. It is important to note that for GBM-4, treatment did not reduce z-axis dispersal. It is possible that in this line, compliance was not effected by treatment, thus allowing cells to penetrate into the scaffold.

Lastly, MEK inhibitor treatment also appears to significantly reduce growth rate of these primary GBM lines in both conventional 2D and in 3D cultures. Other studies have demonstrated in vivo efficacy of PD0325901 in reducing tumor growth in preclinical orthotopic models of glioblastoma [18]. Our study provides compelling evidence that PD0325901 can also reduce dispersal. Growth and dispersal contribute significantly to recurrence. Accordingly, the drug has the potential to significantly delay the onset of recurrence in GBM.

Identifying agents that can contain the primary or recurrent tumor could significantly improve targeted delivery of chemotherapeutic agents and increase the likelihood of total surgical resection. We have previously identified Dexamethasone (Dex) as a potential candidate to reduce dispersal of GBM [1]. Interestingly, the doses required to elicit a dispersal inhibitory response are significantly lower than those typically used to reduce edema [1]. Clinically, MEK inhibitors are generally well tolerated. Commonly occurring toxicities include rash, diarrhea, fatigue, peripheral oedema and acneiform dermatitis. Life-threatening toxicities associated with MEKi are extremely rare. Long-term use is possible providing that adverse events are monitored and dose or treatment schedules are modified, as required [39]. The measureable outcome for MEK inhibitor studies focus on their ability to reduce tumor size. Here, we show an added benefit of one MEK inhibitor as a potential deterrent of tumor cell dispersal. Whereas Dexamethasone readily crosses the blood–brain barrier, some MEK inhibitors, including trametinib, have demonstrated limited brain distribution due to association with the P-glycoprotein efflux transporters found at the blood–brain barrier [19]. Perhaps a strategy in which MEK inhibitors are used as interstitial chemotherapy, followed by continued administration of low-dose Dex, could significantly improve prognosis of this devastating disease.

Conclusions

This study demonstrates that it is possible to impede dispersal of GBM by inhibiting the MAPK/ERK pathway using the MEK inhibitor PD0325901. To our knowledge, this is the first demonstration that the drug can also impede GBM dispersal. Containing the primary or recurrent tumor by interstitial administration of MEK inhibitors could significantly improve delivery of chemotherapeutic agents and increase the likelihood of total surgical resection. This could significantly extend the time of disease-free and overall survival of glioblastoma patients.

Abbreviations

AGM: Astrocyte growth medium; Dex: Dexamethasone; DMSO: dimethyl sulfoxide; ECL: Enhanced chemiluminescence; ECM: Extracellular matrix; EMCC: Electron multiplying charge coupled device; EMEM: Eagle's Minimal Essential Medium; FCS: Fetal calf serum; FNMA: Fibronectin matrix assembly; GBM: Glioblastoma multiforme; GLA: Gamma-linolenic acid; MAPK/ERK: mitogen activated protein kinase/extracellular signal regulated kinase; NHA: Normal human astrocytes; PAGE: polyacrylamide gel electrophoresis; PBS: Phosphate buffered saline; PVDF: polyvinylidine fluoride; SDS: sodium dodecyl sulphate; sFn: Serum fibronectin; TST: Tissue surface tensiometry

Acknowledgements

The authors gratefully acknowledge the efforts of Dr. Joseph Kramer, Director, Confocal Imaging Facility, Rutgers-Robert Wood Johnson Medical School, for assistance in image acquisition and analysis.

Funding

SS was supported by an NIH Institutional Research and Academic Career Development Award K-12 GM093854. MY received funding from the NSF-CMMI. LL was supported by grants from NSF-DMS and from the AFOSR. The study was also supported from research funds from the Department of Surgery-Robert Wood Johnson Medical School to RAF.

Authors' contributions

SS performed and analyzed the dispersal velocity and aggregate spreading assays. DJ performed the immunoblot and immunofluorescence assays. IE generated and analyzed the cell attachment data. PB, CC and JC performed the tissue surface tensiometry assays for measurement of aggregate cohesion and analyzed the data. AM performed the experiments for measurement of aggregate stiffness and viscosity. MY designed the in-house image capture and analysis algorithm and also analyzed the shape relaxation images for extraction of the stiffness and viscosity data. CV conceived, performed and analyzed the cell motility assay. MW generated and analyzed the ex vivo dispersal data. DS, JDZ, LL and HL conceived, designed, and mathematically

solved the solution for extraction of stiffness and viscosity. They also supervised the project at the Departments of Biomedical Engineering (DS, JDZ) and Mechanical and Aerospace Engineering (LL, HL), respectively. RAF conceived the study, supervised the overall project, statistically analyzed the data, generated the figures, interpreted the results, and wrote the manuscript. All authors reviewed and edited the manuscript for intellectual content and have approved the final version.

Competing interest

The authors declare that they have no competing interests.

Author details

[1]Department of Surgery-Rutgers Robert Wood Johnson Medical School, Clinical Academic Building, 125 Paterson Street, New Brunswick, NJ 08901, USA. [2]Rutgers-Department of Biomedical Engineering, 599 Taylor Road, Piscataway, NJ 08854, USA. [3]Rutgers-Department of Mechanical and Aerospace Engineering, 98 Brett Rd, Piscataway Township, NJ 08854, USA. [4]Rutgers-Department of Mathematics, 110 Frelinghuysen Rd, Piscataway, NJ 08854, USA.

References

1. Shannon S, Vaca C, Jia D, Entersz I, Schaer A, Carcione J, Weaver M, Avidar Y, Pettit R, Nair M, et al. Dexamethasone-mediated activation of fibronectin matrix assembly reduces dispersal of primary human glioblastoma cells. PLoS One. 2015;10(8):e0135951.
2. Alves TR, Lima FR, Kahn SA, Lobo D, Dubois LG, Soletti R, Borges H, Neto VM. Glioblastoma cells: a heterogeneous and fatal tumor interacting with the parenchyma. Life Sci. 2011;89(15–16):532–9.
3. Burden-Gulley SM, Qutaish MQ, Sullivant KE, Tan M, Craig SE, Basilion JP, Lu ZR, Wilson DL, Brady-Kalnay SM. Single cell molecular recognition of migrating and invading tumor cells using a targeted fluorescent probe to receptor PTPmu. Int J Cancer. 2013;132(7):1624–32.
4. Kumar S, Weaver VM. Mechanics, malignancy, and metastasis: the force journey of a tumor cell. Cancer Metastasis Rev. 2009;28(1–2):113–27.
5. Jiang WG, Hiscox S, Hallett MB, Horrobin DF, Mansel RE, Puntis MC. Regulation of the expression of E-cadherin on human cancer cells by gamma-linolenic acid (GLA). Cancer Res. 1995;55(21):5043–8.
6. Reinhold WC, Reimers MA, Lorenzi P, Ho J, Shankavaram UT, Ziegler MS, Bussey KJ, Nishizuka S, Ikediobi O, Pommier YG, et al. Multifactorial regulation of E-cadherin expression: an integrative study. Mol Cancer Ther. 2010;9(1):1–16.
7. Montenegro RC, de Vasconcellos MC, Barbosa Gdos S, Burbano RM, Souza LG, Lemos TL, Costa-Lotufo LV, de Moraes MO. A novel o-naphtoquinone inhibits N-cadherin expression and blocks melanoma cell invasion via AKT signaling. Toxicol In Vitro. 2013;27(7):2076–83.
8. Asano K, Duntsch CD, Zhou Q, Weimar JD, Bordelon D, Robertson JH, Pourmotabbed T. Correlation of N-cadherin expression in high grade gliomas with tissue invasion. J Neurooncol. 2004;70(1):3–15.
9. Yamada S, Bu XY, Khankaldyyan V, Gonzales-Gomez I, McComb JG, Laug WE. Effect of the angiogenesis inhibitor cilengitide (EMD 121974) on glioblastoma growth in nude mice. Neurosurgery. 2006;59(6):1304–12. discussion 1312.
10. Jarvelainen H, Sainio A, Koulu M, Wight TN, Penttinen R. Extracellular matrix molecules: potential targets in pharmacotherapy. Pharmacol Rev. 2009;61(2): 198–223.
11. Kostaras X, Cusano F, Kline GA, Roa W, Easaw J. Use of Dexamethasone in patients with high-grade glioma: a clinical practice guideline. Curr Oncol. 2014;21(3):e493–503.
12. LoRusso PM, Krishnamurthi SS, Rinehart JJ, Nabell LM, Malburg L, Chapman PB, DePrimo SE, Bentivegna S, Wilner KD, Tan W, et al. Phase I pharmacokinetic and pharmacodynamic study of the oral MAPK/ERK kinase inhibitor PD-0325901 in patients with advanced cancers. Clin Cancer Res. 2010;16(6):1924–37.
13. Falchook GS, Lewis KD, Infante JR, Gordon MS, Vogelzang NJ, DeMarini DJ, Sun P, Moy C, Szabo SA, Roadcap LT, et al. Activity of the oral MEK inhibitor trametinib in patients with advanced melanoma: a phase 1 dose-escalation trial. Lancet Oncol. 2012;13(8):782–9.

14. Kim KB, Kefford R, Pavlick AC, Infante JR, Ribas A, Sosman JA, Fecher LA, Millward M, McArthur GA, Hwu P, et al. Phase II study of the MEK1/MEK2 inhibitor trametinib in patients with metastatic BRAF-mutant cutaneous melanoma previously treated with or without a BRAF inhibitor. J Clin Oncol. 2013;31(4):482–9.

15. Larkin J, Ascierto PA, Dreno B, Atkinson V, Liszkay G, Maio M, Mandala M, Demidov L, Stroyakovskiy D, Thomas L, et al. Combined vemurafenib and cobimetinib in BRAF-mutated melanoma. N Engl J Med. 2014;371(20):1867–76.

16. Rinehart J, Adjei AA, Lorusso PM, Waterhouse D, Hecht JR, Natale RB, Hamid O, Varterasian M, Asbury P, Kaldjian EP, et al. Multicenter phase II study of the oral MEK inhibitor, CI-1040, in patients with advanced non-small-cell lung, breast, colon, and pancreatic cancer. J Clin Oncol. 2004;22(22):4456–62.

17. Ciuffreda L, Del Bufalo D, Desideri M, Di Sanza C, Stoppacciaro A, Ricciardi MR, Chiaretti S, Tavolaro S, Benassi B, Bellacosa A, et al. Growth-inhibitory and antiangiogenic activity of the MEK inhibitor PD0325901 in malignant melanoma with or without BRAF mutations. Neoplasia. 2009;11(8):720–31.

18. El Meskini R, Iacovelli AJ, Kulaga A, Gumprecht M, Martin PL, Baran M, Householder DB, Van Dyke T, Weaver Ohler Z. A preclinical orthotopic model for glioblastoma recapitulates key features of human tumors and demonstrates sensitivity to a combination of MEK and PI3K pathway inhibitors. Dis Model Mech. 2015;8(1):45–56.

19. Vaidhyanathan S, Mittapalli RK, Sarkaria JN, Elmquist WF. Factors influencing the CNS distribution of a novel MEK-1/2 inhibitor: implications for combination therapy for melanoma brain metastases. Drug Metab Dispos. 2014;42(8):1292–300.

20. See WL, Tan IL, Mukherjee J, Nicolaides T, Pieper RO. Sensitivity of glioblastomas to clinically available MEK inhibitors is defined by neurofibromin 1 deficiency. Cancer Res. 2012;72(13):3350–9.

21. Mehta M, Khan A, Danish S, Haffty BG, Sabaawy HE. Radiosensitization of primary human glioblastoma stem-like cells with Low-dose AKT inhibition. Mol Cancer Ther. 2015;14(5):1171–80.

22. Foty RA, Forgacs G, Pfleger CM, Steinberg MS. Liquid properties of embryonic tissues: measurement of interfacial tensions. Phys Rev Lett. 1994; 72(14):2298–301.

23. Foty RA, Pfleger CM, Forgacs G, Steinberg MS. Surface tensions of embryonic tissues predict their mutual envelopment behavior. Development. 1996;122(5):1611–20.

24. Foty RA, Steinberg MS. The differential adhesion hypothesis: a direct evaluation. Dev Biol. 2005;278(1):255–63.

25. Forgacs G, Foty RA, Shafrir Y, Steinberg MS. Viscoelastic properties of living embryonic tissues: a quantitative study. Biophys J. 1998;74(5):2227–34.

26. Windler-Hart SL, Chen KY, Chenn A. A cell behavior screen: identification, sorting, and enrichment of cells based on motility. BMC Cell Biol. 2005;6(1):14.

27. Sabari J, Lax D, Connors D, Brotman I, Mindrebo E, Butler C, Entersz I, Jia D, Foty RA. Fibronectin matrix assembly suppresses dispersal of glioblastoma cells. PLoS One. 2011;6(9):e24810.

28. Dhillon AS, Hagan S, Rath O, Kolch W. MAP kinase signalling pathways in cancer. Oncogene. 2007;26(22):3279–90.

29. Wakatsuki T, Schwab B, Thompson NC, Elson EL. Effects of cytochalasin D and latrunculin B on mechanical properties of cells. J Cell Sci. 2001;114(Pt 5): 1025–36.

30. Kai F, Laklai H, Weaver VM: Force Matters: Biomechanical Regulation of Cell Invasion and Migration in Disease. Trends Cell Biol. 2016;26(7):486–97.

31. Zhang J, Zahn JD, Lin H. Transient solution for droplet deformation under electric fields. Phys Rev E Stat Nonlin Soft Matter Phys. 2013;87(4):043008.

32. Yu M, Lira RB, Riske KA, Dimova R, Lin H. Ellipsoidal relaxation of deformed vesicles. Phys Rev Lett. 2015;115(12):128303.

33. Darby R. Viscoelastic fluids, and introduction to their properties and behaviour. New York-Basel: Marcel Decker; 1976.

34. Meyers M, Chawla K. Mechanical behavior of materials. Cambridge: Cambridge University Press; 2009.

35. Serres E, Debarbieux F, Stanchi F, Maggiorella L, Grall D, Turchi L, Burel-Vandenbos F, Figarella-Branger D, Virolle T, Rougon G, et al. Fibronectin expression in glioblastomas promotes cell cohesion, collective invasion of basement membrane in vitro and orthotopic tumor growth in mice. Oncogene. 2014;33(26):3451–62.

36. Fenner J, Stacer AC, Winterroth F, Johnson TD, Luker KE, Luker GD. Macroscopic stiffness of breast tumors predicts metastasis. Sci Rep. 2014;4:5512.

37. Garteiser P, Doblas S, Daire JL, Wagner M, Leitao H, Vilgrain V, Sinkus R, Van Beers BE. MR elastography of liver tumours: value of viscoelastic properties for tumour characterisation. Eur Radiol. 2012;22(10):2169–77.

38. DiMilla PA, Stone JA, Quinn JA, Albelda SM, Lauffenburger DA. Maximal migration of human smooth muscle cells on fibronectin and type IV collagen occurs at an intermediate attachment strength. J Cell Biol. 1993; 122(3):729–37.

39. Welsh SJ, Corrie PG. Management of BRAF and MEK inhibitor toxicities in patients with metastatic melanoma. Ther Adv Med Oncol. 2015;7(2):122–36.

7

Overexpression of endothelin B receptor in glioblastoma: a prognostic marker and therapeutic target?

Suhas Vasaikar[1], Giorgos Tsipras[1], Natalia Landázuri[1], Helena Costa[2], Vanessa Wilhelmi[2], Patrick Scicluna[2], Huanhuan L. Cui[2], Abdul-Aleem Mohammad[2], Belghis Davoudi[2], Mingmei Shang[1], Sharan Ananthaseshan[2], Klas Strååt[3], Giuseppe Stragliotto[4], Afsar Rahbar[2], Kum Thong Wong[5], Jesper Tegner[1,6], Koon-Chu Yaiw[2]* and Cecilia Söderberg-Naucler[2]*

Abstract

Background: Glioblastoma (GBM) is the most common malignant brain tumor with median survival of 12-15 months. Owing to uncertainty in clinical outcome, additional prognostic marker(s) apart from existing markers are needed. Since overexpression of endothelin B receptor (ETBR) has been demonstrated in gliomas, we aimed to test whether ETBR is a useful prognostic marker in GBM and examine if the clinically available endothelin receptor antagonists (ERA) could be useful in the disease treatment.

Methods: Data from The Cancer Genome Atlas and the Gene Expression Omnibus database were analyzed to assess ETBR expression. For survival analysis, glioblastoma samples from 25 Swedish patients were immunostained for ETBR, and the findings were correlated with clinical history. The druggability of ETBR was assessed by protein-protein interaction network analysis. ERAs were analyzed for toxicity in in vitro assays with GBM and breast cancer cells.

Results: By bioinformatics analysis, ETBR was found to be upregulated in glioblastoma patients, and its expression levels were correlated with reduced survival. ETBR interacts with key proteins involved in cancer pathogenesis, suggesting it as a druggable target. In vitro viability assays showed that ERAs may hold promise to treat glioblastoma and breast cancer.

Conclusions: ETBR is overexpressed in glioblastoma and other cancers and may be a prognostic marker in glioblastoma. ERAs may be useful for treating cancer patients.

Keywords: Glioblastoma, Endothelin B receptor, Endothelin receptor antagonists

Background

Glioblastoma (GBM; World Health Organization grade IV astrocytoma) is the most common malignant brain tumor with an annual incidence of 3.5 cases per 100,000 worldwide [1]. It is also one of the most lethal human cancers. The median overall survival is 12–15 months with standard treatment [2], and 3–6 months for patients with recurrent GBM [3]. Owing to uncertainty in clinical outcome in individual patients, new prognostic markers are needed for GBM patients, especially those with potential to affect patient outcome through druggable targets.

Endothelins are vasoactive peptides that exert their effects through interactions with the G-protein-coupled receptors endothelin receptor A (ETAR) and endothelin receptor B (ETBR). ETAR is expressed mainly in vascular smooth muscle cells and stromal cells, whereas ETBR is expressed mainly in endothelial cells; ETAR mediates vasoconstriction, and ETBR vasodilatation and also stimulates cell proliferation (reviewed in [4]. Dysregulation of ETBR has been implicated in

* Correspondence: ykcywx@yahoo.com; Cecilia.Naucler@ki.se
Suhas Vasaikar, Giorgos Tsipras and, Natalia Landázuri are contributed equally.
Koon-Chu Yaiw and Cecilia Söderberg-Naucler are senior author.
[2]Cell and Molecular Immunology, Experimental Cardiovascular Unit, Departments of Medicine and Neurology, Center for Molecular Medicine, Karolinska Institutet, SE-171 76 Stockholm, Sweden
Full list of author information is available at the end of the article

cardiovascular disease and linked to a congenital disorder, Hirschsprung's disease (reviewed in [4]). Moreover, ETBR is overexpressed in vulvar cancer [5], clear-cell renal cell carcinoma [6], and esophageal squamous cell carcinoma [7] and is closely associated with disease progression and poor patient survival [5–7]. Consistent with a crucial role for ETBR in tumorigenesis, some ETBR antagonists may be beneficial in treating melanoma or glioma [8–11].

Overexpression of ETBR in GBM was associated with a poor prognosis in a Chinese population [12]. Since ethnicity may play a major role in the pathogenesis of gliomas [13, 14], we investigated whether ETBR overexpression could be detected in patients with GBM and in other cancers outside of China, whether ETBR expression correlates with patient survival (and thus its potential use as a prognostic marker and/or therapeutic target), and whether clinically available endothelin receptor blockers/antagonists have toxic effects on cancer cells in vitro.

Methods

Patient cohort

Formalin-fixed, paraffin-embedded tissue sections were from 25 GBM cases, were selected from our previously studied cohort without prior selection [15]. Demographic information and clinical data with time to tumor progression (TTP) and overall survival (OS) for all GBM cases are shown in Table 1. Ten normal samples from aging control brains (frontal part of brain from men) median age 57 [50-61 yrs] were from the Department of Pathology, University of Malaya Medical Center (ethical number 896.7). The use of patient materials was approved by the Ethics Committee at the Karolinska Institutet and by the Medical Ethics Committee, University of Malaya Medical Center, Malaysia, and conducted in accordance with the Declaration of Helsinki.

ETBR immunohistochemistry

Formalin-fixed, paraffin-embedded sections were analyzed by immunohistochemistry as described but with minor

Table 1 Demographic and available clinical information

Case number	TTP (months)	OS (months)	ETBR expression	Age (years)	Gender	Extent of resection	
						Radical	Partial
K7686-2004	4	5	3+	73	M	No	Yes
K9802-2004	5	5	1+	68	M	Yes	No
K4448-2004	1	14	1+	66	M	No	Yes
K12700-2004	1	5	1+	64	F	Yes	No
K10452-2004	7	10	1+	59	F	Yes	No
K5126-2004	3	7	1+	57	M	Yes	No
K11136-2004	12	20	1+	56	M	Yes	No
K17437-2004	16	17	2+	56	M	Yes	No
K4840-2004	7	20	1+	55	M	Yes	No
K16204-2004	10	11	1+	54	M	Yes	No
K9236-2004	12	15	1+	49	F	Yes	No
K16178-2004	12	13	1+	45	M	Yes	No
K3839-2004	12	14	3+	28	M	Yes	No
K16102-2004	48	48	1+	57	F	Yes	No
K17407-2004	48	48	1+	26	F	Yes	No
K10315-2004	52	52	1+	29	M	Yes	No
K3174-2004	15	19	3+	79	F	Yes	No
K16595/04	17	36	1+	53	F	Yes	No
K1716-2005	7	82	1+	43	M	Yes	No
K3349-2005	3	3	3+	79	F	No	Yes
K8622-2005	9	12	3+	59	F	Yes	No
K9731-2005	4	7	3+	52	F	Yes	No
K15725-2005	2	4	2+	54	M	Yes	No
K16886-2005	4.5	14.5	2+	38	F	No	Yes
K17972-2005	8.5	18	1+	63	F	Yes	No

TTP time to tumor progression, *OS* overall survival; Staining was graded as low (1+) or high (2+ and 3+)

modifications [7]. In brief, the sections were deparaffinized and rehydrated in a graded series of ethanol, and antigen was retrieved with the Decloaking Chamber NxGen (Biocare Medical, Concord, CA, USA) and Antigen Retrieval Citra Plus solution (Biogenex, Emergo Europe, The Hague, The Netherlands) at 110 °C for 15 min. The sections were cooled to room temperature, equilibrated with Tris-buffered saline, pH 7.6, and subjected to a series of blocking steps with protein block (Dako Sweden, Stockholm, Sweden), Fc receptor blocker (Biogenex), and normal horse serum. The sections were then incubated with primary rabbit anti-ETBR (cat. no. E9905; 1:200, Sigma-Aldrich, Stockholm, Sweden) at 4 °C for 16 h, washed three times with Tris-buffered saline, and placed in 3% (v/v) H_2O_2 in water for 15 min at room temperature to quench endogenous peroxidase activity. After three washings with Tris-buffered saline, the sections were incubated with secondary anti-rabbit antibody conjugated to horseradish peroxidase (ImmPRESS kit, Vector Laboratories, Orton Southgate, Peterborough, UK). Immunoreactivity was revealed with diaminobenzidine (Innovex Biosciences, GENTAUR Europe BVBA, Belgium). The sections were then counterstained with hematoxylin, dried, and mounted with xylene-based mounting medium. Positive staining was graded as low or high as described [12].

Analysis of data from the cancer genome atlas (TCGA) and the genome expression omnibus (GEO)

To evaluate the ETBR expression profile in GBM patients, we obtained primary and processed gene expression data for TCGA GBM cohort from The Broad Institute TCGA GDAC Firehose (https://gdac.broadinstitute.org/) using RTCGA (http://rtcga.github.io/RTCGA). Kaplan-Meier survival curves were plotted using the clinical information submitted for GBM patients in TCGA. GEO datasets related to GBM (GSE2223, GSE7696, GSE16011, GSE10878, GSE46016, GSE15824, GSE31262, GSE42656, and GSE50161) were analyzed for ETBR expression normalized to control. Among selected studies GSE2223 (origin: normal brain samples and glioblastoma), GSE7696 (origin: non-tumoral brain samples and glioblastoma samples with radiotherapy or TMZ/radiotherapy, age 27-70 years), GSE10878 (origin: normal tissue and primary glioblastoma tissue, age: 39-76 years), GSE46016 (origin: neural stem cells and human glioblastoma stem cells, age: 33-71 years), GSE15824 (origin: normal brain tissue & astrocytes and primary glioblastoma tissue, age: 35-70 years), GSE31262 (origin: non-tumoral brain tissue and primary glioblastoma tissue, age:33-71 years), GSE42656 (origin: adult control cerebellum and pediatrics glioblastoma, age:1-82 weeks), and GSE50161 (origin: normal brain samples and primary tumor (glioblastoma), age: 35-70 years) were analyzed. Other types of gliomas such as astrocytoma, oligodendroglioma, medulloblastoma were not considered

for the analysis. The data was log2 transformed and then a differential analysis was performed using standard Limma function (R package for the analysis of differential gene expression [16]). The normalized data further scaled between 0 and 1 using formula $Z_i = x_i - \min(x) / \max(x) - \min(x)$, where x represent the expression.

Protein–protein interaction network

Information on proteins that interact with ETBR was obtained with a protein neighborhood analysis tool [17]. The interacting partners were shown with Cytoscape, an online open source software tool to display molecular interaction networks and biological pathways [18]. Gene ontology of ETBR was obtained with a gene set enrichment tool and enrichment scores as described [19].

Proof-of-concept: in vitro cytotoxic assays

To test whether endothelin receptor blockers affect GBM cell growth and toxicity in vitro, three drugs currently in use to treat pulmonary artery hypertension were used—ambrisentan (Letairis/Volibris), which selectively blocks the ETAR, and macitentan (Opsumit) and bosentan (Tracleer), which block both ETAR and ETBR—in standard viability assays with a CellTiter 96 Aqueous One Solution Cell Proliferation Assay system (Promega) as recommended by the manufacturer. We also tested BQ788, which is selective for ETBR, and ACT-132577, the active metabolite of macitentan. The ACT-132577, bosentan, BQ788 and macitentan used in this study were from Medchemexpress LCC (Princeton, NJ, USA), while ambrisentan was from Ark Pharm, Inc. (Libertyville, IL, USA). All the drugs were provided and checked by Medivir, Stockholm, Sweden. To test the effects of the drugs on cancer cells, we used primary GBM cells (GBM30, GBM42, GBM48, GBM392, and GBM398) and three GBM lines (U-251 MG, U-373 MG (Uppsala), and U-343 MGa). To test drug effects on normal cells, we used human umbilical vein endothelial cells (HUVECs, Lonza, CH-3930 Visp, Switzerland), MRC-5 lung fibroblasts (ATCC, LGC Standards, Middlesex, UK), and retinal pigment epithelial cells (a generous gift from Dr. Rich Stanton, Cardiff University). Since the endothelin axis (consisting of endothelins, ETAR, and ETBR) has also been implicated in breast cancer, we also tested the drugs on three breast cancer lines: MCF7, MDA-MA-231, and SK-BR-3. In brief, approximately 1×10^4 cells/well were seeded onto 96-well plates and treated with twofold serial dilutions of drug (0.78–200 µM). Cell viability was assessed on day 6 with a VersaMax ELISA Microplate Reader (Molecular Devices, Wokingham, Berkshire, UK) at an optical density of 490 nm (reference wave length, 650 nm). The optical density of treated cells was expressed as a percentage of untreated cells, which were considered 100% viable.

Statistical analysis

$P < 0.05$ was considered to indicate statistical significance. Survival curves were estimated with the Kaplan–Meier method, and the significance of differences between the curves was determined with the log-rank test. Boxplots were plotted with R programming and analyzed by t test.

Results

Expression data from TCGA and GEO database

To determine whether ETBR is overexpressed in GBM, we analyzed the ETBR mRNA expression in TCGA and GEO databases. In TCGA, mRNA expression data ($n = 171$) demonstrate that the median expression of ETBR was significantly higher in primary (de novo) GBM tumors than in normal aging control brains (Fig. 1a). Similarly, ETBR mRNA expression was higher in patients with untreated primary (de novo) GBM tumor than in tumors from patients treated for primary GBM (from the Affymetrix HuExGeneChip mRNA microarray data, quantile normalized; $n = 517$) (Fig. 1b). Interestingly, patients with untreated primary (de novo) GBM tumors with higher median expression of ETBR tended to have shorter survival compared to those with lower median expression (Fig. 1c). The survival data from GSE7696 and GSE16011 cohorts also showed that patients with over-median expression of ETBR had lower survival rates at 3 years than 5 years, respectively (Additional file 1: Figure S1). In the GEO datasets GSE2223, GSE7696, GSE10878, GSE46016, GSE15824, and GSE31262, ETBR expression was significantly higher in GBM patients than in controls (Fig. 2); no difference of ETBR expression was noted in datasets GSE42656, and GSE50161 (Additional file 1: Figure S2), perhaps mirroring the heterogeneity of the disease.

To further investigate the expression levels of ETBR in other cancers, we analyzed ETBR expression in silico with available datasets. ETBR expression varied among cancer types but was higher in malignant cancer, mixed glioma, GBM, and melanoma (Fig. 3 and Additional file 1: Figure S3). Taken together, these data predicted that overexpression of ETBR may be a prognostic marker for a subset of GBM patients and potentially for other tumor types as well (Additional file 1: Figure S3).

ETBR is overexpressed in GBM

To confirm the higher expression of ETBR shown by the bioinformatics analysis in tissue specimens, we examined tumor tissue specimens obtained from 25 GBM patients we studied in a previous cohort [15] fro ETBR expression. ETBR expression was low in 64% ($n = 16$) and high in 36% ($n = 9$). ETBR was predominantly detected in the cytoplasm of tumor cells and was not found in adjacent nontumor cells, consistent with previous findings [20]. Little or no ETBR immunoreactivity was detected in control brains ($n = 10$) (Fig. 4) and was mainly located in corpora amylacea and occasionally in some arteriole-like structures.

Overexpression of ETBR is correlated with a shorter overall survival

To determine whether ETBR expression levels are of prognostic value for GBM patients, we used the Kaplan-Meier method to analyze the survival of 25 patients with low or high ETBR expression levels. ETBR expression correlated inversely and significantly with the survival times of these GBM patients (Fig. 5). Interestingly, we observed higher expression of ETBR in both 'Classical' and 'Neural' subtypes of GBM according to molecular classification [21] that tended to be correlated with poor overall survival (Additional file 1: Figure S5A-B).

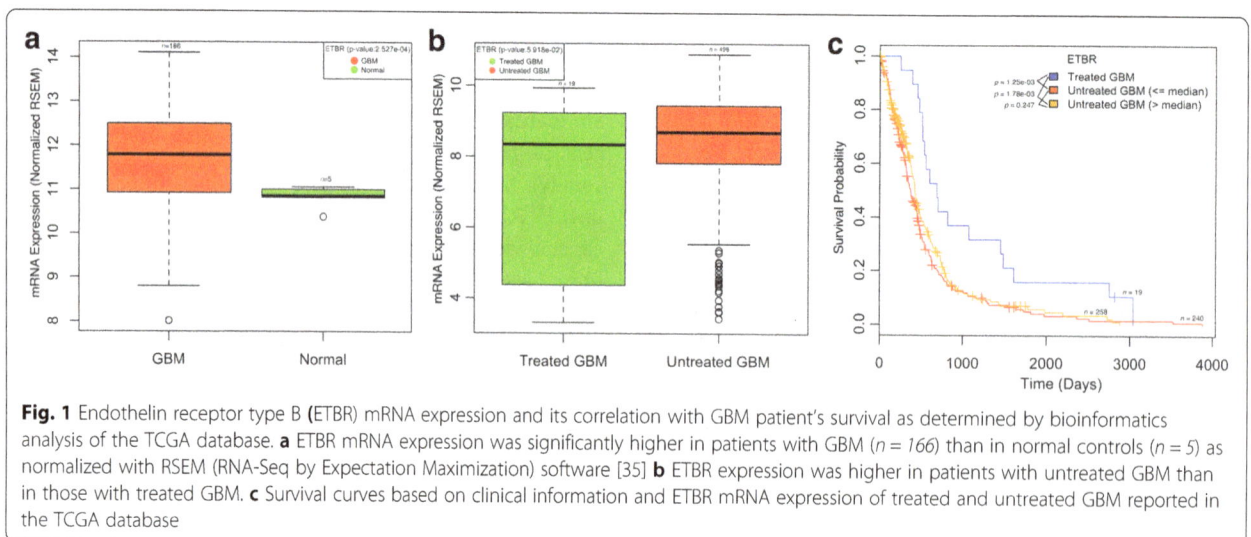

Fig. 1 Endothelin receptor type B (ETBR) mRNA expression and its correlation with GBM patient's survival as determined by bioinformatics analysis of the TCGA database. **a** ETBR mRNA expression was significantly higher in patients with GBM ($n = 166$) than in normal controls ($n = 5$) as normalized with RSEM (RNA-Seq by Expectation Maximization) software [35] **b** ETBR expression was higher in patients with untreated GBM than in those with treated GBM. **c** Survival curves based on clinical information and ETBR mRNA expression of treated and untreated GBM reported in the TCGA database

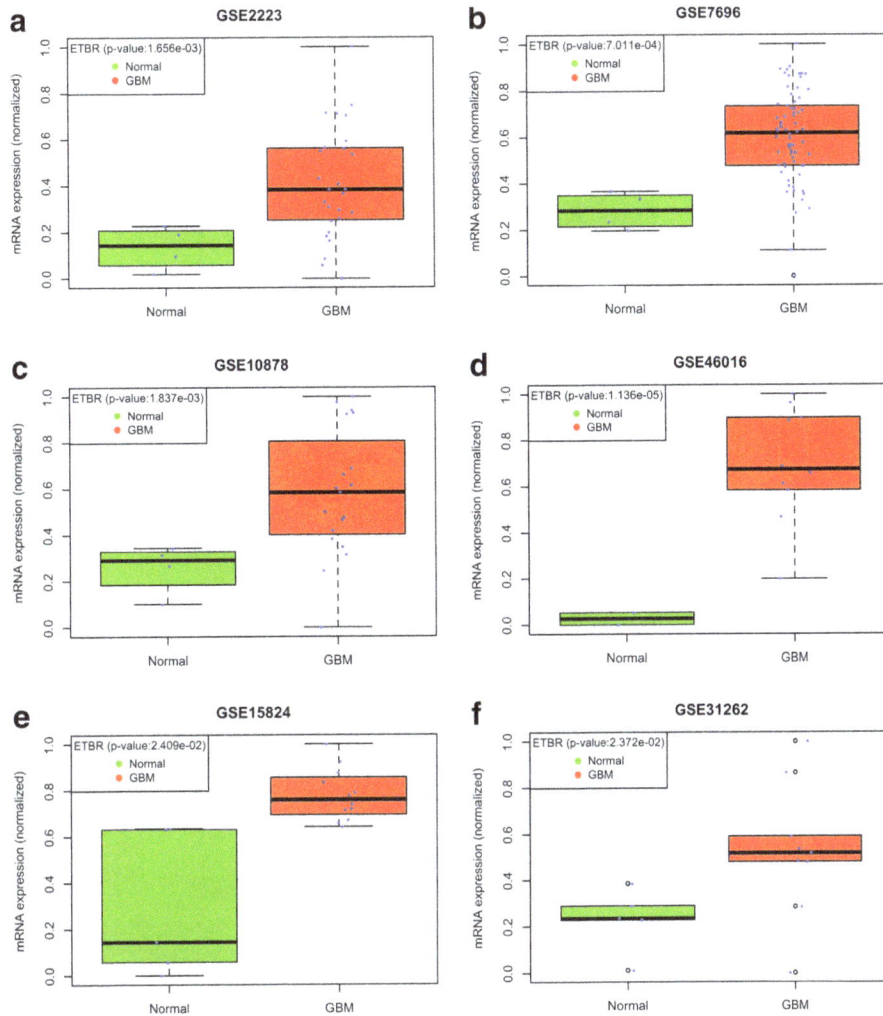

Fig. 2 Normalized ETBR mRNA expression determined by analyzing GEO datasets (**a-f**). ETBR mRNA expression is shown for control (normal) and GBM patients. The signifance obtained from t-test is shown in inset box

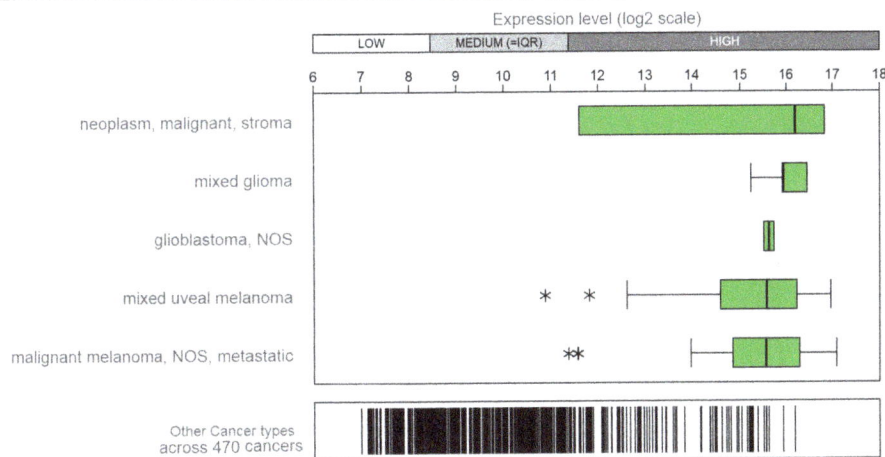

Fig. 3 ETBR expression level in different cancers. The expression level of ETBR in human cancers is shown from Affymetrix Human Genome U133 Plus 2.0 Array. Enrichment of five major cancers in ETBR expression, shown with Genevestigator (http://genevestigator.com/gv/). NOS = Not Otherwise Specified, accordingly to WHO classification of CNS tumors (2016)

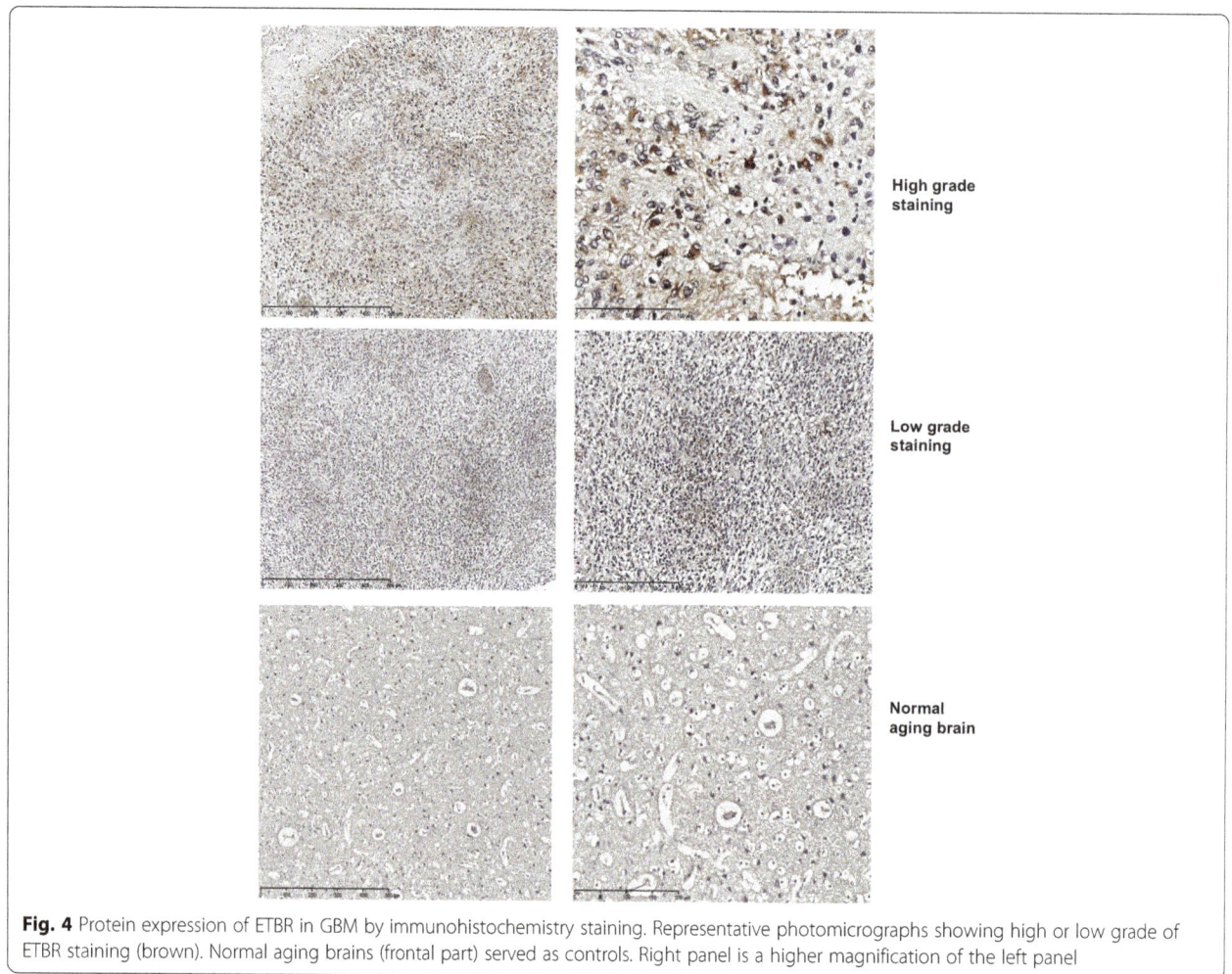

Fig. 4 Protein expression of ETBR in GBM by immunohistochemistry staining. Representative photomicrographs showing high or low grade of ETBR staining (brown). Normal aging brains (frontal part) served as controls. Right panel is a higher magnification of the left panel

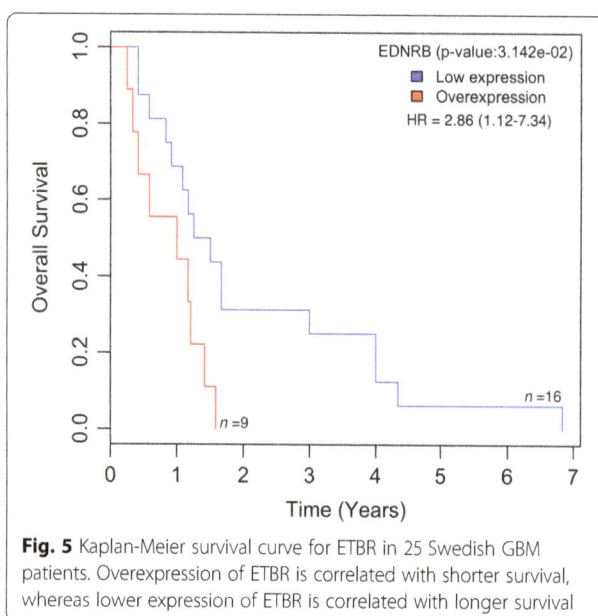

Fig. 5 Kaplan-Meier survival curve for ETBR in 25 Swedish GBM patients. Overexpression of ETBR is correlated with shorter survival, whereas lower expression of ETBR is correlated with longer survival

Druggability of ETBR

Next, we used network neighborhood analysis to examine possible interaction networks and signaling pathways of ETBR. The general structure of ETBR is shown in Fig. 6a. ETBR is known to be expressed on the plasma membrane, in the cytosol and on the nuclear membrane (Fig. 6b). The analysis showed that ETBR potentially interacts with eight proteins: guanine nucleotide-binding protein subunit alpha-11, guanine nucleotide-binding protein subunit alpha-13, caveolin-1, G protein-coupled receptor kinase 6, endothelin-1, endothelin-3, adrenergic beta receptor kinase 1, and nitric oxide synthase 3 (Fig. 6c). Further expansion of protein neighbors showed 175 interacting partners, many of which are involved in cell-cell communications (gap junction, adherens junction), the vascular endothelial growth factor signaling pathway, and calcium signaling that is associated with cancer pathogenesis (Fig. 6d). In addition, the ETBR-interacting proteins (up to second neighbor) acted as signature genes in different cancers; 11 proteins were observed in melanoma, 10 proteins in lung and stomach adenocarcinoma, and 5 proteins in GBM (Additional file

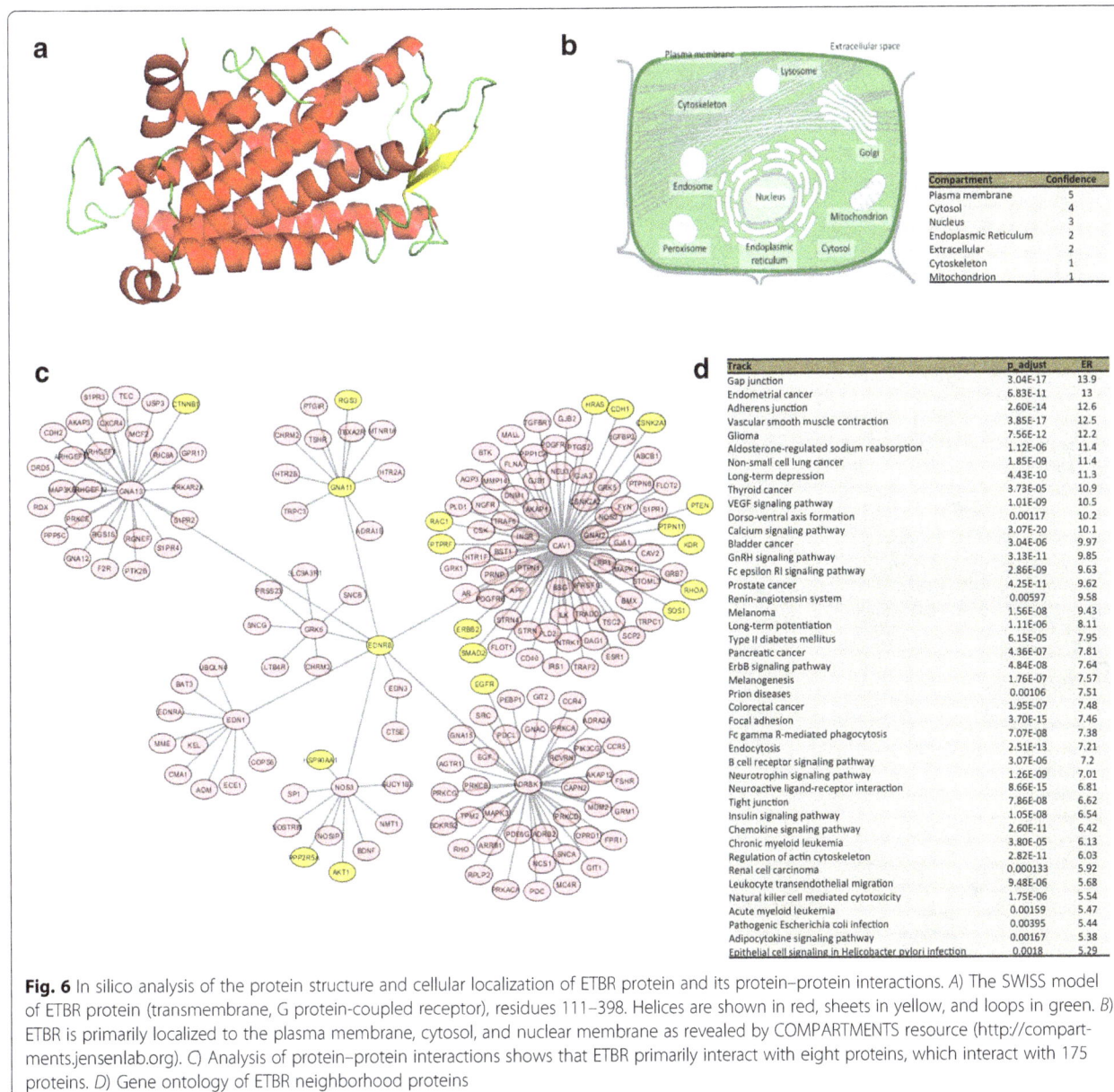

Fig. 6 In silico analysis of the protein structure and cellular localization of ETBR protein and its protein–protein interactions. *A)* The SWISS model of ETBR protein (transmembrane, G protein-coupled receptor), residues 111–398. Helices are shown in red, sheets in yellow, and loops in green. *B)* ETBR is primarily localized to the plasma membrane, cytosol, and nuclear membrane as revealed by COMPARTMENTS resource (http://compartments.jensenlab.org). *C)* Analysis of protein–protein interactions shows that ETBR primarily interact with eight proteins, which interact with 175 proteins. *D)* Gene ontology of ETBR neighborhood proteins

1: Figure S4A) [22]. We also found an association between cancer types and ETBR-interacting proteins (Additional file 1: Figure S4B). Collectively, these data suggest that ETBR is a potential therapeutic target in GBM and other cancers.

In vitro viability assay

To substantiate our prediction that ETBR is a druggable target for GBM and other cancer types, we used a standard viability assay to assess the cytotoxic effects of three clinically available endothelin receptor blockers—macitentan, bosentan, and ambrisentan—on primary GBM cells and GBM and breast cancer cell lines as compared with normal fibroblasts, endothelial and epithelial cells. Macitentan and its active metabolite (ACT-132577) reduced the viability of all GBM primary cells and cell lines tested; the effects were dose dependent (Fig. 7a–h). Bosentan had similar dose-dependent effects (Fig. 7a–c, f–h). In contrast, ambrisentan was not cytotoxic, even at the highest tested dose (Fig. 7d–h), apart from a minor trend toward reduced viability of GBM398 (Fig. 7e). Strikingly, at the highest dose, BQ788 dramatically reduced the viability of primary GBM392 cells and cell line U-343 MGa (Fig. 7a–h). Similar dose-dependent effects in breast cancer cells lines were observed for bosentan and for macitentan and its active metabolite ACT-132577; ambrisentan was not cytotoxic, and BQ788 had a single dramatic effect (Fig. 8a–c). Normal fibroblasts and epithelial cells tolerated ambrisentan and BQ788 well at 100 μM but not at 200 μM (Fig. 8d and e,

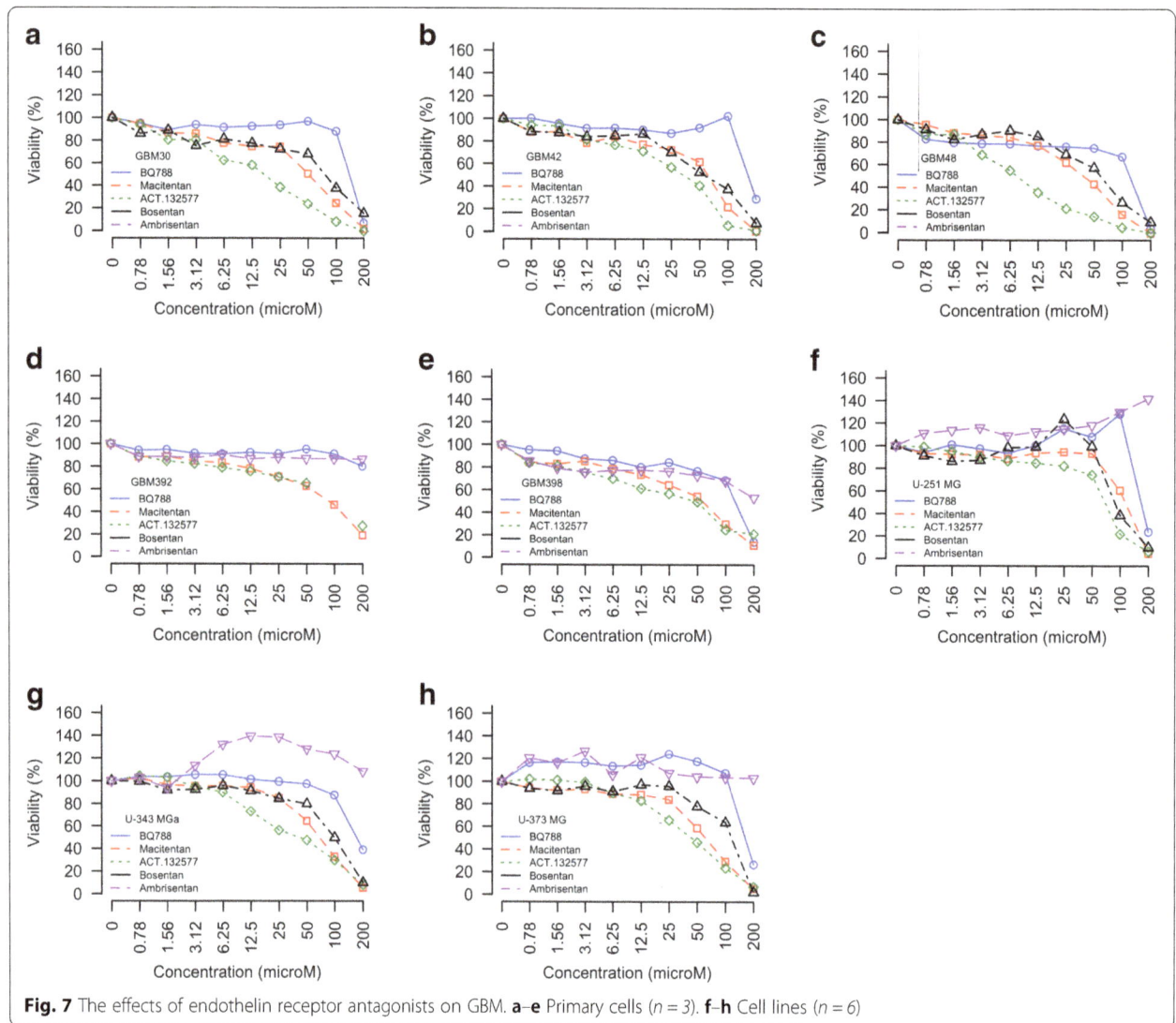

Fig. 7 The effects of endothelin receptor antagonists on GBM. **a–e** Primary cells (n = 3). **f–h** Cell lines (n = 6)

respectively). Macitentan and its active metabolite resulted in 40–50% cell death at 100 μM in both cell types; HUVECs were more sensitive to macitentan and its metabolite (Fig. 8f). Notably, there is a differential baseline expression of ETBR in primary GBM tissues/cells and breast cancer lines compared to that of normal fibroblasts, endothelial and epithelial cells (Additional file 1: Figure S6). These findings suggest the potential feasibility of using endothelin receptor antagonists to treat GBM and breast cancer, and that fine-tuning of the ETAR and ETBR balance is crucial for maximum cytotoxicity while sparing normal cells.

Discussion

In this study, we investigated whether ETBR is overexpressed in GBM tumors in a Swedish patient cohort and assessed the potential usefulness of ETBR as a prognostic marker and drug target for GBMs and other types of

cancer. We found that ETBR is indeed often overexpressed in GBM tumors, with little or no immunoreactivity in control brains. Analysis of expression data from TCGA and a subset of GEO datasets showed that overexpression of ETBR in GBM was correlated with shorter patient survival. Similarly, by examining ETBR expression across 470 cancers, glioma or GBM were again found to have high expression. By mapping the protein neighborhood to ETBR, we found that ETBR is mainly predicted to interact with eight proteins that further interact with 175 additional proteins, many of which are involved in cell-cell communication (gap junction, adherens junction), the vascular endothelial growth factor signaling pathway, and calcium signaling—all of which are associated with cancer pathogenesis. These results support the potential use of ETBR blockers as a targeted therapy for cancer [10].

The endothelin axis has been implicated in the pathogenesis of many types of cancers (reviewed in [23]). In

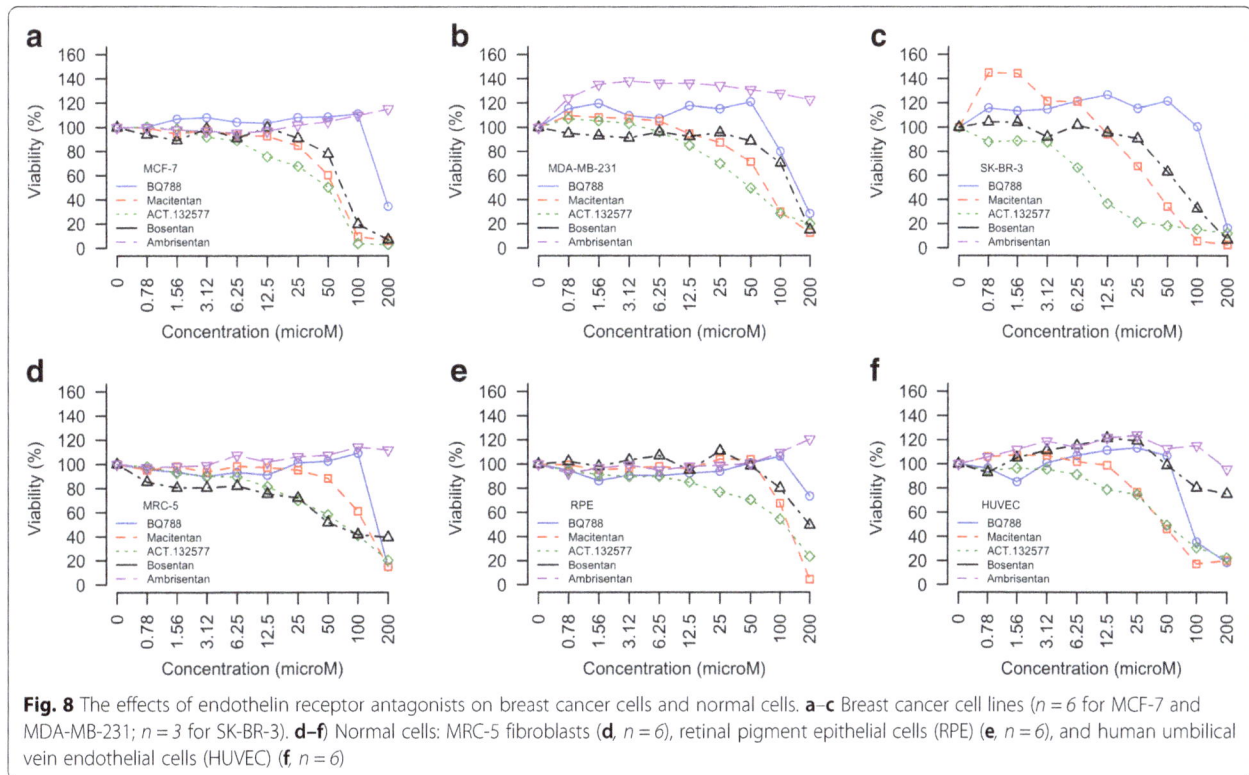

Fig. 8 The effects of endothelin receptor antagonists on breast cancer cells and normal cells. **a–c** Breast cancer cell lines (*n = 6* for MCF-7 and MDA-MB-231; *n = 3* for SK-BR-3). **d–f**) Normal cells: MRC-5 fibroblasts (**d**, *n = 6*), retinal pigment epithelial cells (RPE) (**e**, *n = 6*), and human umbilical vein endothelial cells (HUVEC) (**f**, *n = 6*)

particular, ETBR is overexpresssed in bladder carcinoma [24], melanoma [25], small-cell lung cancer [26], vulvar cancer [5], clear-cell renal cell carcinoma [6], oesophageal squamous cell carcinoma [7], and astrocytoma (including GBM) [12]. ETBR was also earlier reported to be highly expressed in melanoma [25]. Of note, ETBR overexpression was correlated with shorter patient survival or poor patient outcome in small-cell lung cancer, vulvar cancer, clear-cell renal cell carcinoma, esophageal squamous cell carcinoma, and GBM [5–7, 12, 24, 27] and may thereby represent a potential prognostic marker as well as a therapeutic target for several cancer forms. We confirmed this hypothesis in the current study. We assessed the toxicity of ETBR and ETAR blockers for cancer cells of different origins. While Ambrisentan was not cytotoxic to GBM cells or breast cancer cells, the ETBR-selective blocker BQ788, the dual ETBR and ETAR blockers bosentan and macitentan, and the active metabolite of macitentan, ACT-132577 inhibited tumor cell growth to some extent. The affinity of ambrisentan to ETBR is at most 1% of its affinity to ETAR ($IC_{50} = 1$ nM) (reviewed in [28]), and ambrisentan was the least effective of the drugs we tested. We speculate that the ratio between ETAR and ETBR may be crucial for maximum cytotoxic efficiency.

To our knowledge, only two studies have earlier demonstrated overexpression of ETBR in GBM tumors, one study of Han-Chinese patients [12] and one in Japanese patients [29]. Ethnicity is a factor in the pathogenesis of gliomas [13, 14]. Epidemiological data suggest that the incidence of glioma in the United States is higher among whites, followed by blacks, Hawaiians, Chinese or Japanese, Filipinos, and Alaskan natives [30]. The incidence of gliomas is also higher in Scandinavian countries than in Asian countries [30]. The ethnicity difference may be related to or result in alterations in the expression of key proteins. The promoter methylation status of the O^6-methylguanine methyltransferase, a key DNA repair enzyme predicted the outcome of treatments that include an alkylating agent in Caucasian populations but not in Indians [31]. In the present study, we detected higher ETBR immunoreactivity in tumor cells from GBMs of Swedish patients, while little or no ETBR immunoreactivity was detected in adjacent nontumor cells, which consistent with a previous report [20]. ETBR is known to predominantly express by astrocytes, where it helps regulate cell hypertrophy [32]. In normal aging brains, we detected ETBR immunoreactivity in corpora amylacea, which are glycoproteinaceous inclusion bodies associated with aging or neurodegenerative diseases. The significance of this finding is unknown but it is well-known that the corpora amylacea is immunoreactive to various proteins (reviewed in [33]) and recently, to an antibody against a late antigen (MAB8127, Millipore) of human cytomegalovirus, a ubiquitous beta herpesvirus [34].

Our study is limited by the relatively small number of patients. Hence a large-scale patient cohort is needed to further evaluate the usefulness of ETBR as prognostic marker. A future study should also be tailored to better understand the role of ETBR in the pathogenesis of GBM. Nevertheless, our study confirms that ETBR is overexpressed in GBM and other cancer forms and further implicates ETBR as a potentially useful prognostic marker and possibly a therapeutic target for cancer.

Conclusion

This study examined the potential role of ETBR in GBM tumors as well as in other cancer forms. ETBR expression was higher in GBM tumors and several other cancer forms than in control tissues and high ETBR expression was correlated with poor patient outcome. ETBR blockers were in general more toxic to tumor cells than normal cells, which imply a potential benefit of ETBR blockers in cancer therapy.

Additional file

Additional file 1: Figure S1. Survival curves based on clinical information obtained from GSE7696 and GSE16011 for Endothelin receptor type B (ETBR) mRNA expression in GBM. GSE7696 and GSE16011 cohort shows that over-median expression of ETBR has lower survival rate at 3 years than 5 years (http://watson.compbio.iupui.edu/). **Figure S2.** ETBR mRNA expression in GSE42656 (A) and GSE50161 (B). No statistically significant difference was observed for ETBR expression in normal brain tissue compared to that of GBM patients, mirroring heterogeneity of disease. **Figure S3.** Overexpression of ETBR mRNA in different cancers of the TCGA cancer cohort is shown using The Cancer Cell Line Encyclopedia (CCLE, https://portals.broadinstitute.org/ccle). Numbers in parentheses indicate sample size. **Figure S4.** The ETBR-interacting proteins (up to second neighbor) were searched in different cancer signature genes as described [22] A). The number of ETBR-interacting proteins found to be signature genes in various cancer cohorts were shown. B) The association between cancer types and ETBR-interacting proteins suggests a possible role of ETBR in GBM and other cancers. Cancer types are shown with degree-based node shape and surrounding red circles, whereas ETBR-interacting proteins are shown with degree based nodes (orange). **Figure S5.** ETBR expression in different subtypes of GBM (A) and its correlation with survival (B) according to molecular classification [21]. Higher expression of ETBR in both 'Classical' and 'Neural' subtype tended to be correlated with poor overall survival. **Figure S6.** Relative expression of ETBR in various primary GBM cells, breast cancer lines (MCF-7, SKBR3 and MDA-MB-231), fibroblast (MRC-5), endothelial cells (HUVEC) and epithelial cells (RPE) as normalized to MRC-5.

Abbreviations

ERA: Endothelin receptor antagonists; ETAR: Endothelin A receptor; ETBR: Endothelin B receptor; GBM: Glioblastoma

Acknowledgements

We thank all lab members for valuable comments and Stephen Ordway for editorial assistance; Drs. Anna Martinez Casals and Mohsen Karimi Arzenani for the RNA and cDNA derived from GBM tissues, respectively; Anna Ridderstad Wollberg from VINNOVA-BIO-X for excellent coaching; Ylva Terelius, Richard Bethell, Fredrik Öberg and Susana Ayesa Alvarez from Medivir AB for useful technical advice and helped with the procurement and purity analysis of the endothelin antagonists.

Funding

This work was supported by Sten A Olssons Foundation for Research and Culture, Family Erling-Persson Foundation, Torsten Söderberg Foundation, BILTEMA Foundation, IngaBritt and Arne Lundbergs Foundation, Stichting af Jochnick Foundation, Jane and Dan Olssons Research Foundation, Nexttobe,

Swedish Cancer Foundation, Children's Cancer Foundation, Swedish Medical Research Council, Thematic Cardiovascular Research Center and Stockholm County Council, and the Swedish Heart-Lung Foundation, VINNOVA-BIO-X and Medivir AB (all to CSN), Cure cancer /Bota Cancer (to KCY). The funding body had no role in the design of the study and collection, analysis, and interpretation of data and in writing the manuscript.

Authors' contributions

KCY, GT and SV conceived and designed the study; SV, GT, NL, HC, HLC, BD and KCY did the research; VW, AAM, PS, SA, MS, KS, GS, AR, KTW and JT contributed new reagents or analytic tools; SV, GT, CSN and KCY analyzed the data and wrote the paper. All authors read and approved the final manuscript.

Competing interests

A patent application for use of ETBR inhibitors in prevention and treatment of HCMV infection and CMV-related pathologies such as cardiovascular diseases and cancer has been filed (to CSN and KCY).

Author details

[1]Unit of Computational Medicine, Center for Molecular Medicine, Department of Medicine, Karolinska Institutet, Stockholm, Sweden. [2]Cell and Molecular Immunology, Experimental Cardiovascular Unit, Departments of Medicine and Neurology, Center for Molecular Medicine, Karolinska Institutet, SE-171 76 Stockholm, Sweden. [3]Department of Cell and Molecular Biology, Karolinska Institutet, Stockholm, Sweden. [4]Department of Neurosurgery, Karolinska University Hospital, Stockholm, Sweden. [5]Department of Pathology, University of Malaya, Kuala Lumpur, Malaysia. [6]Biological and Environmental Sciences and Engineering Division (BESE), Computer, Electrical and Mathematical Sciences and Engineering Division (CEMSE), King Abdullah University of Science and Technology (KAUST), Thuwal 23955–6900, Kingdom of Saudi Arabia.

References

1. Ohgaki H, Kleihues P. Population-based studies on incidence, survival rates, and genetic alterations in astrocytic and oligodendroglial gliomas. J Neuropathol Exp Neurol. 2005;64(6):479–89.
2. Wen PY, Kesari S. Malignant gliomas in adults. N Engl J Med. 2008;359(5): 492–507.
3. Gruber ML, Buster WP. Temozolomide in combination with irinotecan for treatment of recurrent malignant glioma. Am J Clin Oncol. 2004;27(1):33–8.
4. Mazzuca MQ, Khalil RA. Vascular endothelin receptor type B: structure, function and dysregulation in vascular disease. Biochem Pharmacol. 2012; 84(2):147–62.
5. Eltze E, Bertolin M, Korsching E, Wulfing P, Maggino T, Lelle R. Expression and prognostic relevance of endothelin-B receptor in vulvar cancer. Oncol Rep. 2007;18(2):305–11.
6. Wuttig D, Zastrow S, Fussel S, Toma MI, Meinhardt M, Kalman K, Junker K, Sanjmyatav J, Boll K, Hackermuller J, et al. CD31, EDNRB and TSPAN7 are promising prognostic markers in clear-cell renal cell carcinoma revealed by genome-wide expression analyses of primary tumors and metastases. Int J Cancer. 2012;131(5):E693–704.
7. Tanaka T, Sho M, Takayama T, Wakatsuki K, Matsumoto S, Migita K, Ito M, Hamada K, Nakajima Y. Endothelin B receptor expression correlates with tumour angiogenesis and prognosis in oesophageal squamous cell carcinoma. Br J Cancer. 2014;110(4):1027–33.
8. Bagnato A, Loizidou M, Pflug BR, Curwen J, Growcott J. Role of the endothelin axis and its antagonists in the treatment of cancer. Brit J Pharmacol. 2011;163(2):220–33.
9. Wan X, Zhang LB, Jiang B. Role of endothelin B receptor in oligodendroglioma proliferation and survival: in vitro and in vivo evidence. Mol Med Rep. 2014;9(1):229–34.
10. Asundi J, Reed C, Arca J, McCutcheon K, Ferrando R, Clark S, Luis E, Tien J, Firestein R, Polakis P. An antibody-drug conjugate targeting the endothelin B receptor for the treatment of melanoma. Clin Cancer Res. 2011;17(5):965–75.

11. Kim SJ, Lee HJ, Kim MS, Choi HJ, He J, Wu Q, Aldape K, Weinberg JS, Yung WK, Conrad CA, et al. Macitentan, a dual Endothelin receptor antagonist, in combination with Temozolomide leads to Glioblastoma regression and long-term survival in mice. Clin Cancer Res. 2015;21(20):4630–41.

12. Shen C, Yang L, Yuan X. Endothelin B receptor expression in human astrocytoma: association with clinicopathological variables and survival outcomes. Int J Neurosci. 2011;121(11):626–31.

13. Ratneswaren T, Jack RM, Tataru D, Davies EA. The survival of patients with high grade glioma from different ethnic groups in south East England. J Neuro-Oncol. 2014;120(3):531–6.

14. Chen P, Aldape K, Wiencke JK, Kelsey KT, Miike R, Davis RL, Liu J, Kesler-Diaz A, Takahashi M, Wrensch M. Ethnicity delineates different genetic pathways in malignant glioma. Cancer Res. 2001;61(10):3949–54.

15. Rahbar A, Orrego A, Peredo I, Dzabic M, Wolmer-Solberg N, Straat K, Stragliotto G, Soderberg-Naucler C. Human cytomegalovirus infection levels in glioblastoma multiforme are of prognostic value for survival. J Clin Virol. 2013;57(1):36–42.

16. Ritchie ME, Phipson B, Wu D, Hu Y, Law CW, Shi W, Smyth GK. limma powers differential expression analyses for RNA-sequencing and microarray studies. Nucleic Acids Res. 2015;43(7):e47.

17. Vasaikar SV, Padhi AK, Jayaram B, Gomes J. NeuroDNet - an open source platform for constructing and analyzing neurodegenerative disease networks. BMC Neurosci. 2013;14:3.

18. Smoot ME, Ono K, Ruscheinski J, Wang PL, Ideker T. Cytoscape 2.8: new features for data integration and network visualization. Bioinformatics. 2011;27(3):431–2.

19. Subramanian A, Tamayo P, Mootha VK, Mukherjee S, Ebert BL, Gillette MA, Paulovich A, Pomeroy SL, Golub TR, Lander ES, et al. Gene set enrichment analysis: a knowledge-based approach for interpreting genome-wide expression profiles. P Natl Acad Sci USA. 2005;102(43):15545–50.

20. Egidy G, Eberl LP, Valdenaire O, Irmler M, Majdi R, Diserens AC, Fontana A, Janzer RC, Pinet F, Juillerat-Jeanneret L. The endothelin system in human glioblastoma. Lab Investig. 2000;80(11):1681–9.

21. Verhaak RG, Hoadley KA, Purdom E, Wang V, Qi Y, Wilkerson MD, Miller CR, Ding L, Golub T, Mesirov JP, et al. Integrated genomic analysis identifies clinically relevant subtypes of glioblastoma characterized by abnormalities in PDGFRA, IDH1, EGFR, and NF1. Cancer Cell. 2010;17(1):98–110.

22. Rubio-Perez C, Tamborero D, Schroeder MP, Antolin AA, Deu-Pons J, Perez-Llamas C, Mestres J, Gonzalez-Perez A, Lopez-Bigas N. In silico prescription of anticancer drugs to cohorts of 28 tumor types reveals targeting opportunities. Cancer Cell. 2015;27(3):382–96.

23. Bagnato A, Spinella F, Rosano L. The endothelin axis in cancer: the promise and the challenges of molecularly targeted therapy. Can J Physiol Pharm. 2008;86(8):473–84.

24. Eltze E, Wild PJ, Wulfing C, Zwarthoff EC, Burger M, Stoehr R, Korsching E, Hartmann A. Expression of the endothelin axis in noninvasive and superficially invasive bladder cancer: relation to clinicopathologic and molecular prognostic parameters. Eur Urol. 2009;56(5):837–45.

25. Demunter A, De Wolf-Peeters C, Degreef H, Stas M, van den Oord JJ. Expression of the endothelin-B receptor in pigment cell lesions of the skin - evidence for its role as tumor progression marker in malignant melanoma. Virchows Arch. 2001;438(5):485–91.

26. Blouquit-Laye S, Regnier A, Beauchet A, Zimmermann U, Devillier P, Chinet T. Expression of endothelin receptor subtypes in bronchial tumors. Oncol Rep. 2010;23(2):457–63.

27. de Tayrac M, Aubry M, Saikali S, Etcheverry A, Surbled C, Guenot F, Galibert MD, Hamlat A, Lesimple T, Quillien V, et al. A 4-gene signature associated with clinical outcome in high-grade gliomas. Clin Cancer Res. 2011;17(2):317–27.

28. Vatter H, Seifert V. Ambrisentan, a non-peptide endothelin receptor antagonist. Cardiovasc Drug Rev. 2006;24(1):63–76.

29. Nakashima S, Sugita Y, Miyoshi H, Arakawa F, Muta H, Ishibashi Y, Niino D, Ohshima K, Terasaki M, Nakamura Y, et al. Endothelin B receptor expression in malignant gliomas: the perivascular immune escape mechanism of gliomas. J Neuro-Oncol. 2016;127(1):23–32.

30. Inskip PD, Linet MS, Heineman EF. Etiology of brain tumors in adults. Epidemiol Rev. 1995;17(2):382–414.

31. Jha P, Suri V, Jain A, Sharma MC, Pathak P, Srivastava A, Suri A, Gupta D, Chosdol K, Chattopadhyay P, et al. O6-methylguanine DNA methyltransferase gene promoter methylation status in gliomas and its correlation with other molecular alterations: first Indian report with review of challenges for use in customized treatment. Neurosurgery. 2010;67(6):1681–91.

32. Rogers SD, Peters CM, Pomonis JD, Hagiwara H, Ghilardi JR, Mantyh PW. Endothelin B receptors are expressed by astrocytes and regulate astrocyte hypertrophy in the normal and injured CNS. Glia. 2003;41(2):180–90.

33. Cavanagh JB. Corpora-amylacea and the family of polyglucosan diseases. Brain Res Brain Res Rev. 1999;29(2-3):265–95.

34. Libard S, Popova SN, Amini RM, Karja V, Pietilainen T, Hamalainen KM, Sundstrom C, Hesselager G, Bergqvist M, Ekman S et al: Human Cytomegalovirus Tegument Protein pp65 Is Detected in All Intra- and Extra-Axial Brain Tumours Independent of the Tumour Type or Grade. PLoS One. 2014; 9(9):e108861(1-14).

35. Li B, Dewey CN. RSEM: accurate transcript quantification from RNA-Seq data with or without a reference genome. BMC Bioinformatics. 2011;12:323.

8

Combination of anti-PD-1 therapy and stereotactic radiosurgery for a gastric cancer patient with brain metastasis

Min-joo Ahn[1], Kanghan Lee[1], Kyung Hwa Lee[2], Jin Woong Kim[3], In-Young Kim[4,5*] and Woo Kyun Bae[1,5*]

Abstract

Background: Brain metastases from gastric cancer are difficult to treat and their prognosis is poor. Despite various possible treatments, the survival rate of such patients is still unsatisfactory; therefore, new treatment modalities or combinations of therapies need to be explored.

Case presentation: We herein discuss a case of a 38-year-old man initially diagnosed with a gastric cancer brain metastasis. At first, only stereotactic radiosurgery (SRS) was performed, but it was not effective. After the brain and systemic metastases progressed, SRS and anti-PD-1 therapy were administered in combination, and the brain and intra-abdominal metastatic lesions responded satisfactorily.

Conclusion: The combination of anti-PD-1 therapy and SRS could be effective against gastric cancer with brain metastases.

Keywords: Anti-PD-1 therapy, Stereotactic radiosurgery, Gastric cancer, Brain metastasis

Background

Brain metastases from gastric cancer are uncommon, being diagnosed in fewer than 1% of gastric cancer patients; therefore, the standard treatment has not yet been established [1]. Almost all brain metastases from gastric cancer are observed in advanced-stage disease with concurrent metastasis to other organs. In most cases, the aim of treating metastases is to achieve an appropriate relief of symptoms and assure a good quality of life [2, 3].

PD-1 is a negative co-stimulatory receptor expressed mainly on activated T cells, and downregulates excessive immune responses by binding to its ligands, PD-L1 and PD-L2. PD-L1 is constitutively expressed in various tissues and several kinds of malignancies, including gastric cancer. Binding of PD-1 to PD-L1 inhibits effector T-cell

function, thus resulting in suppression of antitumor response and neoplastic growth. Several studies suggested that PD-L1 expression is significantly upregulated following *Helicobacter pylori* infection and that the resulting decrease in T-cell proliferation can be reversed with anti-PD-L1 antibodies. PD-L1 overexpression was observed in more than 40% of human gastric cancer samples and has been associated with a poor prognosis in several studies [4].

Surgery or stereotactic radiosurgery (SRS) and additional whole brain radiation therapy (WBRT) can be used for patients with a good performance status. However, the role of chemotherapy and radiosensitizers in the treatment of brain metastases from gastric cancer remains undefined. Furthermore, little is known about the safety and outcomes of patients who have received a combination of immune checkpoint blockade therapies and SRS to treat brain metastases of gastric cancer. The present report describes a case in which a patient with advanced gastric cancer with a brain metastasis was successfully treated

* Correspondence: kiy87@chonnam.ac.kr; drwookyun@jnu.ac.kr
[4]Departments of Neurosurgery, Chonnam National University Medical School, Gwangju 501-757, South Korea
[1]Departments of Internal Medicine, Chonnam National University Medical School, Gwangju 501-757, South Korea
Full list of author information is available at the end of the article

with a combination of SRS and immune checkpoint blockade therapy.

Case presentation

A 38-year-old male patient presented to our hospital with right side motor weakness that had started 8 months earlier. He had visited another hospital when the symptoms had started and had been diagnosed with advanced gastric adenocarcinoma with a single metastatic lesion in the left thalamus (Figs. 1a & 2a). He had undergone gamma knife radiosurgery (GKRS) at the other hospital. However, due to brain edema and deterioration of his overall condition, systemic chemotherapy had not been performed.

A physical examination revealed grade 4 motor weakness in the upper and lower right limbs. Laboratory findings revealed mild hypochromic microcytic anemia but were otherwise non-specific. Follow-up abdominal computed tomography (CT) showed aggravation of an advanced gastric malignancy with multiple metastatic regional lymph nodes, and new hepatic, left adrenal, and peritoneal metastases were also observed (Fig. 1b). Follow-up brain magnetic resonance imaging (MRI) showed a mild increase in the size of the metastasis in the left thalamus (Fig. 2b). He was only given palliative treatment and discharged.

Five months later the patient was admitted to our neurosurgery department with a severe headache. A brain MRI showed a slight increase in the previous mass (Fig. 2c) and several newly developed metastases with surrounding edema (Fig. 2d). Repeated GKRS was performed for both recurrent and new lesions. However, his symptoms persisted and his general condition worsened. A pathological examination of the endoscopically biopsied tissue revealed moderately differentiated adenocarcinoma with glandular fusion in a cribriform pattern (Fig. 3a). By immunohistochemistry, the tumor cells were completely negative for PD1, but showed weak to moderate cytoplasmic positivity for PDL1 (Fig. 3b and c). We gave the patient an injection of pembrolizumab (Keytruda) 200 mg.

Two weeks after the injection of pembrolizumab, he returned to our hospital, reporting that his neurological symptoms had dramatically improved and that his headaches no longer occurred. He insisted that the treatment be continued, and after three doses of pembrolizumab, the patient underwent an abdominal CT and brain MRI. The abdominal CT (Fig. 1c) revealed a partial response of the gastric cancer, liver, lymph node, and brain metastases, and the brain MRI showed that the thalamic metastasis had achieved a stable state (Fig. 2e) and that there had been a dramatic reduction of the newly developed brain metastases (Fig. 2f).

The neurological symptoms were markedly improved after 3 doses of pembrolizumab. A follow-up physical examination after treatment revealed grade 3 motor weakness in his right lower limb and grade 4 motor weakness in his upper limb. Although a new brain lesion developed after 7 months of pembrolizumab treatment, his neurological symptoms and signs were not aggravated and he is being treated with systemic chemotherapy and pembrolizumab. The patient is currently still alive and in fair general condition 26 months after the initial diagnosis.

Discussion

Therapy for a metastatic brain tumor includes surgical resection, chemotherapy, and radiation. SRS has become the main therapy for metastatic brain tumors [5]. However, the response to treatment is poor in gastric cancer patients with brain metastasis. Most brain metastases from gastric cancer are detected in the advanced stages of the disease [1, 6]. Therefore, only conservative treatment is performed in many patients. However, appropriate treatment is needed to improve the neurological symptoms of brain metastasis if the progression in other organs can be controlled.

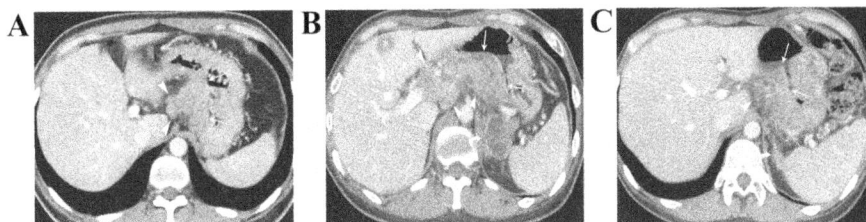

Fig. 1 a. A contrast-enhanced abdominal computed tomography (CT) image shows enhancing gastric cancer (arrows) of the gastric body and conglomerate metastatic lymphadenopathies (arrowheads) along the left gastric chain. **b**. A follow-up contrast-enhanced abdominal CT image demonstrates aggravated gastric cancer of the gastric body (arrows), multiple metastatic lymphadenopathies (arrowheads) in the gastrohepatic space, a hepatic metastasis (asterisk), and left adrenal metastases (curved arrow). **c**. A follow-up contrast-enhanced abdominal CT image after anti-PD-1 therapy shows improving gastric cancer (arrows) of a swollen gastric body and markedly decreased metastatic lymphadenopathies (arrowhead). Note the resolution of the previous metastases in the left adrenal gland (curved arrow)

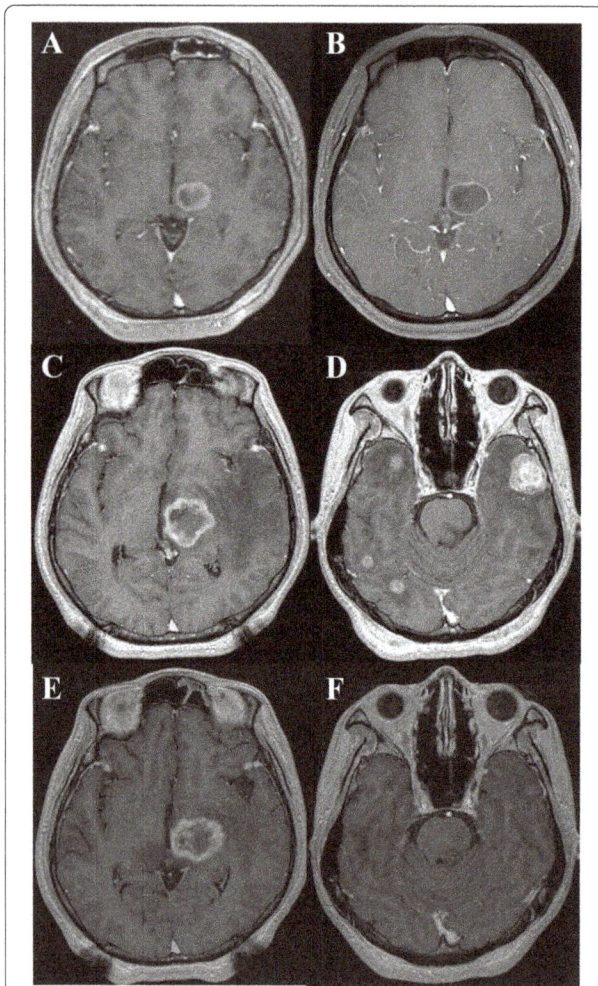

Fig. 2 a. A gadolinium(Gd)-enhanced brain magnetic resonance (MR) image depicts a single metastasis (arrow) in the left thalamus. **b** and **c**. Follow-up Gd-enhanced brain MR images demonstrate tumor progression (arrow) in the left thalamus. **d**. A follow-up gadolinium-enhanced brain MR image shows several new metastases (arrows) with surrounding edema in both cerebral hemispheres. **e** and **f**. Follow-up Gd-enhanced brain MR images after anti-PD-1 therapy demonstrates the stable state of the repeatedly treated thalamic metastasis (arrow) and nearly complete resolution of the newly developed metastases

Preclinical data suggest that PD-L1 expression is significantly upregulated following *Helicobacter pylori* infection and PD-L1 expression has been detected in more than 40% of human gastric cancer samples [4]. Furthermore, anti-PD-1 antibody pembrolizumab treatment showed a 22% overall response in patients with PD-L1-positive recurrent or metastatic adenocarcinoma of the stomach [7]. In our case, since the patient's performance status was poor, he did not receive systemic chemotherapy. Therefore, we checked for anti-PD-L1 expression and selected a combination of SRS and anti-PD-1 therapy. As a result, his neurological function and PS recovered dramatically.

Based on our experience, we believe that a combination of SRS and anti-PD-1 therapy is useful for a brain tumor from gastric cancer. Immune checkpoint inhibitors are revolutionizing the ability to treat metastatic cancer [8]. The interaction between immune checkpoint inhibitors and standard treatments for brain metastases, such as SRS, remains under-investigated [9]. Several retrospective single-institution studies have suggested that ipilimumab in combination with radiation therapy may be more effective than radiotherapy alone for melanoma brain metastases. Knisely et al. reviewed the outcomes of 77 patients with melanoma brain metastases who received SRS as well as ipilimumab. Patients who received combination therapy demonstrated improved survival compared with those who received SRS alone [10]. Another retrospective analysis demonstrated an overall survival benefit of 19.9 months with combination therapy versus 4.0 months for SRS alone, with no associated increase in toxicity after the addition of ipilimumab to SRS [11].

At this point, however, little is known about the safety and outcomes in patients who have received immune checkpoint inhibitors and SRS to treat brain metastases of gastric cancer. In this case, the metastatic lesions of the brain initially showed no response to SRS but showed a partial response after SRS was combined with anti-PD-1 therapy. This effect may be construed as the effect of anti-PD-1 therapy alone, regardless of its combination with SRS. However, several studies have concluded

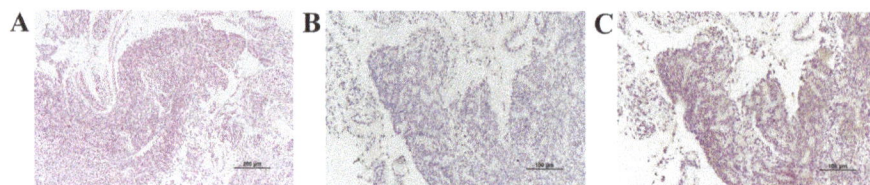

Fig. 3 Pathologic findings of the biopsied gastric tissue. **a** The adenocarcinoma showing fused glands was intermingled with inflammatory exudates and normal mucosal glands (hematoxylin and eosin, original magnification ×100). **b** Immunohistochemistry of PD1 reveals completely negative staining in tumor cells (immunohistochemistry, original magnification ×200). **c** Tumor cells showing cytoplasmic positivity for PDL1 immunostaining (immunohistochemistry, original magnification ×200)

that radiation therapy and immune checkpoint blockade treatment have a synergistic effect on the brain metastases of melanoma and non-small cell lung cancer. The possibility that irradiation can induce neoantigen presentation and upregulate PD-L1 expression has been previously asserted [12].

Here, we present a case in which a patient with advanced gastric cancer and brain metastasis was treated with SRS and anti-PD-1 therapy. The metastatic lesions of the brain showed a partial response after three cycles of anti-PD-1 therapy and SRS. The patient maintained excellent performance status and showed no signs of neurologic toxicities. To the best of our knowledge, this is the first case that reports the successful treatment of a brain metastasis of gastric origin through anti-PD-1 therapy combined with SRS. This case report suggests that the combination of SRS and anti-PD-1 therapy may be an option for patients with gastric cancer who have brain metastases. The main limitation of this study is its retrospective nature. Larger prospective studies are needed to determine if this combination treatment is effective for patients with SRS-unresponsive brain metastases in gastric cancer.

Conclusion
The combination of anti-PD-1 therapy and SRS could be effective against gastric cancer with brain metastases.

Abbreviations
CT: Computed tomography; GKRS: Gamma knife radiosurgery; MRI: Magnetic resonance imaging; SRS: Stereotactic radiosurgery; WBRT: Whole brain radiation therapy

Acknowledgements
Not applicable.

Funding
The authors declare no sources of funding for this study.

Authors' contributions
Substantial contributions to conception and design, acquisition of data, analysis and interpretation of data: MA, KL, KHL, JWK, IK, and WKB. Been involved in drafting manuscript or revising it critically: MA, IK, and WKB. Given final approval for version to be published: MA, KL, KHL, JWK, IK, and WKB. Agree to be accountable: MA, KL, KHL, JWK, IK, and WKB. All authors read and approved the final manuscript.

Competing interests
The authors declare that they have no competing interests.

Author details
[1]Departments of Internal Medicine, Chonnam National University Medical School, Gwangju 501-757, South Korea. [2]Departments of Pathology, Chonnam National University Medical School, Gwangju 501-757, South Korea. [3]Departments of Radiology, Chonnam National University Medical School, Gwangju 501-757, South Korea. [4]Departments of Neurosurgery, Chonnam National University Medical School, Gwangju 501-757, South Korea. [5]Chonnam National University Hwasun Hospital, 160 Ilsim-ri, Hwasun-eup, Hwasun-gun 519-809, South Korea.

References
1. Kasakura Y, Fujii M, Mochizuki F, Suzuki T, Takahashi T. Clinicopathological study of brain metastasis in gastric cancer patients. Surg Today. 2000;30:485–90.
2. Kazda T, Pospisil P, Dolezelova H, Jancalek R, Slampa P. Whole brain radiotherapy: consequences for personalized medicine. Rep Pract Oncol Radiother. 2013;18:133–8.
3. Fernandez G, Pocinho R, Travancinha C, Netto E, Roldao M. Quality of life and radiotherapy in brain metastasis patients. Rep Pract Oncol Radiother. 2012;17:281–7.
4. Kim JW, Nam KH, Ahn SH, Park do J, Kim HH, Kim SH, et al. Prognostic implications of immunosuppressive protein expression in tumors as well as immune cell infiltration within the tumor microenvironment in gastric cancer. Gastric Cancer. 2016;19:42–52.
5. McDermott MW, Sneed PK. Radiosurgery in metastatic brain cancer. Neurosurgery. 2005;57(5 Suppl):S45–53. discusssion S1–4
6. York JE, Stringer J, Ajani JA, Wildrick DM, Gokaslan ZL. Gastric cancer and metastasis to the brain. Ann Surg Oncol. 1999;6:771–6.
7. Muro K, Chung HC, Shankaran V, Geva R, Catenacci D, Gupta S, et al. Pembrolizumab for patients with PD-L1-positive advanced gastric cancer (KEYNOTE-012): a multicentre, open-label, phase 1b trial. Lancet Oncol. 2016;17:717–26.
8. Topalian SL, Hodi FS, Brahmer JR, Gettinger SN, Smith DC, McDermott DF, et al. Safety, activity, and immune correlates of anti-PD-1 antibody in cancer. New Engl J. Medicine. 2012;366:2443–54.
9. Kiess AP, Wolchok JD, Barker CA, Postow MA, Tabar V, Huse JT, et al. Stereotactic radiosurgery for melanoma brain metastases in patients receiving ipilimumab: safety profile and efficacy of combined treatment. Int J Radiat Oncology Biol Phys. 2015;92:368–75.
10. Knisely JP, JB Y, Flanigan J, Sznol M, Kluger HM, Chiang VL. Radiosurgery for melanoma brain metastases in the ipilimumab era and the possibility of longer survival. J Neurosurg. 2012;117:227–33.
11. Silk AW, Bassetti MF, West BT, Tsien CI, Lao CD. Ipilimumab and radiation therapy for melanoma brain metastases. Cancer Med. 2013;2:899–906.
12. D'Souza NM, Fang P, Logan J, Yang J, Jiang W, Li J. Combining radiation therapy with immune checkpoint blockade for central nervous system malignancies. Front Oncol. 2016;6:212.

9

Galectin-1 is a poor prognostic factor in patients with glioblastoma multiforme after radiotherapy

Shang-Yu Chou[1], Shao-Lun Yen[5], Chao-Cheng Huang[2,4] and Eng-Yen Huang[1,3,4,6*] (iD)

Abstract

Background: Galectin-1, a radioresistance marker, was found in our previous study to be a prognostic factor for cervical cancer. The aim of current study is to determine the prognostic significance of the galectin-1 expression level in patients with glioblastoma multiforme (GBM) undergoing adjuvant radiotherapy (RT).

Methods: We included 45 patients with GBM who were treated with maximal safe surgical resection or biopsy alone followed by adjuvant RT of EQD2 (equivalent dose in 2-Gy fractions) > or = 60 Gy for homogeneous treatment. Paraffin-embedded tissues acquired from the Department of Pathology were analyzed using immunohistochemical staining for galectin-1 expression. The primary endpoint was overall survival (OS).

Results: Patients with weak expression had a better median survival (27.9 months) than did those with strong expression (10.7 months; $p = 0.009$). We compared characteristics between weak and strong galectin-1 expression, and only the expression level of galectin-3 showed a correlation. The group with weak galectin-1 expression displayed a 3-year OS of 27.3% and a 3-year cancer-specific survival (CSS) of 27.3%; these values were only 5.9% and 7.6%, respectively, in the group with strong galectin-1 expression ($p = 0.009$ and 0.020, respectively). Cox regression was used to confirm that the expression level of galectin-1 (weak vs. strong) is a significant factor of OS ($p = 0.020$) and CSS ($p = 0.022$). Other parameters, such as the expression level of galectin-3, Eastern Cooperative Oncology Group (ECOG) performance, gender, surgical method, age ≥ 50 years, tumor size, or radiation field were not significant factors.

Conclusion: The expression level of galectin-1 affects survival in patients with GBM treated with adjuvant RT. Future studies are required to analyze the effect of other factors, such as O(6)-methylguanine-DNA methyltransferase (MGMT)-promoter methylation status, in patients with weak and strong galectin-1 expression.

Keywords: Galectin-1, Glioblastoma multiforme, Adjuvant radiotherapy, Radioresistant marker

Background

Glioblastoma multiforme (GBM) is the most common type of brain tumor, accounting for 60% of all malignant primary brain tumors in adults; GBM is also the most malignant type. Although GBM is rare, with an incidence of 2–3 cases per 100,000 patients with primary malignant brain tumors in Europe and North America [1], a significant increase in the incidence of GBM has been observed [2]. In general, the disease progresses rapidly and has a poor outcome. Without treatment, overall survival (OS) in GBM patients is only 3–5 months [3], and despite multimodal aggressive treatment, the median survival of GBM is still only 12 months. Currently, maximal safe surgical resection followed by adjuvant local radiotherapy (RT) and temozolomide (TMZ) is considered the standard treatment for GBM. In 2005, a large clinical trial of 575 participants randomized to treatment with standard RT vs. RT plus TMZ chemotherapy reported that the latter group survived a median of 14.6 months, as opposed to 12.1 months for the former group [4]. Nonetheless, the effectiveness of TMZ is weak in patients without O(6)-methylguanine-DNA methyltransferase (MGMT) promoter methylation [5].

* Correspondence: huangengyen@gmail.com
[1]Departments of Radiation Oncology, Kaohsiung Chang Gung Memorial Hospital, 123 Ta-Pei Road, Niao-Song Dist, Kaohsiung City 83301, Taiwan
[3]Department of Radiation Oncology, Xiamen Chang Gung Hospital, No. 123, Xiafei Rd., Haicang District, Fujian, China
Full list of author information is available at the end of the article

Another possible approach is to target other molecules that can combine with radiation sensitizers to increase the therapeutic effect.

Galectin-1, a lectin that binds to the galactoside moiety of glycoprotein, has been associated with GBM progression via processes of migration [6], invasion [6, 7], angiogenesis [8, 9], and immune escape [10]. We first found galectin-1 to be involved in radioresistance in cervical cancer [11, 12]. However, in contrast to cervical cancer, GBM exhibits high galectin-1 expression [13, 14] and is radioresistant [15, 16]. Therefore, in this study, we sought to investigate role of galectin-1 in determining the outcomes of patients undergoing RT alone without planned concomitant nor adjuvant chemotherapy. The results confirmed our hypothesis that GBM patients with strong galectin-1 expression have poor OS.

Methods

Patients' characteristics

This study was approved by the Institutional Review Board of Chang Gung Memorial Hospital (102-5087B). A total of 63 newly diagnosed GBM patients who were treated at our institution before January 1, 2002, were retrospectively evaluated. Different radiation doses may affect prognosis in GBM patients; Bleehen et al. reported that a survival advantage for patients with grades 3 and 4 astrocytoma was maintained with the high dose of 60 Gy [17]. The current standard dose for GBM at our institution is also 60 Gy, which is according to NCCN guidelines. Hence, we excluded patients with an equivalent dose in 2-Gy fractions (EQD2) < 60 Gy for homogeneous treatment due to poor outcome [17] to exclude the dose effect, which might mask the importance of galectin-1 for prognosis, and selected those with EQD2 ≥ 60 Gy. A total of 45 patients remained and were treated with maximal safe surgical resection or biopsy only followed by adjuvant RT of EQD2 ≥ 60 Gy for homogeneous treatment; the outcomes of these patients were analyzed (Table 1). We chose age ≥ 50 years as a cutoff based on a recursive partitioning analysis (RPA) study [18]; we chose a tumor size ≥ 5 cm as a cutoff because this size is a significant prognostic factor after RT [19]. Brain image analysis by magnetic resonance imaging (MRI) or computed tomography (CT) was performed before treatment. The tumor size was measured in the longest diameter on a T1-weighted axial contrast-enhanced image by brain MRI or axial contrast-enhanced image by brain CT. For multifocal GBM, the sum of the largest axial diameter for all lesions was used to determine the tumor size.

Radiation therapy

Patients were assigned by the radiation oncologist either for whole-brain irradiation (19 patients) followed by

Table 1 Patient characteristics ($n = 45$)

Parameter	Gal-1 expression (weak)	Gal-1 expression (strong)	p value
Age (years)			0.464
< 50	5 (45.5%)	10 (29.4%)	
≥ 50	6 (54.5%)	24 (70.6%)	
Gender			0.732
Female	5 (45.5%)	13 (38.2%)	
Male	6 (54.5%)	21 (61.8%)	
ECOG			1.000
0–2	8 (72.7%)	26 (76.5%)	
3–4	3 (27.3%)	8 (23.5%)	
Tumor size			0.897
< 5 cm	3 (27.3%)	7 (20.6%)	
≥ 5 cm	2 (18.2%)	7 (20.6%)	
Unknown	6 (54.5%)	20 (58.8%)	
OP method			0.525
gross total removal	8 (72.7%)	17 (50.0%)	
subtotal removal + biopsy	3 (27.3%)	14 (41.2%)	
unknown	0 (0%)	3 (8.8%)	
RT field			0.736
Small	7 (63.6%)	19 (55.9%)	
Whole brain	4 (36.4%)	15 (44.1%)	
EQD2 (Gy)			0.987
Mean	66.36	66.38	
SEM	0.67	0.46	

EQD2 equivalent dose in 2-Gy fractions, *OP* operation, *RT* radiotherapy

tumor bed boost or for tumor-site-only irradiation with a small field throughout the entire RT course (26 patients). For the latter, 11 patients were treated with a field-in field (FIF) boost protocol with RT that consisted of daily fractions of 180 cGy applied to a large target volume at the brain tumor site. This was followed by the subsequent application of 70 cGy (total 250 cGy daily) to a reduced field of the tumor bed, for a total dose of 6250–6750 cGy. The remaining 15 patients received conventional RT with 180–200 cGy per day. All RT protocols were administered in five fractions across the week.

For whole-brain irradiation, the photon beams at 6 MV or 10 MV were delivered via two-dimensional RT (2DRT). For tumor-site-only irradiation, three-dimensional conformal RT (3D–CRT) was used. The gross tumor volume (GTV) was defined according to the contrast-enhancing tumor on the CT or MRI images and included the residual tumor, perifocal edema, and entire resection cavity. The GTV plus a safe margin of 2 cm was the clinical target volume (CTV). In the FIF boost protocol, the CTV + 1 cm margin was irradiated as the large target volume, and the CTV alone was irradiated as the boost target volume. For

3D–CRT, the CTV + 3 mm margin was the planning target volume (PTV) for daily setup variation. In the FIF boost protocol, the CTV + 1.3 cm margin was the PTV of the large target.

Tissue microarray construction

Areas showing the histopathologic features of GBM were selected on archival hemolysin and eosin (H&E)-stained sections, and then representative areas of the tumor were marked on the corresponding paraffin block for tissue microarray (TMA) construction. Briefly, after the tissue cylinders were taken from the selected regions of the donor paraffin block, they were punched precisely into a recipient paraffin block using a tissue-arraying instrument. Multiple sections (1 μm thick) were cut and mounted onto microscope slides. The TMA sections were evaluated by the pathologist (SLY), who did not know the outcomes of the patients.

Immunohistochemistry (IHC)

TMA sections were stained with an anti-galectin-1 antibody (1:40, HPA000646; rabbit to human Sigma-Aldrich, St. Louis, MO) using a DAKO REAL EnVision (DAKO, Glostrup, Denmark) and an anti-galectin-3 antibody (Santa Cruz B2C10). The immunostaining patterns for galectin-1 and -3 in the intracellular tumor portion and extracellular stromal portion of the tissue samples were recorded. IHC staining was graded as no, weak, moderate, or strong staining according to the observed intensity (Fig. 1). The staining areas were calculated by the pathologist according to the staining percentage of all tumor cells in each TMA core.

The expression level of galectin-1 can be calculated by multiplying the amount of positively stained tumor cells (%) by the staining intensity of immunoreactive tumor cells. The staining intensity of immunoreactive tumor cells was scored as follows: 0, no staining; 0.5, weak staining; 1, moderate staining; and 2, strong staining (Table 2).

We primarily used a single grader for the immunostaining results. To dramatically reduce intraobserver differences, reference to standard slides, which revealed the reference point of the staining score, was performed before each reading. The grader was completely unaware of the outcome of the patients, and thus bias of the scoring interpretation was negligible. Normal liver tissue was employed as a negative control for galectin staining was and melanoma as a positive control.

Follow-up and statistics

The first brain image analysis, MRI or CT, was obtained for all patients within 2–4 months after the completion of RT and then every 3–6 months or when clinically indicated, such as when new neurologic signs were observed. The optimal cutoffs of galectin-1 and galectin-3 expression for median survival were estimated by univariate analysis with the log-rank test; those for OS, cancer-specific survival (CSS) and progression-free interval were estimated by multivariate analysis with a Cox regression model. OS and CSS were measured beginning on the first day of RT. OS was measured until the date of death from any cause or the last follow-up date, and CSS was defined as a survival measure representing cancer survival until the date of death (in the absence of another cause of death). The progression-free interval indicated the time interval from the first day of RT until the date of tumor progression, as confirmed by follow-up brain CT or MRI or by death.

Results

Univariate and multivariate analyses of treatment outcomes

The median follow-up time was 12 months (range, 1.4–207.0 months). The 3-year OS was 11.1%, and the median survival was 12 months. Multivariate analysis using galectin expression levels as a continuous variable revealed that the expression level of galectin-1 was independent of OS ($p = 0.046$). Fourteen of the 45 patients survived for more than two years. Each patient received an EQD2 ≥ 60 Gy. Among these 14 patients, five patients received whole-brain irradiation followed by tumor bed boost and nine patients got tumor-site-only irradiation; of the latter, two were under the FIF boost protocol and seven conventional RT.

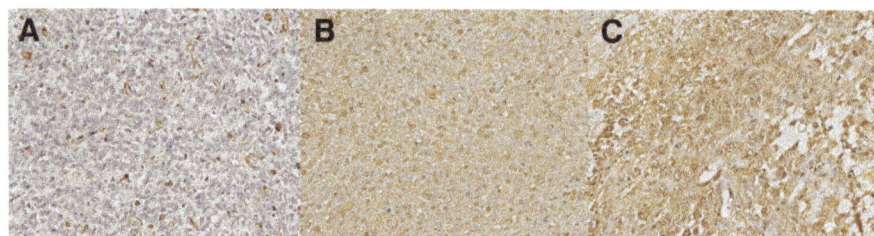

Fig. 1 Representative cases of galectin-1 immunostaining (**a**, **b**, and **c**, respectively). **a** Tumor cells show very faint staining, but the surrounding inflammatory cells and endothelial cells shows strong staining for galectin-1. Original magnification 200X. **b** Tumor cells show moderate nuclear staining. Original magnification 200X. **c** Tumor cells show diffuse strong nuclear staining. Original magnification 200X

Table 2 Staining intensity scores

Staining intensity	No staining	Weak	Moderate	Strong
Score	0	0.5	1	2

We attempted to determine the optimal cutoffs of galectin-1 and galectin-3 expression levels using univariate analysis (Additional file 1). Patients with weak galectin-1 expression (< 35%) had a better median survival (27.9 months) than did those with strong (≥ 35%) galectin-1 expression (10.7 months; $p = 0.009$). Among the 45 patients included, 34 showed strong galectin-1 expression and 11 weak galectin-1 expression. In addition, patients with weak galectin-3 expression (< 15%) had a better median survival (12.1 months) than did those with strong galectin-3 expression (10.7 months; $p = 0.031$). We compared characteristics between weak and strong galectin-1 expression (Table 1) and noted no significant difference. The 3-year OS was 27.3% and 5.9% ($p = 0.009$) (Fig. 2) in patients with weak and strong galectin-1 expression, respectively, and the corresponding CSS was 27.3% and 7.6%, respectively ($p = 0.020$) (Fig. 3).

We applied Cox regression to confirm the role of galectin-1 and again found it to be a significant factor of OS ($p = 0.020$; HR = 2.929; 95% CI 1.180–7.271) (Table 3). Other parameters, such as Eastern Cooperative Oncology Group (ECOG) performance, gender, surgical method, age ≥ 50 years, tumor size ≥ 5 cm, radiation field, and expression level of galectin-3, were not significant factors. CSS was also independent of galectin-1 overexpression ($p = 0.022$; HR = 2.873; 95% CI 1.163–7.101) (Table 4), as was the progression-free rate ($p = 0.037$; HR = 6.080; 95% CI 1.113–33.219) (Table 5).

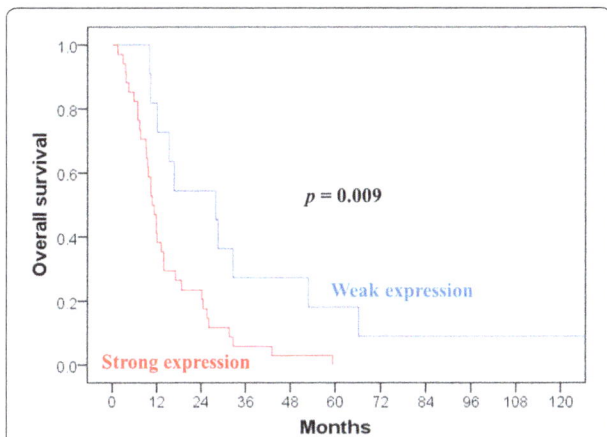

Fig. 2 Overall survival (OS) estimated according to the expression level of galectin-1. The expression level of galectin-1 was a significant factor of OS ($p = 0.009$)

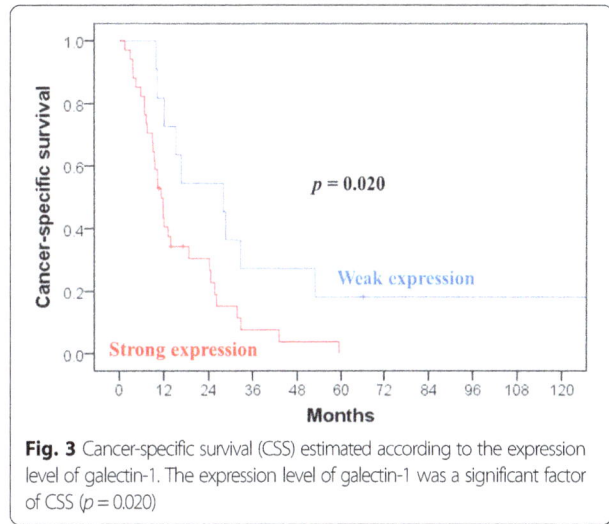

Fig. 3 Cancer-specific survival (CSS) estimated according to the expression level of galectin-1. The expression level of galectin-1 was a significant factor of CSS ($p = 0.020$)

Discussion

Although many molecular targets have been investigated in GBM, few studies have demonstrated the relationship between molecular targets and radiosensitivity. For example, epidermal growth factor receptor (EGFR) plays a role in GBM progression [20] but has no prognostic value in these patients [21]. In addition, EGFRvIII does not affect radiosensitivity in glioblastoma cells [22]. Moreover, the EGFR inhibitor gefitinib is not a radiosensitizer for newly diagnosed GBM [23]. Ras is downstream of EGFR, and k-ras mutations frequently occur in colon cancer. Indeed, ras may play a role in the angiogenic switch in astrocytomas [24] and be involved in chemoradioresistance [25]. TLN-4601, a k-ras inhibitor [26], cannot prevent GBM recurrence [27], and bevacizumab, an anti-vascular endothelial growth factor (VEGF) antibody, was found to be ineffective for treating GBM patients undergoing RT and TMZ in two recent randomized control trials [28, 29].

Galectin-1 is expressed in human gliomas and is associated with poor differentiation [13, 14]. It also functions

Table 3 MVA of OS

Parameters	p value	HR (95% CI)
Age (≥ 50 vs. < 50 years)	0.091	1.904 (0.902–4.018)
Gender (male vs. female)	0.907	1.045 (0.501–2.179)
ECOG (3–4 vs 0–2)	0.330	1.512 (0.658–3.475)
Size (≥ 5 cm vs. < 5 cm)	0.686	0.796 (0.263–2.407)
OP method (non-gross total vs. gross total)	0.887	0.950 (0.465–1.940)
RT field (whole brain vs. small)	0.322	1.510 (0.667–3.417)
Galectin-1 (strong vs. weak)	0.020	2.929 (1.180–7.271)
Galectin-3 (strong vs. weak)	0.478	1.343 (0.594–3.034)

MVA multivariate statistical analysis, *OS* overall survival, *ECOG* Eastern Cooperative Oncology Group, *OP* operation, *RT* radiotherapy

Table 4 MVA of CSS

Parameter	p value	HR (95% CI)
Age (≥ 50 vs. < 50 years)	0.140	1.791 (0.826–3.883)
Gender (male vs. female)	0.822	1.092 (0.506–2.355)
ECOG (3–4 vs 0–2)	0.591	1.273 (0.527–3.075)
Size (≥ 5 cm vs. < 5 cm)	0.701	0.792 (0.241–2.603)
OP method (non-gross total vs. gross total)	0.627	0.831 (0.393–1.755)
RT field (whole brain vs. small)	0.382	1.449 (0.631–3.325)
Galectin-1 (strong vs. weak)	0.022	2.873 (1.163–7.101)
Galectin-3 (strong vs. weak)	0.993	1.004 (0.426–2.364)

MVA multivariate statistical analysis, *CSS* cancer-specific survival, *ECOG* Eastern Cooperative Oncology Group, *OP* operation, *RT* radiotherapy

downstream of the EGFR pathway through H-ras by interacting and activating H-ras to form guanosine triphosphate (GTP). In addition, galectin-1 is involved cancer progression, enhances the migration and invasion of human GBM cells [6, 7] and angiogenesis [8], inhibits the anti-tumor immunity of natural killer (NK) cells [30–32], is involved in glioma chemoresistance [33], and may be considered a biomarker because serum galectin-1 levels are higher in patients with high-grade glioma than in healthy controls [10]. Despite evidence that galectin-1 may be involved in glioma progression in vitro, few animal studies on cancer progression have been performed [7, 13, 14, 31, 32], and only one human study to date reports the role of galectin-1 in glioma prognosis. In this study, Rorive et al. compared the expression level of galectin-1 in high-grade astrocytic tumors from 41 patients (26 with GBM) who survived < 12 months and > 24 months; the expression level of galectin-1 was significantly correlated with survival [13], but no details of treatment modality were reported. In the current study, galectin-1 overexpression was associated with poor survival and short time to progression following RT. To the best of our knowledge, the present study is the first report of the

Table 5 MVA of the progression-free rate

Parameter	p value	HR (95% CI)
Age (≥ 50 vs. < 50 years)	0.159	2.369 (0.712–7.878)
Gender (male vs. female)	0.114	0.320 (0.078–1.312)
ECOG (3–4 vs 0–2)	0.258	2.292 (0.544–9.650)
Size (≥ 5 cm vs. < 5 cm)	0.819	1.213 (0.232–6.350)
OP method (non-gross total vs. gross total)	0.023	7.408 (1.320–41.585)
RT field (whole brain vs. small)	0.609	0.716 (0.202–2.535)
Galectin-1 (strong vs. weak)	0.037	6.080 (1.113–33.219)
Galectin-3 (strong vs. weak)	0.089	0.181 (0.025–1.299)

MVA multivariate statistical analysis, *ECOG* Eastern Cooperative Oncology Group, *OP* operation, *RT* radiotherapy

association of galectin-1 with poor prognosis in GBM patients following RT alone. Thus, targeting galectin-1 has potential in treatment of GBM.

In the past, the entire brain was irradiated as treatment for GBM because malignant gliomas may spread along white matter tracts [34–37]. Subsequent studies found that GBM usually recurs within 2 cm of the initial tumor volume [38, 39], and histologic analysis has shown that perifocal edema often corresponds to parenchyma infiltrated by isolated tumor cells [40]. Therefore, local irradiation, rather than whole-brain RT (WBRT), is the standard radiation treatment for GBM. Because our study was limited by early data prior to 2002, some patients had still been treated with WBRT. In GBM patients, mortality largely occurs due to local recurrence or progression in or adjacent to the resection cavity, as opposed to extracranial metastases. Although the radiation groups included in this study were inhomogeneous, we considered that the local dose is key for outcomes. Accordingly, to exclude an RT regimen effect, we used EQD2 to exclude patients who had received a local dose under 60 Gy.

Currently, the standard treatment for GBM is RT combined with TMZ [4]. Because radiation can induce galectin-1 expression in glioma cells [41], inhibition of galectin-1 expression is important for RT. Danhier et al. reported in an animal study that knockdown of galectin-1 and EGFR using nanocapsules can decrease TMZ resistance in glioblastoma [42]. TMZ also effectively knocks down galectin-1 [9, 43]. Therefore, the combination of TMZ and RT may be successful therapy.

The median survival of our GBM patients was 12.0 months, which was comparable to that in the European Organisation for Research and Treatment of Cancer - National Cancer Institute Canada (EORTC/NCIC) trial (12.1 months) [4]. In patients with and without MGMT methylation and undergoing RT alone, the median survival was 15.3 and 11.8 months [5], respectively. Although TMZ significantly improved the median survival in patients with MGMT methylation (from 15.3 to 21.7 months), this was not observed in those without MGMT methylation (from 11.8 to 12.7 months). In the present study, the median survival of patients with galectin-1 overexpression was 10.7 months, which is very similar to the median survival of patients without MGMT methylation. Despite a median survival of 27.9 months in patients with weak galectin-1 expression, the proportion of this favorable group was low, at 32.4%. Due to the lack of test reagents in our hospital, we failed to obtain the MGMT promotor methylation status, which may affect the efficacy of TMZ. In this study, all the patient received brain RT only without planned concurrent nor adjuvant TMZ. Further analysis of the effect of TMZ in patients with weak and strong galectin-1 expression is encouraged.

Galectin-3 is a common molecule studied in cancer research, especially in colon cancer, whereas only one study [44] involving an animal model has reported that galectin-3 is associated with GBM progression. Regardless, our results do not prove that galectin-3 is a prognostic factor compared with galectin-1. Galectin-1 and galectin-3 are associated with H-ras [45] and K-ras [46] signals, respectively, and H-ras [24, 47–49] but not K-ras is involved in GBM progression. Therefore, further in vitro and in vivo research is encouraged to determine the roles of galectin-1 and -3 in GBM radioresistance.

The limitations of this study are its retrospective nature and limited sample size. According to the national law of human research, informed consent for research should be obtained for work performed in our country after 2002. As we could only include patients before 2002, and the sample size was therefore small. Because these patients were treated a long time ago, almost all were dead, their charts were destroyed, and the time to progression could not be confirmed. Nonetheless, the time to progression and the survival time were correlated in patients who underwent imaging follow-up; not all patients were evaluated for time to progression, yet galectin-1 remained a significant factor of GBM progression after RT. In addition, MGMT promoter methylation is associated with patient response to alkylating agents and OS. Because the proportion of MGMT promoter methylation in the included patients was undetermined, it remains unclear whether galectin-1 expression may affect the importance of the MGMT promoter methylation status for prognosis. Future studies are required to analyze the effect of other factors, such as MGMT methylation promoter status.

Conclusions

Ggalectin-1 expression is a poor prognostic factor for patients with GBM treated with adjuvant RT. Studies investigating the targeting of galectin-1 for radioresistance are encouraged in an effort to treat this aggressive brain tumor.

Abbreviations

2DRT: Two-dimensional RT; 3D–CRT: Three-dimensional conformal RT; CSS: Cancer-specific survival; CTV: Clinical target volume; ECOG: Eastern Cooperative Oncology Group; EGFR: Epidermal growth factor receptor; EQD2: Equivalent dose in 2-Gy fractions; FIF: Field-in-field; GBM: Glioblastoma multiforme; GTP: Guanosine triphosphate; GTV: Gross tumor volume; MGMT: O(6)-methylguanine-DNA methyltransferase; OS: Overall survival; PTV: Planning target volume; RT: Radiotherapy; TMA: Tissue microarray; TMZ: Temozolomide; VEGF: Vascular endothelial growth factor

Acknowledgements
Not applicable.

Funding
This work was partially supported by a grant from the Ministry of Science and Technology Research Project (103–2314-B-182A-065-MY2).
The funding body had no role in the design of the study and collection, analysis, and interpretation of data and in writing the manuscript.

Authors' contributions
SYC and EYH analyzed and collected the patient data and were major contributors in writing the manuscript. SLY and CCH performed the microarray examination of the tissue. All authors read and approved the final manuscript.

Competing interests
The authors declare that they have no competing interests.

Author details
[1]Departments of Radiation Oncology, Kaohsiung Chang Gung Memorial Hospital, 123 Ta-Pei Road, Niao-Song Dist, Kaohsiung City 83301, Taiwan. [2]Department of Pathology, Kaohsiung Chang Gung Memorial Hospital, Chang Gung University College of Medicine, Hospital, 123 Ta-Pei Road, Niao-Song Dist, Kaohsiung City 83301, Taiwan. [3]Department of Radiation Oncology, Xiamen Chang Gung Hospital, No. 123, Xiafei Rd., Haicang District, Fujian, China. [4]School of Traditional Chinese Medicine, Chang Gung University College of Medicine, No. 259, Wenhua 1st Rd., Guishan Dist., Taoyuan City, Taiwan. [5]Department of Pathology, An Nan Hospital, China Medical University, No. 66, Sec.2, Changhe Road, Annan Dist, Tainan City 709, Taiwan. [6]Department of Radiation Oncology, Kaohsiung Chang Gung Memorial Hospital, 123 Ta-Pei Road, Niao-Song Dist, Kaohsiung City 83301, Taiwan.

References
1. Stark AM, Nabavi A, Mehdorn HM, Blomer U. Glioblastoma multiforme-report of 267 cases treated at a single institution. Surg Neurol. 2005;63(2):162–9. discussion 169
2. Dobes M, Khurana VG, Shadbolt B, Jain S, Smith SF, Smee R, Dexter M, Cook R. Increasing incidence of glioblastoma multiforme and meningioma, and decreasing incidence of schwannoma (2000-2008): findings of a multicenter Australian study. Surg Neurol Int. 2011;2:176.
3. Lacroix M, Abi-Said D, Fourney DR, Gokaslan ZL, Shi W, DeMonte F, Lang FF, McCutcheon IE, Hassenbusch SJ, Holland E, et al. A multivariate analysis of 416 patients with glioblastoma multiforme: prognosis, extent of resection, and survival. J Neurosurg. 2001;95(2):190–8.
4. Stupp R, Mason WP, Van Den Bent MJ, Weller M, Fisher B, Taphoorn MJ, Belanger K, Brandes AA, Marosi C, Bogdahn U, et al. Radiotherapy plus concomitant and adjuvant temozolomide for glioblastoma. N Engl J Med. 2005;352(10):987–96.
5. Hegi ME, Diserens AC, Gorlia T, Hamou MF, de Tribolet N, Weller M, Kros JM, Hainfellner JA, Mason W, Mariani L, et al. MGMT gene silencing and benefit from temozolomide in glioblastoma. N Engl J Med. 2005;352(10):997–1003.
6. Jung TY, Jung S, Ryu HH, Jeong YI, Jin YH, Jin SG, Kim IY, Kang SS, Kim HS. Role of galectin-1 in migration and invasion of human glioblastoma multiforme cell lines. J Neurosurg. 2008;109(2):273–84.
7. Toussaint LG 3rd, Nilson AE, Goble JM, Ballman KV, James CD, Lefranc F, Kiss R, Uhm JH. Galectin-1, a gene preferentially expressed at the tumor margin, promotes glioblastoma cell invasion. Mol Cancer. 2012;11:32.
8. Thijssen VL, Postel R, Brandwijk RJ, Dings RP, Nesmelova I, Satijn S, Verhofstad N, Nakabeppu Y, Baum LG, Bakkers J, et al. Galectin-1 is essential in tumor angiogenesis and is a target for antiangiogenesis therapy. Proc Natl Acad Sci U S A. 2006;103(43):15975–80.
9. Le Mercier M, Mathieu V, Haibe-Kains B, Bontempi G, Mijatovic T, Decaestecker C, Kiss R, Lefranc F. Knocking down galectin 1 in human hs683 glioblastoma cells impairs both angiogenesis and endoplasmic reticulum stress responses. J Neuropathol Exp Neurol. 2008;67(5):456–69.
10. Verschuere T, Van Woensel M, Fieuws S, Lefranc F, Mathieu V, Kiss R, Van Gool SW, De Vleeschouwer S. Altered galectin-1 serum levels in patients diagnosed with high-grade glioma. J Neuro-Oncol. 2013;115(1):9–17.

11. Huang EY, Chen YF, Chen YM, Lin IH, Wang CC, Su WH, Chuang PC, Yang KD. A novel radioresistant mechanism of galectin-1 mediated by H-Ras-dependent pathways in cervical cancer cells. Cell Death Dis. 2012;3:e251.

12. Huang EY, Chanchien CC, Lin H, Wang CC, Wang CJ, Huang CC. Galectin-1 is an independent prognostic factor for local recurrence and survival after definitive radiation therapy for patients with squamous cell carcinoma of the uterine cervix. Int J Radiat Oncol Biol Phys. 2013;87(5):975–82.

13. Rorive S, Belot N, Decaestecker C, Lefranc F, Gordower L, Micik S, Maurage CA, Kaltner H, Ruchoux MM, Danguy A, et al. Galectin-1 is highly expressed in human gliomas with relevance for modulation of invasion of tumor astrocytes into the brain parenchyma. Glia. 2001;33(3):241–55.

14. Camby I, Belot N, Rorive S, Lefranc F, Maurage CA, Lahm H, Kaltner H, Hadari Y, Ruchoux MM, Brotchi J, et al. Galectins are differentially expressed in supratentorial pilocytic astrocytomas, astrocytomas, anaplastic astrocytomas and glioblastomas, and significantly modulate tumor astrocyte migration. Brain pathology (Zurich, Switzerland). 2001;11(1):12–26.

15. Tribius S, Pidel A, Casper D. ATM protein expression correlates with radioresistance in primary glioblastoma cells in culture. Int J Radiat Oncol Biol Phys. 2001;50(2):511–23.

16. Hirota Y, Masunaga S, Kondo N, Kawabata S, Hirakawa H, Yajima H, Fujimori A, Ono K, Kuroiwa T, Miyatake S. High linear-energy-transfer radiation can overcome radioresistance of glioma stem-like cells to low linear-energy-transfer radiation. J Radiat Res. 2014;55(1):75–83.

17. Bleehen NM, Stenning SP. A Medical Research Council trial of two radiotherapy doses in the treatment of grades 3 and 4 astrocytoma. The Medical Research Council brain tumour working party. Br J Cancer. 1991;64(4):769–74.

18. Curran WJ Jr, Scott CB, Horton J, Nelson JS, Weinstein AS, Fischbach AJ, Chang CH, Rotman M, Asbell SO, Krisch RE, et al. Recursive partitioning analysis of prognostic factors in three radiation therapy oncology group malignant glioma trials. J Natl Cancer Inst. 1993;85(9):704–10.

19. Jeremic B, Shibamoto Y, Grujicic D, Milicic B, Stojanovic M, Nikolic N, Dagovic A, Aleksandrovic J. Short-course radiotherapy in elderly and frail patients with glioblastoma multiforme. A phase II study. J Neuro-Oncol. 1999; 44(1):85–90.

20. Fan QW, Cheng CK, Gustafson WC, Charron E, Zipper P, Wong RA, Chen J, Lau J, Knobbe-Thomsen C, Weller M, et al. EGFR phosphorylates tumor-derived EGFRvIII driving STAT3/5 and progression in glioblastoma. Cancer Cell. 2013;24(4):438–49.

21. Chakravarti A, Seiferheld W, Tu X, Wang H, Zhang HZ, Ang KK, Hammond E, Curran W Jr, Mehta M. Immunohistochemically determined total epidermal growth factor receptor levels not of prognostic value in newly diagnosed glioblastoma multiforme: report from the radiation therapy oncology group. Int J Radiat Oncol Biol Phys. 2005;62(2):318–27.

22. Struve N, Riedel M, Schulte A, Rieckmann T, Grob TJ, Gal A, Rothkamm K, Lamszus K, Petersen C, Dikomey E, et al. EGFRvIII does not affect radiosensitivity with or without gefitinib treatment in glioblastoma cells. Oncotarget. 2015;6(32): 33867–77.

23. Chakravarti A, Wang M, Robins HI, Lautenschlaeger T, Curran WJ, Brachman DG, Schultz CJ, Choucair A, Dolled-Filhart M, Christiansen J, et al. RTOG 0211: a phase 1/2 study of radiation therapy with concurrent gefitinib for newly diagnosed glioblastoma patients. Int J Radiat Oncol Biol Phys. 2013;85(5):1206–11.

24. Feldkamp MM, Lau N, Rak J, Kerbel RS, Guha A. Normoxic and hypoxic regulation of vascular endothelial growth factor (VEGF) by astrocytoma cells is mediated by Ras. Int J Cancer. 1999;81(1):118–24.

25. Chakravarti A, Chakladar A, Delaney MA, Latham DE, Loeffler JS. The epidermal growth factor receptor pathway mediates resistance to sequential administration of radiation and chemotherapy in primary human glioblastoma cells in a RAS-dependent manner. Cancer Res. 2002;62(15):4307–15.

26. Campbell PM, Boufaied N, Fiordalisi JJ, Cox AD, Falardeau P, Der CJ, Gourdeau H. TLN-4601 suppresses growth and induces apoptosis of pancreatic carcinoma cells through inhibition of Ras-ERK MAPK signaling. J Mol Signal. 2010;5:18.

27. Mason WP, Belanger K, Nicholas G, Vallieres I, Mathieu D, Kavan P, Desjardins A, Omuro A, Reymond D. A phase II study of the Ras-MAPK signaling pathway inhibitor TLN-4601 in patients with glioblastoma at first progression. J Neuro-Oncol. 2012;107(2):343–9.

28. Gilbert MR, Dignam JJ, Armstrong TS, Wefel JS, Blumenthal DT, Vogelbaum MA, Colman H, Chakravarti A, Pugh S, Won M, et al. A randomized trial of bevacizumab for newly diagnosed glioblastoma. N Engl J Med. 2014;370(8):699–708.

29. Chinot OL, Wick W, Mason W, Henriksson R, Saran F, Nishikawa R, Carpentier AF, Hoang-Xuan K, Kavan P, Cernea D, et al. bevacizumab plus radiotherapy-temozolomide for newly diagnosed glioblastoma. N Engl J Med. 2014; 370(8):709–22.

30. Lowenstein PR, Baker GJ, Castro MG. Cracking the glioma-NK inhibitory code: toward successful innate immunotherapy. Oncoimmunology. 2014; 3(11):e965573.

31. Baker GJ, Chockley P, Yadav VN, Doherty R, Ritt M, Sivaramakrishnan S, Castro MG, Lowenstein PR. Natural killer cells eradicate galectin-1-deficient glioma in the absence of adaptive immunity. Cancer Res. 2014;74(18):5079–90.

32. Verschuere T, Toelen J, Maes W, Poirier F, Boon L, Tousseyn T, Mathivet T, Gerhardt H, Mathieu V, Kiss R, et al. Glioma-derived galectin-1 regulates innate and adaptive antitumor immunity. Int J Cancer. 2014;134(4):873–84.

33. Le Mercier M, Lefranc F, Mijatovic T, Debeir O, Haibe-Kains B, Bontempi G, Decaestecker C, Kiss R, Mathieu V. Evidence of galectin-1 involvement in glioma chemoresistance. Toxicol Appl Pharmacol. 2008;229(2):172–83.

34. Kramer S. Tumor extent as a determining factor in radiotherapy of glioblastomas. Acta Radiol Ther Phys Biol. 1969;8(1–2):0567–8064. (Print)):111–117

35. Bull JWDRR. The radiographic localization of intracerebral gliomata. J Fac Radiol Lond. 1957;8:147–57.

36. WE. D. Removal of right cerebral hemisphere for certain tumors with hemiplegia. JAMA. 1928;90:823–5.

37. Matsukado Y Fau - Maccarty CS, Maccarty Cs Fau - Kernohan JW, Kernohan JW: The growth of glioblastoma multiforme (astrocytomas, grades 3 and 4) in neurosurgical practice. Neurosurg 1961, 18(0022–3085 (Print)):636–644.

38. Hochberg Fh Fau - Pruitt A, Pruitt A: Assumptions in the radiotherapy of glioblastoma. Neurology 1980, 30(0028–3878 (Print)):907–911.

39. Wallner KE, Galicich Jh Fau - Krol G, Krol G Fau - Arbit E, Arbit E Fau - Malkin MG, Malkin MG: Patterns of failure following treatment for glioblastoma multiforme and anaplastic astrocytoma. International journal of radiation oncology, biology, physics 1989, 16(0360–3016 (Print)):1045–1409.

40. Kelly Pj Fau - Daumas-Duport C, Daumas-Duport C Fau - Scheithauer BW, Scheithauer Bw Fau - Kall BA, Kall Ba Fau - Kispert DB, Kispert DB: Stereotactic histologic correlations of computed tomography- and magnetic resonance imaging-defined abnormalities in patients with glial neoplasms. Mayo Clinic Proc 1987, 62(0025–6196 (Print)):450–459.

41. Strik HM, Schmidt K, Lingor P, Tonges L, Kugler W, Nitsche M, Rabinovich GA, Bahr M. Galectin-1 expression in human glioma cells: modulation by ionizing radiation and effects on tumor cell proliferation and migration. Oncol Rep. 2007;18(2):483–8.

42. Danhier F, Messaoudi K, Lemaire L, Benoit JP, Lagarce F. Combined anti-Galectin-1 and anti-EGFR siRNA-loaded chitosan-lipid nanocapsules decrease temozolomide resistance in glioblastoma: in vivo evaluation. Int J Pharm. 2015; 481(1–2):154–61.

43. Messaoudi K, Clavreul A, Lagarce F. Toward an effective strategy in glioblastoma treatment. Part I: resistance mechanisms and strategies to overcome resistance of glioblastoma to temozolomide. Drug Discov Today. 2015;20(7):899–905.

44. Ikemori RY, Machado CM, Furuzawa KM, Nonogaki S, Osinaga E, Umezawa K, de Carvalho MA, Verinaud L, Chammas R. Galectin-3 up-regulation in hypoxic and nutrient deprived microenvironments promotes cell survival. PLoS One. 2014;9(11):e111592.

45. Paz A, Haklai R, Elad-Sfadia G, Ballan E, Kloog Y. Galectin-1 binds oncogenic H-Ras to mediate Ras membrane anchorage and cell transformation. Oncogene. 2001;20(51):7486–93.

46. Shalom-Feuerstein R, Plowman SJ, Rotblat B, Ariotti N, Tian T, Hancock JF, Kloog Y. K-ras nanoclustering is subverted by overexpression of the scaffold protein galectin-3. Cancer Res. 2008;68(16):6608–16.

47. Bunda S, Burrell K, Heir P, Zeng L, Alamsahebpour A, Kano Y, Raught B, Zhang ZY, Zadeh G, Ohh M. Inhibition of SHP2-mediated dephosphorylation of Ras suppresses oncogenesis. Nat Commun. 2015;6:8859.

48. Kimmelman AC, Qiao RF, Narla G, Banno A, Lau N, Bos PD, Nunez Rodriguez N, Liang BC, Guha A, Martignetti JA, et al. Suppression of glioblastoma tumorigenicity by the Kruppel-like transcription factor KLF6. Oncogene. 2004;23(29):5077–83.

49. Sonoda Y, Ozawa T, Aldape KD, Deen DF, Berger MS, Pieper RO. Akt pathway activation converts anaplastic astrocytoma to glioblastoma multiforme in a human astrocyte model of glioma. Cancer Res. 2001; 61(18):6674–8.

10

Simultaneous analysis of miRNA-mRNA in human meningiomas by integrating transcriptome: A relationship between PTX3 and miR-29c

Altay Burak Dalan[1†], Sukru Gulluoglu[2,3†], Emre Can Tuysuz[2,3], Aysegul Kuskucu[2], Cumhur Kaan Yaltirik[4], Oguz Ozturk[5], Ugur Ture[4] and Omer Faruk Bayrak[2,6*]

Abstract

Background: Although meningioma is a common disease, there is a lack of understanding of the underlying molecular mechanisms behind its initiation and progression. We used combined miRNA-mRNA transcriptome analysis to discover dysregulated genes and networks in meningiomas.

Methods: Fourteen fresh-frozen meningioma samples and one human meningeal cell line were analyzed by using miRNA and whole transcriptome microarray chips. Data was filtered and analyzed. Candidate miRNAs and mRNAs were selected for validation in fifty-eight patient samples. miRNA and target mRNA relationships were assessed by inhibiting miRNA in meningioma cells. Apoptosis and viability assays were also used as functional tests.

Results: With the whole transcriptome microarray, 3753 genes were found to be dysregulated, and 891 miRNAs were found to be dysregulated as a result of miRNA microarray. Results were combined and analyzed with bioinformatics tools. Top differential pathways included those of inflammation, cancer, and cellular growth and survival. The oncosupressor PTX3 was constitutively low in meningioma samples. Moreover, PTX3 negatively correlated with miR-29c in our samples. Inhibiting miR-29c upregulated the PTX3 level, induced apoptosis of meningioma cells, and decreased cell viability. CABIN1, miR-29c, TMOD1, PTX3, RPL22, SPARCL1 and RELA were correlated with clinicopathological features in patient samples.

Conclusions: Our results present the first integrated mRNA-miRNA analysis in meningiomas. miR-29c-3p and PTX3 are inversely correlated in tissues and meningioma cells, hinting that PTX3 can be regulated by miR-29c-3p. Furthermore, we determined potential clinicopathological markers.

Keywords: meningioma, microarray, miRNA, transcriptome, PTX3, miR-29c

Background

Meningiomas account for 30% of primary brain tumors and occur at a rate of 5 per 100,000 individuals [1]. They originate from cap cells of the arachnoidal membrane [2], and the peak age for occurrence is the seventh decade of life [3]. Meningiomas are generally benign but malignant meningiomas have a high tendency to recur. First choice of treatment is surgery, and predictive biomarkers for meningioma progression that could guide oncologists for treatment alternatives are insufficient.

Although meningiomas are common, there is a lack of understanding of underlying molecular mechanisms behind their initiation and progression. To elucidate some of these mechanisms, we used combined miRNA-mRNA transcriptome analysis to discover novel genes and networks in meningiomas. 14 fresh-frozen meningioma samples were used to integrate miRNA and mRNA

---

* Correspondence: ofbayrak@yeditepe.edu.tr
†Equal contributors
²Department of Medical Genetics, Yeditepe University Medical School, Istanbul, Turkey
⁶Yeditepe Universitesi Hastanesi Genetik Tani Merkezi, Koftuncu Sokak Acıbadem mahallesi Istek Vakfı 3. Kat 34718 No: 57/1, Kadikoy, Istanbul, Turkey
Full list of author information is available at the end of the article

microarray analysis. Herein, we describe integrated analysis of gene networks that might play an important role in the initiation and progression of meningiomas, with emphasis on the downregulation of tumor suppressor PTX3 via miR-29c.

Methods

Sample collection

Fifty-eight fresh samples of meningioma tumor tissue (45 WHO grade 1 and 12 WHO grade 2 and 1 WHO grade 3), acquired from surgery, were immediately transported to the cell culture facility for processing as described below. A portion of these fresh-frozen tissues were used for microarray analysis. Clinical information was collected for each sample, including demographic data, tumor location, treatment options, and prognosis.

Cell cultures

For monolayer culture, two fresh meningioma tissue samples (named as MEN-117 and MEN-141) were minced and grown in culture medium (Dulbecco's Modified Eagle Medium, Gibco) with 10% fetal bovine serum and 1% antibiotics (streptomycin and penicillin) and incubated at 37 °C in a humidified atmosphere (5% CO_2). To prevent loss of character, miRNA transfections of primary cell cultures were done at passage 2. Human meningeal cells (Cat. #1400, ScienCell Laboratories, Carlsbad, California) were cultured according to the provider's protocol and used as the healthy control.

Microarray analysis

Tumor tissues were ground with liquid nitrogen, and TRIzol (ThermoFisher Scientific) was added according to the manufacturer's protocol for total RNA isolation. Whole transcriptome expression profiling was done using Affymetrix Human Gene 2.1 ST Array Strip (Cat no: 902,114, Affymetrix, Santa Clara, CA), which contains over 47,000 transcripts. miRNA microarray analysis was done with the Affymetrix miRNA 4.1 Array Strip (Cat no: 902,404). The chips were used in the GeneAtlas system and the resulting data was analyzed with Transcriptome Analysis Console (TAC) 3 software (Affymetrix).

miRNA and mRNA expression levels

The expression levels of selected miRNAs in patient samples, meningeal cells, and primary cells grown as a monolayer after anti-miRNA transfection were evaluated with real-time polymerase chain reaction (PCR) using miRNA primers obtained from Exiqon (Vedbæk, Denmark). First, cDNA was synthesized from all miRNA samples according to the manufacturer's protocol (Exiqon, Cat. No.: 203,300). Synthesized cDNAs were used as templates for gene-expression analysis through real-time PCR, while mRNA levels were measured using

Taqman primers (ThermoFisher) after cDNA synthesis. Data was analyzed with the $2^{-\Delta\Delta Ct}$ method. For miRNA normalization, 5S RNA was used. For mRNA normalization, GAPDH was used.

Optimiziation of anti-miRNA transfection

Cy3 Dye-Labeled Pre-miR Negative Control #1 (Cat: AM17011, ThermoFisher) was used to evaluate the ability of X-tremeGENE siRNA Transfection Reagent (Roche, Cat. No.: 04476093001) to transfect primary meningioma cells under the fluorescent microscope. After validation, anti-miRNA mimics (Ambion Pre-miR miRNA Precursors PM: 114,065) were transfected into cells. To determine the intracellular functionality of anti-miRs, total RNA isolation and miRNA reverse transcription was done and followed by real-time PCR. The targeted miRNA levels were measured 48 h after transfection. The control groups were the X-tremeGENE group, in which only the transfection reagent and medium were delivered to cells, the scrambled miRNA group (Ambion anti-miR miRNA mimics), and the negative control group, which contained only medium.

Annexin V staining and viability assay

To elucidate the apoptotic effects of hsa-miR-29c-3p and its target PTX3 on primary meningioma cells, annexin V and 7-AAD staining was performed by using apoptosis detection kit I (BD Pharmingen, San Diego, California) 72 h after transfection of anti-miR-29c-3p. Staining was carried out according to the manufacturer's protocol by using BD FACSAria III cell sorter (BD Biosciences).

Cell viability after anti-miR-29c transfection was assessed at day 3 and day 4 with CellTiter 96 Aqueous One Solution Cell Proliferation Assay (MTS) (Promega, Madison, Wisconsin) according to the manufacturer's protocol. Scrambled anti-miR was used as a control. Results were obtained by detecting absorbance at a wavelength of 490 nm with the Elisa microplate reader (BioTek, Winooski, Vermont).

Statistical analysis

The one-way between-subjects ANOVA (unpaired) method was used to evaluate the microarray results. Real-time PCR data was analyzed by using the $2^{-\Delta\Delta Ct}$ method. Spearman's two-tailed correlation test was used to determine correlations of tumor size and mRNA-miRNA levels, and miRNA and mRNA target levels. For other clinicopathological correlations, the two-tailed chi-square test was used. The calculation and interpretation of p values for functions and gene networks (Table 1) was done with a right-tailed Fisher's exact test. All other statistical analyses were done using student's t-test. Differences with p values of less than 0.05 were considered

Table 1 Number and significance range of molecules participating in relevant pathways and molecular and cellular functions in meningioma. Table derived from data compiled from DAVID bioinformatics database. P values were calculated with a right-tailed Fisher's exact test

Gene Network	p-value	Number of Molecules Involved
Inflammatory Response	1.35E-03 – 8.27E-14	182
Cancer	1.28E-03 – 3.20E-11	493
Inflammatory Disease	1.35E-03 – 2.98E-10	161
Cellular Growth	1.23E-03 – 5.70E-18	311
Cell Death-Cell Survival	1.30E-03 – 7.59E-16	265
Cellular Movement	1.34E-03 – 6.11E-15	194
Cellular Development	1.04E-03 – 2.68E-13	257
Cell-Cell Signalling	1.34E-03 – 6.69E-10	157
Immune Cell Traficking	1.06E-03 – 1.95E-09	110

Table 2 Selected mRNAs and miRNAs as a result of microarray analysis. Fold change, the matching miRNA for targeting, fold value of miRNA, and information about targeting has already been validated or predicted with software

mRNA	Fold	Targeting miRNA	miRNA Fold	Targeting Status
PTX3	-337.5	hsa-miR-29c-3p	21.76	Predicted
RPL22	-109.5	hsa-miR-29c-3p	21.76	Validated
CABIN1	-8.76	hsa-miR-4492	53.89	Predicted
RELA	-7.42	hsa-miR-8089	22.13	Predicted
SPARCL1	71.88	N/A		
TMOD1	81.71	N/A		

discussed in this publication have been deposited in NCBI's Gene Expression Omnibus [4] and are accessible through GEO Series accession number GSE88721 (https://www.ncbi.nlm.nih.gov/geo/query/acc.cgi?acc=GSE88721).

statistically significant. The high and low miRNA or gene groups of patients were separated according to the median expression level value. Significant outliers were evaluated for each experiment and removed from analysis.

Results

Differential expression of miRNAs and mRNAs in meningioma

Fourteen meningioma samples and one healthy human meningeal cell line were used to profile miRNA and gene expression (Additional file 1: Table S1). Of 48,226 genes that were checked for expression, 1257 genes were found to be upregulated and 2496 were found to be downregulated as a result of whole transcriptome microarray (Additional file 2: Figure S1). As a result of miRNA microarray, of 6631 miRNAs checked, 580 genes were found to be upregulated and 311 were found to be downregulated (Additional file 3: Figure S2). The results from both microarrays were combined and analyzed by using TAC (Affymetrix), DAVID, KEGG and Reactome software. To increase confidence, fold change (linear) of less than −4 or fold change (linear) greater than 4 and the ANOVA p value (condition pair) less than 0.01 were chosen as selection criteria in both arrays. Deregulated miRNAs and mRNAs were analyzed for their collective effect on important molecular and cellular events (Table 1).

Candidate mRNAs and miRNAs were chosen according to pathways and networks relevant to meningioma, as well as well-matched expression levels of miRNAs and their potential mRNA targets, with the help of web-based databases (mirdb.org/miRDB/, mirtarbase.mbc.nctu.edu.tw, http://targetscan.org/, pictar.mdc-berlin.de, http://www.microrna.org/). The predicted targets were chosen to balance prediction match scores and the relevancy and novelty of the genes in meningioma research (Table 2). The data

Confirmation of microarray data with real-time PCR in patient samples

The levels of selected mRNAs and miRNAs in fifty-eight patient samples, were checked. Among the miRNAs, hsa-miR-8089 could not be detected in any of the samples potentially due to a problem in primer design. Although the microarray result suggested that miR-4492-3p levels are higher in meningioma samples than in the healthy control, we have observed the opposite with real-time PCR (Fig. 1). The level of miR-29c-3p in patient samples and healthy controls was consistent with the microarray (Fig. 1).

RPL22, CABIN1, and RELA levels were not significantly different from the controls (Fig. 1) whereas PTX3, SPARCL1, and TMOD1 levels were in synchrony with the microarray results. These are significant as PTX3 was downregulated and SPARCL1 and TMOD1 were upregulated in patient samples compared with controls.

Anti-miR mimics successfully transfected into cell lines

We assessed the transfection capability of the X-tremeGENE siRNA Transfection Reagent, and the ability of the anti-miR mimics to suppress their target miRNAs in two primary patient-derived meningioma cells. We used Cy3 Labeled Pre-miR Negative Control #1 (ThermoFisher, AM17011) to visualize the presence of anti-miRNA mimic molecules inside the cell 8 h after transfection. Fluorescence microscopy showed that the Cy3-labeled miRNA constructs were successfully transfected into cells (Fig. 2a,b). No fluorescence was detected in the control groups (Fig. 2c,d). Anti-miR mimics were transfected into patient-derived cell lines, and real-time PCR after 48 h revealed that the corresponding anti-miR mimics significantly decreased the level of hsa-miR-29c-3p and hsa-miR-4492-3p (Fig. 2e,f). Levels of hsa-miR-8089 could not be detected.

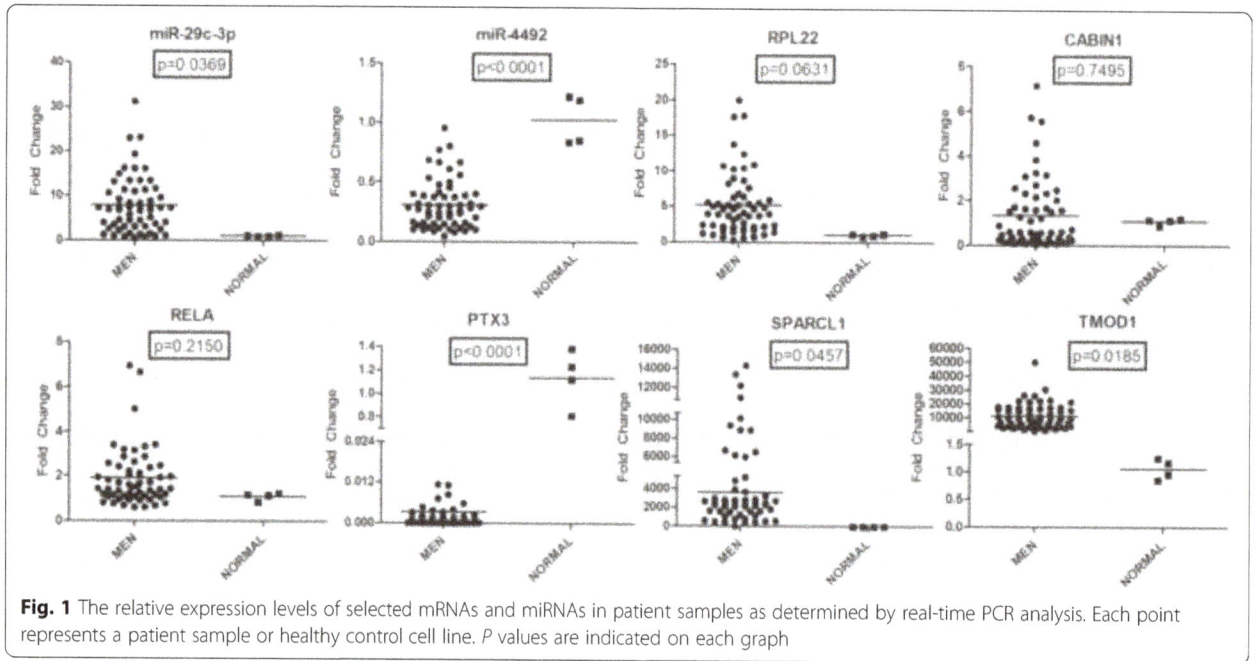

Fig. 1 The relative expression levels of selected mRNAs and miRNAs in patient samples as determined by real-time PCR analysis. Each point represents a patient sample or healthy control cell line. *P* values are indicated on each graph

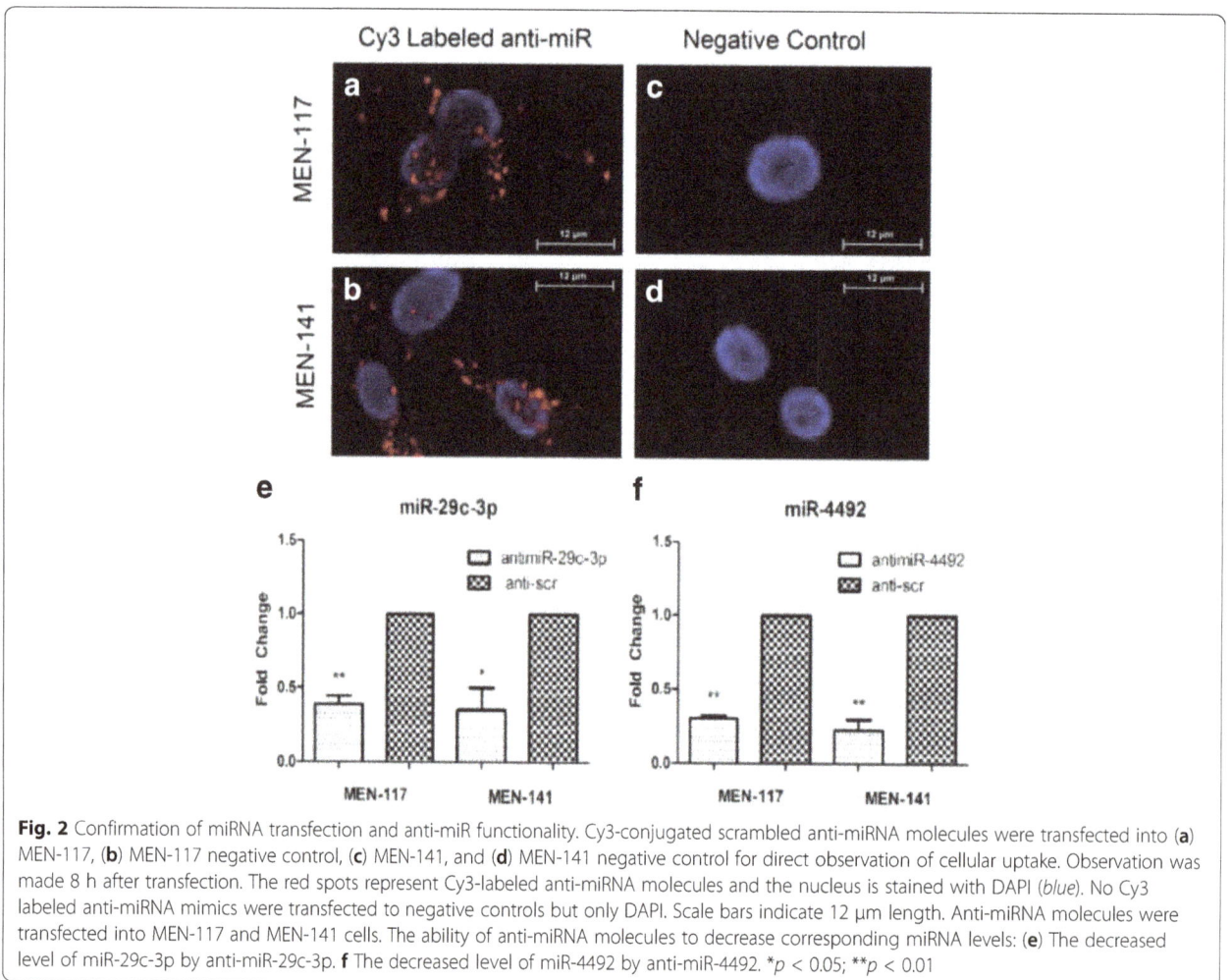

Fig. 2 Confirmation of miRNA transfection and anti-miR functionality. Cy3-conjugated scrambled anti-miRNA molecules were transfected into (**a**) MEN-117, (**b**) MEN-117 negative control, (**c**) MEN-141, and (**d**) MEN-141 negative control for direct observation of cellular uptake. Observation was made 8 h after transfection. The red spots represent Cy3-labeled anti-miRNA molecules and the nucleus is stained with DAPI (*blue*). No Cy3 labeled anti-miRNA mimics were transfected to negative controls but only DAPI. Scale bars indicate 12 μm length. Anti-miRNA molecules were transfected into MEN-117 and MEN-141 cells. The ability of anti-miRNA molecules to decrease corresponding miRNA levels: (**e**) The decreased level of miR-29c-3p by anti-miR-29c-3p. **f** The decreased level of miR-4492 by anti-miR-4492. *$p < 0.05$; **$p < 0.01$

Transfection of anti-hsa-miR-29c-3p increased oncosuppressor PTX3

The expression level of validated target RPL22 and predicted target PTX3 was checked 48 h after anti-miR-29c-3p transfection. We did not observe a significant effect on the RPL22 level compared to the control (Fig. 3a). The PTX3 gene expression level increased significantly in primary cell lines MEN-117 and MEN-141, suggesting a regulation of the gene by miR-29c-3p in meningiomas (Fig. 3b). The expression level of the predicted target of hsa-miR-4492, CABIN1, increased both in MEN-141 and MEN-117 cells (Fig. 3c). Although results for miR-8089 expression level confirmation with real-time PCR could not be obtained we decided to carry on with experiments that are not related to measuring the expression level of the miRNA. The level of RELA consistently increased in both MEN-117 and MEN-141 upon transfection with anti-miR-8089 (Fig. 3d).

Downregulation of hsa-miR-29c-3p decreased cell viability and induced apoptosis in meningioma Cells

To observe the viability and percentage of apoptotic cells, anti-miR molecules against miR-29c-3p were transfected into two meningioma primary culture cells, MEN-117 and MEN-141. MTS cell viability analysis resulted in the decrease of viability of anti-miR-29c transfected cells as compared to controls at day 3. This effect was neutralized at day 4 (Fig. 4a,b).

For flow cytometry analysis, the population for apoptotic cells was chosen as the annexin V-positive and 7AAD- negative cells to eliminate any confusion of late apoptotic and necrotic cells, which are positive for annexin V and 7AAD. The results showed that the anti-miR-29c-3p molecules significantly increased apoptosis after 72 h by 10% in MEN-117 and by 28% in MEN-141 when compared with the anti-scr control (Fig. 4c,d).

Correlation between the level of dysregulated miRNAs and mRNAs with clinicopathological features of meningioma patients

We evaluated the relationships between miR-29c-3p, miR-4492, PTX3, RPL22, CABIN1, RELA, SPARCL1, and TMOD1 levels and the clinicopathological features of meningioma patients including sex, age, tumor grade, tumor volume, calcification, progesterone receptor status, and p53 and Ki67 levels, as well as the correlation between the level of miRNAs and their targets. miR-8089 was excluded since its level of expression could not be determined by real-time PCR. For the chi-square tests, patients were separated into two groups of low and high levels of the corresponding miRNA or mRNA level.

Among the clinical characteristics evaluated, miR-29c-3p was negatively correlated with Ki67 index. PTX3, RPL22, CABIN1 and SPARCL1 expression was negatively correlated with progesterone receptor. RELA and TMOD1 were negatively correlated with calcification (Table 3). PTX3 and RELA were negatively correlated with tumor volume in our cohort (Fig. 5).

Discussion

Since the genomic revolution began, our knowledge about cancers has rapidly improved, leading to the discovery of molecular markers that predict outcomes and

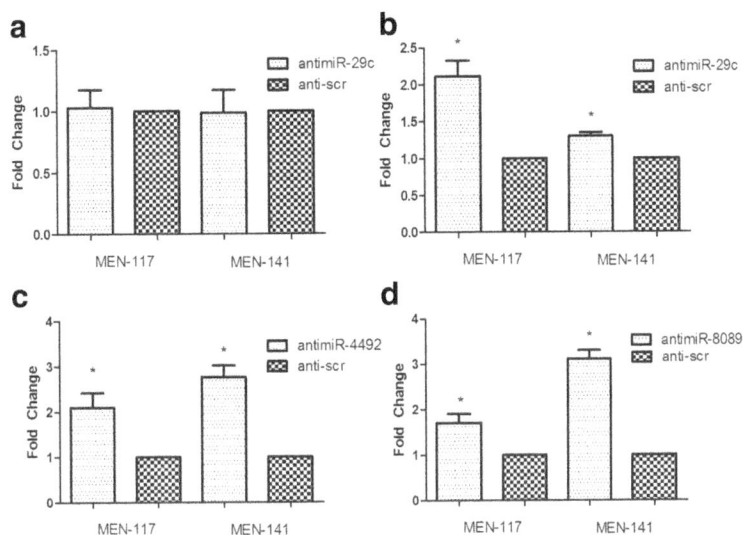

Fig. 3 Target mRNA expression levels after administration of corresponding anti-miRNA molecules. Anti-miRNA molecules of miRNAs, miR-29c-3p, miR-4492, and miR-8089, were administered to MEN-117 and MEN-141, and corresponding target mRNA levels were determined after 48 h. **a** RPL22 as the target of miR-29c-3p. **b** PTX3 as the target of miR-29c-3p. **c** CABIN1 as the target of miR-4492. **d** RELA as the target of miR-8089. *Significant changes ($p < 0.05$)

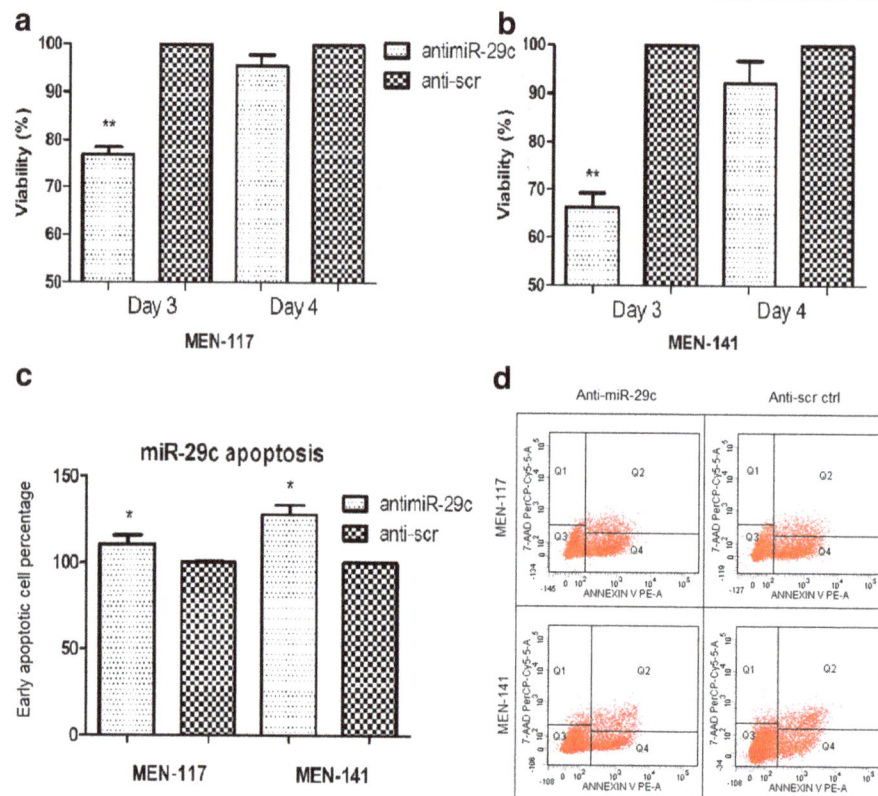

Fig. 4 miR-29c-3p has an anti-proliferative and apoptotic effect on meningioma cells. Anti-scr transfected cells were used as the control groups (**a, b**), and viability was measured with an MTS assay after transfection of miR-29c-3p into meningeal cells for 72 and 96 h. **c** Early apoptosis (annexin V + 7-AAD) rate after transfection of miR-29c-3p into meningeal cells for 72 h. **d** Representative images of Annexin-V/7-AAD staining of meningeal cells after miR-29c-3p transfection for 72 h

help define the best choice for treatment. In the near future, molecular classification and, consequently, personalized therapy is the ultimate goal of treatment for any tumor. Studies using microarray analysis can reveal gene networks that relate to treatment response, clinical outcome, and clinical progression.

Fifteen different subtypes of meningioma have been identified by the World Health Organization (WHO). These subtypes are further classified into three categories: benign (80%), atypical (15%–20%), and malignant (1%–3%) [5]. An atypical meningioma is diagnosed by observing necrosis, sheeting, prominent nucleoli, cellularity, and cell size along with the recent criterion of brain invasion [6].

MicroRNAs (miRNAs) are small, non-coding RNA molecules that are about 22 nucleotides long. There is growing interest in miRNAs with respect to their role in the initiation and progression of cancer, but studies of the miRNA profile of meningiomas are limited in number. In one study, 60 sporadic meningiomas and three healthy arachnoidal tissue samples were used in a whole genome array to find that miR-200a down regulation was associated with tumor growth, epithelial-to-

mesenchymal transition status, and Wnt signaling [7]. miR-145, which decreased proliferation and induced apoptosis in vitro and in vivo, was downregulated in atypical and anaplastic meningiomas when compared with benign meningiomas and this molecule [8].

Previous studies using microarrays led to the discovery of important dysregulated mRNA molecules and altered pathways, such as IGF2, Wnt, PI3K, MAPK, MMP12, and TGF-β [9–12]. But few studies of the miRNA profiling of meningiomas have been conducted. A number of miRNAs have been found to be dysregulated. These include miR-145, let-7d, miR-335, miR-98, miR-181a, miR-200a, miR-373*, miR-575, miR-335, miR-96-5p, miR-190a, miR-29c-3p, and miR-219-5p [7, 8, 13, 14]. But only two of these studies incorporated microarray data. In addition, no common miRNA has been identified in any two of these studies, reflecting the lack of well-designed studies in this field of research.

Our microarray data defined three miRNAs that can play a role in gene networks and that are potentially important for meningioma initiation and progression. To the best of our knowledge, there is no previous integrated miRNA-mRNA study of meningiomas that uses

Table 3 Correlation between the expression level of selected miRNAs and mRNAs with clinicopathological features. Selected miRNAs and mRNAs were analyzed with Spearman's non-parametric correlation test and the chi-square test for age, sex, WHO grade, calcification, progesterone receptor status, p53 status, and Ki67 index. Significant results are shown here

Molecule Name	Clinicopathological Features	High	Low	Total	p-Value
miR-29c-3p	Ki67 index				
	>7	12	19	31	0.0471
	≤7	17	10	27	
PTX3	Progesterone Receptor				
	Positive	16	25	41	0.0002
	Negative/Focal Positive/Nuclear Positive	11	0	11	
RPL22	Progesterone Receptor				
	Positive	19	22	41	0.0361
	Negative/Focal Positive/Nuclear Positive	9	2	11	
CABIN1	Progesterone Receptor				
	Positive	14	27	41	0.0004
	Negative/Focal Positive/Nuclear Positive	10	1	11	
SPARCL1	Progesterone Receptor				
	Positive	16	25	41	0.0022
	Negative/Focal Positive/Nuclear Positive	10	1	11	
RELA	Calcification				
	Positive	17	25	42	0.0447
	Negative	10	4	14	
TMOD1	Calcification				
	Positive	17	25	42	0.0447
	Negative	10	4	14	

microarray data. In addition, ours is the first study in which a miRNA and mRNA expression profiles have been observed in the same samples. Combining the data from the two most up-to-date arrays provided us with valuable information on potential gene networks in the disease about inflammatory responses, cancer, cellular growth and survival, cellular movement and development, cell-to-cell signaling and immune cell trafficking. A limitation to our study is the usage of one healthy human cell line due to unavailability of more commercial cell lines and ethical difficulty in acquiring healthy meningeal tissue from patients du to ethical responsibilities. In further studies the number of healthy controls should be increased and should not be limited to only cell lines but also healthy meningeal tissue.

In this study, we found that miR-29c-3p is upregulated in meningiomas, whereas its predicted target PTX3 is downregulated. Inhibiting miR-29c-3p has increased the expression level of PTX3 in primary meningioma cells, indicating a potential targeting of PTX3 by miR-29c.

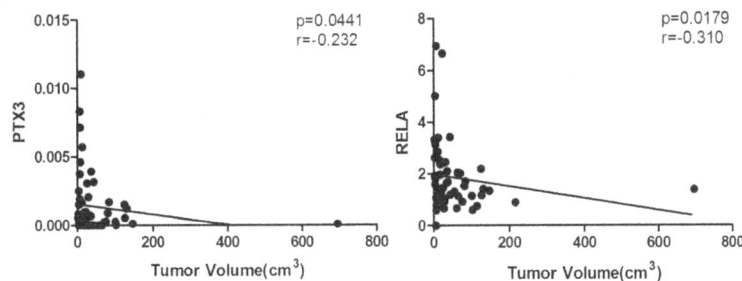

Fig. 5 Correlation between the expression level of selected PTX3 and RELA with tumor volume. Selected miRNAs and mRNAs were analyzed with Spearman's non-parametric correlation test for tumor volume. Significant results are shown here. PTX3 and RELA expressions are indicative of lower tumor volume in the meningioma cohort

miR-29c-3p was found to be downregulated when compared with adjacent tissue in meningioma. In the same study, lower miR-29c was associated with advanced clinical stages of meningioma which is in synchrony with our finding that lower miR-29c is associated with a higher ki67 index [14]. The miR-29 family members miR-29a, miR-29b, and miR-29c have diverse roles in cancer [15] by inhibiting tumorigenesis [16], promoting cancer cell apoptosis [17], and suppressing cell proliferation [18]. On the other hand, the miR-29 family can induce an epithelial-to-mesenchymal transition acting as drivers of tumor growth and metastasis [19]. In our study, the downregulation of miR-29c decreased cell viability and increased apoptosis.

PTX3 plays a role in inflammation, both endogenously and exogenously, with dual effects on the process [20, 21]. PTX3 is considered a tumor suppressor gene that plays a role in tumor-promoting inflammation in cancer [22]. Our data show that the tumor suppressor PTX3 is constitutively downregulated in meningiomas. PTX3 level was negatively correlated with tumor volume and progesterone receptor level in our cohort which supports the argument that the gene can act as a tumor suppressor for meningioma. Progesterone level relates to the WHO grade and Ki67 status of meningiomas, as previously reported [23]. Furthermore, our microarray data show the altered expression of hundreds of molecules that take part in inflammatory pathways. These findings suggest that the emerging cancer hallmark of tumor-promoting inflammation is potentially a driving force in the initiation and progression of meningiomas with PTX3 potentially taking part in the process.

We also assessed relationship between the selected miRNAs and mRNAs and clinicopathological features. High TMOD1 and RELA levels were associated with low calcification in our patient group. Calcification is considered predictive of outcome in meningioma patients. The level of calcification in tumors seen on magnetic resonance images is used to determine the treatment strategy for the tumor. Calcification in meningiomas is associated with a low growth rate, suggesting a conservative treatment option [24]. RELA level is also associated with a lower tumor volume in our cohort. RPL22, CABIN1 and SPARCL1 levels were also negatively correlated with the progesterone receptor level, a relation similar to that of PTX3.

The level of miR-4492 was found to be upregulated in our microarray data. However real-time PCR confirmation tests revealed that this miRNAs was significantly downregulated not only in the group that microarray analysis was conducted but also in our extended cohort. This is probably due to an error in the microarray design for the particular miRNA which is relatively recently discovered. This result shows that microarray assessments may not always be indicative of the level of expression and confirmation with real-time PCR is crucial to detect the expression level.

Conclusions

Our study presents valuable integrated data about mRNA and miRNA expression in meningioma samples. Markers that can play a role in meningioma pathophysiology and tumor-promoting inflammation have been determined, and the results reveal that the relationship between miR-29c-3p and PTX3 can be one of the driving forces in meningioma pathology. Further studies of these gene networks can produce translational information, leading to a better understanding of the initiation and progression of meningiomas and perhaps introducing alternative treatment approaches for the disease.

Abbreviations

WHO: World health organization; miRNA: micro RNA; PCR: Polymerase Chain Reaction; ANOVA: Analysis of variance

Acknowledgements

We would like to thank Julie Yamamoto for her editorial assistance.

Funding

This study was supported by Yeditepe University, Istanbul.

Authors' contributions

BD and SG carried out microarrays. Cell culturing and flow cytometry was done by ECT. Tumor samples and patient data were acquired by CKY and UT. SG, BD and OFB performed the statistical analysis. BD, SG, AK and OO were involved in writing and editing the manuscript. BD and OFB and designed the study and provided financial support for this work. All authors read and approved the final manuscript.

Competing interests

The authors declare that they have no competing interests.

Author details

[1]Department of Biochemistry, Yeditepe University Medical School, Istanbul, Turkey. [2]Department of Medical Genetics, Yeditepe University Medical School, Istanbul, Turkey. [3]Department of Biotechnology, Institute of Science, Yeditepe University, Istanbul, Turkey. [4]Department of Neurosurgery, Yeditepe University Medical School, Istanbul, Turkey. [5]Department of Molecular Medicine, Capa School of Medicine, Istanbul University, Istanbul, Turkey. [6]Yeditepe Universitesi Hastanesi Genetik Tani Merkezi, Koftuncu Sokak Acıbadem mahallesi Istek Vakfi 3. Kat 34718 No: 57/1, Kadikoy, Istanbul, Turkey.

References

1. Shibuya M. Pathology and Molecular Genetics of Meningioma: Recent Advances. Neurol Med Chir (Tokyo). 2015;55(Suppl 1):14–27.

2. Kalamarides M, Stemmer-Rachamimov AO, Niwa-Kawakita M, Chareyre F, Taranchon E, Han ZY, Martinelli C, Lusis EA, Hegedus B, Gutmann DH, et al. Identification of a progenitor cell of origin capable of generating diverse meningioma histological subtypes. Oncogene. 2011;30(20):2333–44.

3. Riemenschneider MJ, Perry A, Reifenberger G. Histological classification and molecular genetics of meningiomas. Lancet Neurol. 2006;5(12):1045–54.

4. Edgar R, Domrachev M, Lash AE. Gene Expression Omnibus: NCBI gene expression and hybridization array data repository. Nucleic Acids Res. 2002; 30(1):207–10.

5. Bi WL, Abedalthagafi M, Horowitz P, Agarwalla PK, Mei Y, Aizer AA, Brewster R, Dunn GP, Al-Mefty O, Alexander BM, et al. Genomic landscape of intracranial meningiomas. J Neurosurg. 2016;125(3):525–35.

6. Louis DN, Perry A, Reifenberger G, von Deimling A, Figarella-Branger D, Cavenee WK, Ohgaki H, Wiestler OD, Kleihues P, Ellison DW. The 2016 World Health Organization Classification of Tumors of the Central Nervous System: a summary. Acta Neuropathol. 2016;131(6):803–20.

7. Saydam O, Shen Y, Wurdinger T, Senol O, Boke E, James MF, Tannous BA, Stemmer-Rachamimov AO, Yi M, Stephens RM, et al. Downregulated microRNA-200a in meningiomas promotes tumor growth by reducing E-cadherin and activating the Wnt/beta-catenin signaling pathway. Mol Cell Biol. 2009;29(21):5923–40.

8. Kliese N, Gobrecht P, Pachow D, Andrae N, Wilisch-Neumann A, Kirches E, Riek-Burchardt M, Angenstein F, Reifenberger G, Riemenschneider MJ, et al. miRNA-145 is downregulated in atypical and anaplastic meningiomas and negatively regulates motility and proliferation of meningioma cells. Oncogene. 2013;32(39):4712–20.

9. Watson MA, Gutmann DH, Peterson K, Chicoine MR, Kleinschmidt-DeMasters BK, Brown HG, Perry A. Molecular characterization of human meningiomas by gene expression profiling using high-density oligonucleotide microarrays. Am J Pathol. 2002;161(2):665–72.

10. Sasaki T, Hankins GR, Helm GA. Comparison of gene expression profiles between frozen original meningiomas and primary cultures of the meningiomas by GeneChip. Neurosurgery. 2003;52(4):892–8. discussion 898-899

11. Wrobel G, Roerig P, Kokocinski F, Neben K, Hahn M, Reifenberger G, Lichter P. Microarray-based gene expression profiling of benign, atypical and anaplastic meningiomas identifies novel genes associated with meningioma progression. Int J Cancer. 2005;114(2):249–56.

12. Carvalho LH, Smirnov I, Baia GS, Modrusan Z, Smith JS, Jun P, Costello JF, McDermott MW, Vandenberg SR, Lal A. Molecular signatures define two main classes of meningiomas. Mol Cancer. 2007;6:64.

13. Kim Y, Kim H, Park D, Jeoung D. miR-335 Targets SIAH2 and Confers Sensitivity to Anti-Cancer Drugs by Increasing the Expression of HDAC3. Mol Cells. 2015;38(6):562–72.

14. Zhi F, Zhou G, Wang S, Shi Y, Peng Y, Shao N, Guan W, Qu H, Zhang Y, Wang Q, et al. A microRNA expression signature predicts meningioma recurrence. Int J Cancer. 2013;132(1):128–36.

15. Jiang H, Zhang G, Wu JH, Jiang CP. Diverse roles of miR-29 in cancer (review). Oncol Rep. 2014;31(4):1509–16.

16. Fabbri M, Garzon R, Cimmino A, Liu Z, Zanesi N, Callegari E, Liu S, Alder H, Costinean S, Fernandez-Cymering C, et al. MicroRNA-29 family reverts aberrant methylation in lung cancer by targeting DNA methyltransferases 3A and 3B. Proc Natl Acad Sci U S A. 2007;104(40):15805–10.

17. Bargaje R, Gupta S, Sarkeshik A, Park R, Xu T, Sarkar M, Halimani M, Roy SS, Yates J, Pillai B. Identification of novel targets for miR-29a using miRNA proteomics. PLoS One. 2012;7(8):e43243.

18. Matsuo M, Nakada C, Tsukamoto Y, Noguchi T, Uchida T, Hijiya N, Matsuura K, Moriyama M. MiR-29c is downregulated in gastric carcinomas and regulates cell proliferation by targeting RCC2. Mol Cancer. 2013;12:15.

19. Gebeshuber CA, Zatloukal K. Martinez J: miR-29a suppresses tristetraprolin, which is a regulator of epithelial polarity and metastasis. EMBO Rep. 2009; 10(4):400–5.

20. Daigo K, Mantovani A, Bottazzi B. The yin-yang of long pentraxin PTX3 in inflammation and immunity. Immunol Lett. 2014;161(1):38–43.

21. Kunes P, Holubcova Z, Kolackova M, Krejsek J. Pentraxin 3(PTX 3): an endogenous modulator of the inflammatory response. Mediat Inflamm. 2012;2012:920517.

22. Bonavita E, Gentile S, Rubino M, Maina V, Papait R, Kunderfranco P, Greco C, Feruglio F, Molgora M, Laface I, et al. PTX3 is an extrinsic oncosuppressor regulating complement-dependent inflammation in cancer. Cell. 2015; 160(4):700–14.

23. Roser F, Nakamura M, Bellinzona M, Rosahl SK, Ostertag H, Samii M. The prognostic value of progesterone receptor status in meningiomas. J Clin Pathol. 2004;57(10):1033–7.

24. Rubin G, Herscovici Z, Laviv Y, Jackson S, Rappaport ZH. Outcome of untreated meningiomas. Isr Med Assoc J. 2011;13(3):157–60.

11

Curcumin decreases malignant characteristics of glioblastoma stem cells via induction of reactive oxygen species

Zachary C. Gersey[1], Gregor A. Rodriguez[1], Eric Barbarite[1], Anthony Sanchez[1], Winston M. Walters[1], Kelechi C. Ohaeto[1], Ricardo J. Komotar[1] and Regina M. Graham[1,2*]

Abstract

Background: Glioblastoma Multiforme (GBM) is the most common and lethal form of primary brain tumor in adults. Following standard treatment of surgery, radiation and chemotherapy, patients are expected to survive 12–14 months. Theorized cause of disease recurrence in these patients is tumor cell repopulation through the proliferation of treatment-resistant cancer stem cells. Current research has revealed curcumin, the principal ingredient in turmeric, can modulate multiple signaling pathways important for cancer stem cell self-renewal and survival.

Methods: Following resection, tumor specimens were dissociated and glioblastoma stem cells (GSCs) were propagated in neurosphere media and characterized via immunocytochemistry. Cell viability was determined with MTS assay. GSC proliferation, sphere forming and colony forming assays were conducted through standard counting methods. Reactive oxygen species (ROS) production was examined using the fluorescent molecular probe CM-H2DCFA. Effects on cell signaling pathways were elucidated by western blot.

Results: We evaluate the effects of curcumin on patient-derived GSC lines. We demonstrate a curcumin-induced dose-dependent decrease in GSC viability with an approximate IC_{50} of 25 μM. Treatment with sub-toxic levels (2.5 μM) of curcumin significantly decreased GSC proliferation, sphere forming ability and colony forming potential. Curcumin induced ROS, promoted MAPK pathway activation, downregulated STAT3 activity and IAP family members. Inhibition of ROS with the antioxidant N-acetylcysteine reversed these effects indicating a ROS dependent mechanism.

Conclusions: Discoveries made in this investigation may lead to a non-toxic intervention designed to prevent recurrence in glioblastoma by targeting glioblastoma stem cells.

Keywords: Glioblastoma, Stem cell, STAT3, Curcumin, Reactive oxygen species, Brain tumor, Natural product

Background

Glioblastoma multiforme (GBM) is the most common and deadly primary malignant brain tumor. GBM comprises about 15% of all intracranial tumors in adults ages 40–75 [1]. The tumor is exceptionally aggressive, with a mean survival of less than 15 months and a 5-year survival rate of 9.8% after standard therapy of resection, radiation and temozolomide chemotherapy [2, 3]. Despite numerous efforts, there has been stagnation in the advancement in treatment of this disease. The lack of improvement in survival rates of glioblastoma has led to the identification of novel therapeutic mechanisms such as targeting cancer stem cells (CSCs), also known as tumor initiating cells or cancer stem-like cells, in order to eradicate this lethal disease.

CSCs are small subset of cells within tumors that have stem-cell-like characteristics that allow them to sustain and repopulate the cancer [4]. The unique qualities of CSCs allow them to evade the chemotherapy and radiation that destroys the bulk of the tumor, eventually leading to the recurrence of disease. This idea has led researchers in search for targeted therapies that will eliminate CSCs and therefore prevent the relapse of cancer

* Correspondence: rgraham@med.miami.edu
[1]Department of Neurosurgery, University of Miami Miller School of Medicine, Miami, Florida, USA
[2]Department of Neurological Surgery, University of Miami Brain Tumor Initiative (UMBTI) Research Laboratory, Lois Pope LIFE Center, 2nd Floor, 1095 NW 14th Terrace, Miami, Florida 33136, USA

[4]. A compound that has shown promising anti-CSC properties is the natural phenol curcumin.

Curcumin is the principal curcuminoid in the Indian plant turmeric that has been used for thousands of years in Asian medicine to treat inflammatory conditions. Curcumin has also been shown to have antineoplastic properties including inhibition of proliferation, inducing apoptosis, inhibiting invasion and metastasis and decreasing angiogenesis in multiple tumors including glioblastoma [5–8]. Specifically, curcumin targets CSCs in vitro and in vivo in several cancers, including breast, colorectal, esophageal and glioma [9–13]. It is proposed that these effects are made through curcumin's ability to induce reactive oxygen species [14–20].

Reactive oxygen species (ROS) are natural products formed by the metabolism of oxygen whose regulation plays an essential role in normal cell signaling and homeostasis [21]. The dysregulation of ROS has been implicated in many diseases such as dementia, cardiovascular disease, as well as cancer [22–24]. Current research also suggests that ROS have anti-neoplastic effects on CSCs and that these effects are brought about through the modulation of several molecular pathways including Mitogen-activated protein kinases (MAPKs) and Janus kinas (JAK)- Signal Transducer and Activator of Transcription (STAT3) signaling cascades [25–32]. Aberrations of the MAPKs and JAK-STAT3 pathways have been shown to be critical in the tumorgenesis and maintenance of GBM [33–37].

In this study, we assess the effects of curcumin on glioblastoma stem cells (GSCs) and propose the molecular mechanisms behind such effects.

Methods
Cells and cell culture
Human Glioblastoma Multiforme (GBM) tissue was obtained from five adult patients from the University of Miami Department of Neurosurgery diagnosed with WHO-IV gliomas based on the World Health Organization (WHO) classification of tumors of the Central Nervous System. Patients or guardians provided written informed consent prior to tumor sample retrieval. Samples were named Glio3, Glio4, Glio9, Glio11 and Glio14. GBM stem-like cell lines were generated as previously described [38]. Briefly, tumors were mechanically and enzymatically dissociated, red blood cells were removed using Red Cell Lysis buffer (SigmaAldrich, St. Louis, MO), Cells were filtered and plated in a 3:1 ratio of Dulbecco's Modified Eagle's medium (DMEM): F12 (Gibco, Carlsbad, Ca) media supplemented with 1% penicillin and streptomycin (penn/strep), 20 ng/ml each of human epidermal growth factor and human fibroblast growth factor, and 2% Gem21 NeuroPlex Serum-Free Supplement (Gemini Bioscience, Sacramento, CA); a formulation consistent for the

generation of neurospheres. The GBM cell lines U87, U251 and U235 were purchased from ATCC (Manassas, VA) and were maintained in RPMI media supplemented with 10% FBS and 1% penn/strep. These established GBM cell lines grew in an adherent fashion. All cell lines were routinely tested for mycoplasma using LookOut mycoplasma PCR detection kit (SigmaAldrich, St. Louis, MO) according to the manufacturer's instructions and were maintained at 37 °C in a humidified 5% CO_2 incubator.

Immunofluorescence
To evaluate stem cell marker expression, neurospheres were dissociated mechanically or enzymatically with Accutase (Gemini Bioscience, Sacramento, CA). To facilitate adherence, cells were plated on poly-L-lysine/laminin coated four-well plates in neurosphere media. Cells were fixed in 4% paraformaldehyde, blocked and permeabilized with a 5% bovine serum albumin (BSA) with 0.6% Triton-× 100 and then treated with the primary antibodies Nestin (Abcam, Cambridge, MA), Sox2, Musashi 1, CD44, Bmi-1 (Cell Signaling Technology, Danvers, MA), CD133 (Biorbyt, Cambridge, UK) and A2B5 (A2B5 clone 105, ATCC, Manassas, VA). A "no primary control" was included for all antibodies tested for all cell lines. For these, the cells were incubated with only the antibody diluent (2.5% BSA, 0.3% triton, balance PBS). Cells were then treated with a fluorochrome-conjugated secondary antibody followed by Prolong Gold Antifade Reagent with DAPI (Thermo Fisher Scientific, Waltham, MA). Samples were examined under an EVOS FLoid Cell Imaging Station fluorescent microscope (Thermo Fisher Scientific, Waltham, MA).

MTS assay
Viability was determined using the CellTiter 96® AQueous One Solution Cell Proliferation Assay (MTS) assay (Promega Madison, WI). Cells were seeded into 96-well plates using a modified neurosphere media containing 5% FBS at a density of 10,000 cells per well in 100 μl of cell culture media. Following treatment, media was aspirated and 100 μl of a 1:5 solution of MTS to cell culture media was added to each well and incubated for 1–4 h. Optical density was measured at 490 nm using BoiTek Synergy HT plate reader. To examine the effect of temozolomide (Sigma-Aldrich, St. Louis, MO), GBM stem cells were treated with 100 μM for 72 h or U87 cells were treated with 10–100 μM. Data is represented as the average of 3 separate experiments in which the viability was calculated as the percent of non-treated cells. To determine the effect of curcumin, cells were treated with increasing concentrations of curcumin (Sigma-Aldrich, St. Louis, MO) for 72 h. The IC_{50}, the concentration of curcumin at which 50% of cells were non-viable, was

determined for a minimum of 3 separate experiments. Data is presented as the average IC_{50} for each cell line examined.

Proliferation assay

To determine the effect on cell proliferation 100,000 cells were plated in 10 ml of neurosphere media (100 mm dish for Glio9, and T25 flask for Glio3). Curcumin was added at a concentration of 2.5 μM on day 0. Cells were counted on days 4, 7 and 10 using Orflo Technologies Cell Counter Moxi z (Ketchum, ID). Experiments were done in triplicate.

Sphere forming assay

The effect of curcumin on clonogenic growth potential was determined using sphere-forming assays. Single cells were seeded at 50–100 cells per well in a 96-well plate and treated with 2.5 μM of curcumin on day 0. Spheres were manually counted under microscopy on day 14. All experiments were done in triplicate.

Colony forming assay

Colony counting was performed to determine colony forming potential of the adherent GSC line. Cells were plated at 200 cells per well in 6-wells plates and treated with 2.5 μM of curcumin at day 0. Colonies were stained with 0.01% crystal violet (Sigma-Aldrich, St. Louis, MO) and counted under microscopy on day 14. Cell clusters of less than 50 cells were not considered colonies and therefore were not counted. Experiments were done in triplicate.

ROS assay

Curcumin-induced ROS was visualized and quantitated using the general oxidative stress indicator CM-H2DCFDA (Thermo Fisher Scientific, Waltham, MA). CM-H2DCFDA passively diffuses into cells and reacts with ROS to yield a fluorescent adduct. For quantification, cells were split into 96-well plates in cell culture media with the addition of 5% FBS to cause adherence to the well bottoms. Samples were treated with 25 μM of curcumin in phenol red free media for 30 min, 4 h, and 24 h. Cells were incubated with 0.5 μM CM-H2DCFDA in PBS for 5 min subsequently washed in PBS and read at an excitation of 495 nm and an emission of 525 nm using BoiTek Synergy HT plate reader. Data is presented as fold change from non-treated cells. Curcumin-induced ROS activity was also examined using fluorescent microscopy. Dissociated GSCs were plated in neurosphere media on poly-L-lysine/laminin coated four-well plates. CM-H2DCFDA fluorescence was evaluated at 1, 6 and 24 h post curcumin (25 μM) treatment. Images were obtained using the EVOS FLoid Cell Imaging Station fluorescent microscope (Thermo Fisher Scientific, Waltham, MA).

Western blot analysis

Neurospheres cultures, Glios 3, 4, 11 and 14 were plated and treated as neurospheres ranging in size from 100–300 μm as determined by light microscopy. At 8 or 24 h of treatment, the effect of curcumin, N-acetylcysteine (NAC, Sigma-Aldrich, St. Louis, MO) or the combination of curcumin and NAC on protein levels was determined by western blot analysis.

Our method for western blot analysis has previously described [39]. Briefly, GSCs were lysed in RIPA buffer, protein concentrations determined by using BCA protein assay and 20 μg of protein was loaded onto 8, 12 or 15% polyacrylamide gel (BioRad Hercules, CA) gels for electrophoresis and subsequently transferred onto nitrocellulose membranes. The membranes were then blocked for 1 h in 5% non-fat milk (Biorad, Hercules, CA) at room temperature (RT) and incubated with the primary antibody diluted in 2.5% BSA overnight. All primary antibodies were purchased from Cell Signaling (Danvers, MA) except for alpha-tubulin, which was purchased from Abcam (Cambridge, UK) and STAT3, which was purchased from Santa Cruz Biotechnology (Dallas, TX). Membranes were then incubated at room temperature with anti-mouse or anti-rabbit secondary antibodies for 1 h. Blots were developed using SuperSignal™ West Pico Chemiluminescent Substrate (Thermo Scientific Waltham, MA).

Statistical analysis

Significance was determined using Student's t-tests for all pairwise comparisons of the different treatments that were tested. The results are presented as the mean ± standard error mean (SEM). Significance was set at $p < 0.05$.

Results

Human GBM-derived cell lines display cancer stem cell characteristics

In neurosphere media four out of five cell lines formed spheres, where as the Glio9 grew in an adherent fashion (Fig. 1a). Since there is no definitive marker for GBM stem cells, we examined the expression of multiple putative cancer stem cell markers by immunocytochemistry [40–45]. Except for Glio9 the cell lines demonstrated expression of all markers examined (Fig. 1a). Negative controls for each antibody are shown in Additional file 1: Figure S1A. No SOX2 expression was observed in Glio9. Recently it has been shown that GBM stem cells can be further classified into subgroups, proneural and mesenchymal. These differ both morphologically (neurosphere verse a more adherent phenotype) and in stem cell marker expression [46]. The adherent fashion and the lack of SOX2 expression suggests that glio9 falls into the mesenchymal subgroup. In order to determine if our patient derived cell lines exhibited the cancer stem cell

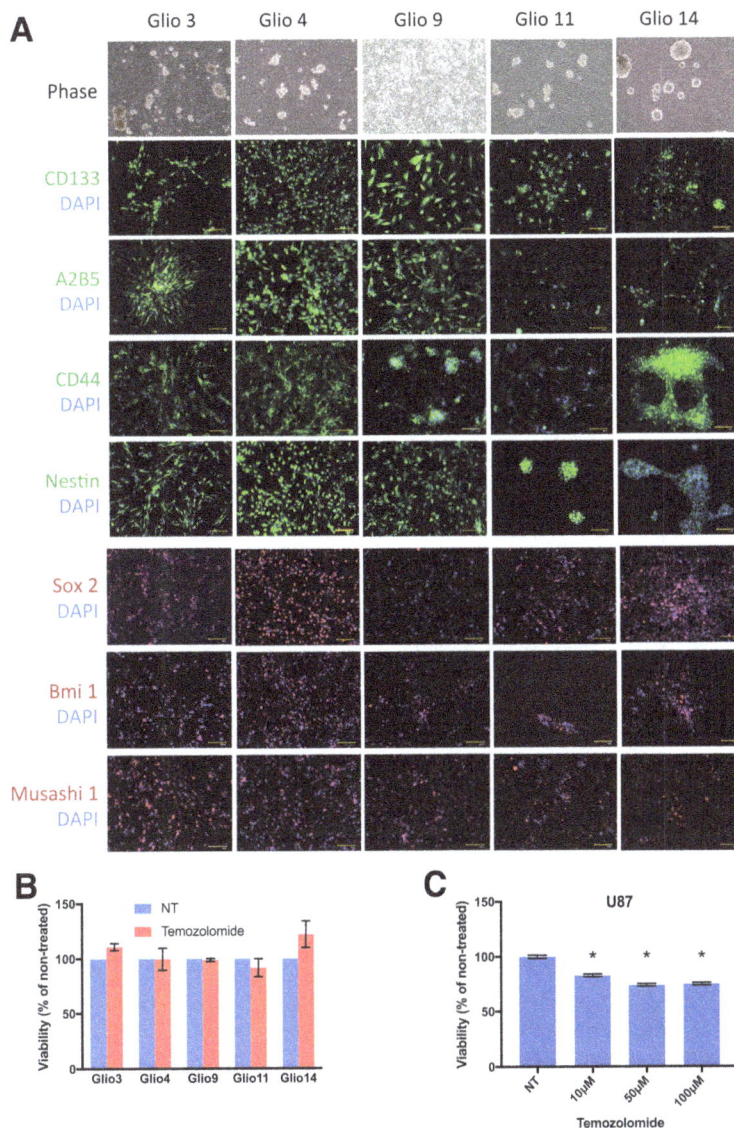

Fig. 1 Patient-derived GBM Stem Cells and Characterization of GBM Stem Cell Lines. **a** Glio 3, 4, 9, 11, 14 immunostaining. Cells are positive for stem cell markers CD133, A2B5, CD44, Nestin, SOX2, Bmi 1 and musashi. Cell nuclei were counterstained with DAPI. Scale bar: 100 μm. **b** GBM stem cell lines were treated with100μm temozolomide and viability determined after 72 h with MTS assay. Results displayed as percent viable cells compared to untreated controls. **c** U87 cells were treated with temozolomide at concentrations shown and viability determined at 72 h with MTS assay. *$p < 0.001$ compared to non-treated controls (NT)

property of chemoresistance [47], we treated five cell lines with 100 μM temozolomide, the chemotherapeutic agent of choice for GBM. We chose a concentration of 100 μM since this is well above the reported (approximately 10 μM) peak levels in cerebral spinal fluid and brain tissue of treated GBM patients [48, 49]. Our results demonstrate that temozolomide had no significant effect on the viability of these GBM cell lines compared to non-treated controls (Fig. 1b). In contrast, the non-GBM stem cell line U87 was sensitive to temozolomide treatment at doses as low as 10 μM, the lowest dose examined (Fig. 1c). These data suggest that our patient-derived GBM cell

lines demonstrate progenitor cell properties consistent with glioblastoma stem cells (GSCs).

Curcumin decreases viability of glioblastoma stem cells and non-stem cells

Several reports have demonstrated that curcumin has anti-neoplastic effects on glioblastoma cells [9, 50–52]. To determine the effect of curcumin on GSC viability we treated five GSC cell lines with increasing concentrations of curcumin for 72 h. In all cell lines analyzed, curcumin demonstrated a does-dependent decrease in viability (Fig. 2a). All cell lines reached levels less than

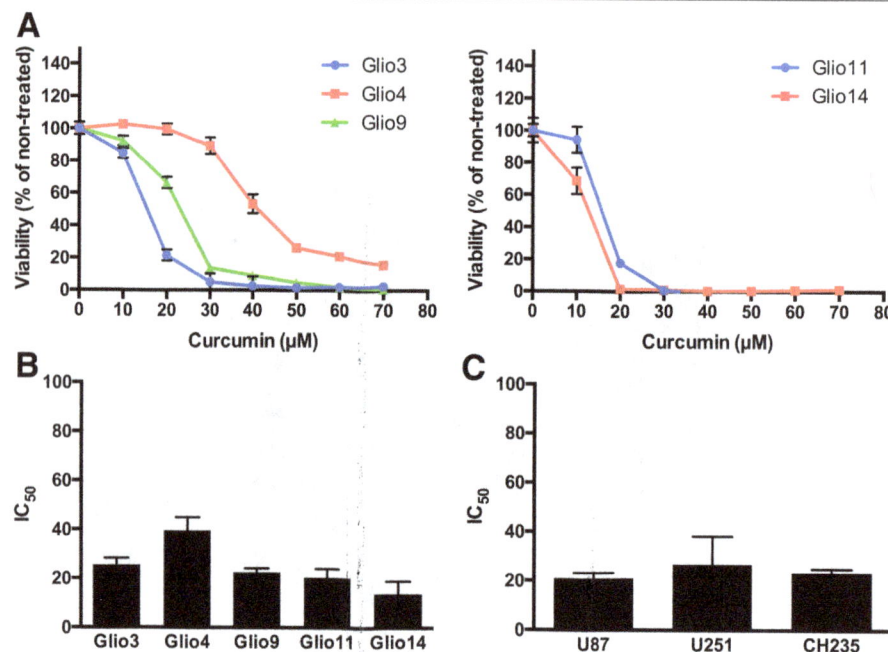

Fig. 2 Effect of curcumin on GBM Stem Cell Lines and non-stem Cell Lines. **a** GBM stem cells were treated with increasing concentrations of curcumin and viability was assessed 72 h later with MTS assay. **b** MTS viability assay was used to determine concentrations needed to induce 50% cell death (IC$_{50}$) in GBM stem cell lines. **c** MTS viability assay was used to determine concentrations needed to induce 50% cell death (IC$_{50}$) in GBM non-stem cell lines

20% viability at 70 μM curcumin—the highest concentration tested. The concentration of curcumin at which 50% of cells were non-viable is known as the IC$_{50}$. The IC$_{50}$s were as follows: Glio3 25.5 μM (SEM: 2.7 μM), Glio4 39.5 μM (SEM: 5.4 μM), Glio9 22.5 μM (SEM: 1.7 μM), Glio11 20.3 μM (SEM: 3.7 μM), and Glio14 13.9 μM (SEM: 5.0 μM) (Fig. 2b). We also verified that curcumin decreases the viability of GBM non-stem cells using the established GBM cell lines U87, U251 and CH235. The IC$_{50}$s of these common GBM cell lines were 30.0 μM (SEM: 2.2 μM) for U87, 26.8 μM (SEM: 11.5 μM) for U251, and 23.4 μM (SEM: 1.6 μM) for CH235 (Fig. 2c). Taken together, these results show that curcumin has a does-dependent effect on the viability of both GBM stem cells and non-stem cells.

Curcumin inhibits proliferation, sphere-forming ability and colony-forming potential of glioblastoma stem cells

Cancer stem cells are marked by their ability to proliferate indefinitely and by their sphere- and colony-forming potential at the single cell level in vitro [53, 54]. We chose to carry out the remainder of the experiments in this study using Glio3, a non-adherent GSC cell line, and Glio9, an adherent GSC cell line, due to their similar IC$_{50}$s and differing adherence patterns. In order to determine if curcumin affects the proliferative ability of GSCs, we plated Glio3 and Glio9 at 1×10^5 cells and treated with 2.5 μM curcumin on day 0. Curcumin treated Glio3

showed a statistically significant decrease in cell number on days 7 and 10 ($p < 0.05$) compared to non-treated controls, whereas Glio9 showed a non-significant decrease in cell number on days 7 and 10 (Fig. 3a). To investigate whether curcumin has an effect on the sphere-forming capacity of GSCs, we seeded the non-adherent cell line Glio3 at 50–100 cells per well and treated it with 2.5 μM curcumin on day 0. Spheres were counted on day 14. Glio3 demonstrated a 60% decrease in sphere formation when treated with curcumin compared to non-treated controls ($p <0.05$) (Fig. 3b). The adherent cell line Glio9 was used to determine if curcumin affects the colony-forming ability of GSCs. Glio9 was plated at 200 cells per well and 2.5 μM curcumin was treated at day 0. On day 14, the curcumin treated cells showed a dramatic 95% reduction in colony number compared to non-treated controls ($p < 0.05$) (Fig. 3c). These data show that low doses of curcumin inhibit proliferation, sphere-forming and colony-forming potentials of GSCs.

Curcumin induces ROS in glioblastoma stem cells

Curcumin has been demonstrated to induce reactive oxygen species (ROS) in various cancer cell lines [55–57]. To determine if curcumin has the same effect on GSCs we used the molecular probe CM-H2DCFDA, a general oxidative stress indicator, to measure ROS via fluorescence in two cell lines. Under fluorescence microscopy, Glio9

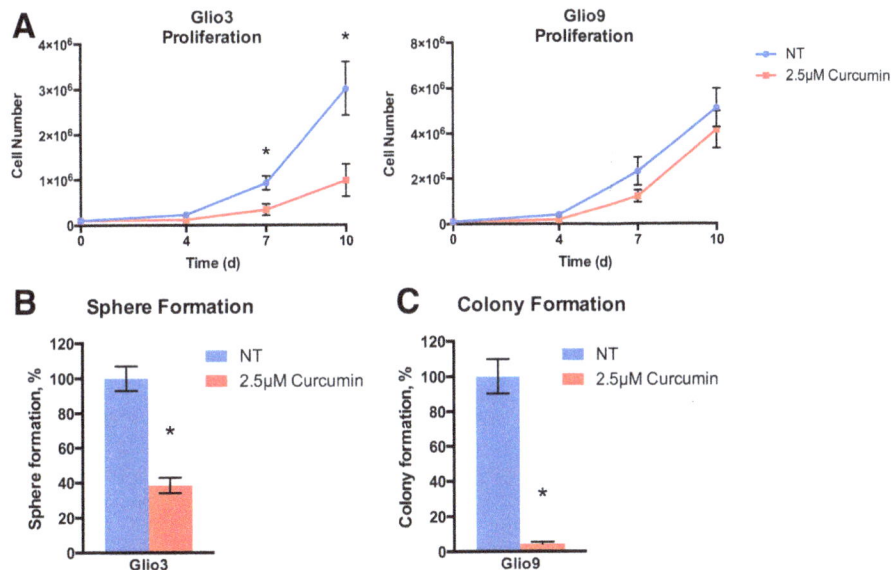

Fig. 3 Curcumin decreases proliferation, sphere forming ability and colony forming potential in GSC cell lines. **a** Glio3 and Glio9 GSCs were plated at 1×10⁵ cells initially and treated with 2.5 µM curcumin on day 0. Cells were counted using Orflo Technologies Cell Counter Moxi z on days 4, 7 and 10. **b** Glio3 GSCs were seeded at 50–100 cells per well in a 96-well plate and treated with 2.5 µM curcumin on day 0. Spheres were counted on day 14. **c** Glio9 GSCs were plated at 200 cells and treated with 2.5 µM curcumin at day 0. Colonies were stained with crystal violet and counted on day 14. *$p < 0.05$, non-treated controls (NT) vs. curcumin treated

showed an induction of ROS at the 1 and 6 h time points after treatment with 25 µM curcumin with a return to control levels at 24 h (Fig. 4a). After quantification, a one time treatment of 25 µM curcumin was shown to significantly induce ROS in Glio3 and Glio9 with a peak increase of approximately 6–8 fold relative fluorescence at 4 h post-treatment relative to non-treated controls ($p < 0.05$). ROS were shown to decrease 24 h post-treatment (Fig. 4b). These data suggest that curcumin may cause its effects in GSCs via induction of ROS.

Curcumin induces MAPK activation, inactivates STAT3 and downregulates the STAT3 downstream target Survivin in glioblastoma stem cells

Studies have demonstrated that ROS can induce the activation of multiple signaling pathways including the MAPK pathways in several cell types [58, 59]. We used western blot analysis to determine curcumin's, and potentially ROS activation's, modulation on different signaling pathways. Following 8 h of 25 µM curcumin treatment, the phosphorylated (activated) form of ERK, p38 and c-jun (as an indicator of JNK activation) was increased in the GSCs Glio3 and Glio9 (Fig. 5a). This was also demonstrated in all other GSC cell lines (Additional file 2: Figure S2), ERK has been shown to cause the repression of STAT3 activity via dephosphorylation at the Tyr705 position and phosphorylation at the Ser727 location [60]. Here we show that treatment with curcumin decreases the Tyr705 phosphorylated form of STAT3 and increases the Ser727 form in Glio3 and Glio9 (Fig. 5b). When STAT3 is

dephosphorylated at the Tyr705 position and phosphorylated at the Ser727 position it is rendered inactive and is incapable of translocating to the nucleus to carry out its downstream effects. We also demonstrate the decreased expression of STAT3's downstream target Survivin as well as the other anti-apoptosis proteins IAP1 and IAP2 (Glio9 only) in these GSCs (Fig. 5c). These results suggest that curcumin induces the activation of MAPKs and the inhibition of STAT3 activity in GSCs.

N-acetylcysteine rescues curcumin-induced effects on glioblastoma stem cells

N-acetylcysteine (NAC) is an antioxidant shown to decrease ROS [61, 62]. To test whether ROS induction was truly the mechanism for curcumin's anti-malignant effects on GSCs, we conducted a cell viability assay and western blot analysis to determine if NAC could rescue curcumin's effects on GSCs. We treated cells with 5 mM NAC, 25 µM curcumin, and a combination of both treatments and viability was determined at 72 h. Treatment with NAC alone had no significant effect on viability on all cell lines except for Glio4, which showed an 18.7% increase in viability ($p < 0.05$). Treatment with curcumin alone showed significant decreases in viability in all cell lines compared to non-treated controls ($p < 0.001$). When cells were pretreated with NAC to prevent ROS induction, cell viability was significantly rescued in all cell lines compared to curcumin only treated cells ($p < 0.001$) (Fig. 6a). To determine if NAC treatment reverses curcumin's effects on signaling pathways in Glio3 and Glio9, cells were treated

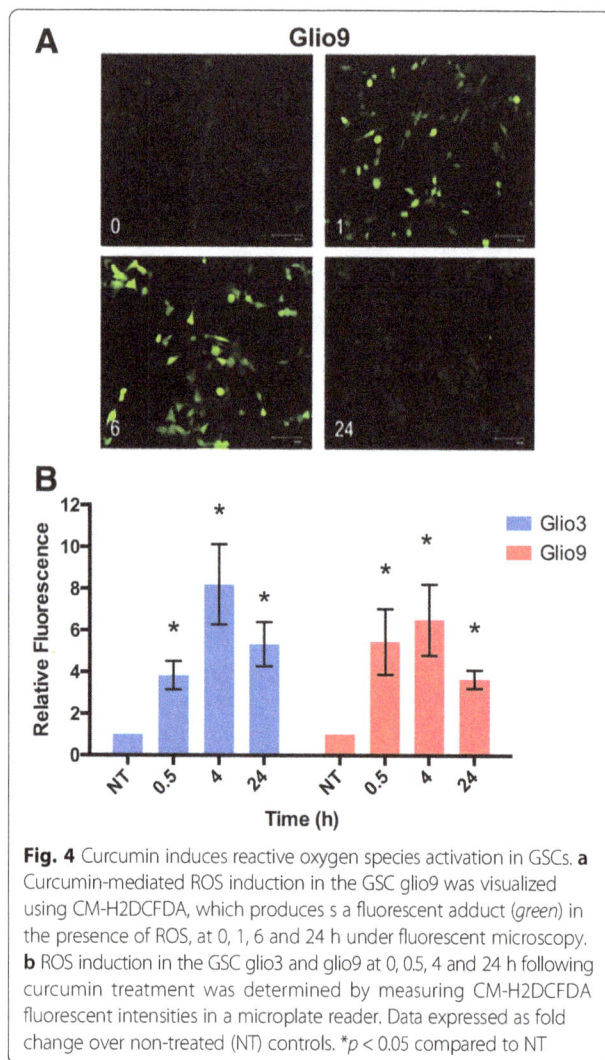

Fig. 4 Curcumin induces reactive oxygen species activation in GSCs. **a** Curcumin-mediated ROS induction in the GSC glio9 was visualized using CM-H2DCFDA, which produces s a fluorescent adduct (*green*) in the presence of ROS, at 0, 1, 6 and 24 h under fluorescent microscopy. **b** ROS induction in the GSC glio3 and glio9 at 0, 0.5, 4 and 24 h following curcumin treatment was determined by measuring CM-H2DCFDA fluorescent intensities in a microplate reader. Data expressed as fold change over non-treated (NT) controls. *$p < 0.05$ compared to NT

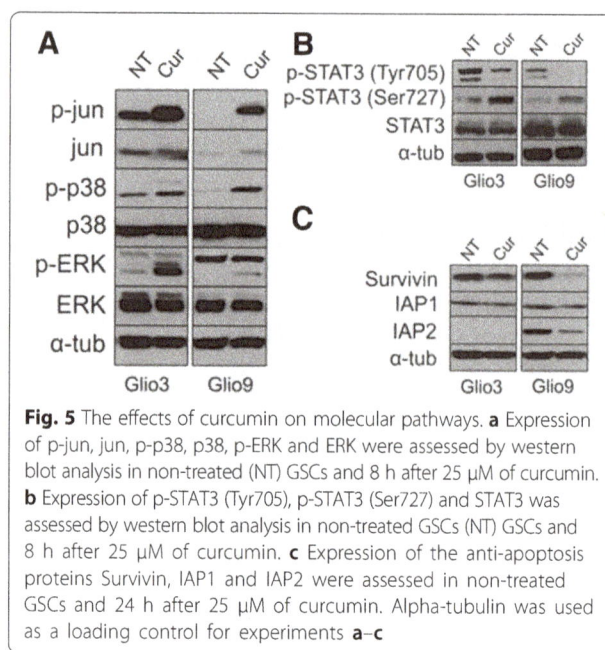

Fig. 5 The effects of curcumin on molecular pathways. **a** Expression of p-jun, jun, p-p38, p38, p-ERK and ERK were assessed by western blot analysis in non-treated (NT) GSCs and 8 h after 25 µM of curcumin. **b** Expression of p-STAT3 (Tyr705), p-STAT3 (Ser727) and STAT3 was assessed by western blot analysis in non-treated GSCs (NT) GSCs and 8 h after 25 µM of curcumin. **c** Expression of the anti-apoptosis proteins Survivin, IAP1 and IAP2 were assessed in non-treated GSCs and 24 h after 25 µM of curcumin. Alpha-tubulin was used as a loading control for experiments **a–c**

with 5 mM NAC, 25 µM curcumin, and a combination of both treatments for 8 h. Western blot analysis indicates that NAC reversed the curcumin-induced MAPK activation (Fig. 6b) and STAT3 deactivation—signified by an increase in p-STAT3 (Tyr705) and a decrease in p-STAT3 (Ser727) (Fig. 6c). This was also demonstrated in all GSC cell lines at the Tyr705 position (Additional file 3: Figure S3). These data demonstrate that ROS induction may be the mechanism behind curcumin's anti-cancer effects.

Discussion

A growing body of evidence indicates that GSCs are responsible for tumor formation, progression and recurrence and that targeting these cells may be paramount in the eradication of GBM [63, 64]. Studying GSCs from patient derived GBM samples is the best model of disease in humans, as it has been shown that established, indefinitely passaged GBM cell lines do not predict clinical drug efficacy and are not representative of patient tumors [65]. Here we demonstrate the anti-neoplastic

effects of curcumin, a blood brain barrier permeable compound shown to be non-toxic to normal astrocytes and neurons, on patient derived GSCs [66, 67].

In this study we demonstrate through a neurosphere growth pattern (with the exception of the adherent Gio9), chemoresistance and the expression of all tested stem cell markers (with the exception of SOX2 in Glio9) in all cell lines that our samples are indeed GSCs (Fig. 1). Due to its adherent nature and lack of SOX2 expression, we hypothesize that Glio9 is of the mesenchymal GBM subtype [46, 68]. We show that curcumin decreases viability of GSCs in a dose dependent manner (Fig. 2) and that low doses of curcumin inhibit proliferation, sphere formation and colony formation of GSCs (Fig. 3). Experiments at doses this low are lacking from the GBM literature. We have shown that treatment with curcumin induces ROS activity (Fig. 4) and that pretreatment with the antioxidant n-acetylcysteine reverses curcumin's effects on viability and molecular pathways (Fig. 6). It has been shown that the ERK pathway is inducible through ROS [58, 59] and that activated ERK can cause repression of STAT3 and downregulation of its downstream targets though an inhibition of its tyrosine 705 phosphorylation and activation of its serine 727 phosphorylation [60]. Although more work needs to be done, our data suggests that curcumin may exert its effects through this mechanism via induction of ROS.

The role of ROS in cancer is dichotomist in nature. Low levels of ROS have been shown to promote cancer through stimulation of cell proliferation, increased cell survival and amplified angiogenesis through activation of several pathways including NF-κB [69–71]. High levels

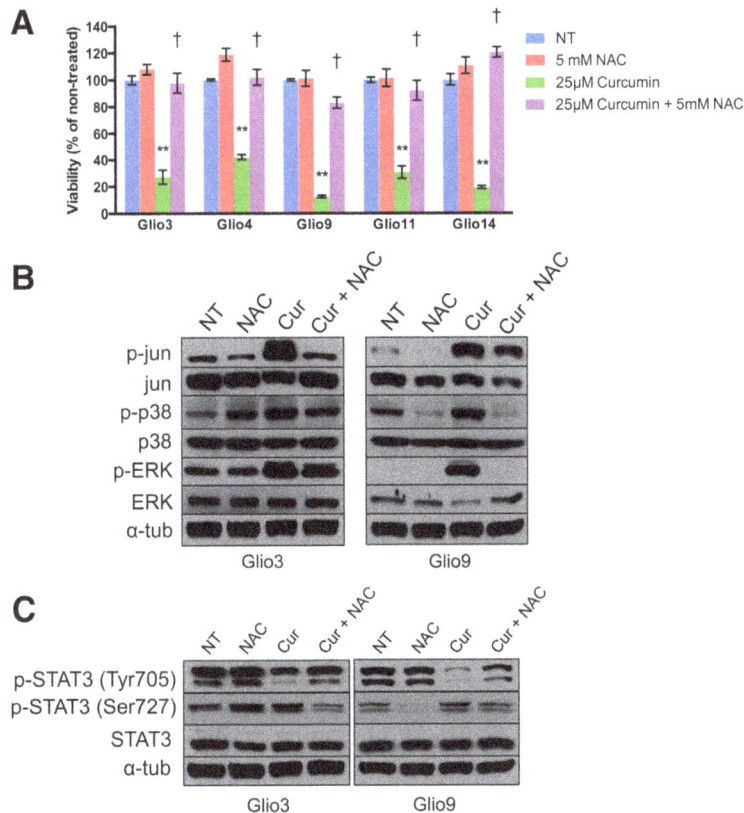

Fig. 6 N-acetylcysteine (NAC) rescues curcumin-induced decrease in viability and modulation of molecular pathways in multiple GSC cell lines. **a** GSCs were treated with 5 mM NAC alone, 25uM curcumin alone or 5 mM NAC and 25uM curcumin in combination. Viability was assessed at 72 h using the MTS assay. Results displayed as percent viable cells compared to untreated controls (NT). **b** Expression of p-jun, jun, p-p38, p38, p-ERK and ERK was assessed in non-treated (NT), 5 mM NAC treated, 25 μM curcumin treated, and pretreated 5 mM NAC followed by 25 μM curcumin treated GSCs after 8 h. **c** Expression of p-STAT3 (Tyr705), p-STAT3 (Ser727) and STAT3 was assessed in non-treated (NT), 5 mM NAC treated, 25 μM curcumin treated, and pretreated 5 mM NAC followed by 25 μM curcumin treated GSCs after 8 h. Alpha-tubulin was used as a loading control. **P < 0.001 vs. NT. †P < 0.001 vs. 25 μM Curcumin

of ROS have been shown to have anti-cancer effects by inducing cell cycle arrest and apoptosis via several mechanisms including Rac-1/NADPH oxidase pathway induction [72, 73]. CSCs have been shown to have lower intracellular ROS content due to increased expression of free radical scavenging systems [74]. Although this may indicate CSC ROS resistance, several studies have demonstrated ROS-induced targeting of CSCs. Induction of ROS through niclosamide treatment in AML, parthenolide treatment in AML and CML, and arsenic trioxide treatment in PML (promyelocytic leukemia) target CSCs [75–77]. In this study we demonstrate that curcumin-induced ROS targets glioblastoma stem cells.

Curcumin has been shown to be an effective CSC targeting molecule in glioma as well as other tumor types [9–12] while maintaining a minimal side effect profile even at high doses of 12 g/day [78]. The main hurdle facing curcumin as a potential chemotherapeutic agent is its bioavailability [14]. When dosed orally, unformulated curcumin has been shown to reach peak plasma levels of

<2 μM in humans [79]. In order to overcome this limitation, researchers have formulated several bioavailable forms of curcumin. Nano-emulsion curcumin, thermacurcumin (curcumin within colloidal nanoparticles), and curcumin within N-trimethyl chitosan coated solid lipid nanoparticles have been shown to reach peak plasma levels of 12.6 μM, 4.6 μM, and 3.28 μM respectively in rodent models [80–82]. In this study we demonstrate that 2.5 μM of curcumin inhibits the self-renewal properties of GSCs. In order to target GSC viability at curcumin levels of 25 μM (Fig. 6) and above, alternative routes of administration must be considered. Polymeric drug and convection-enhanced delivery systems have been shown to deliver high local concentrations of active agents while decreasing systemic toxicities in GBM and may serve to circumvent the bioavailability issues facing curcumin [83]. Currently curcumin is being evaluated clinically for neurological diseases including bi-polar disorder and Alzheimer's disease as well as for multiple cancers, however clinical trials are needed to determine

the potential of curcumin alone and in combination with radiotherapy and or chemotherapy for GBM patients.

Conclusions

In summary, we have found that curcumin targets glioblastoma stem cells though the induction of ROS, potentially through downregulation of STAT3 activity. The importance of STAT3 in GBM has previously been described [84]. Specifically, inhibition of STAT3 signaling decreased GSC survival both in culture and in orthotopic xenograft models [85]. Furthermore, levels of STAT3's downstream target, Survivin correlate with astrocytoma grade and may be predictive of poor patient survival [86, 87]. We show that low doses of curcumin inhibit the self-renewal properties of GSCs—an important characteristic for a chemotherapy targeting GBM relapse—and that curcumin decreases GSC viability in a dose dependent manner. These findings indicate that curcumin may be a safe future chemotherapeutic agent for the treatment of glioblastoma and further studies are warranted.

Additional files

Additional file 1: Figure S1. No primary controls for stem cell immunofluorescence shown in Fig. 1a. For control staining, antibody diluent without primary antibody was used, followed by the secondary antibody. Cells were counterstained with DAPI to identify nucleus. No stem cell marker fluorescence was observed in control cells. Scale bar: 100 μm.

Additional file 2: Figure S2. The effects of curcumin on MAPKs in additional GBM stem cell lines. Expression of p-jun, jun, p-p38, p38, p-ERK and ERK were assessed by western blot analysis in non-treated (NT) GSCs and 8 h after 25 μM of curcumin. Alpha-tubulin was used as a loading control for all experiments.

Additional file 3: Figure S3. N-acetylcysteine (NAC) rescues curcumin-induced p-STAT3 (Tyr705) activation in additional GBM stem cell lines. Expression of p-STAT3 (Tyr705) and STAT3 was assessed in non-treated (NT), 5 mM NAC treated, 25 μM curcumin treated, and pretreated 5 mM NAC followed by 25 μM curcumin treated GSCs after 8 h. Alpha-tubulin was used as a loading control.

Abbreviations

AML: Acute myeloid leukemia; ATCC: American type culture collection; BCA: Bicinchoninic acid; BSA: Bovine serum albumin; CML: Chronic myeloid leukemia; DAPI: 4',6-diamidino-2-phenylindole; DMEM: Dulbecco's modified Eagle's medium; ERK: Extracellular signal–regulated kinases; FBS: Fetal bovine serum; GBM: Glioblastoma multiforme; GSCs: Glioblastoma stem cells; IAP: Inhibitor of apoptosis protein; JAK: Janus kinase; JNK: Jun N-terminal kinases; MAPK: Mitogen-activated protein kinases; NAC: N-acetylcysteine; NADPH: Nicotinamide adenine dinucleotide phosphate; NF-κB: Nuclear factor kappa-light-chain-enhancer of activated B cells; PCR: Polymerase chain reaction; PML: Promyelocytic leukemia; Rac-1: Ras-related C3 botulinum toxin substrate 1; ROS: Reactive oxygen species; RPMI: Roswell Park Memorial Institute; SEM: Standard error of the mean; STAT3: Signal transducer and activator of transcription 3; WHO: World health organization

Acknowledgements

We would like to thank our wonderful laboratory volunteers Beatriz Hawkins, Amelia Bahamonde, Nicolas de Cordoba and Sumedh Shah for their contributions to our research efforts.

Funding

University of Miami Brain Tumor Initiative (UMBTI) and the Mystic Force Foundation provided salary support for RMG and cost of all materials/reagents required for this work.

Authors' contributions

ZCG conducted experiments, analyzed data and contributed to writing the manuscript. GAR conducted experiments and analyzed data. ERB conducted experiments and analyzed data. AS conducted experiments and analyzed data. WMW conducted experiments and analyzed data. KCO conducted experiments. RJK analyzed data and contributed to writing the manuscript. RMG conducted experiments, analyzed data and contributed to writing the manuscript. All authors read and approved the final manuscript.

Competing interests

The authors declare that they have no competing interests.

References

1. Iacob G, Dinca EB. Current data and strategy in glioblastoma multiforme. J Med Life. 2009;2:386–93.
2. Spratt DE, Folkert M, Zumsteg ZS, Chan TA, Beal K, Gutin PH, Pentsova E, Yamada Y. Temporal relationship of post-operative radiotherapy with temozolomide and oncologic outcome for glioblastoma. J Neurooncol. 2014;116:357–63.
3. Sundar SJ, Hsieh JK, Manjila S, Lathia JD, Sloan A. The role of cancer stem cells in glioblastoma. Neurosurg Focus. 2014;37:E6.
4. Tan BT, Park CY, Ailles LE, Weissman IL. The cancer stem cell hypothesis: a work in progress. Lab Invest. 2006;86:1203–7.
5. Perry MC, Demeule M, Regina A, Moumdjian R, Beliveau R. Curcumin inhibits tumor growth and angiogenesis in glioblastoma xenografts. Mol Nutr Food Res. 2010;54:1192–201.
6. Liao H, Wang Z, Deng Z, Ren H, Li X. Curcumin inhibits lung cancer invasion and metastasis by attenuating GLUT1/MT1-MMP/MMP2 pathway. Int J Clin Exp Med. 2015;8:8948–57.
7. Sobolewski C, Muller F, Cerella C, Dicato M, Diederich M. Celecoxib prevents curcumin-induced apoptosis in a hematopoietic cancer cell model. Mol Carcinog. 2015;54:999–1013.
8. Zhang X, Wang R, Chen G, Dejean L, Chen QH. The Effects of Curcumin-based Compounds on Proliferation and Cell Death in Cervical Cancer Cells. Anticancer Res. 2015;35:5293–8.
9. Hossain M, Banik NL, Ray SK. Synergistic anti-cancer mechanisms of curcumin and paclitaxel for growth inhibition of human brain tumor stem cells and LN18 and U138MG cells. Neurochem Int. 2012;61:1102–13.
10. Almanaa TN, Geusz ME, Jamasbi RJ. Effects of curcumin on stem-like cells in human esophageal squamous carcinoma cell lines. BMC Complement Altern Med. 2012;12:195.
11. Lin L, Liu Y, Li H, Li PK, Fuchs J, Shibata H, Iwabuchi Y, Lin J. Targeting colon cancer stem cells using a new curcumin analogue, GO-Y030. Br J Cancer. 2011;105:212–20.
12. Charpentier MS, Whipple RA, Vitolo MI, Boggs AE, Slovic J, Thompson KN, Bhandary L, Martin SS. Curcumin targets breast cancer stem-like cells with microtentacles that persist in mammospheres and promote reattachment. Cancer Res. 2014;74:1250–60.

13. Rodriguez GA, Shah AH, Gersey ZC, Shah SS, Bregy A, Komotar RJ, Graham RM. Investigating the therapeutic role and molecular biology of curcumin as a treatment for glioblastoma. Ther Adv Med Oncol. 2016;8:248–60.

14. Shehzad A, Wahid F, Lee YS. Curcumin in cancer chemoprevention: molecular targets, pharmacokinetics, bioavailability, and clinical trials. Arch Pharm (Weinheim). 2010;343:489–99.

15. Padhye S, Chavan D, Pandey S, Deshpande J, Swamy KV, Sarkar FH. Perspectives on chemopreventive and therapeutic potential of curcumin analogs in medicinal chemistry. Mini Rev Med Chem. 2010;10:372–87.

16. Sarkar FH, Li Y, Wang Z, Padhye S. Lesson learned from nature for the development of novel anti-cancer agents: implication of isoflavone, curcumin, and their synthetic analogs. Curr Pharm Des. 2010;16:1801–12.

17. Shehzad A, Lee YS. Molecular mechanisms of curcumin action: signal transduction. Biofactors. 2013;39:27–36.

18. Chang PY, Peng SF, Lee CY, Lu CC, Tsai SC, Shieh TM, Wu TS, Tu MG, Chen MY, Yang JS. Curcumin-loaded nanoparticles induce apoptotic cell death through regulation of the function of MDR1 and reactive oxygen species in cisplatin-resistant CAR human oral cancer cells. Int J Oncol. 2013;43:1141–50.

19. Liu H, Zhou BH, Qiu X, Wang HS, Zhang F, Fang R, Wang XF, Cai SH, Du J, Bu XZ. T63, a new 4-arylidene curcumin analogue, induces cell cycle arrest and apoptosis through activation of the reactive oxygen species-FOXO3a pathway in lung cancer cells. Free Radic Biol Med. 2012;53:2204–17.

20. Chung SS, Vadgama JV. Curcumin and epigallocatechin gallate inhibit the cancer stem cell phenotype via down-regulation of STAT3-NFkappaB signaling. Anticancer Res. 2015;35:39–46.

21. Devasagayam TP, Tilak JC, Boloor KK, Sane KS, Ghaskadbi SS, Lele RD. Free radicals and antioxidants in human health: current status and future prospects. J Assoc Physicians India. 2004;52:794–804.

22. Kaur U, Banerjee P, Bir A, Sinha M, Biswas A, Chakrabarti S. Reactive oxygen species, redox signaling and neuroinflammation in Alzheimer's disease: the NF-kappaB connection. Curr Top Med Chem. 2015;15:446–57.

23. Kornfeld OS, Hwang S, Disatnik MH, Chen CH, Qvit N, Mochly-Rosen D. Mitochondrial reactive oxygen species at the heart of the matter: new therapeutic approaches for cardiovascular diseases. Circ Res. 2015;116:1783–99.

24. Saito S, Lin YC, Tsai MH, Lin CS, Murayama Y, Sato R, Yokoyama KK. Emerging roles of hypoxia-inducible factors and reactive oxygen species in cancer and pluripotent stem cells. Kaohsiung J Med Sci. 2015;31:279–86.

25. Chang Z, Xing J, Yu X. Curcumin induces osteosarcoma MG63 cells apoptosis via ROS/Cyto-C/Caspase-3 pathway. Tumour Biol. 2014;35:753–8.

26. Kaushik G, Kaushik T, Yadav SK, Sharma SK, Ranawat P, Khanduja KL, Pathak CM. Curcumin sensitizes lung adenocarcinoma cells to apoptosis via intracellular redox status mediated pathway. Indian J Exp Biol. 2012;50:853–61.

27. Li PM, Li YL, Liu B, Wang WJ, Wang YZ, Li Z. Curcumin inhibits MHCC97H liver cancer cells by activating ROS/TLR-4/caspase signaling pathway. Asian Pac J Cancer Prev. 2014;15:2329–34.

28. Yu T, Ji J, Guo YL. MST1 activation by curcumin mediates JNK activation, Foxo3a nuclear translocation and apoptosis in melanoma cells. Biochem Biophys Res Commun. 2013;441:53–8.

29. Kobayashi CI, Suda T. Regulation of reactive oxygen species in stem cells and cancer stem cells. J Cell Physiol. 2012;227:421–30.

30. Li X, Wang K, Ren Y, Zhang L, Tang XJ, Zhang HM, Zhao CQ, Liu PJ, Zhang JM, He JJ. MAPK signaling mediates sinomenine hydrochloride-induced human breast cancer cell death via both reactive oxygen species-dependent and -independent pathways: an in vitro and in vivo study. Cell Death Dis. 2014;5:e1356.

31. Jung SN, Shin DS, Kim HN, Jeon YJ, Yun J, Lee YJ, Kang JS, Han DC, Kwon BM. Sugiol inhibits STAT3 activity via regulation of transketolase and ROS-mediated ERK activation in DU145 prostate carcinoma cells. Biochem Pharmacol. 2015;97:38–50.

32. Chae IG, Kim DH, Kundu J, Jeong CH, Kundu JK, Chun KS. Generation of ROS by CAY10598 leads to inactivation of STAT3 signaling and induction of apoptosis in human colon cancer HCT116 cells. Free Radic Res. 2014;48:1311–21.

33. Cha JH, Choi YJ, Cha SH, Choi CH, Cho WH. Allicin inhibits cell growth and induces apoptosis in U87MG human glioblastoma cells through an ERK-dependent pathway. Oncol Rep. 2012;28:41–8.

34. Dutra-Oliveira A, Monteiro RQ, Mariano-Oliveira A. Protease-activated receptor-2 (PAR2) mediates VEGF production through the ERK1/2 pathway in human glioblastoma cell lines. Biochem Biophys Res Commun. 2012;421:221–7.

35. Liu Z, Jiang Z, Huang J, Huang S, Li Y, Yu S, Yu S, Liu X. miR-7 inhibits glioblastoma growth by simultaneously interfering with the PI3K/ATK and Raf/MEK/ERK pathways. Int J Oncol. 2014;44:1571–80.

36. Sherry MM, Reeves A, Wu JK, Cochran BH. STAT3 is required for proliferation and maintenance of multipotency in glioblastoma stem cells. Stem Cells. 2009;27:2383–92.

37. Rahaman SO, Harbor PC, Chernova O, Barnett GH, Vogelbaum MA, Haque SJ. Inhibition of constitutively active Stat3 suppresses proliferation and induces apoptosis in glioblastoma multiforme cells. Oncogene. 2002;21:8404–13.

38. Pastori C, Daniel M, Penas C, Volmar CH, Johnstone AL, Brothers SP, Graham RM, Allen B, Sarkaria JN, Komotar RJ, et al. BET bromodomain proteins are required for glioblastoma cell proliferation. Epigenetics. 2014;9:611–20.

39. Graham RM, Hernandez F, Puerta N, De Angulo G, Webster KA, Vanni S. Resveratrol augments ER stress and the cytotoxic effects of glycolytic inhibition in neuroblastoma by downregulating Akt in a mechanism independent of SIRT1. Exp Mol Med. 2016;48:e210.

40. Gotte M, Wolf M, Staebler A, Buchweitz O, Kelsch R, Schuring AN, Kiesel L. Increased expression of the adult stem cell marker Musashi-1 in endometriosis and endometrial carcinoma. J Pathol. 2008;215:317–29.

41. Prince ME, Sivanandan R, Kaczorowski A, Wolf GT, Kaplan MJ, Dalerba P, Weissman IL, Clarke MF, Ailles LE. Identification of a subpopulation of cells with cancer stem cell properties in head and neck squamous cell carcinoma. Proc Natl Acad Sci U S A. 2007;104:973–8.

42. Jin X, Jin X, Jung JE, Beck S, Kim H. Cell surface Nestin is a biomarker for glioma stem cells. Biochem Biophys Res Commun. 2013;433:496–501.

43. Anido J, Saez-Borderias A, Gonzalez-Junca A, Rodon L, Folch G, Carmona MA, Prieto-Sanchez RM, Barba I, Martinez-Saez E, Prudkin L, et al. TGF-beta Receptor Inhibitors Target the CD44(high)/Id1(high) Glioma-Initiating Cell Population in Human Glioblastoma. Cancer Cell. 2010;18:655–68.

44. Tchoghandjian A, Baeza N, Colin C, Cayre M, Metellus P, Beclin C, Ouafik L, Figarella-Branger D. A2B5 cells from human glioblastoma have cancer stem cell properties. Brain Pathol. 2010;20:211–21.

45. Brescia P, Ortensi B, Fornasari L, Levi D, Broggi G, Pelicci G. CD133 is essential for glioblastoma stem cell maintenance. Stem Cells. 2013;31:857–69.

46. Mao P, Joshi K, Li J, Kim SH, Li P, Santana-Santos L, Luthra S, Chandran UR, Benos PV, Smith L, et al. Mesenchymal glioma stem cells are maintained by activated glycolytic metabolism involving aldehyde dehydrogenase 1A3. Proc Natl Acad Sci U S A. 2013;110:8644–9.

47. Malik B, Nie D. Cancer stem cells and resistance to chemo and radio therapy. Front Biosci (Elite Ed). 2012;4:2142–9.

48. Portnow J, Badie B, Chen M, Liu A, Blanchard S, Synold TW. The neuropharmacokinetics of temozolomide in patients with resectable brain tumors: potential implications for the current approach to chemoradiation. Clin Cancer Res. 2009;15:7092–8.

49. Ostermann S, Csajka C, Buclin T, Leyvraz S, Lejeune F, Decosterd LA, Stupp R. Plasma and cerebrospinal fluid population pharmacokinetics of temozolomide in malignant glioma patients. Clin Cancer Res. 2004;10:3728–36.

50. Shi L, Fei X, Wang Z. Demethoxycurcumin was prior to temozolomide on inhibiting proliferation and induced apoptosis of glioblastoma stem cells. Tumour Biol. 2015;36:7107–19.

51. Zhuang W, Long L, Zheng B, Ji W, Yang N, Zhang Q, Liang Z. Curcumin promotes differentiation of glioma-initiating cells by inducing autophagy. Cancer Sci. 2012;103:684–90.

52. Lim KJ, Bisht S, Bar EE, Maitra A, Eberhart CG. A polymeric nanoparticle formulation of curcumin inhibits growth, clonogenicity and stem-like fraction in malignant brain tumors. Cancer Biol Ther. 2011;11:464–73.

53. Singh SK, Clarke ID, Terasaki M, Bonn VE, Hawkins C, Squire J, Dirks PB. Identification of a cancer stem cell in human brain tumors. Cancer Res. 2003;63:5821–8.

54. Lobo NA, Shimono Y, Qian D, Clarke MF. The biology of cancer stem cells. Annu Rev Cell Dev Biol. 2007;23:675–99.

55. Picone P, Nuzzo D, Caruana L, Messina E, Scafidi V, Di Carlo M. Curcumin induces apoptosis in human neuroblastoma cells via inhibition of AKT and Foxo3a nuclear translocation. Free Radic Res. 2014;48:1397–408.

56. Rana C, Piplani H, Vaish V, Nehru B, Sanyal SN. Downregulation of PI3-K/Akt/PTEN pathway and activation of mitochondrial intrinsic apoptosis by Diclofenac and Curcumin in colon cancer. Mol Cell Biochem. 2015;402:225–41.

57. Ko YC, Lien JC, Liu HC, Hsu SC, Ji BC, Yang MD, Hsu WH, Chung JG. Demethoxycurcumin induces the apoptosis of human lung cancer NCI-H460 cells through the mitochondrial-dependent pathway. Oncol Rep. 2015;33:2429–37.

58. Keshari RS, Verma A, Barthwal MK, Dikshit M. Reactive oxygen species-induced activation of ERK and p38 MAPK mediates PMA-induced NETs release from human neutrophils. J Cell Biochem. 2013;114:532–40.

59. McCubrey JA, Lahair MM, Franklin RA. Reactive oxygen species-induced activation of the MAP kinase signaling pathways. Antioxid Redox Signal. 2006;8:1775–89.

60. Jain N, Zhang T, Fong SL, Lim CP, Cao X. Repression of Stat3 activity by activation of mitogen-activated protein kinase (MAPK). Oncogene. 1998;17:3157–67.

61. Zhu Y, Paul P, Lee S, Craig BT, Rellinger EJ, Qiao J, Gius DR, Chung DH. Antioxidant inhibition of steady-state reactive oxygen species and cell growth in neuroblastoma. Surgery. 2015;158:827–36.

62. Sun Y, Pu LY, Lu L, Wang XH, Zhang F, Rao JH. N-acetylcysteine attenuates reactive-oxygen-species-mediated endoplasmic reticulum stress during liver ischemia-reperfusion injury. World J Gastroenterol. 2014;20:15289–98.

63. Zhu Z, Khan MA, Weiler M, Blaes J, Jestaedt L, Geibert M, Zou P, Gronych J, Bernhardt O, Korshunov A, et al. Targeting self-renewal in high-grade brain tumors leads to loss of brain tumor stem cells and prolonged survival. Cell Stem Cell. 2014;15:185–98.

64. Chen J, Li Y, Yu TS, McKay RM, Burns DK, Kernie SG, Parada LF. A restricted cell population propagates glioblastoma growth after chemotherapy. Nature. 2012;488:522–6.

65. Lee J, Kotliarova S, Kotliarov Y, Li A, Su Q, Donin NM, Pastorino S, Purow BW, Christopher N, Zhang W, et al. Tumor stem cells derived from glioblastomas cultured in bFGF and EGF more closely mirror the phenotype and genotype of primary tumors than do serum-cultured cell lines. Cancer Cell. 2006;9:391–403.

66. Zanotto-Filho A, Braganhol E, Edelweiss MI, Behr GA, Zanin R, Schroder R, Simoes-Pires A, Battastini AM, Moreira JC. The curry spice curcumin selectively inhibits cancer cells growth in vitro and in preclinical model of glioblastoma. J Nutr Biochem. 2012;23:591–601.

67. Purkayastha S, Berliner A, Fernando SS, Ranasinghe B, Ray I, Tariq H, Banerjee P. Curcumin blocks brain tumor formation. Brain Res. 2009; 1266:130–8.

68. Sathyan P, Zinn PO, Marisetty AL, Liu B, Kamal MM, Singh SK, Bady P, Lu L, Wani KM, Veo BL, et al. Mir-21-Sox2 Axis Delineates Glioblastoma Subtypes with Prognostic Impact. J Neurosci. 2015;35:15097–112.

69. Schreck R, Albermann K, Baeuerle PA. Nuclear factor kappa B: an oxidative stress-responsive transcription factor of eukaryotic cells (a review). Free Radic Res Commun. 1992;17:221–37.

70. Rabbani ZN, Spasojevic I, Zhang X, Moeller BJ, Haberle S, Vasquez-Vivar J, Dewhirst MW, Vujaskovic Z, Batinic-Haberle I. Antiangiogenic action of redox-modulating Mn (III) meso-tetrakis (N-ethylpyridinium-2-yl) porphyrin, MnTE-2-PyP (5+), via suppression of oxidative stress in a mouse model of breast tumor. Free Radic Biol Med. 2009;47:992–1004.

71. Burdon RH, Gill V, Rice-Evans C. Oxidative stress and tumour cell proliferation. Free Radic Res Commun. 1990;11:65–76.

72. Sahu RP, Zhang R, Batra S, Shi Y, Srivastava SK. Benzyl isothiocyanate-mediated generation of reactive oxygen species causes cell cycle arrest and induces apoptosis via activation of MAPK in human pancreatic cancer cells. Carcinogenesis. 2009;30:1744–53.

73. Chung YM, Bae YS, Lee SY. Molecular ordering of ROS production, mitochondrial changes, and caspase activation during sodium salicylate-induced apoptosis. Free Radic Biol Med. 2003;34:434–42.

74. Diehn M, Cho RW, Lobo NA, Kalisky T, Dorie MJ, Kulp AN, Qian D, Lam JS, Ailles LE, Wong M, et al. Association of reactive oxygen species levels and radioresistance in cancer stem cells. Nature. 2009;458:780–3.

75. Ito K, Bernardi R, Morotti A, Matsuoka S, Saglio G, Ikeda Y, Rosenblatt J, Avigan DE, Teruya-Feldstein J, Pandolfi PP. PML targeting eradicates quiescent leukaemia-initiating cells. Nature. 2008;453:1072–8.

76. Guzman ML, Rossi RM, Karnischky L, Li X, Peterson DR, Howard DS, Jordan CT. The sesquiterpene lactone parthenolide induces apoptosis of human acute myelogenous leukemia stem and progenitor cells. Blood. 2005;105:4163–9.

77. Jin Y, Lu Z, Ding K, Li J, Du X, Chen C, Sun X, Wu Y, Zhou J, Pan J. Antineoplastic mechanisms of niclosamide in acute myelogenous leukemia stem cells: inactivation of the NF-kappaB pathway and generation of reactive oxygen species. Cancer Res. 2010;70:2516–27.

78. Lao CD, Ruffin MT, Normolle D, Heath DD, Murray SI, Bailey JM, Boggs ME, Crowell J, Rock CL, Brenner DE. Dose escalation of a curcuminoid formulation. BMC Complement Altern Med. 2006;6:10.

79. Cheng AL, Hsu CH, Lin JK, Hsu MM, Ho YF, Shen TS, Ko JY, Lin JT, Lin BR, Ming-Shiang W, et al. Phase I clinical trial of curcumin, a chemopreventive agent, in patients with high-risk or pre-malignant lesions. Anticancer Res. 2001;21:2895–900.

80. Ramalingam P, Ko YT. Enhanced oral delivery of curcumin from N-trimethyl chitosan surface-modified solid lipid nanoparticles: pharmacokinetic and brain distribution evaluations. Pharm Res. 2015;32:389–402.

81. Sasaki H, Sunagawa Y, Takahashi K, Imaizumi A, Fukuda H, Hashimoto T, Wada H, Katanasaka Y, Kakeya H, Fujita M, et al. Innovative preparation of curcumin for improved oral bioavailability. Biol Pharm Bull. 2011;34:660–5.

82. Zhongfa L, Chiu M, Wang J, Chen W, Yen W, Fan-Havard P, Yee LD, Chan KK. Enhancement of curcumin oral absorption and pharmacokinetics of curcuminoids and curcumin metabolites in mice. Cancer Chemother Pharmacol. 2012;69:679–89.

83. Zhou J, Atsina KB, Himes BT, Strohbehn GW, Saltzman WM. Novel delivery strategies for glioblastoma. Cancer J. 2012;18:89–99.

84. Kim JE, Patel M, Ruzevick J, Jackson CM, Lim M. STAT3 Activation in Glioblastoma: Biochemical and Therapeutic Implications. Cancers (Basel). 2014;6:376–95.

85. Stechishin OD, Luchman HA, Ruan Y, Blough MD, Nguyen SA, Kelly JJ, Cairncross JG, Weiss S. On-target JAK2/STAT3 inhibition slows disease progression in orthotopic xenografts of human glioblastoma brain tumor stem cells. Neuro Oncol. 2013;15:198–207.

86. Shirai K, Suzuki Y, Oka K, Noda SE, Katoh H, Suzuki Y, Itoh J, Itoh H, Ishiuchi S, Sakurai H, et al. Nuclear survivin expression predicts poorer prognosis in glioblastoma. J Neurooncol. 2009;91:353–8.

87. Kajiwara Y, Yamasaki F, Hama S, Yahara K, Yoshioka H, Sugiyama K, Arita K, Kurisu K. Expression of survivin in astrocytic tumors: correlation with malignant grade and prognosis. Cancer. 2003;97:1077–83.

12

Metabolomic profiling identifies distinct phenotypes for ASS1 positive and negative GBM

Lina Mörén[1], Richard Perryman[2], Tim Crook[3], Julia K. Langer[2], Kevin Oneill[2], Nelofer Syed[2*] and Henrik Antti[1*] [iD]

Abstract

Background: Tumour cells have a high demand for arginine. However, a subset of glioblastomas has a defect in the arginine biosynthetic pathway due to epigenetic silencing of the rate limiting enzyme argininosuccinate synthetase (ASS1). These tumours are auxotrophic for arginine and susceptible to the arginine degrading enzyme, pegylated arginine deiminase (ADI-PEG20). Moreover, ASS1 deficient GBM have a worse prognosis compared to ASS1 positive tumours. Since altered tumour metabolism is one of the hallmarks of cancer we were interested to determine if these two subtypes exhibited different metabolic profiles that could allow for their non-invasive detection as well as unveil additional novel therapeutic opportunities.

Methods: We looked for basal metabolic differences using one and two-dimensional gas chromatography-time-of-flight mass spectrometry (1D/2D GC-TOFMS) followed by targeted analysis of 29 amino acids using liquid chromatography-time-of-flight mass spectrometry (LC-TOFMS). We also looked for differences upon arginine deprivation in a single ASS1 negative and positive cell line (SNB19 and U87 respectively). The acquired data was evaluated by chemometric based bioinformatic methods.

Results: Orthogonal partial least squares-discriminant analysis (OPLS-DA) of both the 1D and 2D GC-TOFMS data revealed significant systematic difference in metabolites between the two subgroups with ASS1 positive cells generally exhibiting an overall elevation of identified metabolites, including those involved in the arginine biosynthetic pathway. Pathway and network analysis of the metabolite profile show that ASS1 negative cells have altered arginine and citrulline metabolism as well as altered amino acid metabolism. As expected, we observed significant metabolite perturbations in ASS negative cells in response to ADI-PEG20 treatment.

Conclusions: This study has highlighted significant differences in the metabolome of ASS1 negative and positive GBM which warrants further study to determine their diagnostic and therapeutic potential for the treatment of this devastating disease.

Keywords: Glioblastoma, Epigenetics, ASS1, Arginine, ADI-PEG20, Metabolomics, Chemometrics

Background

Glioblastoma (GBM) is the most common and most lethal primary brain tumour affecting adults of all ages. Despite improvements in imaging, surgical techniques, radiotherapy and chemotherapy the prognosis remains poor with a median overall survival typically around 12 months in optimally treated patients. This poor survival is attributed to the highly invasive nature of GBM, making complete surgical resection almost impossible resulting in tumour recurrence in most cases. In addition, these tumours exhibit a high degree of radio and chemo resistance [1, 2].

Extensive profiling of GBM has led to a greater understanding of the underlying biology of this disease. For example, the majority of genomic lesions identified to date lie in three core signalling pathways (receptor tyrosine kinase/RAS/phosphatidylinosintol 3 kinase (RTK/RAS/PI3K), p53 and retinoblastoma (RB) [3]. Hence

* Correspondence: n.syed@imperial.ac.uk; henrik.antti@umu.se
[2]John Fulcher Neuro-Oncology Laboratory, Imperial College London, London, UK
[1]Department of Chemistry, Umeå University, SE 901 87 Umeå, Sweden
Full list of author information is available at the end of the article

aberrant signalling through these pathways is likely to be essential for the development of GBM. Furthermore, these studies have identified four distinct molecular subclasses of GBM based on the enrichment of specific molecular alterations (proneural, classical, mesenchymal and neural). Interestingly, these subclasses were shown to have different responses to standard therapies [4].

This wealth of information has led to the development of several molecularly targeted therapies for GBM, some of which have shown promise in preclinical and clinical settings. However, most have failed to show promise in improving outcomes and hence the standard of care for GBM patients remains the same [5, 6].

Since cancer cells have a high reliance on glucose and amino acids to support their increased growth rate, one strategy to target them is the removal of an essential metabolic resource. This strategy has been successfully employed for the treatment of acute lymphoid leukaemia where asparaginase is the standard therapy in combination with chemotherapy for this cancer [7, 8].

From the initial observation that mycoplasma infection can kill cancer cells and spare normal cells [9] and the subsequent discovery that this was due an arginine degrading enzyme found in mycoplasma, arginine deiminase (ADI) [10, 11], there has been an explosion in the use of arginine deprivation as a therapeutic strategy for numerous cancers.

Arginine is a nonessential amino acid that fuels an array of metabolic reactions including nitric oxide synthesis, polyamines and amino acids such as glutamine and proline, all of which are important regulators of cell growth and survival [12]. Arginine is synthesized from aspartate and citrulline by two closely coupled enzymes of the urea cycle, argininosuccinate synthetase (ASS) and argininosuccinate lyase (ASL) with the former being the rate limiting step [13]. Healthy adults predominantly obtain arginine from dietary intake and from intracellular protein degradation but can also synthesize it when required and the level of synthesis is sufficient to meet their energy demands [14]. Tumour cells due to their rewired metabolism have a greater requirement for arginine and make use of the extracellular pools [15, 16]. Cancers that have reduced expression of ASS/ASL and unable to synthesise arginine become highly dependent on these pools and therefore susceptible to arginine deprivation therapy using arginine degrading enzymes [12, 17]. Although the mechanism of ASS/ASL downregulation is not completely understood, there is strong evidence for both promoter methylation and hypoxia-inducible factor-1α mediated transcriptional repression in some cancers [18, 19] and further mechanisms are likely to exist. Two enzymes that are continually being evaluated for their effectiveness in degrading arginine are: ADI-PEG20 (a pegylated form of ADI to reduce

immunogenicity in humans and extend half-life) and recombinant human arginase 1 [20–23]. ADI-PEG20 degrades arginine to citrulline and ammonia and arginase 1 degrades it to ornithine and urea. Since the first reports of arginine deprivation in melanoma [24] and hepatocellular carcinoma (HCC) [25], the list of cancer types that are amenable to this therapeutic strategy is constantly growing and includes prostate, breast, ovarian, lung, sarcoma and malignant pleural mesothelioma to name but a few including our own study in GBM [26, 27]. Since most of these studies have used ADI-PEG20 to degrade arginine, this enzyme has been extensively evaluated [28]. Many of these studies revealed mechanistic insights into the molecular effects of arginine deprivation in ASS deficient tumours identifying additional vulnerabilities prompting the use of other agents in combination with this strategy to achieve more effective killing. For example the use of TRAIL in mesothelioma [29], cisplatin in multiple tumour types [28], chloroquine in sarcomas [30] and 5FU in HCC [31].

In contrast, given the diverse role of arginine in numerous metabolic pathways there are far fewer studies investigating the metabolic effects of arginine deprivation and to our knowledge no studies have been performed in GBM. One such study includes our own study in bladder cancer where we observed ASS negative cells had increased uptake of thymidine which becomes suppressed upon ADI-PEG20 treatment. Since thymidine can be imaged by positron emission tomography, its reduced uptake can serve as a biomarker of response to therapy [32]. Similarly, Locke et al. [33] through their metabolomic analysis identified that ASS1 negative mesothelioma have a dependency for polyamine metabolism and that ADI-PEG20 decreases polyamine metabolites. Thus, this finding provides a dual synthetic lethal strategy for ASS negative mesothelioma with ADI-PEG20 and inhibition of polyamine synthesis. Another study by Kremer et al. [34] identified a potential synthetic lethal interaction with ADI-PEG20 and glutamine inhibition in sarcoma, as a consequence of discovering up-regulation of glutamine anerplerosis and serine biosynthesis upon ADI-PEG20 therapy. To our knowledge, there are no studies specifically looking at basal metabolic differences between ASS negative and positive GBM tumours.

Metabolic reprogramming manifested as altered nutrient uptake and use has been proposed to be a hallmark of cancer. Since this reprogramming is thought to be essential for rapid cancer cell proliferation, a metabolomic analysis of cancer metabolism will paint a broad picture of the altered pathways and their interactions with each other. Metabolomics is the profiling of metabolites within a cell, the levels of which integrate the effects of gene regulation, post-transcriptional regulation, pathway interactions, and environmental perturbations [35, 36]. Thus, this downstream synthesis of diverse signals ultimately makes metabolites and patterns thereof direct molecular readouts of cell status that reflect a meaningful physiological phenotype.

Combined with bioinformatic approaches that consider the multivariate interaction between multiple variables (i.e. chemometric bioinformatics), metabolomics can aid to detect patterns of metabolites as biomarkers (latent biomarkers) to better map and predict complex metabolic events [37, 38].

The present study was carried out to investigate our hypothesis that metabolomic analysis, represented here by 1D and 2D GC-TOFMS combined with chemometric bioinformatics, can discriminate between ASS1 positive and ASS1 negative GBM cell lines and potentially identify metabolic biomarkers for the non-invasive detection of these subtypes and unveil additional novel targets for their treatment. Novel treatment strategies are desperately needed as currently there are no effective therapies for this devastating tumour.

Methods
Cell culture
All GBM cell lines used in this study are negative for the IDH1 mutation (previously sequenced in our lab) and were obtained from ATCC. ASS negative (LN229, SNB19, GAMG) and ASS positive (U118, T98G, U87) GBM cell lines were plated into 6 replicate wells of a 6 well plate at a density of 1.5×10^5 cells/well in 3 ml of DMEM or MEM media (T98G) containing 10% fetal calf serum (FCS). Supernatants and cell pellets were collected 48 h after plating and stored at -80 °C until required. Control wells containing media alone were included for normalization purposes.

ADI-PEG20 treatment
SNB19 and U87 cells, cultured in DMEM + 10% FBS and normal human astrocytes, cultured in speciality media provided by lonza were seeded in replicates ($n = 12$) at 8×10^4 cells per well in 6-well dishes (Corning, NY, USA). 24 h post seeding, cells were washed with phosphate buffered saline (PBS) and cultured in the presence or absence of ADI-PEG20 (1 µg/ml) in media containing, 1 mM citrulline and 10% fetal FBS. ADI-PEG20 was added at the start of the experiment and no fresh media was added to any of the experimental plates before harvesting. ADI-PEG20 treated and untreated media ($n = 3$) was included for normalization purposes. 48 h after ADI-PEG20 treatment replicate samples for each condition ($n = 3$) were harvested, collecting both spent media and cells for GC-TOFMS metabolomic analysis. Additional replicates ($n = 3$) of each condition were collected for total cell count determination.

Analytical strategy
In an attempt to cover a large proportion of the metabolome and to detect and identify overlapping compounds, samples were screened for metabolites using both 1D and 2D GC-TOFMS. The results obtained from this initial screen were verified by a targeted amino acid analysis using LC-TOFMS.

Sample preparation
Frozen samples (supernatants and cell pellets) were thawed at room temperature and 900 µl of extraction solution (90% methanol, 10% water, 7 internal standards (Salicylic acid, myristic acid, hexadecanoic acid, cholesterol, succinic acid, glutamic acid och sucrose; 7 ng/µl)) were added to 100 µl of supernatant and to the cell pellet. Two tungsten beads were also added to the pellets. Samples were extracted using a MM301 vibration Mill (Retsch GmbH & Co. KG, Haan, Germany) for 2 min at 30 Hz and placed on ice for 2 h and centrifuged for 15 min at 14,000 rpm at 4 °C. 200 µl of the supernatants were transferred to vials and evaporated to complete dryness before being stored at -80 °C. Before 1D and 2D GC-TOFMS analysis the samples were methoxymated with 30 µl of methoxyamine solution in pyridine (15 µg/µl) first at 70 °C for 1 h and then at room temperature for 16 h. Thereafter, the samples were trimethylsilylated with 30 µl of MSTFA at room temperature for 1 h before the addition of 30 µl of heptane (containing 0.5 µg of methyl stearate). Prior to analysis, the samples were randomized and analysed together with a series of n-alkanes (C_{12}-C_{32}) to allow retention indexes to be calculated.

For the ADI-PEG20 experiment, samples were randomized, defrosted at room temperature and vortexed. For the cell media fraction, 200 µl were transferred to individual microcentrifuge tubes. A quality control sample was prepared from a pool of each sample, and 200 µl were transferred to individual microcentrifuge tubes. 1.5 ml of methanol was added to each sample, mixed for 5 min and spun at 10,000 g for 10 min at 4 °C. 1.3 ml of supernatant was transferred to individual silylated glass tubes and evaporated to dryness at 40 °C under nitrogen gas in a concentration evaporator (Turbovap LV, Biotage, Uppsala, Sweden).

For the cellular fraction, 200 µl cell lysate was transferred to individual microcentrifuge tubes and 1.3 ml extraction mixture (water:MeOH [2:10]) was added, giving a final methanol concentration of 80% together with the cell lysate. Samples were vortexed for 5 min for cellular disruption and extracted on ice for 20 min, following centrifugation at 4 °C at 17,500 g for 10 min. 1.4 ml supernatant was transferred to silylated glass tubes and dried at 40 °C under nitrogen gas with a concentration evaporator.

Both individual and pooled standards were prepared, making a stock solution in water (10 mg/ml). Individual samples were diluted in methanol (0.005 mg/ml), and 100 µl were transferred to silylated glass tubes. Pooled standards were diluted to 300 µl water containing metabolite standards and 200 µl methanol.

GC-TOFMS

One µl sample was injected splitless by an Agilent 7683 Series autosampler (Agilent, Atlanta, GA) into an Agilent 6980 GC equipped with a 10 m × 0.18 mm i.d. fused-silica capillary column chemically bonded with 0.18 µm DB5-MS stationary phase (J&W Scientific, Folsom, CA). The injector temperature was 270 °C. Helium was used as carrier gas with a constant flow rate of 1 ml/min. The purge time was 60 s at a purge flow rate of 20 ml/min and an equilibration time of 1 min per analysis. Initially, the column temperature was kept at 70 °C for 2 min and then increased to 320 °C at 30 °C/min, where it was kept for 2 min. The column efflu-ent was introduced into the ion source of a Pegasus III TOFMS (Leco Corp., St Joseph, MI). The transfer line temperature was 250 °C and the ion source temperature 200 °C. Ions were generated by a 70 eV electron beam at a current of 2.0 mA. Masses were acquired from m/z 50 to 800 at a rate of 30 spectra/s, and the acceleration voltage was turned on after a solvent delay of 165 s.

The acquired data was exported to MATLAB 7.11.0 (R2014b) (Mathworks, Natick, MA) as NetCDF files. An in-house script was used for alignment, peak detection, mass spectrum deconvolution, mass spectra library search for identification and calculation of peak height/area. To identify the detected compounds, the mass spectral pro-files and retention indices were compared to spectra in an in-house spectra library established at Swedish Metabolo-mics Centre (SMC) (www.swedishmetabolomicscentre.se).

For the ADI-PEG20 treatment experiment, samples were subjected to GC-TOFMS on a Pegasus GC-TOFMS (Leco Corp., St Joseph, MI, USA), connected with an Agilent 7890 gas chromatograph, using a fused silica capillary column (Agilent J&W Scientific), with 0.25 µm thickness and open split interface. Under helium as carrier gas, samples were injected, with constant temperatures for injection (220 °C), transfer (280 °C), ion source (250 °C). Primary oven temperatures were programmed at 70 °C for 0.2 min, raised to 270 °C for 5 min and further increased to 310 °C for 11 min. 70 eV electron beams were used for the ionization and masses were recorded from 40 to 600 m/z at a rate of 20 spectra/s with the detector voltage set at 1650 V.

Gas chromatograms were baseline corrected, de-convoluted, noise-reduced, smoothed, library matched and areas were calculated with ChromaTOF software (LecoCorp. v 4.4). Signal-to-noise ratio above 150 were analysed. Putative analyte identities were found by comparing MS spectra with RI of the US National Insti-tute of Science and Technology (NIST) library, as well as the Fiehn library, Golm Metabolome Database, Human Metabolome Database and in-house databases.

2D GC-TOFMS

The samples were analysed on a Pegasus 4D (Leco Corp., St Joseph, MI, USA) equipped with an Agilent 6890 gas chromatograph (Agilent Technologies, Palo Alto, GA, USA), a secondary gas chromatograph oven, a quad-jet thermal modulator, and a time-of-flight mass spectrom-eter. Leco's ChromaTOF software was used for setup and data acquisition. The column set used for the GCxGC separation was a polar BPX-50 (30 m × 0.25 mm × 0.25 µm; SGE, Ringwood, Australia) as first-dimension column and a non-polar VF-1MS (1.5 m × 0.15 mm × 0.15 µm; J&W Scientific Inc., Folsom, CA, USA) for the second-dimension column. Splitless injection of 1 µl sam-ple aliquots was performed with an Agilent 7683B auto sampler at an injection temperature of 270 °C (2 respect-ively 5 pre/post-wash cycles were used with hexane). The purge time was 60 s with a rate of 20 ml/min and helium was used as carrier gas with a flow rate of 1 ml/min. The temperature program for the primary oven started with an initial temperature of 60 °C for 2 min, followed by a temperature increase of 4 °C/min up to 300 °C and where the temperature was held for 2 min. The secondary oven maintained the same temperature program but with an offset of + 15 °C compared to the primary oven. The modulation time was 5 s with a hot pulse time of 0.8 s and a 1.7 s cooling time between the stages. The MS transfer line had a temperature of 300 °C and the ion source 250 °C. 70 eV electron beams were used for the ionization and masses were recorded from 50 to 550 m/z at a rate of 100 spectra/s with detector voltage set at 1780 V.

Baseline correction, peak detection, mass spectrum deconvolution, mass spectra library search for identification and calculation of peak height/area was done in Leco's ChromaTOF software. For peak picking a signal-to-noise ratio of 10 was used. The library search was performed against publicly available mass spectral libraries from US National Institute of Science and Technology (NIST) and from the Max Planck Institute in Golm [39] together with in-house libraries established at SMC. csv-files (comma-separated values) containing peak information for each of the samples was exported. The csv-files were imported into the data processing software Guineu (1.0.3 VTT; Espoo, Finland) [40] for alignment and filtering.

Amino acid analysis

Derivatization of amino acids was achieved using the AccQ-Tag kit obtained from Waters (Millford, MA) as specified in the manufacturer's instructions. An amino acid standard mixture including 29 amino acids was prepared and diluted into eight concentrations ranging from 20 pmol to 0.1 pmol. An internal standard, norvaline [10 pmol/μl] was added to each sample and the amino-acid standards mixture. The samples were analysed on a Waters Acquity UPLC system coupled to a Micromass LCT Premier mass spectrometer (Waters, Millford, MA) operated in W-mode. The acquired data was exported as NetCDF files. MATLAB 7.11.0 (R2014b) (Mathworks, Natick, MA) was used with an in-house script for alignment and extraction of the integrated peak area for each amino acid.

Pattern recognition and statistical analysis

The data from the cell pellet and the cell supernatant from the different analytical methods were analysed separately. Prior to any data analysis, data from the cell medium was subtracted from the cell supernatant data to minimize the influence of the cell medium in further investigations. Data from the amino acid analysis data was normalized to the internal standard norvaline.

A chemometric bioinformatics approach using pattern recognition based on multivariate projection methods was used to detect systematic patterns in the data associated with ASS1 status and the corresponding response to ADI-PEG20 treatment. In this way patterns of co-varying metabolites can be detected and evaluated both predictively as latent biomarkers and mechanistically by comparing the involved metabolites to known biochemical pathways.

To obtain an initial overview of the systematic variation in the data and detect deviating samples (outliers), the data was analysed using principal component analysis (PCA) [41], an unsupervised multivariate projection method focusing on the maximum variation in the data (not shown). Thereafter, to investigate potential differences between ASS positive and ASS negative cell lines as well as to evaluate the effect of arginine deprivation therapy by ADI-PEG20, OPLS-DA [42] was used. OPLS-DA is a supervised multivariate analysis method where the systematic pattern differences between pre-defined classes in the data are examined. Variable selection was used to extract metabolites responsible for the separation in the calculated OPLS-DA models. Model weight values (w*), i.e. variable contribution values for the pre-defined sample class separations, were extracted and metabolites with low w*- values ($|w^*| < 0.05$), i.e. variables unrelated to the class separation were discarded [43]. All OPLS-DA models were validated using cross-validation and p-values for the cross-validated model were calculated using ANOVA [44]. A univariate p-value for each metabolite was calculated using the Mann-Whitney U-test.

Pathway and network analysis

Identified metabolites were subjected to pathway analysis using the software Ingenuity Pathway Analysis (IPA). Accession numbers of detected metabolites (HMDB, PubChem, and KEGG Identifiers) were listed in MS Excel and imported into IPA to map the canonical pathways and generate networks of interacting biological entities. Data were submitted as fold change values (ratios) between ASS positive and ASS negative cells. Comprehensive pathway and network analyses were performed. Downstream biological processes were scored in accordance to the ontology support using Ingenuity Knowledge Base (www.ingenuity.com).

Results

GC-TOFMS analysis reveals metabolic differences between ASS negative and ASS positive GBM

We previously demonstrated that ASS negative GBM (deficient in the arginine biosynthetic pathway) can be targeted by arginine deprivation therapy using ADI-PEG20 whereas ASS positive GBM are unaffected due to their ability to endogenously synthesize arginine [27]. (It is important to note that these cells were negative for the IDH1 mutation (previously screened in our lab), a feature that can significantly impact on the metabolome. In an attempt to identify additional metabolic vulnerabilities between these two subgroups of GBM, we profiled the metabolome of a panel of ASS negative (LN229, SNB19 and GAMG) and ASS positive (U118 and T98G) GBM cell lines using 1D and 2D GC-TOFMS. GBM cells were cultured for 48 h as described in materials and methods and both the cell supernatants and cell pellets were harvested for analysis.

Using 1D GC-TOFMS, we identified 76 and 83 unique metabolites in the supernatant and cell pellet respectively by comparing mass spectra and retention indices to existing and available compound libraries. In contrast, using 2D GC-TOFMS a greater number of peaks were retained in both fractions (815 in supernatant and 317 in cell pellet) after filtering in Guineu (1.0.3 VTT; Espoo, Finland). Of these peaks we could adequately identify 89 unique metabolites in the supernatants and 83 in cell pellets.

The data generated using both 1D and 2D GC-TOFMS was subjected separately to multivariate analysis by means of OPLS-DA to model systematic differences in metabolite patterns between ASS positive and ASS negative cell lines. This supervised multivariate projection method allows for a division of the variation in the data into a predictive part which is related to a specified difference i.e. ASS1 status, and an orthogonal part which is unrelated to this difference. These variation sources can be overviewed and interpreted on the sample level in the OPLS-DA scores and on the variable level (contributing metabolite patterns) in the OPLS-DA loadings. This analysis revealed a clear systematic difference between ASS1 positive and ASS1 negative cell lines using both 1D and 2D GC-TOFMS data in both the cell pellet and supernatant

(Fig. 1). Further analysis of the metabolites contributing to this difference revealed an elevation of those involved in the arginine biosynthetic pathway in ASS positive cells compared to ASS negative cells (Tables 1 and 2). Moreover, ANOVA of the cross validated model showed a statistical significance in the pattern of extracted metabolites i.e. 1D GC-TOFMS cell supernatant, $p = 1.84*10^{-5}$ (63 metabolites), 1D GC-TOFMS cell pellet, $p = 0.03$ (50 metabolites), 2D GC-TOFMS cell supernatant $p = 0.0007$ (180 metabolites), 2D GC-TOFMS cell pellet, $p = 0.004$ (122 metabolites). This analysis also revealed a large number of metabolite differences that were unrelated to the arginine metabolic pathway. This is shown in Tables 1 and 2 which summarizes all identified metabolites, their p-values and the metabolic pathway they belong to.

Amino acid analysis

We next proceeded to validate some of the metabolites identified in our global screen using LC-MS by specifically targeting a selection of 29 amino acids. We included those involved in the arginine biosynthetic pathway

primarily to determine if we could detect differences in this pathway between ASS positive and ASS negative cell lines, in line with our hypothesis. As well as successfully detecting all 29 amino acids by LC-MS, we were by means of OPLS-DA also able to detect metabolite differences that were related to the arginine biosynthetic pathway in these cell lines (Fig. 2). In the cell supernatant, glutamic acid, proline, ornithine, arginine and citrulline where elevated in ASS positive cell lines, all of which are included in the arginine biosynthetic pathway. Ammonia and leucine where elevated in the ASS negative cell lines. In the cell pellet, ammonia, glutamic acid, ornithine, arginine and citrulline were elevated in the ASS positive cell lines, all of which are included in the arginine biosynthetic pathway. Serine, glycine, GABA, tyrosine, methionine, valine, isoleucine and N-acetylornithine were elevated in the ASS negative cell lines.

The final cross-validated OPLS-DA score plot based on the pattern of these 29 amino acids showed the same class separation as detected using the global GC-TOFMS screening (supernatant $p = 0.01$, pellet $p = 0.2$).

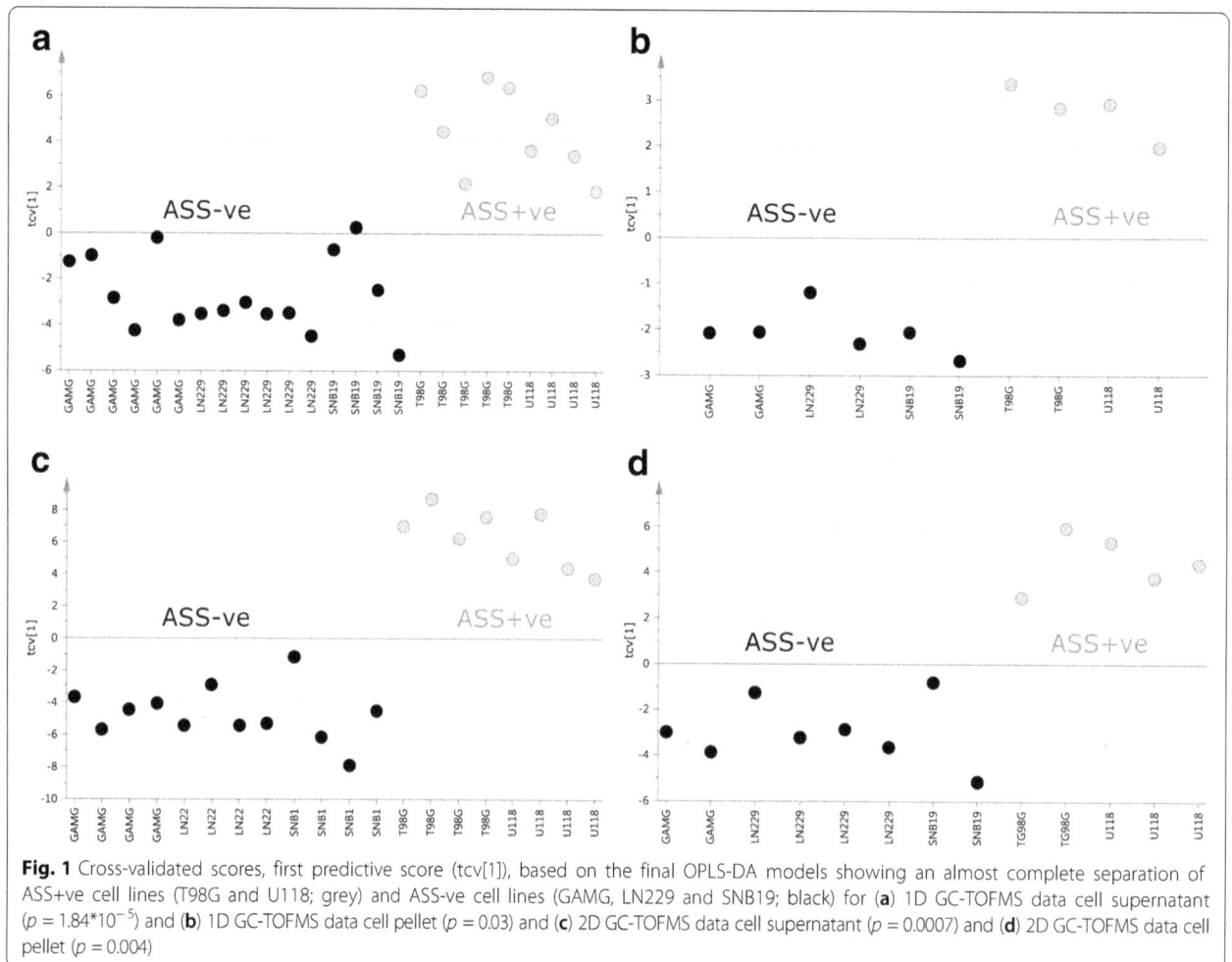

Fig. 1 Cross-validated scores, first predictive score (tcv[1]), based on the final OPLS-DA models showing an almost complete separation of ASS+ve cell lines (T98G and U118; grey) and ASS-ve cell lines (GAMG, LN229 and SNB19; black) for (**a**) 1D GC-TOFMS data cell supernatant ($p = 1.84*10^{-5}$) and (**b**) 1D GC-TOFMS data cell pellet ($p = 0.03$) and (**c**) 2D GC-TOFMS data cell supernatant ($p = 0.0007$) and (**d**) 2D GC-TOFMS data cell pellet ($p = 0.004$)

Table 1 Metabolites affected in the cell supernatant

Pathway	Metabolite	1D GC-MS	p-value	2D GC-MS	p-value	AA Analysis	p-value
Alanine And Aspartate Metabolism	Aspargine	↑	0.000			↑	0.002
	Alanine	↑	0.000			↑	0.007
	Aspartic Acid			↑	0.029	↓	0.135
Amino Sugar Metabolism	N-Acetyl Glucosamine	↑	0.000				
	N-Acetyl Mannosamine	↑	0.000				
Beta-Alanine Metabolism	Pantothenic Acid	↓	0.292	↑	0.009		
Citric Acid Cycle	Succinic Acid	↑	0.010				
Creatine Metabolism	Creatinine	↑	0.003				
	Cystein					↑	0.121
Cysteine And Methionine Metabolism	Cystein (2 Derivative)					↑	0.005
	Cystine	↑	0.005			↑	0.003
	Methionine	↑	0.003			↑	0.044
Fatty Acid Biosynthesis	3-Hydroxybutyric Acid			↑	0.004		
	Butanoic Acid			↑	0.000		
	Hexadecanoic Acid	↓	0.200				
	Fructose-1- Phosphate	↑	0.050				
Fructose And Mannose Degradation	Mannose	↓	0.020				
	Fructose	↑	0.011				
Galactose Metabolism	Galactose	↓	0.225				
Glutamate Metabolism	Glutamic Acid	↑	0.000			↑	0.247
	GABA					↑	0.001
	Glutamine	↑	0.000	↑	0.009		
Glutathione Metabolism	Pyroglutamic Acid	↑	0.000				
Glycerolipid Metabolism	Ethanolamine	↑	0.010				
Glycine, Serine And Threonine Metabolism	Glycine	↑	0.068	↑	0.012	↑	0.152
	Sarcosine	↑	0.000				
	Serine			↑	0.007	↑	0.020
	Threonine	↑	0.017			↑	0.155
Glycolysis. Gluconeogenesis.	Glucose	↓	0.143				
Pyruvate Metabolism	Glyceric Acid	↑	0.000				
	Lactic Acid	↑	0.002				
	Malic Acid	↑	0.039				
Histidine Metabolism	Histidine			↑	0.033	↑	0.027
Homocysteine Degradation	3-Methyl-2-Ketobutyric Acid			↑	0.000		
Inositol Metabolism	Inositol	↑	0.002				
Lysine Metabolism	Lysine	↑	0.044	↑	0.008	↑	0.191
	Lysine (2 Derivative)					↑	0.027
Nicotinate And Nicotinamide Metabolism	Nicotinamide	↑	0.021	↑	0.001		
	Arabinose	↑	0.003				
Nucleotide Sugar. Pentose Metabolism	Arabitol	↑	0.000				
Nucleotide Sugars Metabolism	Xylose	↑	0.004				
Pentose Phosphate Pathway	Gluconic Acid 1.4-Lactone	↑	0.034				
	Ribofuranose			↑	0.013		
	Ribose	↑	0.000	↑	0.028		
	Sedoheptulose-7-Phosphate	↑	0.276				

Table 1 Metabolites affected in the cell supernatant *(Continued)*

Pathway	Metabolite	1D GC-MS	p-value	2D GC-MS	p-value	AA Analysis	p-value
Phenylalanine Metabolism	Phenylalanine	↑	0.000	↑	0.022		
Purine Metabolism	Allantoin	↑	0.051				
Pyrimidine Metabolism	Uracil	↓	0.024				
Riboflavin Metabolism	Ribitol	↑	0.000				
Sugar. Sugar Substitute. Starch	Erythritol	↑	0.002				
Tryptophan Metabolism	Tryptophan					↑	0.035
Tyrosine Metabolism	Tyrosine	↑	0.034	↑	0.010	↑	0.052
Urea Cycle. Arginine and Proline Metabolism	Ammonia					↓	0.038
	Arginine	↑	0.015	↑	0.010	↑	0.070
(Arginine biosynthetic pathway)	Argininosuccinate	↑	0.021				
	Asymetrical-N.N- Dimethylarginine	↑	0.018				
	Citrulline					↑	0.098
	Citrulline (Arginine)	↑	0.016				
	Citrulline (Ornithine)	↑	0.019				
	Hydroxyproline			↑			
	Ornithine (2 Derivative)					↑	0.000
	Ornithine	↑	0.006			↑	0.156
	Proline	↑	0.000			↑	0.000
	Urea	↑	0.058	↑	0.001		
	2-Keto-3-Methylvaleric Acid			↑	0.002		
Valine. Leucine And Isoleucine Degradation	2-Oxoisocaproic Acid	↑	0.002	↑	0.000		
	Isoleucine	↑	0.008	↑	0.033	↓	0.373
	Leucine	↑	0.056			↓	0.253
	Valine	↑	0.010	↑	0.002	↓	0.132
Other	2-Aminobutyric Acid	↑	0.000				
	2-Deoxy-Galactose	↑	0.002				
	Allothreonine	↑	0.010	↑	0.000		
	Cellotriose	↓	0.224				
	Ellagic Acid	↓	0.293				
	Gluconic Acid	↓	0.095				
	Isoerythritol	↑	0.000				
	Mannitol	↓	0.031				
	Pentanoic Acid			↑	0.000		
	Propanoic Acid			↑	0.001		
	Silanamine			↑	0.021		
	Sorbose	↑	0.002				
	Xylitol	↑	0.000				

↑ Elevated in ASS+ve cell lines, ↓ lowered in ASS+ve cell lines. *p*-values was calculated using a Mann-Whitney U-test

ASS positive and ASS negative GBM have different metabolic responses to arginine deprivation induced by ADI-PEG20 treatment

To investigate the metabolic response of these different GBM cell populations to arginine deprivation, a representative ASS negative (SNB19) and ASS positive (U87) cell line was treated with or without the arginine degrading enzyme, ADI-PEG20 (1 μg/ml) for 48 h and both supernatants and cell pellets were analysed by 1D GC-TOFMS. We included normal human astrocytes (non-tumour cells), and media alone in this analysis. The data generated from the 1D–GC-TOFMS analysis of the cell supernatants was subjected to OPLS-DA in order to obtain an overview of the metabolic variation between the samples. As can be seen in Fig. 3, the second predictive component, shows a unique effect in the ASS

Table 2 Metabolites affected in the cell pellet

Pathway	Metabolite	1D GC-MS	p-value	2D GC-MS	p-value	AA Analysis	p-value
Alanine And Aspartate Metabolism	Aspargine	↑	0.097			↑	0.077
	Alanine	↑	0.051	↑	0.274	↑	0.274
	Aspartic Acid			↑	0.068	↑	0.356
	Beta-Alanine	↑	0.511	↑	0.354		
Linoleic Acid Metabolism	Linoleic Acid			↑	0.324		
Amino Sugar Metabolism	N-Acetyl Glucosamine	↓	0.080				
Beta-Alanine Metabolism	Pantothenic Acid			↓	0.080		
Citric Acid Cycle	Alpha-Ketoglutaric Acid	↓	0.127	↓	0.047		
	Citric Acid			↓	0.263		
	Fumaric Acid			↑	0.329		
Creatine Metabolism	Creatinine	↓	0.165	↓	0.042		
	Cysteine	↓	0.113			↑	0.200
Cysteine And Methionine Metabolism	Methionine			↓	0.382	↓	0.619
Dipeptide	Glycylvaline	↑	0.168				
Fatty Acid Biosynthesis	Dodecanoic Acid	↓	0.649				
	Hexadecanoic Acid	↓	0.336				
	Mannose	↓	0.252				
Fructose And Mannose Degradation	Sorbitol-6-Phosphate (Fragment)	↑	0.600				
Galactose Metabolism	Galactose	↓	0,407				
Glutamate Metabolism	Glutamic Acid	↑	0.535			↑	0.195
	Glutamine	↑	0.651			↑	0.412
	GABA					↓	0.466
Glutathione Metabolism	Pyroglutamic Acid	↓	0.366	↓	0.125		
Glycerol Phosphate Shuttle	Glycerol-2-Phosphate	↑	0.184				
	Glycerol-3-Phosphate	↑	0.005	↑	0.003		
Glycerolipid Metabolism	Ethanolamine	↑	0.658				
	Serine			↓	0.081	↓	0.553
Glycine, Serine And Threonine Metabolism	Glycine	↓	0.487	↓	0.085	↓	0.157
	Threonine			↓	0.301	↑	0.033
	Sarcosine	↑	0.197				
Glycolysis, Gluconeogenesis, Pyruvate Metabolism	Fructose-6-Phosphate	↑	0.103				
	Glucose	↓	0.341				
Glycolysis, Gluconeogenesis, Pyruvate Metabolism	Glucose-6-Phosphate	↑	0.174				
	Glyceric Acid	↑	0.011				
	Glyceric Acid-2-Phosphate			↑	0.227		
	Glyceric Acid-3-Phosphate	↑	0.320	↑	0.228		
	Pyruvic Acid	↓	0.049	↓	0.000		
Homocysteine Degradation	3-Methyl-2-Ketobutyric Acid			↑	0.051		
Inositol Metabolism	Inositol	↓	0.066				
Lysine Metabolism	Lysine			↓	0.128	↑	0.404
	Lysine 2 Derivative					↑	0.128
	2-Amino-Adipic Acid			↑	0.043		
Nicotinate And Nicotinamide Metabolism	Nicotinamide			↓	0.371		
Nucleotide Sugar, Pentose Metabolism	Arabitol	↑	0.294				

Table 2 Metabolites affected in the cell pellet *(Continued)*

Pathway	Metabolite	1D GC-MS	p-value	2D GC-MS	p-value	AA Analysis	p-value
Oxidative Phosphorylation	Pyrophosphate			↑	0.377		
Pentose Phosphate Pathway	Erythrose-4-Phosphate			↑	0.007		
	Glucaric Acid 1,4 Lactone	↓	0.622				
	Ribofuranose			↓	0.213		
	Ribose			↓	0.359		
	Ribose-5-Phosphate	↑	0.137				
Polyamine Metabolism	Putrescine	↓	0.653				
	Spermidine	↑	0.244				
Purine Metabolism	Adenine			↓	0.265		
	Hypoxanthine			↑	0.119		
Pyrimidine Metabolism	Uracil	↑	0.445				
	Uridine	↑	0.001				
Sugar, Sugar Substitute, Starch	Erythritol			↓	0.270		
Taurine And Hypotaurine Metabolism	Taurine					↑	0.282
Tryptophan Metabolism	Tryptophan					↑	0.104
Tyrosine Metabolism	Tyrosine			↓	0.221	↓	0.759
Urea Cycle, Arginine and	Ammonia					↑	0.258
Proline Metabolism	Arginine	↑	0.251			↑	0.502
(Arginine biosynthetic pathway)	Asymetrical-N,N-Dimethylarginine	↑	0.253				
	Citrulline (Arginine)	↑	0.247				
	Citrulline (Ornthine)	↑	0.193				
	Citrulline					↑	0.122
	N-Acetylornithine					↓	0.370
	Ornithine	↑	0.313	↑	0.219	↑	0.010
	2-Oxoisocaproic Acid	↑	0.600				
Valine, Leucine And Isoleucine Degradation	Isoleucine			↓	0.156	↓	0.550
	Leucine			↓	0.367		
	Valine					↓	0.085
Other	1,2-Ethandimine			↓	0.007		
	1,3,5-Trioxepane			↓	0.085		
	1-Mo nostearoylgly cer o l			↓	0.373		
	2-Pyrrolidone-5-Carboxylic Acid			↓	0.179		
	Aminomalonic Acid			↓	0.252		
	Cadaverine	↑	0.289				
	Cellotriose	↑	0.042				
	Dihydroxyacetonephosphate	↑	0.096	↑	0.195		
	Elaidic Acid			↑	0.165		
	Glucopyranose			↑	0.198		
	N-Acetyl Glutamyl Phosphate					↑	0.362
	Nonanoic Acid	↓	0.264	↓	0.144		
	Phosphoric Acid			↑	0.013		
	Pyrazine			↓	0.179		
	Stearic Acid			↑	0.357		
	Xylitol	↓	0.233				

↑ Elevated in ASS+ve cell lines, ↓ lowered in ASS+ve cell lines. *p*-values was calculated using a Mann-Whitney U-test

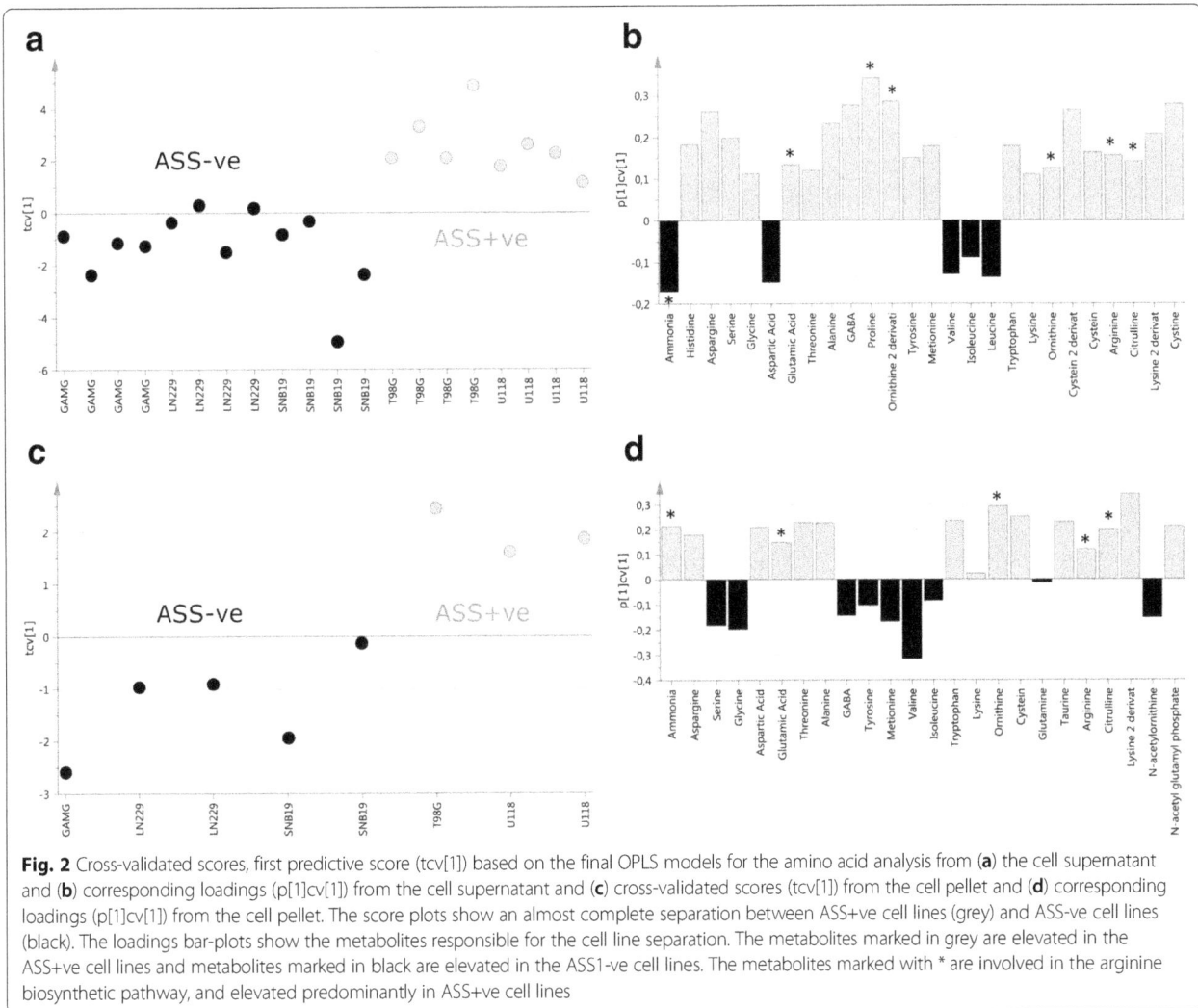

Fig. 2 Cross-validated scores, first predictive score (tcv[1]) based on the final OPLS models for the amino acid analysis from (**a**) the cell supernatant and (**b**) corresponding loadings (p[1]cv[1]) from the cell supernatant and (**c**) cross-validated scores (tcv[1]) from the cell pellet and (**d**) corresponding loadings (p[1]cv[1]) from the cell pellet. The score plots show an almost complete separation between ASS+ve cell lines (grey) and ASS-ve cell lines (black). The loadings bar-plots show the metabolites responsible for the cell line separation. The metabolites marked in grey are elevated in the ASS+ve cell lines and metabolites marked in black are elevated in the ASS1-ve cell lines. The metabolites marked with * are involved in the arginine biosynthetic pathway, and elevated predominantly in ASS+ve cell lines

negative cells in response to ADI-PEG20 treatment ($p = 0.001$), while the ASS positive cells and normal astrocytes remain unchanged in that direction (metabolite signature). The first predictive component showed a difference associated with ADI-PEG20 treatment in astrocytes suggesting a general unspecific increase in metabolite concentration in those cells after treatment (not shown).

Pathway and network analysis

To identify pathways that are most significantly altered between ASS negative and ASS positive cells, we performed pathway analysis using the IPA software of all the metabolite alterations detected using all three analytical methods. The analysis revealed the signalling and metabolic pathways and biological processes that are most significantly perturbed between these cells such as transfer of ribonucleic acid charging, super pathway of citrulline metabolism, arginine degradation VI, citrulline biosynthesis, arginine degradation I, proline biosynthesis

II, urea cycle, glycine degradation, asparagine biosynthesis 1 and glutamate receptor signalling. These hits were consistent between all three datasets in the supernatant. In summary, these results indicate an alteration in citrulline and arginine metabolism between these two populations. Similar patterns were observed in the cell pellets with transfer ribonucleic acid charging being amongst the top 10 hits. Interestingly, large shifts in amino acid metabolism were observed in the extract, particularly with the amino acids alanine and glycine. The degradation of arginine in ASS negative cells to its respective products is decreased and α-ketoglutarate levels are concurrently increased, possibly due to lack of ornithine amino transferase activity. In the greater context of citrulline biosynthesis, the convergence of multiple pathways for citrulline production is observed. Decreases in both alanine and glutamate with corresponding increases in α-ketoglutarate and pyruvate suggests that ASS negative cells are converting less pyruvate to alanine which is one of the by-products of high

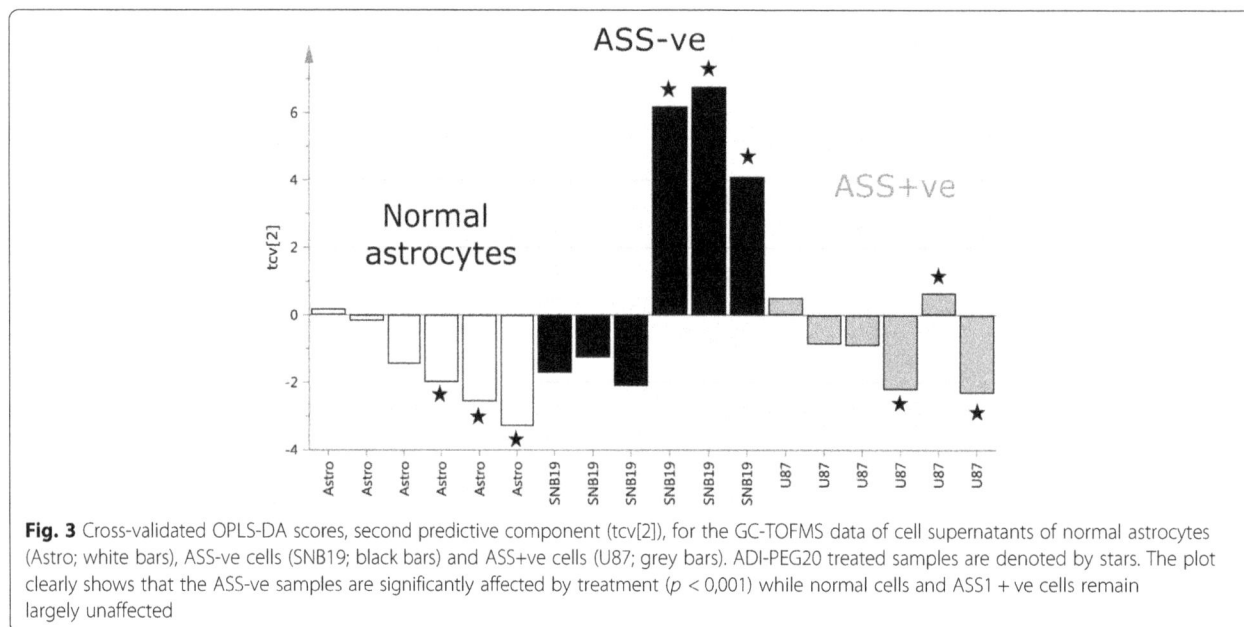

Fig. 3 Cross-validated OPLS-DA scores, second predictive component (tcv[2]), for the GC-TOFMS data of cell supernatants of normal astrocytes (Astro; white bars), ASS-ve cells (SNB19; black bars) and ASS+ve cells (U87; grey bars). ADI-PEG20 treated samples are denoted by stars. The plot clearly shows that the ASS-ve samples are significantly affected by treatment ($p < 0,001$) while normal cells and ASS1 + ve cells remain largely unaffected

glycolytic flux. There were clear changes in the metabolic intermediates generated by the breakdown of glutamine to fumarate in ASS negative versus ASS positive cells. Hence increased flux in these reactions may be due to increased levels of glutaminosis in ASS negative cells with glutamine being used to fuel the TCA cycle. A complete summary of the observed metabolite changes can be found in Fig. 4 and in Tables 1 and 2.

Discussion

GBM is a fatal primary brain tumour for which there is no cure. Although numerous targeted therapeutic strategies have shown promise in pre-clinical models, none of these have successfully translated to the clinical setting.

We previously identified a new treatment option for a subset of primary GBM based on their inability to synthesize arginine, a semi-essential amino acid. We further showed that this inability was due to the transcriptional down-regulation of ASS1, the rate limiting step of arginine biosynthesis. This defect rendered GBM amenable to arginine deprivation therapy using the arginine degrading enzyme ADI-PEG20 [27]. Since ADI-PEG20 depletes blood arginine, this therapeutic strategy therefore potentially overcomes the limitations imposed by the blood brain barrier. An understanding of how ADI-PEG20 effects arginine levels in the CSF would help to advance our knowledge of how arginine deprivation affects the central nervous system and we plan to include such analysis in future clinical trials in GBM patients. Nevertheless, we have preliminary data showing regression of an intracranial GBM tumour in a xenograft mouse model after weekly intramuscular injections of ADI-PEG20 (manuscript in preparation).

Arginine is synthesized by the sequential action of two urea cycle enzymes, ASS1 and ASL. ASS1 converts citrulline and aspartate into argininosuccinate, with citrulline being derived from ornithine and recycled arginine and aspartate from the tricarboxylic acid (TCA) cycle. ASL then cleaves argininosuccinate into arginine and fumarate which can enter the TCA cycle. These enzymes thus participate in both the urea and TCA cycle. A deficiency in either gene will therefore lead to an accumulation of upstream metabolites i.e. citrulline and aspartate and a deficiency of downstream metabolites i.e. arginine and fumarate. Fumarate is an important intermediate in the TCA cycle for the generation of energy and arginine is a substrate for the generation of many metabolites that have key roles in numerous metabolic pathways which include cell signalling (NO, agamate), survival (NO) and proliferation (polyamines, proline). A deficiency in ASS1 would therefore have additional consequences on other pathways that rely on the substrates generated by ASS1 which may manifest an altered metabolic phenotype.

Since metabolomics allows for the global assessment of cellular states, this study was carried out to determine if ASS negative and ASS positive GBM have distinct basal metabolic phenotypes that could be exploited for their non-invasive detection in vivo and reveal new therapeutic strategies for the treatment of these GBM phenotypes. GBM is an extremely vascular and infiltrative tumour and complete surgical resection is often not possible. Since ADI-PEG20 has been shown to have anti-angiogenic effects, treating susceptible patients with ADI-PEG20 prior to surgery may help to reduce tumour growth and allow for more successful resection. It is

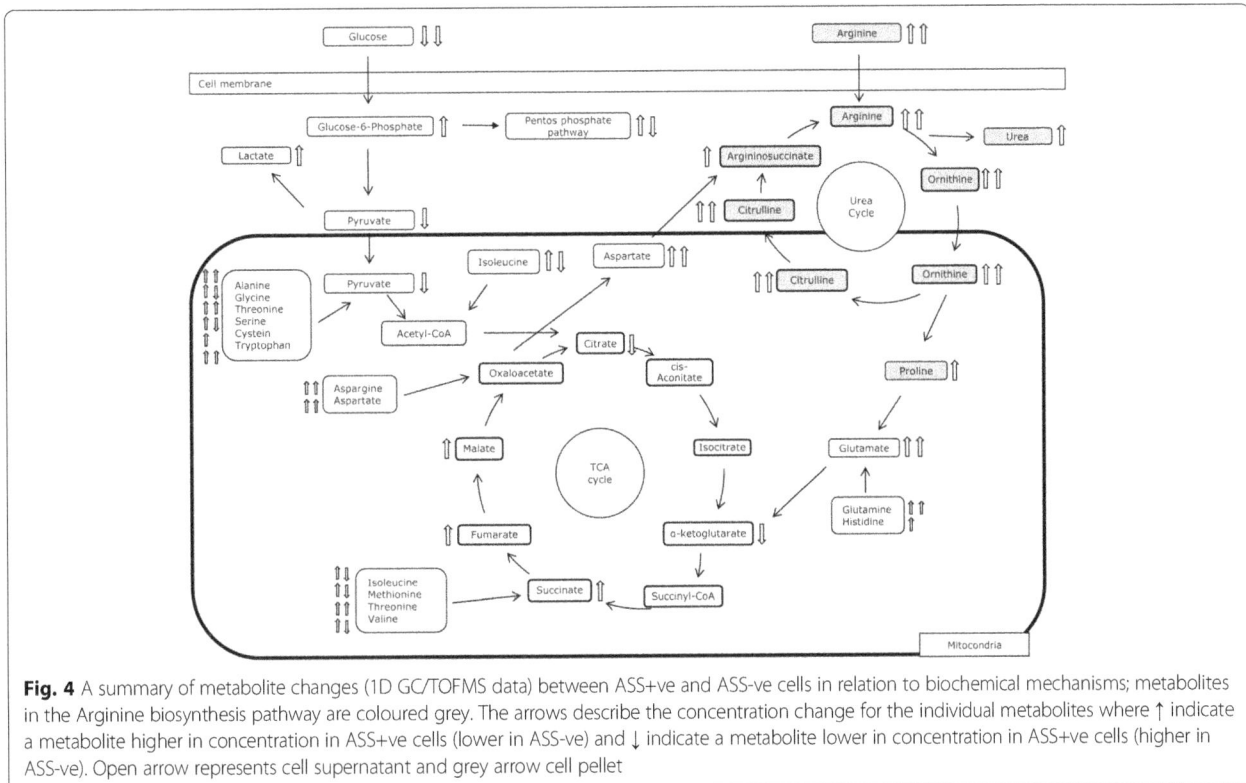

Fig. 4 A summary of metabolite changes (1D GC/TOFMS data) between ASS+ve and ASS-ve cells in relation to biochemical mechanisms; metabolites in the Arginine biosynthesis pathway are coloured grey. The arrows describe the concentration change for the individual metabolites where ↑ indicate a metabolite higher in concentration in ASS+ve cells (lower in ASS-ve) and ↓ indicate a metabolite lower in concentration in ASS+ve cells (higher in ASS-ve). Open arrow represents cell supernatant and grey arrow cell pellet

important to note that the GBM cells used in this study were primary GBM cell lines (not having progressed from a lower grade counterpart) and not mutated for IDH1. IDH1 mutations are more common in low grade gliomas and in secondary GBM and predict longer survival [45]. However, 10% of primary GBM do present with this mutation, a feature that is known to influence the metabolome [46].

OPLS analysis of both the 1D and 2D GC-TOFMS data revealed clear systemic differences between these two populations of GBM cells. As hypothesized, an analysis of metabolites contributing to this difference identified an upregulation of those involved in the arginine biosynthetic pathway in ASS positive cells compared to their negative counterparts. Interestingly, these cells also exhibited an upregulation of numerous other metabolites which may be consistent with the fact that arginine is a substrate for many metabolites such as proline and creatine. This upregulation in metabolite levels was observed predominantly in the supernatant and not in the cell pellet where the distribution of elevated versus decreased metabolites was much more equivalent. In addition to mannose, galactose and glucose several other metabolites are decreased in the cell pellet in the ASS positive cell lines. Pyruvic acid, citrate and α-keto-glutaric acid, metabolites included in the initial steps of the citric acid cycle, are decreased in ASS positive cell lines.

Using pathway analysis to assess the biological significance of altered pathways between these two cell populations, it was clear that ASS negative cells have significantly altered arginine and citrulline metabolism in addition to large differences in amino acid metabolism.

This study provides methodological proof of concept for how metabolomics can be used in combination with other omics methodologies, in this case epigenetics, to generate a more detailed molecular characterization of GBM in terms of detecting and verifying specific molecular subgroups and suggest metabolic markers or rather marker patterns for the diagnosis and treatment of these GBM subgroups. It is a logical assumption that alterations in the genome or epigenome with effect on the phenotype would be reflected in the metabolome, which makes the characterization of the metabolome highly useful in order to filter out the relevant changes to the genome. In addition, altered metabolites or metabolic patterns are potentially markers for non-invasive diagnosis of new tumour subgroups, e.g. by magnetic resonance spectroscopy (MRS), and affected metabolic pathways can be used to reveal novel treatment targets for these. Our results show significant metabolite pattern changes between ASS positive and ASS negative cell lines and in relation to the specific treatment effect of arginine deprivation to ASS negative cells accentuate the strength of using metabolomics as a method to support and verify alterations in the epigenome. This highlights the possibility to develop and evaluate more efficient diagnostics and treatments within specific tumour types guided by more detailed molecular evidence as compared to the current standard, something that would not have been feasible without using the strategy of using metabolomics as a complement to one or more omics descriptions. An important part of this work is the bio-informatics approach based on chemometric or multi-variate techniques which allowed us to extract metabolite patterns differentiating ASS positive and ASS negative cells as well as for the specific treatment effect in ASS negative cells. These metabolite patterns could potentially be refined into novel diagnostic markers, so called latent biomarkers, utilizing the strength in the correlation between co-varying metabolites as opposed to the traditional way of only considering single markers for diagnosis. From our results we could verify the differences between ASS positive and ASS negative cell lines related to the arginine biosynthesis pathway. However, our extracted metabolite pattern also included other significantly changing metabolites, something that could be of value both diagnostically as well as for pondering treatment options also for ASS positive tumours or other options for ASS negative tumours targeting other pathways. From a diagnosis point of view an interesting avenue to explore is the development of a non-invasive diagnosis of molecular tumour subgroups, in this case ASS positive and ASS negative GBM, by the use of MRS or similar techniques. If successful this would be a valuable contribution to the clinical practice. Interestingly, our differentiating metabolite pattern contained a number of metabolites detectable by MR spectroscopy in brain tumours (Tables 1 and 2), including glucose [47], glutamate [48], glutamine [49] and glycine [50]. Thus, it would be of high interest to investigate the diagnostic potential of such a metabolite pattern in vivo in an animal model, something that we aim to do in the near future. Another interesting prospect for the proposed methodology would be to do a more comprehensive screening of the GBM epigenome in combination with metabolomics analysis to construct a detailed map of the molecular subgroups of GBM that can be used to navigate towards improved diagnosis and development of tailored treatments based on molecular evidence.

Conclusion

In conclusion we were able to verify our hypothesis that the metabolome contains systematic information discriminating between ASS1 positive and negative GBM cell lines and that there is a potential of identifying metabolite biomarkers for the non-invasive detection of these subtypes in addition to unveiling novel treatment targets. The study provides proof of concept for how metabolomics data combined with chemometric bio-informatics can be used to detect metabolite pattern changes, i.e. latent biomarkers, associated with alterations in the genome. Thus, providing a tool for detection of tumour subgroups based on specific molecular evidence.

Abbreviations

ADI-PEG20: Pegylated arginine deiminase; ASL: Argininosuccinate lyase; ASS1: Argininosuccinate synthetase; DMEM: Dulbecco's modified eagle medium; FCS: Fetal calf serum; GBM: Glioblastoma multiforme; GC-TOFMS: Gas chromatography-time-of-flight mass spectrometry; GCxGC: Two-dimensional gas chromatography; HCC: Hepatocellular carcinoma; IDH1: Isocitrate dehydrogenase 1; IPA: Ingenuity pathway analysis; LC-TOFMS: Liquid chromatography-time-of-flight mass spectrometry; MEM: Minimum essential media; MS: Mass spectrometry; OPLS-DA: Orthogonal partial least squares-discriminant analysis; PCA: Principal component analysis; PI3K: Phosphatidylinosintol 3 kinase; RB: Retinoblastoma; RTK: Receptor tyrosine kinase

Funding

This work was funded by the Swedish Cancer Society (HA), the Swedish Research Council (HA) and by the Brain Tumour Research Campaign, London which formed part of the Grassini PhD studentship (NS).

Authors' contributions

LM performed lab works and analyses in the metabolomics studies of untreated cells, analyzed the metabolomics data and co-wrote the paper. RP performed the IPA analysis and helped in interpreting the results. TC assisted in the design of the paper and in the critical analysis of the data. JL performed the cell culture experiments and the metabolomics analysis involving ADI-PEG20 treated cells. KO helped in the initial design of the study. NS is the principal investigator at Imperial College, London who initiated the study and co-wrote the paper. HA is the principal investigator at Umeå university, Umeå who designed the metabolomics study of untreated cells, took part in analyzing the metabolomics data and co-wrote the paper. All authors read and approved the final manuscript.

Competing interests

The authors declare that they have no competing interests.

Author details

[1]Department of Chemistry, Umeå University, SE 901 87 Umeå, Sweden. [2]John Fulcher Neuro-Oncology Laboratory, Imperial College London, London, UK. [3]St Luke's Cancer Centre, Royal Surrey County Hospital, Guildford, Surrey, UK.

References

1. Maher EA, Furnari FB, Bachoo RM, Rowitch DH, Louis DM, Cavenee WK, et al. Malignant glioma: genetics and biology of a grave matter. Genes Dev. 2001;15(11):1311–33. https://doi.org/10.1101/gad.891601.

2. Alifieris C, Trafalis DT. Glioblastoma multiforme: pathogenesis and treatment. Pharmacol Ther. 2015;152:63–82. https://doi.org/10.1016/j.pharmthera.2015.05.005.

3. Crespo I, Vital AL, Gonzalez-Tablas M, del Carmen Patino M, Otero A, Lopes MC, et al. Molecular and genomic alterations in glioblastoma multiforme. Am J Pathol. 2015;185(7):1820–33. https://doi.org/10.1016/j.ajpath.2015.02.023.

4. Verhaak RGW, Hoadley KA, Purdom E, Wang V, Qi Y, Wilkerson MD, et al. Integrated genomic analysis identifies clinically relevant subtypes of glioblastoma characterized by abnormalities in PDGFRA, IDH1, EGFR, and NF1. Cancer Cell. 2010;17(1):98–110. https://doi.org/10.1016/j.ccr.2009.12.020.

5. Polivka J Jr, Polivka J, Rohan V, Topolcan O, Ferda J. New molecularly targeted therapies for glioblastoma multiforme. Anticancer Res. 2012;32(7): 2935–46.

6. Cloughesy TF, Cavenee WK, Mischel PS. Glioblastoma: from molecular pathology to targeted treatment. Annu Rev Pathol. 2014;9:1–25. https://doi.org/10.1146/annurev-pathol-011110-130324.

7. Okada S, Hongo T, Yamada S, Watanabe C, Fujii Y, Ohzeki T, et al. In vitro efficacy of L-asparaginase in childhood acute myeloid leukaemia. Br J Haematol. 2003;123(5):802–9. https://doi.org/10.1046/j.1365-2141.2003.04703.x.

8. Buaboonnam J, Cao X, Pauley JL, Pui C-H, Ribeiro RC, Rubnitz JE, et al. Sequential administration of methotrexate and asparaginase in relapsed or refractory pediatric acute myeloid leukemia. Pediatr Blood Cancer. 2013; 60(7):1161–4. https://doi.org/10.1002/pbc.24470.

9. Kenny GE, Pollock ME. Mammalian cell cultures contaminated with pleuropneumonia-like organisms. I. Effect of pleuropneumonia-like organisms on growth of established cell strains. J Infect Dis. 1963;112:7–16. No abstract available

10. Kraemer PM, Defendi V, Hayflick L, Manson LA. Mycoplasma (pplo) strains with lytic activity for murine lymphoma cells in vitro. Proc Soc Exp Biol Med. 1963;112:381–7.

11. Schimke RT, Berlin CM, Sweeney EW, Carroll WR. The generation of energy by the arginine dihydrolase pathway in Mycoplasma hominis 07. J Biol Chem. 1966;241(10):2228–36. No abstract available

12. Delage B, Fennell DA, Nicholson L, McNeish I, Lemoine NR, Crook T, et al. Arginine deprivation and argininosuccinate synthetase expression in the treatment of cancer. Int J Cancer. 2010;126(12):2762–72. https://doi.org/10.1002/ijc.25202.

13. Husson A, Brasse-Lagnel C, Fairand A, Renouf S, Lavoinne A. Argininosuccinate synthetase from the urea cycle to the citrulline-NO cycle. Eur J Biochem. 2003;270(9):1887–99. Review

14. Choi BS, Martinez-falero IC, Corset C, Munder M, Modolell M, Muller I, Kropf P. Differential impact of l-arginine deprivation on the activation and effector functions of t cells and macrophages. J Leukoc Biol. 2009;85(2):268–77. https://doi.org/10.1189/jlb.0508310. Epub 2008 Nov 13

15. Dillon BJ, Prieto VG, Curley SA, Ensor CM, Holtsberg FW, Bomalaski JS, Clark MS. Incidence and distribution of argininosuccinate synthetase deficiency in human cancers: a method for identifying cancers sensitive to arginine deprivation. Cancer. 2004;100(4):826–33.

16. Wheatley DN, Kilfeather R, Stitt A, Campbell E. Integrity and stability of the citrulline-arginine pathway in normal and tumour cell lines. Cancer Lett. 2005;227(2):141–52.

17. Feun LG, Kuo MT, Savaraj N. Arginine deprivation in cancer therapy. Curr Opin Clin Nutr Metab Care. 2015;18(1):78–82. https://doi.org/10.1097/MCO.0000000000000122. Review

18. Szlosarek PW, Klabatsa A, Pallaska A, Sheaff M, Smith P, Crook T, et al. In vivo loss of expression of argininosuccinate synthetase in malignant pleural mesothelioma is a biomarker for susceptibility to arginine depletion. Clin Cancer Res. 2006;12:7126–31.

19. Tsai WB, Aiba I, Lee SY, Feun L, Savaraj N, Kuo MT. Resistance to arginine deiminase treatment in melanoma cells is associated with induced argininosuccinate synthetase expression involving c-Myc/HIF-1alpha/Sp4. Mol Cancer Ther. 2009;8:3223–33.

20. Feun LG, Kuo MT, Savaraj N. Arginine deprivation in cancer therapy. Curr Opin Clin Nutr Metab Care. 2015;18(1):78–82. https://doi.org/10.1097/mco.0000000000000122.

21. Han RZ, Xu GC, Dong JJ, Ni Y. Arginine deiminase: recent advances in discovery, crystal structure, and protein engineering for improved properties as an anti-tumor drug. Appl Microbiol Biotechnol. 2016;100(11):4747–60. https://doi.org/10.1007/s00253-016-7490-z. Epub 2016 Apr 18. Review

22. Yau T, Cheng PN, Chan P, Chen L, Yuen J, Pang R, Fan ST, Wheatley DN, Poon RT. Preliminary efficacy, safety, pharmacokinetics, pharmacodynamics and quality of life study of pegylated recombinant human arginase 1 in patients with advanced hepatocellular carcinoma. Investig New Drugs. 2015;33(2):496–504. https://doi.org/10.1007/s10637-014-0200-8. Epub 2015 Feb 10

23. Fung MKL, Chan GC. Drug-induced amino acid deprivation as strategy for cancer therapy. J Hematol Oncol. 2017;10(1):144. https://doi.org/10.1186/s13045-017-0509-9. Review

24. Savaraj N, You M, Wu C, Wangpaichitr M, Kuo MT, Feun LG. Arginine deprivation, autophagy, apoptosis (AAA) for the treatment of melanoma. Curr Mol Med. 2010;10(4):405–12. Review

25. Lam TL, Wong GK, Chong HC, Cheng PN, Choi SC, Chow TL, Kwok SY, Poon RT, Wheatley DN, Lo WH, Leung YC. Recombinant human arginase inhibits proliferation of human hepatocellular carcinoma by inducing cell cycle arrest. Cancer Lett. 2009;277(1):91–100. https://doi.org/10.1016/j.canlet.2008.11.031. Epub 2009 Jan 12

26. Qiu F, Huang J, Sui M. Targeting arginine metabolism pathway to treat arginine-dependent cancers. Cancer Lett. 2015;364(1):1–7. https://doi.org/10.1016/j.canlet.2015.04.020. Epub 2015 Apr

27. Syed N, Langer J, Janczar K, Singh P, Lo Nigro C, Lattanzio L, et al. Epigenetic status of argininosuccinate synthetase and argininosuccinate lyase modulates autophagy and cell death in glioblastoma. Cell Death Dis. 2013;4 https://doi.org/10.1038/cddis.2012.197.

28. Phillips MM, Sheaff MT, Szlosarek PW. Targeting arginine-dependent cancers with arginine-degrading enzymes: opportunities and challenges. Cancer Res Treat. 2013;45(4):251–62. https://doi.org/10.4143/crt.2013.45.4.251. Epub 2013 Dec 31. Review

29. Wangpaichitr M, Wu C, Bigford G, Theodoropoulos G, You M, Li YY, Verona-Santos J, Feun LG, Nguyen DM, Savaraj N. Combination of arginine deprivation with TRAIL treatment as a targeted-therapy for mesothelioma. Anticancer Res. 2014;34(12):6991–9.

30. Bean GR, Kremer JC, Prudner BC, Schenone AD, Yao JC, Schultze MB, Chen DY, Tanas MR, Adkins DR, Bomalaski J, Rubin BP, Michel LS, Van Tine BA. A metabolic synthetic lethal strategy with arginine deprivation and chloroquine leads to cell death in ASS1-deficient sarcomas. Cell Death Dis. 2016;7(10):e2406. https://doi.org/10.1038/cddis.2016.232.

31. Thongkum A, Wu C, Li Y, Wangpaichitr M, Navasumrit P, Parnlob V, Sricharunrat T, Bhudhisawasdi V, Ruchirawat M, Savaraj N, et al. Int J Mol Sci. 2017;18(6) https://doi.org/10.3390/ijms18061175.

32. Allen MD, Luong P, Hudson C, Leyton J, Delage B, Ghazaly E, Cutts R, Yuan M, Syed N, Lo Nigro C, Lattanzio L, Chmielewska-Kassassir M, Tomlinson I, Roylance R, Whitaker HC, Warren AY, Neal D, Frezza C, Beltran L, Jones LJ, Chelala C, Wu BW, Bomalaski JS, Jackson RC, Lu YJ, Crook T, Lemoine NR, Mather S, Foster J, Sosabowski J, Avril N, Li CF, Szlosarek PW. Prognostic and therapeutic impact of argininosuccinate synthetase 1 control in bladder cancer as monitored longitudinally by PET imaging. Cancer Res. 2014;74(3):896–907. https://doi.org/10.1158/0008-5472.CAN-13-1702. Epub 2013 Nov 27

33. Locke M, Ghazaly E, Freitas MO, Mitsinga M, Lattanzio I, Lo Nigro C, Nagano A, Wang J, Chelala C, Szlosarek P, Martin SA. Inhibition of the polyamine synthesis pathway is synthetically lethal with loss of argininosuccinate synthase 1. Cell Rep. 2016;16(6):1604–13. https://doi.org/10.1016/j.celrep.2016.06.097. Epub 2016 Jul 21

34. Kremer JC, Prudner BC, Lange SE, Bean GR, Schultze MB, Brashears CB, Radyk MD, Redlich N, Tzeng SC, Kami K, Shelton L, Li A, Morgan Z, Bomalaski JS, Tsukamoto T, McConathy J, Michel LS, Held JM, Van Tine BA. Arginine deprivation inhibits the warburg effect and upregulates glutamine anerplerosis and serine biosynthesis in ASS1-deficient cancers. Cell Rep. 2017;18(4):991–1004. https://doi.org/10.1016/j.celrep.2016.12.077.

35. Fiehn O. Metabolomics - the link between genotypes and phenotypes. Plant Mol Biol. 2002;48(1–2):155–71. https://doi.org/10.1023/a:1013713905833.

36. Nicholson JK, Lindon JC, Holmes E. 'Metabonomics': understanding the metabolic responses of living systems to pathophysiological stimuli via multivariate statistical analysis of biological NMR spectroscopic data. Xenobiotica. 1999;29(11):1181–9.

37. Jonsson P, Johansson ES, Wuolikainen A, Lindberg J, Schuppe-Koistinen I, Kusano M, et al. Predictive metabolite profiling applying hierarchical multivariate curve resolution to GC-MS datas - a potential tool for multi-parametric diagnosis. J Proteome Res. 2006;5(6):1407–14. https://doi.org/10.1021/pr0600071.

38. Trygg J, Holmes E, Lundstedt T. Chemometrics in metabonomics. J Proteome Res. 2007;6(2):469–79. https://doi.org/10.1021/pr060594q.

39. MaxPlanckInstitute. http://gmd.mpimp-golm.mpg.de/.

40. Castillo S, Mattila I, Miettinen J, Oresic M, Hyotylainen T. Data analysis tool for comprehensive two-dimensional gas chromatography/time-of-flight mass spectrometry. Anal Chem. 2011;83(8):3058–67. https://doi.org/10.1021/ac103308x.

41. Wold S, Esbensen K, Geladi P. Principal component analysis. Chemom Intell Lab Syst. 1987;2(1–3):37–52.

42. Trygg J, Wold S. Orthogonal projections to latent structures (O-PLS). J Chemom. 2002;16(3):119–28. https://doi.org/10.1002/cem.695.

43. Moren L, Bergenheim AT, Ghasimi S, Brannstrom T, Johansson M, Antti H. Metabolomic screening of tumor tissue and serum in glioma patients reveals diagnostic and prognostic information. Meta. 2015;5(3):502–20. https://doi.org/10.3390/metabo5030502.

44. Eriksson L, Trygg J, Wold S. CV-ANOVA for significance testing of PLS and OPLS (R) models. J Chemom. 2008;22(11–12):594–600. https://doi.org/10.1002/cem.1187.

45. SongTao Q, Lei Y, Si G, YanQing D, HuiXia H, XueLin Z, LanXiao W, Fei Y. IDH mutations predict longer survival and response to temozolomide in secondary glioblastom. Cancer Sci. 2012;103(2):269–73. https://doi.org/10.1111/j.1349-7006.2011.02134.x. Epub 2011 Nov 28

46. Izquierdo-Garcia JL, Viswanath P, Eriksson P, Cai L, Radoul M, Chaumeil MM, Blough M, Luchman HA, Weiss S, Cairncross JG, Phillips JJ, Pieper RO, Ronen SM. IDH1 mutation induces reprogramming of pyruvate metabolism. Cancer Res. 2015;75(15):2999–3009. https://doi.org/10.1158/0008-5472.CAN-15-0840. Epub 2015 Jun 4

47. Herholz K, Heindel W, Luyten PR, Denhollander JA, Pietrzyk U, Voges J, et al. In vivo imaging of glucose consumption and lactate concentration in human gliomas. Ann Neurol. 1992;31(3):319–27. https://doi.org/10.1002/ana.410310315.

48. Bartha R, Megyesi JF, Watling CJ. Low-grade glioma: correlation of short echo time H-1-MR spectroscopy with Na-23 MR imaging. Am J Neuroradiol. 2008;29(3):464–70. https://doi.org/10.3174/ajnr.A0854.

49. Kallenberg K, Bock HC, Helms G, Jung K, Wrede A, Buhk JH, et al. Untreated glioblastoma multiforme: increased myo-inositol and glutamine levels in the contralateral cerebral hemisphere at proton MR spectroscopy. Radiology. 2009;253(3):805–12. https://doi.org/10.1148/radiol.2533071654.

50. Choi C, Ganji SK, DeBerardinis RJ, Dimitrov IE, Pascual JM, Bachoo R, et al. Measurement of glycine in the human brain in vivo by H-1-MRS at 3 T: application in brain tumors. Magn Reson Med. 2011;66(3):609–18. https://doi.org/10.1002/mrm.22857.

13

Prognostic significance of E-cadherin and N-cadherin expression in Gliomas

Myung-Giun Noh[1], Se-Jeong Oh[1], Eun-Jung Ahn[2], Yeong-Jin Kim[2], Tae-Young Jung[2], Shin Jung[2], Kyung-Keun Kim[3], Jae-Hyuk Lee[1], Kyung-Hwa Lee[1*] and Kyung-Sub Moon[2*]

Abstract

Background: Epithelial-mesenchymal transition (EMT), principally involving an E-cadherin to N-cadherin shift, linked to tumor invasion or metastasis, and therapeutic resistance in various human cancer. A growing body of recent evidence has supported the hypothesis that EMT play a crucial role in the invasive phenotype of gliomas. To evaluate the prognostic connotation of EMT traits in glioma, expression of E-cadherin and N-cadherin was explored in a large series of glioma patients in relation to patient survival rate.

Methods: Expressions of E- and N-cadherin were examined using immunohistochemical analysis in 92 glioma cases diagnosed at our hospital. These markers expressions were also explored in 21 cases of fresh frozen glioma samples and in glioma cell lines by Western blot analysis.

Results: Expression of E-cadherin was observed in eight cases (8.7%) with weak staining intensity in the majority of the immunoreactive cases (7/8). Expression of N-cadherin was identified in 81 cases (88.0%) with high expression in 64 cases (69.5%). Fresh frozen tissue samples and glioma cell lines showed similar results by Western blot analysis. There was no significant difference in either overall survival (OS) or progression-free survival (PFS) according to E-cadherin expression ($P > 0.05$). Although the OS rates were not affected by N-cadherin expression levels ($P = 0.138$), PFS increased in the low N-cadherin expression group with marginal significance ($P = 0.058$). The survival gains based on N-cadherin expression levels were significantly augmented in a larger series of publicly available REMBRANDT data ($P < 0.001$).

Conclusions: E- and N-cadherin, as representative EMT markers, have limited prognostic value in glioma. Nonetheless, the EMT process in gliomas may be compounded by enhanced N-cadherin expression supported by unfavorable prognostic outcomes.

Keywords: E-cadherin, Epithelial-mesenchymal transition, Glioma, N-cadherin, Prognosis, Survival

Background

Infiltrative tendency is such a prominent feature of malignant gliomas that tumor cells migrate far from the tumoral epicenter through the surrounding parenchyma [1, 2]. In addition to cytological atypia and mitotic activity that are needed for histopathological definition of lower-grade gliomas, microvascular proliferation and/or necrosis are specific defining attributes of glioblastoma, which is the most malignant primary brain tumor [3]. Even lower-grade gliomas assorted as World Health Organization (WHO) grade II to III are characterized by propensity for diffuse infiltration and for the malignant transformation to higher-grade tumors. The hurdle in therapeutic resistance of gliomas is intimately connected to the infiltrative phenotype. The infiltrative feature is an essential part of the clinical aggravation of malignant glioma, making surgical resection incomplete and promoting regrowth of residual tumor cells [1–3]. Infiltrative phenotypes in epithelial

* Correspondence: mdkaylee@chonnam.ac.kr; moonks@chonnam.ac.kr
[1]Department of Pathology, Chonnam National University Hwasun Hospital and Medical School, 322 Seoyang-ro, Hwasun-eup, Hwasun-gun, Jeollanam-do 519-763, South Korea
[2]Department of Neurosurgery, Chonnam National University Hwasun Hospital and Medical School, 322 Seoyang-ro, Hwasun-eup, Hwasun-gun, Jeollanam-do 519-763, South Korea
Full list of author information is available at the end of the article

malignancies have been unequivocally linked to the phenomenon of epithelial-mesenchymal transition (EMT) that manifests as tumor recurrence, metastasis and therapeutic intractability [4]. By contrast, only recently has the EMT process in non-epithelial tumors been highlighted as an important player in tumor progression [5–7]. Considering that the various downstream pathways of EMT are related with cancer invasion or metastasis, and therapeutic resistance in non-epithelial human cancer, EMT/EMT-like process can be addressed as a possible therapeutic target [8].

EMT, as a complicated cellular machinery provoked by various circumstantial factors, leads cellular and biochemical acquisition of motile mesenchymal properties from immobile epithelial cells [9]. In recent glioma research, EMT have been named as a key player of tumor progression and invasion. In this respect, the recently defined mesenchymal subgroup of glioblastomas reinforce the idea that the EMT-like process has prognostic consequence for malignant brain tumors [10, 11]. In line with the regulation of stem cell features, EMT may contribute to tumor progression and chemoresistance, and in tumor relapse after treatment as well [8].

Although the contribution of EMT in glioma progression is not as clear as that in epithelial malignancies, glial-mesenchymal transition as a counterpart of EMT has been revealed as an essential process in glioma invasion [12–16]. EMT principally involves an E-cadherin to N-cadherin shift. Still, the clinical impact of E- and N-cadherin including their effect on patient survival rates remains unknown. It is conceivable that expression of E-cadherin and N-cadherin affects the clinical aspect of glioma patients in terms of survival rates. This study assessed the expression of the classic EMT markers in human glioma samples including formalin-fixed paraffin embedded tissues, fresh frozen glioma samples and human and mouse glioma cell lines, and analyzed the implication in the context of patient survival by comparing the data with the statistics from the large cohort NCI Repository for Molecular Brain Neoplasia Database (REMBRANDT).

Methods

Glioma cell lines and human glioma tissue specimens

U118, U87, T98G, U343, and U251 human glioma cells lines were from ATCC (Manassas, VA, USA). The GL261 mouse glioma cell line was a gift from Dr. Maciej S. Lesniak at University of Chicago. All cells were maintained and cultured as described previously [12].

Ninety two glioma specimens were obtained from the patient who underwent surgical resection at Chonnam National University Hwasun Hospital between 2007 and 2012. WHO classification of the central nervous system was used for diagnostic criteria [3]. Frozen samples [$N = 20$; 8 low-grade (WHO grades I/II) and 12 high-grade (WHO grades III/IV)] were handled as previously described [12]. Samples obtained within 30 min after surgical resection were frozen immediately using liquid nitrogen. The specimens were stored at −80 °C until used. Clinicopathological data were based on the medical records. Radiological findings, such as size and location of tumor, peritumoral edema, and cystic or necrotic changes were obtained from preoperative magnetic resonance imaging (MRI). Overall survival (OS) and progression-free survival (PFS) were determined as previously described [12]. The endpoint of OS was the date of death/the last follow-up visit. The endpoint of PFS was the date of recurrence/progression/death. The Chonnam National University Hwasun Hospital Institutional Review Board approved this study (CNUHH-2016-081), and written informed consent was obtained from patients or their legal surrogates for using resected glioma samples.

Tissue microarray construction and immunohistochemistry

Areas with a high cellularity were selected for tissue microarrays. Immunohistochemical staining was performed as described previously [12]. E-cadherin (1:50 dilution; DAKO, Glostrup, Denmark; Catalogue No. M3612) and N-cadherin (1:500 dilution; Abcam, Cambridge, UK; Catalogue No. ab12221) antibodies were applied into a Bond-max autostainer system (Leica Microsystems, Bannockburn, IL, USA). Antigen retrieval was carried out using citrate buffer at pH 6.0. Negative controls were prepared without using primary antibodies.

All immunostained slides were evaluated twice by two independent observers (NMG and LKH) with no knowledge of the clinical details. E- and N-cadherin immunohistochemistry showed cytoplasmic positivity in glioma cells and sometimes stained the cytoplasmic borders. The intensity of staining was initially classified into 4 grades: 0, no immunoreaction; 1, weak positivity; 2, moderate positivity; and 3, strong reactivity. With N-cadherin staining, cases of grades 0 and 1 positivity were grouped as a low-expression, and cases of grades 2 and 3 as a high-expression for statistical convenience. Two pathologists re-evaluated cases with discordant staining intensity together and made concessions for such cases.

Western blot analysis

Western blot analysis was performed as described [12]. After extraction and quantification of protein from glioma cells and tissues, proteins (30 μg) were resolved by 10% polyacrylamide gel electrophoresis. The proteins were electrotransferred onto nitrocellulose membranes, blocked by 3% skimmed milk, and followed by sequential incubation with primary antibodies (E-cadherin, 1:500 dilution, mouse host; N-cadherin, 1:500 dilution, rabbit host; Actin, 1:10,000, mouse host, BD Transduction Laboratories, San Jose, CA, USA, Catalogue No. 612656). Protein level was measured by electrochemiluminescence (ECL) system (Pierce Biotechnology, Rockford, IL USA).

Patient datasets and data analysis from REMBRANDT

The past NCI REMBRANDT (used to be at https://caintegrator.nci.nih.gov/rembrandt/login.do, and currently housed in Georgetown University's G-DOC System at https://gdoc.georgetown.edu/gdoc/) provided de-identified open data on 343 glioma patients through to May 13, 2014. The correlations between E- or N-cadherin expression and OS were checked in samples from the patients as described previously [12]. The construction of graphs was based on the data according to Affymetrix reporters 219,330 at the Highest Geometric Mean Intensity and related survival. Upregulated, downregulated, or intermediate group represented $\geq$ 2-fold changes in E- or N-cadherin level in comparison with the level of nonglioma samples. Survival differences in groups were estimated by the log-rank test.

Statistical analyses

All data were analyzed with IBM SPSS Statistics program version 23.0 for Window (Armonk, NY, USA), as previously described [12]. For relationships between E- or N-cadherin expression and WHO tumor grades, chi-square test or Fisher's exact probability test was used. The effect of single variables on OS or PFS was estimated by univariate and multivariate analyses. Cox's proportional hazards model was applied to find out the independent prognostic factors. A certain variable that could be influenced by other variables, e.g., postoperative adjuvant therapy, was ruled out from the model. The level of significance was set at $P < 0.05$.

Results

Clinical presentation

This series of 92 cases included 42 male patients (45.7%) and 50 female patients (54.3%). The mean age at the time of histological diagnosis was 47.2 years (range: 2 to 84 years). Fifty eight patients (63.0%) underwent gross total resection and 34 patients (37%) underwent subtotal to partial resection. Forty-four patients (47.8%) received concomitant radiation therapy and chemotherapy. The clinicopathological features of our cases are summarized in Table 1.

Table 1 Clinicopathologic features of the patients

Variable		Number	Percent
Age (year)	<60	63	68.5%
	≥60	29	31.5%
Sex	Male	42	45.7%
	Female	50	54.3%
WHO grade	I	6	6.5%
	II	28	30.4%
	III	14	15.2%
	IV	44	47.8%
Tumor size	< 4.5 cm	49	53.3%
	≥ 4.5 cm	43	46.7%
Location	Non-eloquent area	45	48.9%
	Near eloquent area	47	51.1%
Edema	None to minimal	42	45.7%
	Moderate to severe	50	54.3%
Cystic change	None	40	43.5%
	Present	52	56.5%
Resection degree	Partial to subtotal	34	37.0%
	Gross total	58	63.0%
Postoperative adjuvant therapy	CT + RT	44	47.8%
	CT alone	1	1.1%
	RT alone	20	21.7%
	None	27	29.3%

Expression of E- and N-cadherin in gliomas

Expression of E- and N-cadherin in gliomas was explored according to WHO tumor grades. E-cadherin expression was observed in eight cases of glioma (Fig. 1a & b). Of 34 low-grade gliomas, three cases showed E-cadherin expression; two cases showed weak expression and one case of subependymal giant cell astrocytoma (SEGA) showed strong expression (Fig. 1b). Five cases out of 58 high-grade gliomas showed E-cadherin immunopositivity, although the staining intensity was weak in all five cases. The correlation between presence of E-cadherin expression and WHO tumor grades (low-grade vs. high-grade) was not significant statistically ($P = 0.973$, Table 2).

N-cadherin was expressed in the majority of the glioma cases (cases with staining intensity 1 through 3, 81/92, 88.0%), regardless of the staining intensity (Fig. 1c & d). No expression was found in 6 of 58 high-grade (10.3%) and 5 of 34 low-grade gliomas (14.7%). When the cases were categorized into low-expression group and high-expression group, low expression of N-cadherin was observed in 28 cases (30.5%). N-cadherin was highly expressed in 64 cases (69.5%). Of 58 high-grade tumors, 17 cases displayed

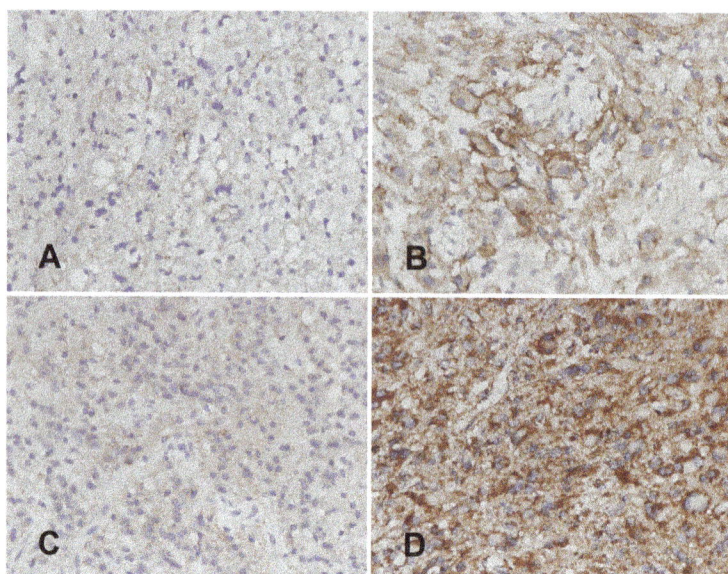

Fig. 1 Immunohistochemical findings using E- and N-cadherin antibodies. Most tumor cells showed no to mild expression of E-cadherin (**a**), and only one case displayed strong positivity along the cytoplasmic borders (**b**). Immunohistochemical analysis for N-cadherin showed from mild (**c**) to strong (**d**) positivity in the cytoplasm of the tumor cells

low expression of N-cadherin and 41 cases showed high expression. N-cadherin expression was not significantly associated with WHO tumor grades, either ($P = 0.759$).

The expressions of E- and N-cadherin were similarly demonstrated by Western blot analysis in the fresh frozen tissues (Fig. 2). Compared to N-cadherin expression, which was detected in the majority of the glioma samples, the number of cases with E-cadherin expression was much smaller. Also, the positive reaction rates of E- and N-cadherin did not differ significantly according to the tumor grades. Five glioma cell lines including U118, T98G, U343, U251 and GL261 showed N-cadherin expression bands by Western blot analysis.

OS and PFS

Median OS of all patients was 44.8 months (95% confidence interval (CI): 37.8–51.8 months). The clinical variables of age and WHO tumor grade were significantly associated with longer survival in univariate analysis (both $P < 0.001$) (Fig. 3, Table 3) and multivariate analysis ($P = 0.002$ and $P = 0.004$, respectively). Smaller tumor size was marginally associated with longer survival by univariate analysis ($P = 0.086$) but did not show statistical significance by multivariate analysis ($P = 0.151$). Sex, location, peritumoral edema, cystic or necrotic change, resection degree and E- and N-cadherin expression were not significantly associated with survival benefit. OS by low

Table 2 Immunohistochemical expression of E- and N-cadherin in association with WHO tumor grade

Marker	Staining intensity	No. (%)	WHO grade				P value
			Low (I-II)		High (III-IV)		
E-cadherin	0	84 (91.3%)	31	31 (36.9%)	53	53 (63.1%)	0.973
	1	7 (7.6%)	2	3 (37.5%)	5	5 (62.5%)	
	2	0 (0.0%)	0		0		
	3	1 (1.1%)	1		0		
N-cadherin	0	11 (12.0%)	5	11 (39.3%)	6	17 (60.7%)	0.759
	1	17 (18.5%)	6		11		
	2	30 (32.6%)	9	23 (35.9%)	21	41 (64.1%)	
	3	34 (37.0%)	14		20		

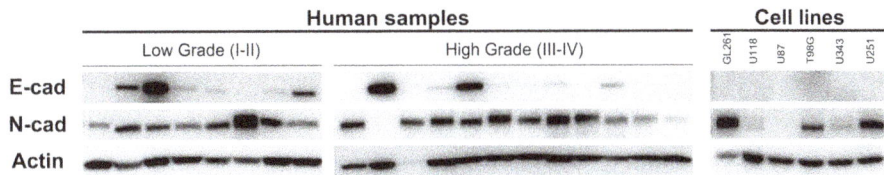

Fig. 2 E- and N-cadherin expression in human glioma samples and glioma cell lines. Western blot analysis demonstrated that the majority of human gliomas, both low- and high grades, displayed N-cadherin expression while a small number of gliomas are positive for E-cadherin and that the proportion of positive cases were similar in both groups. Similarly, 5glioma cell lines (U118, U251, T98G, U343, GL261) showed positive bands for N-cadherin

N-cadherin expression was not statistically significant either by univariate analysis or multivariate analysis (both $P > 0.05$). However, patients with low N-cadherin expression showed longer survival than patients with high expression (49.8 months vs. 42.0 months, Fig. 3 and Table 3).

PFS was also analyzed in the context of clinical variables. Similarly to the results of OS analysis, only younger age and lower WHO tumor grades showed statistical significance with relevance to the survival benefit by both univariate and multivariate analyses (Fig. 4 and Table 4, all $P < 0.05$). Interestingly,

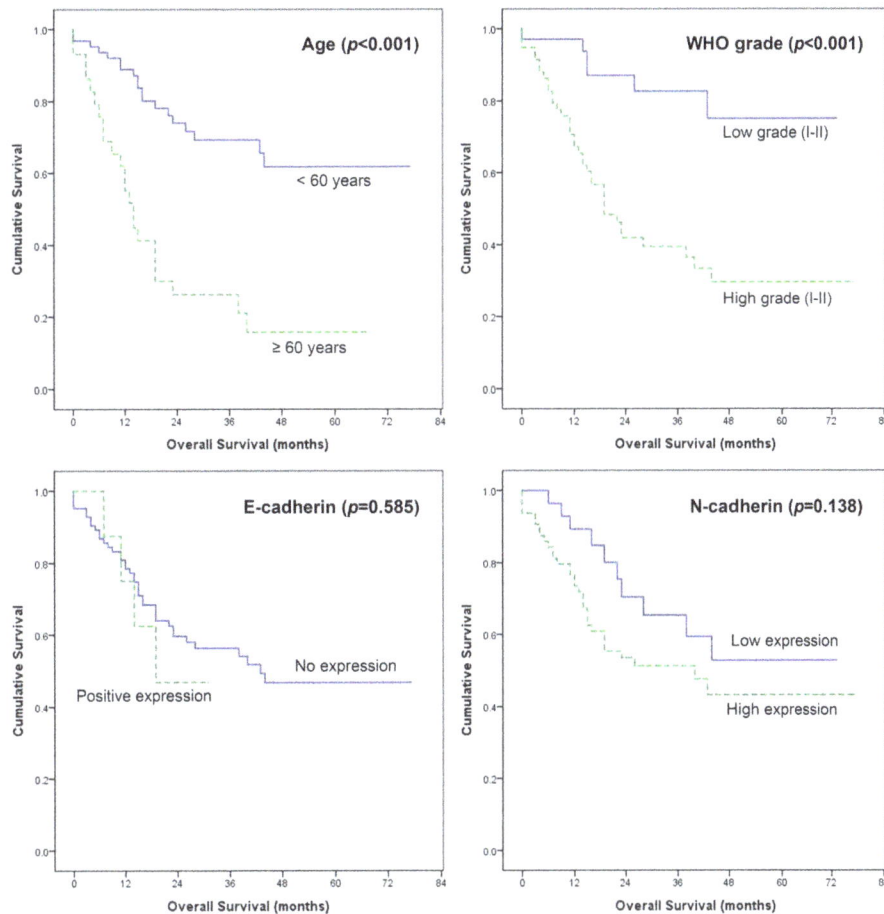

Fig. 3 Kaplan–Meier estimates of overall survival according to age, tumor grades and E- and N-cadherin expression level. Age ($P < 0.001$) and WHO tumor grade ($P < 0.001$) showed statistically significance. Expression of E-cadherin and N-cadherin was not related with overall survival of glioma patients

Table 3 Univariate and multivariate analysis for overall survival predictors in patients with glioma

Characteristics		No	Mean (months)	P-value (univariate)	P-value (multivariate)	Hazard ratio
Age	<60	63	55.4	<0.001	0.002	1
	≥60	29	22.5			2.982
Sex	M	42	43.5	0.962	0.672	1
	F	50	44.7			0.855
WHO grade	Low (I-II)	34	60.7	<0.001	0.004	1
	High (III-IV)	58	34.2			4.016
Tumor size	<4.5	49	50.0	0.086	0.151	1
	≥4.5	43	37.8			1.752
Location	Non-eloquent area	45	31.7	0.141	0.487	1
	Near eloquent area	47	38.4			1.290
Edema	None/minimal	42	35.6	0.581	0.280	1
	Moderate/severe	50	34.4			0.675
Cystic change	None	40	37.5	0.941	0.870	1
	Present	52	34.6			1.062
Resection degree	Partial/subtotal	34	33.6	0.959	0.455	1
	Gross total	58	36.8			1.303
E-cadherin	No	84	45.4	0.585	0.780	1
	Positive	8	21.5			1.181
N-cadherin	Low	28	49.8	0.138	0.456	1
	High	64	42.0			1.362

smaller tumor size showed significantly longer PFS (P = 0.046) and low N-cadherin expression was marginally associated with survival benefit (P = 0.058) by univariate analysis, although both variables did not prove to be independent prognostic factors by multivariate analysis (P = 0.255 and P = 0.463, respectively). Increased PFS gap between the low N-cadherin expression group and high-expression group compared to OS curves are shown in Fig. 4.

Assessment of 343 glioma patients in the REMBRANDT cohort showed that levels of N-cadherin expression were significantly correlated with OS gaps. Comparison between up-regulated or intermediate N-cadherin expression groups and all glioma group showed statistically significant survival differences (Fig. 5; all $P < 0.001$). With up-regulated N-cadherin expression, OS was significantly shortened. However, significant OS gaps were not related to E-cadherin level, similar to our glioma cohort data.

Discussion

In the present study, expression of the representative EMT markers, E- and N-cadherin, was investigated in a series of gliomas consisting of WHO grade I through IV tumors to explore the clinical implication with regard to patient survival. Epithelial phenotypes

indicated by E-cadherin expression were rarely identified in both low-grade and high-grade tumors, as intuitively expected in non-epithelial malignancies. In comparison, mesenchymal phenotypes denoted by N-cadherin expression were observed in the majority of gliomas through grade I through IV. Although the survival benefit in terms of PFS in the patient group with down-regulated N-cadherin expression showed marginal significance, the survival advantage in the patient group with low N-cadherin expression was increased in the larger REMBRANDT cohort. The current results suggest that the gain of mesenchymal traits in gliomas is boosted by increased N-cadherin expression that is not balanced by E-cadherin alteration.

Glial tumors that lack epithelial phenotypes intrinsically have been observed to rearrange the cytoskeleton, dissimilar to classical EMT of epithelial tumors manifested by E-cadherin to N-cadherin shift [8, 13]. Similar to our data, a prior study reported that the majority of glioblastomas did not show intrinsic E-cadherin expression in a previous study [14]. It has been a very rare occasion to encounter malignant gliomas with E-cadherin expression [17].

Malignant glioma is notable for biological heterogeneity and extreme fatalness, which is fairly

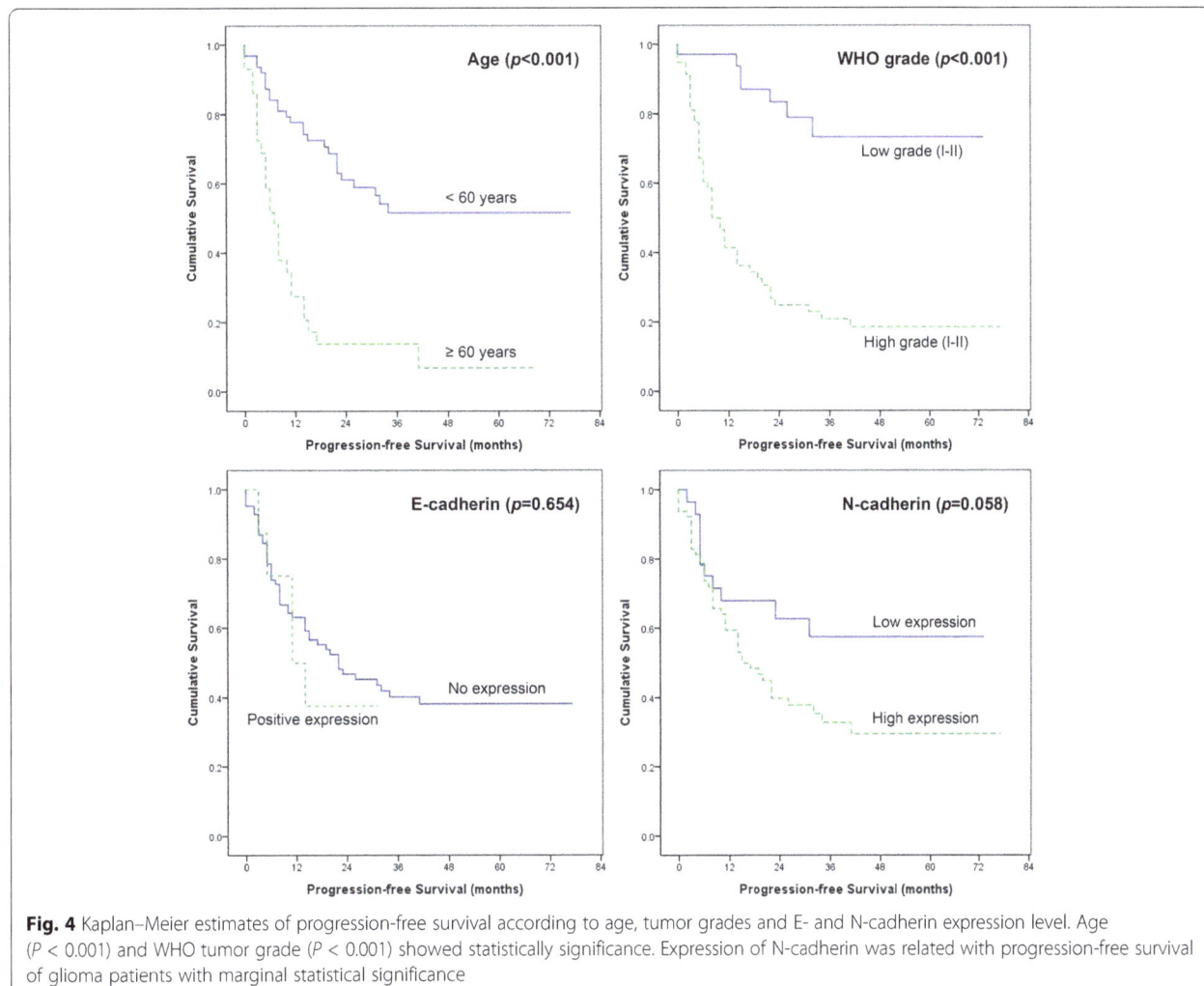

Fig. 4 Kaplan–Meier estimates of progression-free survival according to age, tumor grades and E- and N-cadherin expression level. Age ($P < 0.001$) and WHO tumor grade ($P < 0.001$) showed statistically significance. Expression of N-cadherin was related with progression-free survival of glioma patients with marginal statistical significance

connected to its infiltrative attribute. [1, 2]. EMT is a crucial component in early developmental course, tissue repair process and restructuring [18], and takes an important part of tumor advancement [19] and metastasis [4]. Certain transcription factors such as Slug, Snai1, Twist and matrix metalloproteinases, have been reported to be implicated in EMT, and to promote glioma cell migration and invasion [19–22]. Epithelial cell plasticity is rigorously redirected to display increased mesenchymal cadherins including N-cadherin or cadherin-11 and to convert immotile parent epithelial cells to motile cells with enhanced invasive properties [23, 24].

In cancerous transformations, the acquisition of EMT traits is closely linked to the proceeding of dedifferentiation and gain of stem cell status [4]. As supported by important experimental findings in epithelial malignancies including colon, pancreatic and breast cancer, induction of EMT can co-induce stem cell properties, thereby connecting cell motility and

stem cell-like programs [4, 25, 26]. Malignant gliomas turned out to have cancer stem cell population recently [27]. However, the co-existence of stem cell and EMT features during the progression of glioblastoma has been described lately [9]. Aside from metastasis, which is rare in gliomas, dedifferentiated phenotype in the residual tumor cell population at the invasive front is coupled with malignant transformation in the recurrent tumor. Despite removal of extensive tumor volume based on grossly detectable levels, microscopic foci of remnant tumor cells beyond the resection margins bring about eventual tumor recurrence, not infrequently accompanied by advance into a higher-grade glioma. With the most infiltrative phenotype of the cells in the invasion front far off the resection margins, the tumor cells are prone to proliferate and to progress after a variable dormant period by means of stem cell characteristics in the remaining population. A previous study reported the enhanced expression of stem cell factors

Table 4 Univariate and multivariate analysis for progression-free survival predictors in patients with glioma

Characteristics		No	Mean (months)	P-value (univariate)	P-value (multivariate)	Hazard ratio
Age	<60	63	47.0	<0.001	0.002	1
	≥60	29	13.4			2.673
Sex	M	42	33.1	0.623	0.432	1
	F	50	38.1			0.775
WHO grade	Low (I-II)	34	58.8	<0.001	<0.001	1
	High (III-IV)	58	22.7			5.278
Tumor size	<4.5	49	43.0	0.046	0.255	1
	≥4.5	43	28.4			1.487
Location	Non-eloquent area	45	42.3	0.549	0.913	1
	Near eloquent area	47	44.1			0.966
Edema	None/minimal	42	41.4	0.800	0.794	1
	Moderate/severe	50	45.0			0.920
Cystic change	None	40	45.8	0.840	0.954	1
	Present	52	42.1			1.019
Resection degree	Partial/subtotal	34	42.8	0.746	0.473	1
	Gross total	58	44.4			1.248
E-cadherin	No	28	46.5	0.654	0.838	1
	Positive	64	31.7			1.111
N-cadherin	Low	68	38.2	0.058	0.463	1
	High	24	24.9			1.333

in paired primary and recurrent glioma samples by unsupervised clustering analysis of gene expression profiling [28]. The concurrence of a stem cell status with EMT features in glioblastoma, either via the β–catenin pathway or KITENIN mediation, has been recently described [12, 13].

Increased mesenchymal traits are considered to be a pivotal molecular event that leads to enhanced malignancy in gliomas [8]. Based on genome-scale analysis of large cohorts of glioblastomas, four different subgroups were identified that are dependent on neural differentiation [10, 11]. Glioblastomas categorized into the mesenchymal subtype displayed by far shorter overall and progression-free survival periods, related with extensive aggressiveness indicated by multifocality or therapeutic resistance against radio- and chemo-therapy [11]. Accordingly, the clinical consequence of invasive phenotype induced by EMT is evident. A previous study proposed that a small population of glioma cells undergo molecular events that bring about cytoskeletal reorganization and apoptotic resistance. As a result, the tumor cells become highly motile and invasive and then evolve into the treatment-resistant condition [8]. Compared to metastases of most carcinomas in which the eventual process recapitulate the organization of the

primary tumors [29], the evolutional changes in glioma progression do not involve the organization represented by restoration of E-cadherin expression. Instead, glioma progression seems to incorporate strengthened mesenchymal phenotypes in relevance to up-regulated N-cadherin expression and resultant therapeutic resistance. In addition, glioblastoma clusters other than the mesenchymal subtype acquire mesenchymal traits over recurrent episodes [11]. An evolutional change with increased mesenchymal phenotype appears to be a frequent episode with regard to disease progression, alike cancer cells using EMT mechanism during the advance to a more aggressive status [8, 30]. However, further investigation needs be performed to reveal the relation between N-cadherin or other EMT markers/inducers and key parameters for new 2016 WHO glioma classification, such as IDH1 mutation, 1p/19q co-deletion or MGMT promoter methylation [31].

Conclusions

The present study shows that E- and N-cadherin expressions in glioma have limited value as a survival predictor. However, N-cadherin expression showed prognostic implication with marginal significance in our glioma cohort and by far more significant

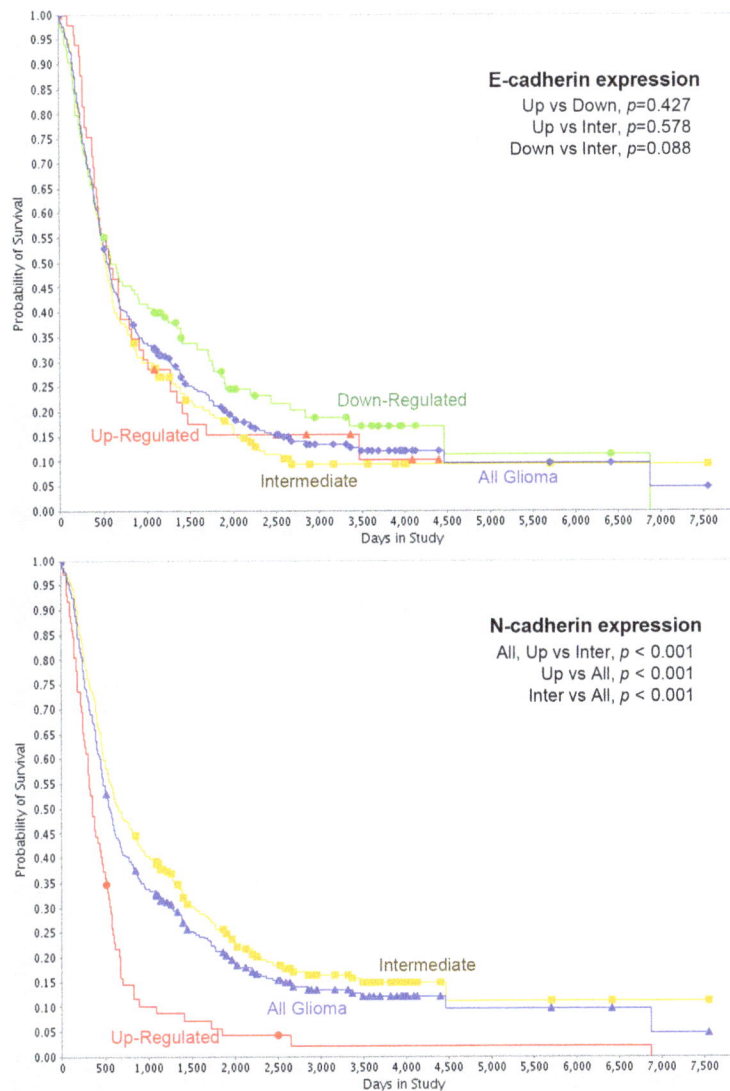

Fig. 5 Kaplan–Meier survival analysis according to E-cadherin and N-cadherin expression levels in a cohort of 343 glioma patients in the REMBRANDT database. Overall survival was significantly shorter in patients with high than intermediate N-cadherin expression (*P* < 0.001)

prognostic meaning in the larger REMBRANDT data. The EMT process accompanied by enhanced N-cadherin expression may contribute the biological aggressiveness in glioma by increased mesenchymal phenotype that is supported by variably unfavorable prognostic outcome.

Abbreviations
EMT: Epithelial-mesenchymal transition; IHC: Immunohistochemistry; MRI: Magnetic resonance imaging; OS: Overall survival; PFS: Progression-free survival

Acknowledgements
Not applicable.

Funding
This work was supported by Chonnam National University Hospital Biomedical Research Institute (HCRI14024-1, HCRI15014-21), partly by Basic Science Research Program through the National Research Foundation of

Korea (NRF) funded by the Minist (2016R1A2B1014597, 2016R1C1B2007494). There was no role of the funding bodies in the design of the study, in collection, analysis, and interpretation of data or in writing the manuscript.

Authors' contributions
KHL and KSM designed this study. MGN, SJO and EJA carried out the experimental studies. MGN, KHL and KSM drafted the manuscript. KHL and KSM carried out the statistical analysis. YJK, TYJ, SJO and SJ carried out the acquisition and analysis of clinical data. KKK, EJA and JHL carried out the interpretation of clinical and experimental data. YJK, TYJ, SJ, KKK and JHL revised the manuscript for critical points. All authors read and approved the final manuscript.

Competing interests
The authors declare that they have no competing interests.

Author details
[1]Department of Pathology, Chonnam National University Hwasun Hospital and Medical School, 322 Seoyang-ro, Hwasun-eup, Hwasun-gun, Jeollanam-do 519-763, South Korea. [2]Department of Neurosurgery, Chonnam National University Hwasun Hospital and Medical School, 322 Seoyang-ro, Hwasun-eup, Hwasun-gun, Jeollanam-do 519-763, South Korea. [3]Medical Research Center of Gene Regulation and Center for Creative Biomedical Scientists, Chonnam National University Medical School, Gwangju, South Korea.

References
1. Louis DN, Ohgaki H, Wiestler OD, Cavenee WK, Burger PC, Jouvet A, Scheithauer BW, Kleihues P. The 2007 WHO classification of tumours of the central nervous system. Acta Neuropathol. 2007;114(2):97–109.
2. Rousseau A, Mokhtari K, Duyckaerts C. The 2007 WHO classification of tumors of the central nervous system - what has changed? Curr Opin Neurol. 2008;21(6):720–7.
3. Kleihues P, Louis DN, Wiestler OD, Burger PC, Scheithauer BW. WHO grading of tumours of the central nervous system. In: Louis DN, Ohgaki H, Wiestler OD, Cavenee WK, editors. WHO classification of tumours of the central nervous system. 4th ed. Lyon: International Agency for Research on Cancer; 2007. p. 10–1.
4. Brabletz T. To differentiate or not–routes towards metastasis. Nat Rev Cancer. 2012;12(6):425–36.
5. Nagaishi M, Paulus W, Brokinkel B, Vital A, Tanaka Y, Nakazato Y, Giangaspero F, Ohgaki H. Transcriptional factors for epithelial-mesenchymal transition are associated with mesenchymal differentiation in gliosarcoma. Brain Pathol. 2012;22(5):670–6.
6. Guo Y, Zi X, Koontz Z, Kim A, Xie J, Gorlick R, Holcombe RF, Hoang BH. Blocking Wnt/LRP5 signaling by a soluble receptor modulates the epithelial to mesenchymal transition and suppresses met and metalloproteinases in osteosarcoma Saos-2 cells. J Orthop Res. 2007; 25(7):964–71.
7. Cosset E, Hamdan G, Jeanpierre S, Voeltzel T, Sagorny K, Hayette S, Mahon FX, Dumontet C, Puisieux A, Nicolini FE, Maguer-Satta V. Deregulation of TWIST-1 in the CD34+ compartment represents a novel prognostic factor in chronic myeloid leukemia. Blood. 2011;117(5):1673–6.
8. Kahlert UD, Nikkhah G, Maciaczyk J. Epithelial-to-mesenchymal(–like) transition as a relevant molecular event in malignant gliomas. Cancer Lett. 2013;331(2):131–8.
9. Kalluri R, Weinberg RA. The basics of epithelial-mesenchymal transition. J Clin Invest. 2009;119(6):1420–8.
10. Phillips HS, Kharbanda S, Chen R, Forrest WF, Soriano RH, Wu TD, Misra A, Nigro JM, Colman H, Soroceanu L, Williams PM, Modrusan Z, Feuerstein BG, Aldape K. Molecular subclasses of high-grade glioma predict prognosis, delineate a pattern of disease progression, and resemble stages in neurogenesis. Cancer Cell. 2006;9(3):157–73.
11. Verhaak RG, Hoadley KA, Purdom E, Wang V, Qi Y, Wilkerson MD, Miller CR, Ding L, Golub T, Mesirov JP, Alexe G, Lawrence M, O'Kelly M, Tamayo P, Weir BA, Gabriel S, Winckler W, Gupta S, Jakkula L, Feiler HS, Hodgson JG, James CD, Sarkaria JN, Brennan C, Kahn A, Spellman PT, Wilson RK, Speed TP, Gray JW, Meyerson M, Getz G, Perou CM, Hayes DN, Cancer Genome Atlas Research Network. Integrated genomic analysis identifies clinically relevant subtypes of glioblastoma characterized by abnormalities in PDGFRA, IDH1, EGFR, and NF1. Cancer Cell. 2010;17(1):98–110.
12. Lee KH, Ahn EJ, Oh SJ, Kim O, Joo YE, Bae JA, Yoon S, Ryu HH, Jung S, Kim KK, Lee JH, Moon KS. KITENIN promotes glioma invasiveness and progression, associated with the induction of EMT and stemness markers. Oncotarget. 2015;6(5):3240–53.
13. Kahlert UD, Maciaczyk D, Doostkam S, Orr BA, Simons B, Bogiel T, Reithmeier T, Prinz M, Schubert J, Niedermann G, Brabletz T, Eberhart CG, Nikkhah G, Maciaczyk J. Activation of canonical WNT/beta-catenin signaling enhances in vitro motility of glioblastoma cells by activation of ZEB1 and other activators of epithelial-to-mesenchymal transition. Cancer Lett. 2012;325(1):42–53.
14. Mikheeva SA, Mikheev AM, Petit A, Beyer R, Oxford RG, Khorasani L, Maxwell JP, Glackin CA, Wakimoto H, Gonzalez-Herrero I, Sánchez-García I, Silber JR, Horner PJ, Rostomily RC. TWIST1 promotes invasion through mesenchymal change in human glioblastoma. Mol Cancer. 2010;9:194.
15. Qi S, Song Y, Peng Y, Wang H, Long H, Yu X, Li Z, Fang L, Wu A, Luo W, Zhen Y, Zhou Y, Chen Y, Mai C, Liu Z, Fang W. ZEB2 mediates multiple pathways regulating cell proliferation, migration, invasion, and apoptosis in glioma. PLoS One. 2012;7(6):e38842.
16. Yang HW, Menon LG, Black PM, Carroll RS, Johnson MD. SNAI2/slug promotes growth and invasion in human gliomas. BMC Cancer. 2010;10:301.
17. Lewis-Tuffin LJ, Rodriguez F, Giannini C, Scheithauer B, Necela BM, Sarkaria JN, Anastasiadis PZ. Misregulated E-cadherin expression associated with an aggressive brain tumor phenotype. PLoS One. 2010;5(10):e13665.
18. Kalluri R, Neilson EG. Epithelial-mesenchymal transition and its implications for fibrosis. J Clin Invest. 2003;112(12):1776–84.
19. Thiery JP. Epithelial-mesenchymal transitions in tumour progression. Nat Rev Cancer. 2002;2(6):442–54.
20. Kang Y, Massague J. Epithelial-mesenchymal transitions: twist in development and metastasis. Cell. 2004;118(3):277–9.
21. Qiao B, Johnson NW, Gao J. Epithelial-mesenchymal transition in oral squamous cell carcinoma triggered by transforming growth factor-beta1 is snail family-dependent and correlates with matrix metalloproteinase-2 and -9 expressions. Int J Oncol. 2010;37(3):663–8.
22. Radisky ES, Radisky DC. Matrix metalloproteinase-induced epithelial-mesenchymal transition in breast cancer. J Mammary Gland Biol Neoplasia. 2010;15(2):201–12.
23. Tran NL, Nagle RB, Cress AE, Heimark RL. N-Cadherin expression in human prostate carcinoma cell lines. An epithelial-mesenchymal transformation mediating adhesion withStromal cells. Am J Pathol. 1999;155(3):787–98.
24. Zeisberg M, Neilson EG. Biomarkers for epithelial-mesenchymal transitions. J Clin Invest. 2009;119(6):1429–37.
25. Morel AP, Lievre M, Thomas C, Hinkal G, Ansieau S, Puisieux A. Generation of breast cancer stem cells through epithelial-mesenchymal transition. PLoS One. 2008;3(8):e2888.
26. Mani SA, Guo W, Liao MJ, Eaton EN, Ayyanan A, Zhou AY, Brooks M, Reinhard F, Zhang CC, Shipitsin M, Campbell LL, Polyak K, Brisken C, Yang J, Weinberg RA. The epithelial-mesenchymal transition generates cells with properties of stem cells. Cell. 2008;133(4):704–15.
27. Singh SK, Hawkins C, Clarke ID, Squire JA, Bayani J, Hide T, Henkelman RM, Cusimano MD, Dirks PB. Identification of human brain tumour initiating cells. Nature. 2004;432(7015):396–401.
28. Kwon SM, Kang SH, Park CK, Jung S, Park ES, Lee JS, Kim SH, Woo HG. Recurrent Glioblastomas reveal molecular subtypes associated with mechanistic implications of drug-resistance. PLoS One. 2015;10(10):e0140528.
29. Brabletz T, Jung A, Spaderna S, Hlubek F, Kirchner T. Opinion: migrating cancer stem cells - an integrated concept of malignant tumour progression. Nat Rev Cancer. 2005;5(9):744–9.
30. Iwadate Y. Epithelial-mesenchymal transition in glioblastoma progression. Oncol Lett. 2016;11(3):1615–20.
31. Louis DN, Perry A, Reifenberger G, von Deimling A, Figarella-Branger D, Cavenee WK, Ohgaki H, Wiestler OD, Kleihues P, Ellison DW. The 2016 World Health Organization classification of tumors of the central nervous system: a summary. Acta Neuropathol. 2016;131(6):803–20.

14

Enhanced expression of Vastatin inhibits angiogenesis and prolongs survival in murine orthotopic glioblastoma model

Yi Li[1], Jun Li[1], Yat Ming Woo[2], Zan Shen[3], Hong Yao[4], Yijun Cai[1], Marie Chia-mi Lin[1] and Wai Sang Poon[1*]

Abstract

Background: Antiangiogenic therapies are considered promising for the treatment of glioblastoma (GB). The non-collagenous C-terminal globular NC1 domain of type VIII collagen a1 chain, Vastatin, is an endogenous antiangiogenic polypeptide. Sustained enhanced expression of Vastatin was shown to inhibit tumour growth and metastasis in murine hepatocellular carcinoma models. In this study, we further explored the efficacy of Vastatin in the treatment of GB xenografts.

Method: Treatment of Vastatin was carried out using a nanopolymer gene vector PEI600-CyD-Folate (H1). Antiangiogenic effect of Vastatin was tested in vitro by using co-culture system and conditioned medium. An orthotopic GB murine model was established to examine the in vivo therapeutic effect of Vastatin alone treatment and its combination with temozolomide.

Results: Vastatin gene transfection mediated by H1 could target tumour cells specifically and suppress the proliferation of microvessel endothelial cells (MECs) through a paracrine inhibition manner. Enhancing Vastatin expression by intracerebral injection of H1-Vastatin significantly prolonged animal survival from 48 to 75 days in GB murine model, which was comparable to the effect of Endostatin, the most studied endogenous antiangiogenic polypeptide. The diminished presence of CD34 positive cells in the GB xenografts suggested that Vastatin induced significant antiangiogenesis. Moreover, a synergistic effect in extending survival was detected when H1-Vastatin was administered with temozolomide (TMZ) in GB chemoresistant murine models.

Conclusion: Our results suggest, for the first time, that Vastatin is an antiangiogenic polypeptide with significant potential therapeutic benefit for GB. H1-Vastatin gene therapy may have important implications in re-sensitizing recurrent GB to standard chemotherapeutic agents.

Keywords: Vastatin, Glioblastoma, Antiangiogenesis, Gene therapy, Chemoresistance

Background

Glioblastoma (GB) is a lethal and aggressive human malignancy, accounting for over 60% of high-grade primary brain tumours [1, 2]. In spite of significant technological advances in neurosurgery, anaesthesia, intensive care and oncology in the last few decades, GB remains incurable with a median overall survival of 15 months after its first diagnosis [3, 4]. Antiangiogenesis is a therapeutic strategy aiming at the suspension of tumour cells in a state of dormancy by disrupting their blood supply [5]. As hypervascularity, characterized by endothelial proliferation, is a hallmark of GB, antiangiogenic therapies are naturally considered potential oncologic treatment options [6]. Studies focused on this therapeutic strategy have led to the development and approval of bevacizumab, a recombinant humanized monoclonal antibody against vascular endothelial growth factor (VEGF), for recurrent GB [7]. However, such clinical trials have produced inconsistent results and the overall benefits of bevacizumab on GB patients are being challenged [8–10]. Moreover, bevacizumab was not recommended for newly diagnosed GB due

* Correspondence: wpoon@surgery.cuhk.edu.hk
[1]Brain Tumor Centre, Department of Surgery, The Chinese University of Hong Kong, Hong Kong, China
Full list of author information is available at the end of the article

to its limited survival benefit and common adverse events [11, 12]. Thus there is an urgent need to develop novel alternative antiangiogenic agents with more convincing therapeutic effects.

Vastatin is the C-terminal non-triple-helical (NC1) domain of the type VIII collagen α1 chain. It is an endogenous polypeptide that initially discovered to inhibit the proliferation and migration of bovine aortic endothelial cells [13]. Our recent study proved that Vastatin, which is normally expressed in normal liver tissue, was distinctly absent in hepatocellular carcinoma (HCC) and possessed antiangiogenic properties. Through interfering with proliferation and metabolism of endothelial cells, Vastatin inhibited tumour growth and prevented metastasis in HCC-bearing rats [14]. Concurrently a recombinant form of Vastatin, rhEDI-8 t, was discovered to be an angiogenesis inhibitor with potential therapeutic benefits for retinopathy-related neovascularization [15]. Since collagen VIII expression is known to be increased in brain tumours and participates in angiogenesis, we are interested in determining whether Vastatin could be used for the treatment of other hypervascular malignancies such as GB [16].

An ideal cancer therapeutic agent should be able to maintain predominantly high concentrations in the tumour thereby minimizing systemic adverse effects. We previously developed a polyplex-forming plasmid delivery agent, Folate-PEI600-CyD (H1). H1 formed nanoparticles with plasmid DNA and showed high affinity to cancer cells through binding to the folate receptors that enriched on cancer cell surface. It had high transfection efficiency especially on GB cells like U87 and U138 [17–19]. More importantly, H1 demonstrated low cytotoxicity and had little effect on normal cells. In the present study we aimed to test the feasibility of using H1 delivered Vastatin gene for treatment of GB xenografts. We report for the first time that enhancing Vastatin expression by H1 mediated gene transfection induced antiangiogenesis and prolonged survival of GB bearing mice, suggesting a promising treatment candidate for future GB drug development.

Methods
Cell lines and Cell culture
The murine tumour-derived microvessel endothelial cells (MECs) SVEC4-10EE2 and human GB cell lines U87MG were purchased from American Type Culture Collection (ATCC). They were maintained in either Minimum Essential Medium (MEM; Gibco) or Dulbecco's modified Eagle's medium (DMEM; Gibco) with 10% fetal-bovine-serum (FBS; Gibco) supplementation at 37 °C, 5% CO_2, and used for test within 20 passages after purchase.

GB cells with acquired TMZ resistance (ATR) were derived from U87MG cells through chronic exposure to TMZ. U87MG cells were first incubated in DMEM containing 20 μM TMZ for 2 weeks, then subcultured into DMEM with 200 μM TMZ. Cells that managed to survive and proliferate in this medium for more than five passages were then collected. The final generated cells were considered resistant to TMZ treatment and named U87-ATR.

Preparation of H1/DNA Polyplexes
Plasmid pORF-EGFP, pORF-Endostatin and pORF-Vastatin were constructed by inserting DNA fragments encoding EGFP, Endostatin and Vastatin into the multiple cloning sites of the pORF-mcs expression vector (InvivoGen). The secretion of Vastatin and Endostatin protein were mediated by the Igk leader. The encoded gene was further confirmed by DNA sequencing.

The PEI600-CyD-Folate (H1) gene vector was synthesized as previously reported [18]. H1 polymer solution was added to pDNA solution in equal volumes to form the polyplexes. The ratio between the amount of nitrogen in PEI and the amount of phosphate in DNA (N/P ratio) was predetermined at 20. The polyplex suspension was allowed to incubate at room temperature for 15 min before being used for transfection or injection.

Orthotopic GB Murine Model
Animal studies were performed in accordance with the protocol approved by the Animal Experimentation Ethics Committee of the Chinese University of Hong Kong (CUHK). Female nude mice, 6 to 8 weeks old, were purchased from the laboratory animal services center in CUHK. To establish the murine orthotopic GB model, animals were anaesthetised with ketamine:xylazine (100 mg/kg:10 mg/kg.body weight) and mounted into a stereotaxic frame (Stoelting Co.). A burr hole located 0.5 mm anterior to the coronal suture and 1.2 mm right to the sagittal suture was created. U87MG GB cells or U87-ATR cells were harvested and resuspended in phosphate buffered saline (PBS) to a concentration of 1×10^5 cells/μL. The needle of a Hamilton microsyringe was inserted through the burr hole to a depth of 2.5 mm where the right striatum is located. A total of 2×10^5 cells were slowly injected into this area at a rate of 0.2 μL/min. The needle was slowly withdrawn 5 min after cell injection. The mice were then kept within far infrared lighting cabinets until recovery.

Gene Expression Test
Total 15 mice bearing U87MG xenografts were used for detection of gene expression after H1-Vastatin treatment. Treatments were performed by intracerebral injecting the H1-Vastatin polyplexes to the same location of tumour cell inoculation and ventricle nearby. A 20 μL volume of H1-Vastatin solution was injected into each mouse at a rate of 0.5 μL/min. This process was performed twice, on day 7 and day 14 post cell-inoculation, to achieve a total

dosage of 20 μg plasmid DNA. Mice were sacrificed on day 7 (1 h after the first treatment), 10, 14 (1 h after the second treatment), 17 and 21, with 3 mice each time. The right hemispheres were isolated immediately for measurement of Vastatin mRNA level. Total RNA was extracted from brain tissues using TRIzol® Reagent (Invitrogen) and then reverse transcribed to cDNA with SuperScript® II Reverse Transcriptases (Invitrogen). The cDNA was then subjected to PCR assay and gel electrophoresis. The following primer sequences were used: Vastatin (forward:5'-AAC TAC AAC CCG CAG ACA GG -3'; reverse:5'- TGA ATA GAG CAA CCC ACA CG -3'); Collagen VIII α1 (forward: 5'- ACT CTG TCA GAC TCA TTC AGG C -3'; reverse: 5'- CAA AGG CAT GTG AGG GAC TTG -3'); and GAPDH (forward:5'- GAA TCT ACT GGC GTC TTC ACC -3'; reverse:5'-GTC ATG AGC CCT TCC ACG ATG C -3').

Animal survival tests

Total 28 mice bearing U87MG xenografts were used to study the survival benefit of H1-Vastatin single treatment. On day 7 after model establishment, the mice were randomized into four groups, 7 mice for each group, and treated with H1-Vastatin, H1-Endostatin, H1-EGFP or PBS respectively. Treatments were performed using the same protocol for H1-Vastatin in gene expression test. The behaviors and survival of these mice were monitored daily. Mouse was sacrificed and recorded as dead when it lost over 20% of its body weight or exhibited serious behavioral disorders like seizures and limb weakness. The animal survivals after model establishment will be summarized in Kaplan-Meier survival curves.

To test the sensitivities of different model to TMZ treatment, 10 mice bearing U87MG xenografts and 10 mice bearing U87-ATR xenografts were used. On day 7 after model establishment, 5 mice with U87MG xenografts and 5 mice with U87-ATR xenografts were scheduled to be treated with TMZ, while the other 10 mice treated with PBS. TMZ was administered via intraperitoneal (i.p.) injection at a dose of 50 mg/kg/day. TMZ powder was first dissolved in dimethyl sulfoxide (DMSO; Sigma) and diluted with PBS before injection. This treatment was performed five times per week and lasted for 2 weeks. The behaviors and survival of animals were monitored daily as mentioned above.

To examine the combination effect of H1-Vastatin and TMZ, 20 mice bearing U87-ATR xenografts were used. On day 7 after model establishment, the mice were randomized into four groups, 5 mice for each group, and treated with H1-EGFP + PBS, H1-EGFP + TMZ, H1-Vastatin + PBS, or H1-Vastatin + TMZ respectively. Treatment of H1-DNA and TMZ were performed using the same protocols mentioned above. The first TMZ administration was carried out 1 h after the first H1-DNA treatment on day 7.

The behaviors and survival of animal were monitored and recorded daily.

Histology study

Nine mice bearing U87MG xenografts were used for histological study and microvessel density (MVD) analysis. On day 7 after model establishment, animals were divided into three groups, three mice in each group, and received the treatment of H1-Vastatin, H1-EGFP or PBS. All these mice were sacrificed on day 42. Whole brain tissues were collected and processed through 10% formalin fixation and paraffin embedding. The tissue blocks were then cut at 5 μm thickness with a microtome for histological analysis. Tumour structure assessment was performed using Hematoxylin & Eosin (H&E) staining. Angiogenesis in tumour tissues was detected by immunohistochemical staining using rabbit anti-CD34 primary antibody (Abcam) and HRP-linked anti-rabbit secondary antibody (Cell Signaling Technology), in accordance with a previous publication [20]. MVD was calculated by counting the percentage of CD34 positive cells in five randomly chosen high-power fields from each tumour.

Cell proliferation assay

For proliferation assays, 2×10^4 U87MG cells or 2×10^5 SVEC4-10EE2 MECs were seeded in a six-well plate and allowed to adhere. Twenty-four hours later, these cells were treated with H1/Vastatin or H1/EGFP (N/P ratio = 20) for 6 h at a dosage of 10 μg DNA per well and then incubated in DMEM with 10% FBS. Cell viability was assessed 2, 4, or 7 days later by trypan blue exclusion and viable cells were counted manually [21]. In the co-culture system, 2×10^5 MECs were seeded in a six-well plate while 2×10^5 U87MG cells were seeded onto the inner surface of the PET membrane located at the base of the Falcon™ culture insert (BD Biosciences). The insert was then placed into the six-well plate where the MECs were seeded. H1/Vastatin or H1/EGFP treatment was added to the inner surface of the insert for 6 h. Proliferation assays were carried out by counting the viable MECs at the same aforementioned time points.

To evaluate the inhibitory effects of secreted Vastatin on MEC proliferation, conditioned media were used. In brief, 2×10^6 U87MG or SVEC4-10EE2 cells were seeded in 100 mm culture dishes, treated with H1-Vastatin or H1-EGFP at a dose of 10 μg DNA per dish for 8 h, then incubated in DMEM with 10% FBS for 96 h. The conditioned media were collected and centrifuged at 600 g, 4 °C for 10 min. SVEC4-10EE2 MECs were seeded in a 96-well plate at a density of 5000 cells per well. After cell attachment, the media were changed to serial dilutions of conditioned media with 10% FBS. Seven days later, 3-(4,5-dimethyl-2-thiazolyl)-2,5-diphenyl-2H-tetrazolium bromide (MTT) was added to the media and incubated for 2 h. The media were then changed to dimethyl sulfoxide (DMSO) and assessed by colorimetric analysis at 570 nm.

In vitro temozolomide resistance testing

For proliferation inhibition, 2000 U87MG or U87-ATR cells were seeded into each well of a 96-well plate and treated with increasing concentrations of TMZ. MTT assays were used to examine cell viability 4 days later. For clonogenic survival assays, U87MG or U87-ATR cells were seeded into a six-well plate at a density of 500 cells per well. The media were then changed to DMEM containing 10% FBS and 100 μM TMZ for incubation. On day 14 the number of colonies containing more than 50 cells were counted.

Statistical analysis

Mice survival was analysed with PASW Statistics Version 18 (SPSS Inc., Chicago, Illinois). Comparisons in proliferation tests and MVD analysis were conducted by one-way analysis of variance or two-tailed Student's t test. Comparisons of animal survivals were performed using Log-rank test. $P < 0.05$ was considered statistically significant.

Results

H1-Vastatin transfected GB cells and inhibited MECs proliferation through paracrine suppression

The H1 gene vector was designed specifically to target tumour cells [18]. We proposed that H1 mediated gene transfection could restrict the expression and secretion of therapeutic agents in tumour areas and prevent systemic side effects. To prove this idea, GB U87MG cells and mouse MECs SVEC4-10EE2 were treated with either H1-Vastatin or H1-EGFP in culture. Only U87MG cells treated by H1-Vastain showed enhanced Vastatin mRNA levels (Fig. 1a), which was consistent with previous report that H1-DNA nanoparticles transfected cancer cells specifically. We further conducted a series of proliferation tests on days 2, 4 and 7 after the cells received H1-Vastatin treatment. As anticipated, H1-Vastatin showed no significant influence on cell viability of either U87MG or MECs (Fig. 1b, *left and middle*). However in a U87MG and MECs trans-well co-culture system, the proliferation of MECs was significantly inhibited on day 7 post-transfection (Fig. 1b, *right*; $P < 0.05$). This has demonstrated that the expression and secretion of Vastatin from H1-Vastatin transfected U87MG cells was necessary for inducing proliferation inhibition in MECs. Then we collected conditioned media (CM) from different culture groups on day 4 post-treatment. MECs SVEC4-10EE2 were seeded into a 96-well plate and incubated in serial dilutions of these CM. Proliferation test was performed 1 week later. Cell viabilities from different culture conditions were normalized to the NO CM culture group to generate an inhibition curve (Fig. 1c). The results

showed that CM collected form H1-Vastatin treated U87MG reduced MECs proliferation in a dose-dependent way, while CM from H1-Vastatin treated MECs or H1-EGFP treated U87MG had no such effect. This further supported our anticipation that H1-Vastatin could induce Vastatin secretion from tumour cells and suppress MECs proliferation by paracrine inhibition.

Administration of H1-Vastatin prolonged survival in GB-bearing mice

The therapeutic benefit of H1-Vastatin was studied on GB-bearing mice and compared with PBS, EGFP and Endostatin. An orthotopic GB model was established by intracranial inoculation of U87MG cells into the nude mice. Intracerebral injections of H1-Vastatin, H1-Endostatin, H1-EGFP or PBS were performed on day 7 and day 14 after cells inoculation. Sustained expression enhancement of intracranial Vastatin level was observed after H1-Vastatin treatment (Fig. 2a). H1-Vastatin successfully prolonged animal survival from a median of 48 days (PBS treated group) to 75 days ($P < 0.01$, $n = 7$ for each group; Fig. 2b). The animal survival was also significantly extended in the Endostatin treated group (median survival of 64 days; $P < 0.01$ against the PBS treated group). H1-EGFP caused no significant difference on animal survival (median survival of 51 days), suggesting that the vector per se did not interfere with the test. However, no significant difference in animal survival was detected between the Vastatin group and the Endostatin group. These results imply that Vastatin has a potent anti-tumour activity in this GB model, and is comparable to the well studied endogenous antiangiogenic agent Endostatin.

Administration of H1-Vastatin decreased microvessel density (MVD) in GB-bearing mice

For histological assessment, mice bearing GB xenografts were treated with PBS, H1-EGFP or H1-Vastatin respectively ($n = 3$ for each group). The animals were sacrificed at day 42 post tumour cell inoculation. The brain tissues were then fixed in formalin, embedded into paraffin blocks and processed for slicing and staining. Angiogenesis was detected by immunohistochemical staining against cells expressing CD34, a protein marker for blood vessel endothelial cells. Results showed that H1-Vastatin significantly reduced CD34+ cells in brain tumours (Fig. 3a). Microvessel density in the H1-Vastatin treated group (7.3 ± 1.9) was significantly lower than those in the PBS (13.7 ± 1.8, $P < 0.05$) and H1-EGFP (14.5 ± 2.9, $P < 0.05$) treated groups (Fig. 3b). These results indicated that Vastatin induced angiogenesis inhibition and eliminated tumor microvessels in the orthotopic GB model, which could be the underlying mechanism of its survival benefits.

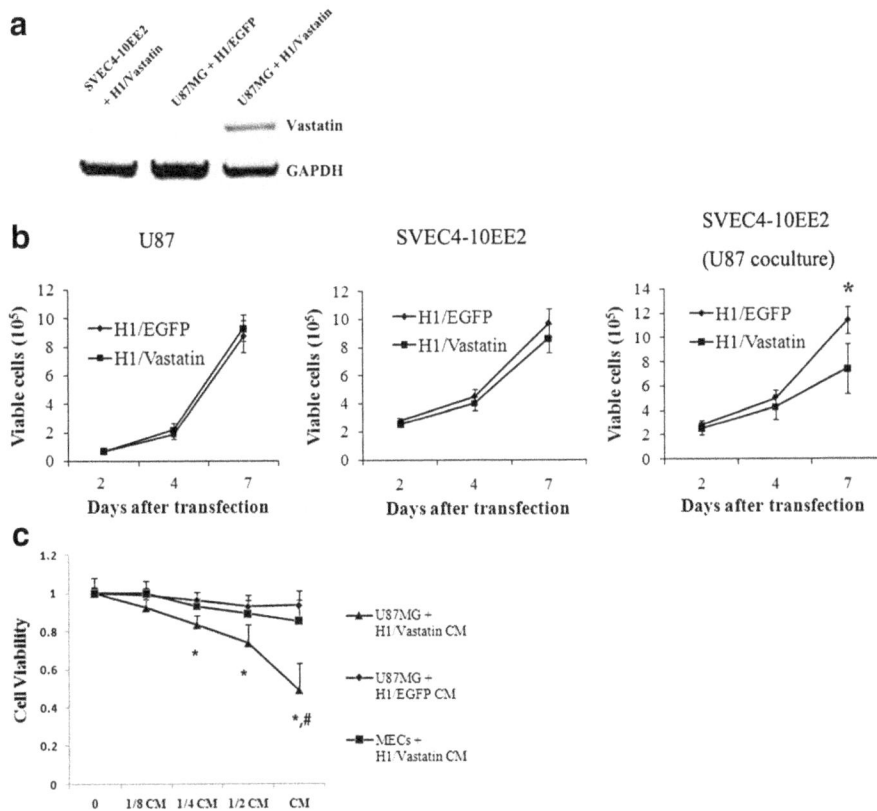

Fig. 1 H1-Vastatin transfectd tumour cells specifically and suppressed MECs proliferation through paracrine inhibition. **a** H1 mediated gene transfections targeted only the tumour cells. Enhanced transcription level of Vastatin was only detected in the H1-Vastatin treated U87MG cells. **b** Proliferation curves of cells treated by H1-Vastatin or H1-EGFP. H1-Vastatin did not affected the proliferation of U87MG cells or MECs in separate culture condition. In the U87MG and MECs co-culure system, H1-Vastatin significantly suppressed the MECs growth on day 7 post treatment ($P < 0.05$). **c** Inhibition curves showing effects of different conditioned media (CM) on MECs proliferation. Conditioned medium from H1-Vastatin treated U87MG cells significantly decreased the cell viability of MECs in a dosage dependant way (* $P < 0.05$ against CM from H1-EGFP treated U87MG cells; # $P < 0.05$ against CM from H1-Vastatin treated MECs), suggesting Vastatin secreted by tumour cells inhibited neovascularization in paracrine manner

H1-Vastatin synergized with TMZ in chemoresistant GB model

TMZ is an alkylating agent which damages tumor cell DNA and triggers cell death. It has been demonstrated to confer moderate survival benefits for GB patients. To test whether H1-Vastatin could facilitate current management of GB, we performed a combined treatment of Vastatin and TMZ on GB orthotopic model. We also established a TMZ resistant GB model, since intrinsic and acquired chemoresistance are the main clinical challenges encountered in TMZ therapy. To induce a stable TMZ resistant cell line, U87MG cells were exposed to TMZ containing medium for a long term incubation. The generated cells, named U87-ATR, were confirmed to be TMZ resistant in both proliferation and survival assays (Fig. 4a). Nude mice intracranially inoculated with U87-ATR cells had significantly shorter survival (median survival of 25 days, $n = 5$) than those with U87MG cells (median survival of 50 days; $P < 0.05$). TMZ was found extremely effective in treating U87MG bearing mice,

with all the animals in this group survived the total duration of 100 days. In contrast, mice with U87-ATR xenografts showed no significant response to TMZ treatment (median survival of 29 days; Fig. 4c). Our results further showed that H1-Vastatin was effective in the treatment of this TMZ resistant model, and significantly extended the median survival from 23 days of the H1-EGFP treated group to 34 days (Fig. 4d; $n = 5$, $P < 0.05$). More interestingly, a synergistic effect was noted between H1-Vastatin and TMZ, which further prolonged the median survival to 54 days ($P < 0.01$ against H1-EGFP treated group; $P < 0.05$ against H1-Vastatin single treatment group).

Discussion

Angiogenesis is the physiological process by which new blood vessels develop from pre-existing vessels. In normal tissues, it is precisely regulated by a series of angiogenic stimulators and inhibitors. In the state of tumour growth, the balance between the stimulators and inhibitors is

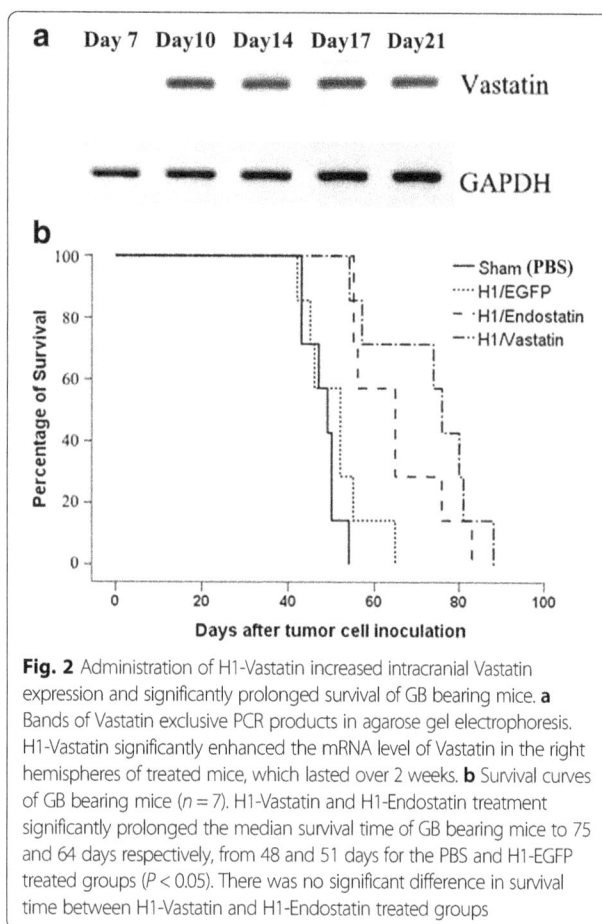

Fig. 2 Administration of H1-Vastatin increased intracranial Vastatin expression and significantly prolonged survival of GB bearing mice. **a** Bands of Vastatin exclusive PCR products in agarose gel electrophoresis. H1-Vastatin significantly enhanced the mRNA level of Vastatin in the right hemispheres of treated mice, which lasted over 2 weeks. **b** Survival curves of GB bearing mice (n = 7). H1-Vastatin and H1-Endostatin treatment significantly prolonged the median survival time of GB bearing mice to 75 and 64 days respectively, from 48 and 51 days for the PBS and H1-EGFP treated groups (P < 0.05). There was no significant difference in survival time between H1-Vastatin and H1-Endostatin treated groups

tipped, towards an "angiogenic switch" [22]. VEGF is one of these stimulators and plays a predominant role in regulating tumour angiogenesis. A humanized monoclonal antibody against VEGF, bevacizumab, has been shown to exhibit treatment response resulting in a longer progression-free survival in GB patients [23, 24]. However, angiogenic inhibitors like bevacizumab which target a single pathway often encounter rapid onset resistance through alternative pathways [25]. Studies that aimed to overcome this resistance have suggested the utilization of a combination of single-pathway targeted antiangiogenic agents [26]. Another alternative is to use broad-spectrum antiangiogenic agents. Endostatin, for example, is a 20-kDA C-terminal cleavage fragment of collagen type XVIII and possesses the broadest anti-cancer spectrum. It targets angiogenesis regulatory genes that comprise of more than 12% of the human genome [27]. Approved by the State Food and Drug Administration of the People's Republic of China, Endostatin is currently a treatment option for non-small-cell lung cancer. Several reports also suggest that Endostatin might be effective in inhibiting tumour growth in malignant glioma in animal models [28–30].

Endostatin represents a group of endogenous angiogenic inhibitors that are fragments of larger extracellular matrix

(ECM) molecules. During angiogenesis, the breakdown of the ECM is a prerequisite for the initiation of sprouting. Endogenous antiangiogenic components are released during this process and act as focal natural feedback [15]. Among them are the NC1 domains cleaved from collagen molecules. Endostatin is the NC1 domain of collagen XVIII. Others include Arresten, Canstatin and Tumstatin from collagen IV, Restin from collagen XVα1, and Vastatin from collagen VIII [13, 31–34]. They form a family collectively referred to as collagen-derived antiangiogenic factors (CDAFs). In cancer studies CDAFs have been reported to be effective in suppressing tumour progression, both in vitro and in vivo [35–37]. Furthermore, these endogenous inhibitors, having been demonstrated to be safe, acting on multiple proangiogenic pathways, are therefore attractive therapeutic candidates [38, 39].

Vastatin is a CDAF from type VIII collagen. Type VIII collagen is present in the ECM of sclera, skin and the renal glomerulus participating in their vascularization [40]. In contrast, Vastatin, contributes to the suppression of ocular neovascularization [15]. The potential of Vastatin in tumour treatment is not fully explored, even though type VIII collagen is highly expressed in selected solid tumours. As far as we know, we are the first to introduce Vastatin into preclinical malignant tumour studies. In our previous report, Vastatin is absent in human HCC, and rAAV-Vastatin infection effectively inhibits proliferation, migration and microvessel formation activities in MECs [14]. In this study we further demonstrate that Vastatin can inhibit angiogenesis and may be of therapeutic benefit in GB. Mechanism studies from our previous HCC research showed that Vastatin inhibited cellular metabolism, Notch and AP-1 signaling pathways [14]. Considering this result was from an in vitro study using MECs not specifically originated from HCC, we believed it could also be used for explaining the Vastatin induced antiangiogenesis in the GB model. The Notch signaling pathway in tumour angiogenesis is well-characterized. In general, delta-like ligand 4 (Dll4) interacts with Notch receptors and reduces VEGF signal transduction on stalk cells during sprouting, which contributes to the structural and functional integrity of newly formed vessels [41]. Inhibition of Dll4 and Notch signaling leads to functionally compromised vessels and suppresses tumour growth [42]. This may help to explain why Vastatin aggravated necrosis in our previous HCC study [14]. Changes in the degree of necrosis was not so obvious in current GB study, probably because the nature of the tumour inherently exhibits an abundance of necrosis as a hallmark feature. In GB, the Notch ligands provided by endothelial cells were also shown to be important for maintaining cancer stem-like cells (CSLCs) [43]. Inhibition of Notch signaling may cause growth inhibition of GSCs [44], which we believed was a possible mechanism underlying Vastatin's anti-glioma effect and

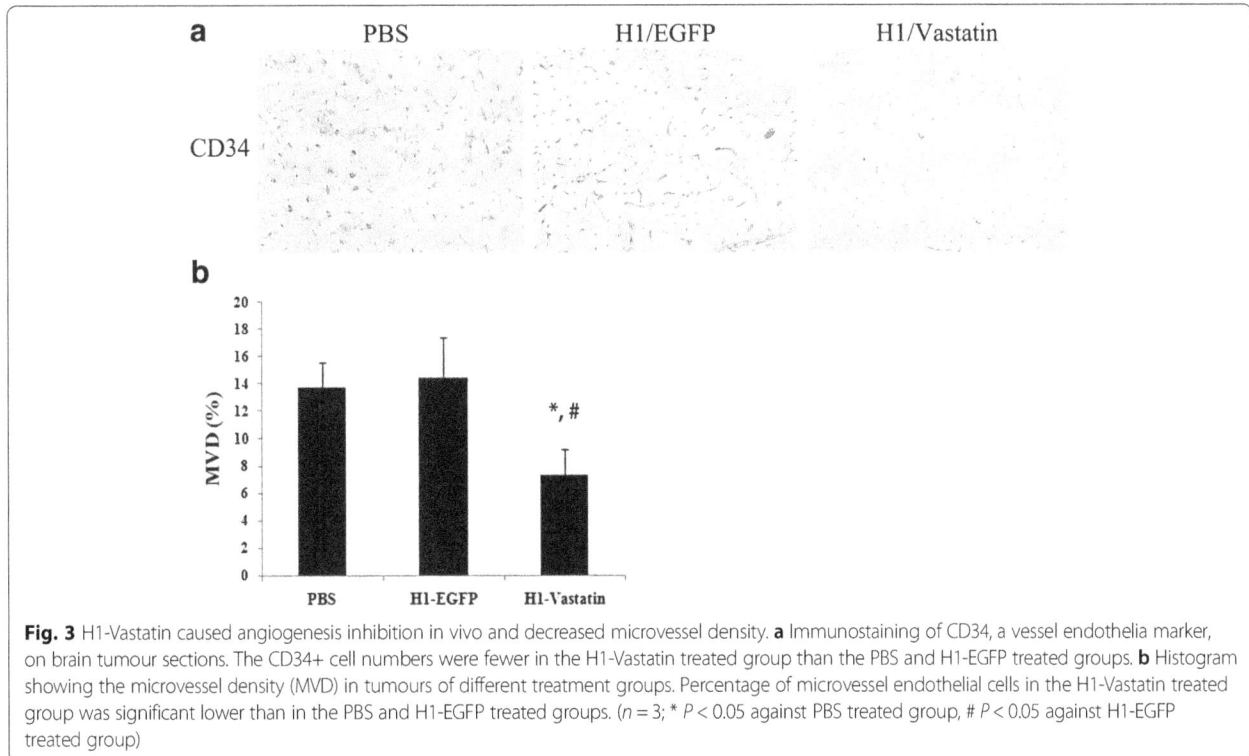

Fig. 3 H1-Vastatin caused angiogenesis inhibition in vivo and decreased microvessel density. **a** Immunostaining of CD34, a vessel endothelia marker, on brain tumour sections. The CD34+ cell numbers were fewer in the H1-Vastatin treated group than the PBS and H1-EGFP treated groups. **b** Histogram showing the microvessel density (MVD) in tumours of different treatment groups. Percentage of microvessel endothelial cells in the H1-Vastatin treated group was significant lower than in the PBS and H1-EGFP treated groups. ($n = 3$; * $P < 0.05$ against PBS treated group, # $P < 0.05$ against H1-EGFP treated group)

distinguished Vastatin from traditional antiangiogenic agents. Unlike Notch signaling, the down-regulation of AP-1 and cell metabolism pathways seems to have a more direct influence on reducing MEC viability. AP-1 is a transcription factor that regulates a wide range of cellular processes, including cell growth, differentiation and apoptosis. In GB, it mediates anoxia induced up-regulation of interleukin-8 (IL-8), a tumourigenic and proangiogenic chemokine [45]. In addition, AP-1 is involved in epidermal growth factor receptor (EGFR) mediated TMZ resistance [46]. Although we did not investigate the relationship between endothelium metabolism and antiangiogenic therapies, it was generally accepted that insufficient nutrients metabolism would lead to cell cycle arrest and apoptosis [47]. This is substantiated by evidence showing that enhanced glucose and glutamine metabolism in proliferating endothelial cells promotes tumour angiogenesis [48]. Altogether these findings depict a multi-targeted antiangiogenic pattern for Vastatin and considerably promotes its potential as an effective therapy for GB.

Safety is a primary concern in the treatment of brain tumours. Vastatin has been proven to be generally safe for systemic administration in previous HCC study [14]. However in this report, we highlighted the feasibility of recruiting H1 for local administration of antiangiogenic therapeutics. H1 induces endocytosis by binding to folate receptors that are highly expressed on certain tumour cell surfaces but not MECs [18]. Both the co-culture and conditioned medium test results imply that H1-Vastatin

induced inhibition of MECs proliferation can be achieved by Vastatin secreted from adjacent GB tumour cells. In other words, H1-Vastatin selectively infects GB cells, restricting its antiangiogenic effects to the vicinity of the tumor thereby reducing the possibility of systemic adverse effects. Our observations that no deleterious effects were detected during the subsequent animal study is consistent with this hypothesis. This type of paracrine inhibition is also compatible with the "angiogenic switch" theory and restores the balance between angiogenic stimulators and inhibitors in the perivascular tumor microenvironment.

Whether antiangiogenic treatments could promote or attenuate chemotherapies is controversial, since changes in vascular integrity and permeability might complicate the passing of medications across the blood brain barrier. Clinical studies have combined bevacizumab with different cytotoxic chemotherapeutic agents in the treatment of either primary or recurrent GB. The results, unfortunately, were negative [12, 49, 50]. Nevertheless, the present study showed H1-Vastatin had a significant synergistic effect with TMZ in a chemoresistant GB murine model. This might be explained by the difference in anti-angiogenic mechanisms of bevacizumab and Vastatin, especially with regards to the Notch signaling regulation. Notch ligands expressed by endothelial cells are crucial for maintaining self-renewal of cancer stem cells [43]. Notch signaling pathway inhibition coupled with TMZ has been proven to exert an anti-glioma stem cell effect [51]. Moreover, the negative Notch-1 expression state was associated with

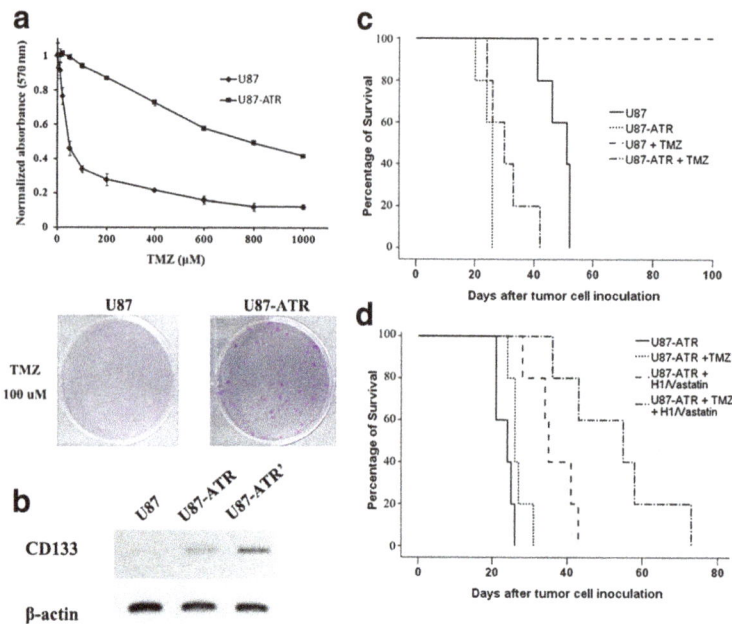

Fig. 4 Vastatin synergized with temozolomide in GB chemoresistant model. **a** TMZ resistance of U87-ATR cells. U87-ATR had a much higher half inhibited dosage of TMZ (>800 μM) than U87MG (<50 μM) in the proliferation test (*upper*). More U87-ATR than U87MG cells survived the treatment of 100 μM TMZ and formed cell colonies (*lower*). **b** U87-ATR cells showed enhanced cancer stem cell property by expression of CSC marker CD133. U87-ATR' were cells amplified from a single cell clone which was picked out from TMZ treated U87-ATR. **c** Survival curves showing that GB model established using U87-ATR had a much shorter survival time (25 days) than using U87MG cells (50 days, $P < 0.05$), and did not respond to TMZ treatment ($n = 5$). **d** Survival curves of TMZ resistance GB animals treated by H1-Vastatin and/or TMZ ($n = 5$). H1-Vastatin significantly prolonged the median survival of animals bearing U87-ATR xenografts to 34 days ($P < 0.05$). The combination of TMZ and H1-Vastatin showed even better therapeutic effects, with median survival extended to 54 days ($P < 0.01$ against H1-EGFP treated group; $P < 0.05$ against H1-Vastatin single treatment group). This result suggested Vastatin synergized with TMZ and restored the sensitivity of chemoresistant mice to TMZ treatments

longer patient survival [52]. During the development of our mouse model, we introduced a group of cells with acquired TMZ resistance from original U87MG cells. These U87-ATR cells exhibited significant stem cell properties as evidenced by the high expression of cancer stem cell marker CD133 (Fig. 4b). The synergistic effect between Vastatin and TMZ in U87-ATR bearing mice might possibly be mediated by the suppression of Notch signaling in MECs, which subsequently lead to the eradication of perivascular niches for U87-ATR and other chemoresistant cancer stem like cells. However, it is one of our limitations that we did not show a direct inhibition effect of Vastatin treated MECs on U87-ATR cells, due to the lack of efficient cell-cell interaction model as well as the complications caused by the paracrine angiogenesis inhibition strategy. Studies to further investigate the synergistic effect between Vastatin and TMZ are ongoing, which we believe will help to discover the underlying mechanisms not just limited to a single pathway.

Conclusion

We report for the first time that Vastatin can induce antiangiogenesis and prolong survival in mice bearing GB orthotopic xenografts. We also confirm that H1-Vastatin

offers a safe and efficient targeting method for GB antiangiogenic therapeutic tests. More importantly, a synergistic treatment effect is observed when Vastatin is coupled with TMZ therapy, which leads to the resensitization of initial chemoresistant GB model to TMZ treatment. At present, there is no effective treatment for patients with recurrent GB. Our results regarding the anti-tumor effects of Vastatin bear potential clinical therapeutic significance. The limitation of this study was that only used one animal model with one GB cell line were employed. Future studies should confirm these findings in models with more cell lines and different animals. Studies are also needed to further elucidate the pharmacological properties of Vastatin and its toxicological profile. In addition, combination effect of Vastatin and radiotherapy should be tested, since radiotherapy is a first-line treatment to GB patient and radioresistance is related to CSCs as well.

Abbreviations
AP-1: Activator protein-1; ATR: Acquired temozolomide resistance; CDAF: Collagen-derived antiangiogenic factor; CM: Conditioned medium; CSC: Cancer stem cell; ECM: Extracellular matrix; EGFP: Enhanced Green Fluorescent Protein; GB: Glioblastoma; HCC: Hepatocellular carcinoma; MEC: Microvessel endothelial cell; MVD: Microvessel density; PBS: Phosphate buffered saline; PEI: Polyethylenimine; rAAV: Recombinant adeno-associated virus; TMZ: Temozolomide; VEGF: Vascular endothelial growth factor

Acknowledgements
We are grateful to Prof. Gong Chen and his team, Ms Jennifer Siu and Mr Johnny SZE for their technical assistance in H1 and plasmids preparation and cell culture.

Funding
This work was supported by the General Research Fund (CUHK 772910) from the Research Grants Council, Hong Kong. Otto Wong Brain Tumour Centre of the Chinese University of Hong Kong had partially supported a Research Assistant and laboratory consumables.

Authors' contributions
YL designed this study, performed the experiments, analyzed data and prepared the manuscript; JL and YC designed this the study and participated in the cellular studies; HY and ZS participated in the nanoparticle preparation and animal treatment design; YW advised on clinical backgrounds and helped preparing this manuscript; ML and WP gave professional advices on study design and clinical backgrounds. All authors have read and approved the manuscript.

Competing interest
The authors declare that they have no competing interests.

Author details
[1]Brain Tumor Centre, Department of Surgery, The Chinese University of Hong Kong, Hong Kong, China. [2]Department of Neurosurgery, Kwong Wah Hospital, Hong Kong, China. [3]Department of Oncology, Affiliated 6th People's Hospital, Shanghai Jiaotong University, Shanghai, China. [4]Jiangsu Eng. Lab of Cancer Biotherapy, Xuzhou Medical College, Xuzhou, China.

References
1. Dolecek TA, Propp JM, Stroup NE, Kruchko C. CBTRUS statistical report: primary brain and central nervous system tumors diagnosed in the United States in 2005-2009. Neuro Oncol. 2012;14 Suppl 5:v1–49.
2. Wen PY, Kesari S. Malignant gliomas in adults. N Engl J Med. 2008;359(5):492–507.
3. Van Meir EG, Hadjipanayis CG, Norden AD, Shu HK, Wen PY, Olson JJ. Exciting new advances in neuro-oncology: the avenue to a cure for malignant glioma. CA Cancer J Clin. 2010;60(3):166–93.
4. Johnson DR, Leeper HE, Uhm JH. Glioblastoma survival in the United States improved after Food and Drug Administration approval of bevacizumab: a population-based analysis. Cancer. 2013;119(19):3489–95.
5. Folkman J. Tumor angiogenesis: therapeutic implications. N Engl J Med. 1971;285(21):1182–6.
6. Gilbert MR. Antiangiogenic therapy for glioblastoma: complex biology and complicated results. J Clin Oncol. 2016;34(14):1567–9.
7. Norden AD, Young GS, Setayesh K, Muzikansky A, Klufas R, Ross GL, Ciampa AS, Ebbeling LG, Levy B, Drappatz J, et al. Bevacizumab for recurrent malignant gliomas: efficacy, toxicity, and patterns of recurrence. Neurology. 2008;70(10):779–87.
8. Pope WB, Xia Q, Paton VE, Das A, Hambleton J, Kim HJ, Huo J, Brown MS, Goldin J, Cloughesy T. Patterns of progression in patients with recurrent glioblastoma treated with bevacizumab. Neurology. 2011;76(5):432–7.
9. Junck L. Bevacizumab antiangiogenic therapy for glioblastoma. Neurology. 2011;76(5):414–5.
10. Wick W, Weller M, van den Bent M, Stupp R. Bevacizumab and recurrent malignant gliomas: a European perspective. J Clin Oncol. 2010;28(12):e188–189. author reply e190-182.
11. Gilbert MR, Dignam JJ, Armstrong TS, Wefel JS, Blumenthal DT, Vogelbaum MA, Colman H, Chakravarti A, Pugh S, Won M, et al. A randomized trial of bevacizumab for newly diagnosed glioblastoma. N Engl J Med. 2014;370(8):699–708.
12. Chinot OL, Wick W, Mason W, Henriksson R, Saran F, Nishikawa R, Carpentier AF, Hoang-Xuan K, Kavan P, Cernea D, et al. Bevacizumab plus radiotherapy-temozolomide for newly diagnosed glioblastoma. N Engl J Med. 2014; 370(8):709 22.
13. Xu R, Yao ZY, Xin L, Zhang Q, Li TP, Gan RB. NC1 domain of human type VIII collagen (alpha 1) inhibits bovine aortic endothelial cell proliferation and causes cell apoptosis. Biochem Biophys Res Commun. 2001;289(1):264–8.
14. Shen Z, Yao C, Wang Z, Yue L, Fang Z, Yao H, Lin F, Zhao H, Sun YJ, Bian XW, et al. Vastatin, an Endogenous Antiangiogenesis Polypeptide That Is Lost in Hepatocellular Carcinoma, Effectively Inhibits Tumor Metastasis. Mol Ther. 2016;24(8):1358–68.
15. Zhang L, Shen X, Lu Q, Zhou Q, Gu J, Gan R, Zhang H, Sun X, Xie B. A potential therapeutic strategy for inhibition of ocular neovascularization with a new endogenous protein: rhEDI-8t. Graefe's Arch Clin Exp Ophthalmology. 2012;250(5):731–9.
16. Paulus W, Sage EH, Liszka U, Iruela-Arispe ML, Jellinger K. Increased levels of type VIII collagen in human brain tumours compared to normal brain tissue and non-neoplastic cerebral disorders. Br J Cancer. 1991;63(3):367–71.
17. Yao H, Ng SS, Huo LF, Chow BK, Shen Z, Yang M, Sze J, Ko O, Li M, Yue A, et al. Effective melanoma immunotherapy with interleukin-2 delivered by a novel polymeric nanoparticle. Mol Cancer Ther. 2011;10(6):1082–92.
18. Yao H, Ng SS, Tucker WO, Tsang YK, Man K, Wang XM, Chow BK, Kung HF, Tang GP, Lin MC. The gene transfection efficiency of a folate-PEI600-cyclodextrin nanopolymer. Biomaterials. 2009;30(29):5793–803.
19. Hu BG, Liu LP, Chen GG, Ye CG, Leung KK, Ho RL, Lin MC, Lai PB. Therapeutic efficacy of improved alpha-fetoprotein promoter-mediated tBid delivered by folate-PEI600-cyclodextrin nanopolymer vector in hepatocellular carcinoma. Exp Cell Res. 2014;324(2):183–91.
20. Liu XM, Zhang QP, Mu YG, Zhang XH, Sai K, Pang JC, Ng HK, Chen ZP. Clinical significance of vasculogenic mimicry in human gliomas. J Neurooncol. 2011;105(2):173–9.
21. Shen Z, Yang ZF, Gao Y, Li JC, Chen HX, Liu CC, Poon RT, Fan ST, Luk JM, Sze KH, et al. The kringle 1 domain of hepatocyte growth factor has antiangiogenic and antitumor cell effects on hepatocellular carcinoma. Cancer Res. 2008;68(2):404–14.
22. Ribatti D. Endogenous inhibitors of angiogenesis: a historical review. Leuk Res. 2009;33(5):638–44.
23. Cloughesy T. FDA accelerated approval benefits glioblastoma. Lancet Oncol. 2010;11(12):1120.
24. Kreisl TN, Kim L, Moore K, Duic P, Royce C, Stroud I, Garren N, Mackey M, Butman JA, Camphausen K, et al. Phase II trial of single-agent bevacizumab followed by bevacizumab plus irinotecan at tumor progression in recurrent glioblastoma. J Clin Oncol. 2009;27(5):740–5.
25. Norden AD, Drappatz J, Wen PY. Antiangiogenic therapies for high-grade glioma. Nat Rev Neurol. 2009;5(11):610–20.
26. Moreno Garcia V, Basu B, Molife LR, Kaye SB. Combining antiangiogenics to overcome resistance: rationale and clinical experience. Clin Cancer Res. 2012;18(14):3750–61.
27. Abdollahi A, Hahnfeldt P, Maercker C, Grone HJ, Debus J, Ansorge W, Folkman J, Hlatky L, Huber PE. Endostatin's antiangiogenic signaling network. Mol Cell. 2004;13(5):649–63.
28. Read TA, Sorensen DR, Mahesparan R, Enger PO, Timpl R, Olsen BR, Hjelstuen MH, Haraldseth O, Bjerkvig R. Local endostatin treatment of gliomas administered by microencapsulated producer cells. Nat Biotechnol. 2001;19(1):29–34.
29. Peroulis I, Jonas N, Saleh M. Antiangiogenic activity of endostatin inhibits C6 glioma growth. Int J Cancer. 2002;97(6):839–45.
30. Schmidt NO, Ziu M, Carrabba G, Giussani C, Bello L, Sun Y, Schmidt K, Albert M, Black PM, Carroll RS. Antiangiogenic therapy by local intracerebral microinfusion improves treatment efficiency and survival in an orthotopic human glioblastoma model. Clin Cancer Res. 2004;10(4):1255–62.
31. Colorado PC, Torre A, Kamphaus G, Maeshima Y, Hopfer H, Takahashi K, Volk R, Zamborsky ED, Herman S, Sarkar PK, et al. Anti-angiogenic cues from vascular basement membrane collagen. Cancer Res. 2000;60(9):2520–6.
32. Kamphaus GD, Colorado PC, Panka DJ, Hopfer H, Ramchandran R, Torre A, Maeshima Y, Mier JW, Sukhatme VP, Kalluri R. Canstatin, a novel matrix-derived inhibitor of angiogenesis and tumor growth. J Biol Chem. 2000; 275(2):1209–15.
33. Maeshima Y, Colorado PC, Kalluri R. Two RGD-independent alpha vbeta 3 integrin binding sites on tumstatin regulate distinct anti-tumor properties. J Biol Chem. 2000;275(31):23745–50.
34. John H, Radtke K, Standker L, Forssmann WG. Identification and characterization of novel endogenous proteolytic forms of the human angiogenesis inhibitors restin and endostatin. Biochim Biophys Acta. 2005;1747(2):161–70.

35. Monboisse JC, Oudart JB, Ramont L, Brassart-Pasco S, Maquart FX. Matrikines from basement membrane collagens: a new anti-cancer strategy. Biochim Biophys Acta. 2014;1840(8):2589–98.

36. Oliveira-Ferrer L, Wellbrock J, Bartsch U, Penas EM, Hauschild J, Klokow M, Bokemeyer C, Fiedler W, Schuch G. Combination therapy targeting integrins reduces glioblastoma tumor growth through antiangiogenic and direct antitumor activity and leads to activation of the pro-proliferative prolactin pathway. Mol Cancer. 2013;12(1):144.

37. Thevenard J, Ramont L, Mir LM, Dupont-Deshorgue A, Maquart FX, Monboisse JC, Brassart-Pasco S. A new anti-tumor strategy based on in vivo tumstatin overexpression after plasmid electrotransfer in muscle. Biochem Biophys Res Commun. 2013;432(4):549–52.

38. Chen Z, Guo W, Cao J, Lv F, Zhang W, Qiu L, Li W, Ji D, Zhang S, Xia Z, et al. Endostar in combination with modified FOLFOX6 as an initial therapy in advanced colorectal cancer patients: a phase I clinical trial. Cancer Chemother Pharmacol. 2015;75(3):547–57.

39. Herbst RS, Hess KR, Tran HT, Tseng JE, Mullani NA, Charnsangavej C, Madden T, Davis DW, McConkey DJ, O'Reilly MS, et al. Phase I study of recombinant human endostatin in patients with advanced solid tumors. J Clin Oncol. 2002;20(18):3792–803.

40. Shuttleworth CA. Type VIII collagen. Int J Biochem Cell Biol. 1997;29(10):1145–8.

41. Phng LK, Gerhardt H. Angiogenesis: a team effort coordinated by notch. Dev Cell. 2009;16(2):196–208.

42. Noguera-Troise I, Daly C, Papadopoulos NJ, Coetzee S, Boland P, Gale NW, Lin HC, Yancopoulos GD, Thurston G. Blockade of Dll4 inhibits tumour growth by promoting non-productive angiogenesis. Nature. 2006;444(7122): 1032–7.

43. Zhu TS, Costello MA, Talsma CE, Flack CG, Crowley JG, Hamm LL, He X, Hervey-Jumper SL, Heth JA, Muraszko KM, et al. Endothelial cells create a stem cell niche in glioblastoma by providing NOTCH ligands that nurture self-renewal of cancer stem-like cells. Cancer Res. 2011;71(18): 6061–72.

44. Saito N, Fu J, Zheng S, Yao J, Wang S, Liu DD, Yuan Y, Sulman EP, Lang FF, Colman H, et al. A high Notch pathway activation predicts response to gamma secretase inhibitors in proneural subtype of glioma tumor-initiating cells. Stem Cells. 2014;32(1):301–12.

45. Brat DJ, Bellail AC, Van Meir EG. The role of interleukin-8 and its receptors in gliomagenesis and tumoral angiogenesis. Neuro Oncol. 2005;7(2):122–33.

46. Munoz JL, Rodriguez-Cruz V, Greco SJ, Ramkissoon SH, Ligon KL, Rameshwar P. Temozolomide resistance in glioblastoma cells occurs partly through epidermal growth factor receptor-mediated induction of connexin 43. Cell Death Dis. 2014;5:e1145.

47. Mason EF, Rathmell JC. Cell metabolism: an essential link between cell growth and apoptosis. Biochim Biophys Acta. 2011;1813(4):645–54.

48. Polet F, Feron O. Endothelial cell metabolism and tumour angiogenesis: glucose and glutamine as essential fuels and lactate as the driving force. J Intern Med. 2013;273(2):156–65.

49. Lai A, Tran A, Nghiemphu PL, Pope WB, Solis OE, Selch M, Filka E, Yong WH, Mischel PS, Liau LM, et al. Phase II study of bevacizumab plus temozolomide during and after radiation therapy for patients with newly diagnosed glioblastoma multiforme. J Clin Oncol. 2011;29(2):142–8.

50. Hasselbalch B, Lassen U, Hansen S, Holmberg M, Sorensen M, Kosteljanetz M, Broholm H, Stockhausen MT, Poulsen HS. Cetuximab, bevacizumab, and irinotecan for patients with primary glioblastoma and progression after radiation therapy and temozolomide: a phase II trial. Neuro Oncol. 2010; 12(5):508–16.

51. Yahyanejad S, King H, Iglesias VS, Granton PV, Barbeau LM, van Hoof SJ, Groot AJ, Habets R, Prickaerts J, Chalmers AJ, et al. NOTCH blockade combined with radiation therapy and temozolomide prolongs survival of orthotopic glioblastoma. Oncotarget. 2016;7(27):41251–64.

52. Saito N, Aoki K, Hirai N, Fujita S, Iwama J, Hiramoto Y, Ishii M, Sato K, Nakayama H, Harashina J, et al. Effect of Notch expression in glioma stem cells on therapeutic response to chemo-radiotherapy in recurrent glioblastoma. Brain Tumor Pathol. 2015;32(3):176–83.

15

Adjuvant stereotactic fractionated radiotherapy to the resection cavity in recurrent glioblastoma – the GlioCave study (NOA 17 – ARO 2016/3 – DKTK ROG trial)

Christoph Straube[1,7]* (iD), Hagen Scherb[2], Jens Gempt[3], Jan Kirschke[4], Claus Zimmer[4], Friederike Schmidt-Graf[5], Bernhard Meyer[3] and Stephanie E. Combs[1,6,7]

Abstract

Background: Glioblastoma relapses in the vast majority of cases within 1 year. Maximum safe resection of the recurrent glioblastoma can be offered in some cases. Re-irradiation has been established for the treatment of recurrent glioblastoma, too. In both cases, adjuvant treatment, mostly using temozolomide, can improve PFS and OS after these interventions. However, combining gross tumor resection and adjuvant re-radiotherapy to the resection cavity has not been tested so far.

Methods/Design: In the multicenter two-armed randomized Phase II GlioCave Study, fractionated stereotactic radiotherapy to the resection cavity, after gross tumor resection of recurrent glioblastoma, will be compared to observation. Depending on the size of the target volume, a total dose of 46 Gy in 2 Gy per fraction or a total dose if 36 Gy in 3 Gy per fraction will be applied. Progression free survival will be the primary endpoint of the study.

Discussion: Adjuvant treatment after gross tumor resection of recurrent glioblastoma is currently deemed to be limited to chemotherapy. However, re-irradiation has proven safety and tolerability in the treatment of macroscopic disease. Performing re-irradiation as an adjuvant measure after gross tumor resection has not been tested so far. The GlioCave Study will investigate the efficacy and the safety profile of this approach.

Keywords: Glioblastoma, Recurrence, Re-irradiation, Gross total resection, Randomized trial, NOA, PFS

Background

Glioblastomas (GBM) refer to the most frequent and most aggressive primary brain tumors in adults; they are associated with a significant treatment resistance, in the primary situation as well as in the case of recurrence [1, 2]. Offering an extensive trimodal course of therapies, containing surgery, postoperative radiochemotherapy as well as adjuvant chemotherapy, survival still remains at a poor level. When first published from a randomized study in 2005, the radiochemotherapy regimen with temozolomide (TMZ) elevated median survival from 12.1 to 14.6 months [3]. However, despite extensive research, only minor progress has been achieved since almost 10 years [4–8].

In the vast majority of cases, GBM recurs within 1 year [3], and in most cases recurrence occurs locally [9]. Currently no standard of care can be defined for the treatment of relapsed GBM so far [10]. Thus, patients are treated within individual concepts, mostly based on retrospective studies or small, non-randomized trials [11].

Re-irradiation, especially when modern techniques such as radiosurgery (RS) or fractionated stereotactic radiotherapy (FSRT) has been established in the clinical

* Correspondence: Christoph.Straube@mri.tum.de
[1]Klinik für RadioOnkologie und Strahlentherapie, Technische Universität München (TUM), Ismaninger Straße 22, 81675 Munich, Germany
[7]Deutsches Konsortium für Translationale Krebsforschung (DKTK) - Partner Site Munich, 81675 Munich, Germany
Full list of author information is available at the end of the article

routine and can be considered a safe and effective alternative for the treatment of recurrent glioblastoma [12–15]. Median overall and progression free survival ranges around 12 and 5 months, respectively, which is comparable to surgery [15, 16]. Generally, re-irradiation is applied in cases with macroscopic tumor remnants, not exceeding a maximum diameter of 4 cm; however, there is much controversy on the ideal target volume, the rationale for imaging during the treatment planning process, as well as to the ideal timepoint of re-irradition. In all cases surgery is evaluated in the case of recurrence, thus is must be discussed whether re-irradiation is only applicable in cases with tumor remnants. To overcome these limitations, it is worth considering multimodal concepts also for recurrent glioblastoma in order to achieve a prolongation of progression free survival.

As a first step, surgery is feasible especially if the tumor recurs in a not eloquent region, in patients with good physical performance status and if the recurrent tumor has a low tumor volume [17]. Furthermore, younger age might be a factor for better outcome [18], yet the prognostic value of second surgery is currently discussed controversially [19, 20].

Combinations of surgery and adjuvant systemic therapy as well as Re-irradiation with concurrent or adjuvant chemotherapy have been reported from several centers [21–24]. Especially the latter was able to achieve median overall survival of up 15 months, counting from the date of radiosurgery, in some series [16]. If only systemic therapy is possible in recurrent GBM due to its location, an early time point after former radiotherapy or the size, then it is associated with an overall survival of 6–8 month [11, 16].

Re-irradiation after surgery was reported to be superior to surgery alone in one prospective cohort, increasing OS from 13 weeks with surgery alone to 34 weeks with surgery plus chemotherapy or radiotherapy as adjuvant treatment [25]. Unfortunately, no target volumes were reported in these series. However, there is no data from randomized trials comparing observation after complete resection to an adjuvant treatment in the same situation. Bimodal local strategies combining complete resection followed by a second course radiotherapy have been reported in the context of brachytherapy, too. The median survival in several studies ranged from 52 weeks to 64 weeks after gross total resection with concurrent implantation of permanent ^{125}Iodine seeds [26, 27]. No case of re-surgery for radionecrosis was reported in these two series, rendering adjuvant radiotherapy after GTR of a recurrent GBM as a safe treatment approach. Within a context of high dose rate brachytherapy, the GliaSite system was tested after maximal safe resection of recurrent glioblastoma in small series, gaining an overall survival of 9–13 months [19, 28]. Low dose rate as well as high dose rate brachytherapy are applied

directly after surgery, thereby precluding sufficient MRI-based planning. Thus, residual tumor might have received only insufficient doses in this series. This would explain remarkably early progressive disease (16 weeks) described in Larson et al. in 2004 [26].

Within the present GlioCave study, we will investigate the impact of radiotherapy as an adjuvant treatment to patients that underwent gross tumor resection of a recurrent GBM.

Methods/Design
Study design
GlioCave is a two-armed randomized multicentre open label phase II trial. Patients fulfilling the inclusion criteria will be 1:1 randomized into two arms (Fig. 1):

Arm A – Experimental Arm.

Postoperative stereotactic fractionated radiotherapy to a Total Dose of 46 Gy, 2 Gy single dose or 36 Gy in 3 Gy fractions depending in the size and location of the target volume.

Arm B – Standard Arm.

Observation
Up to 24th April 2017, the study is active in two sides (Munich, Dresden). Activation of more sides is currently under preparation (Regensburg, Heidelberg, Cologne).

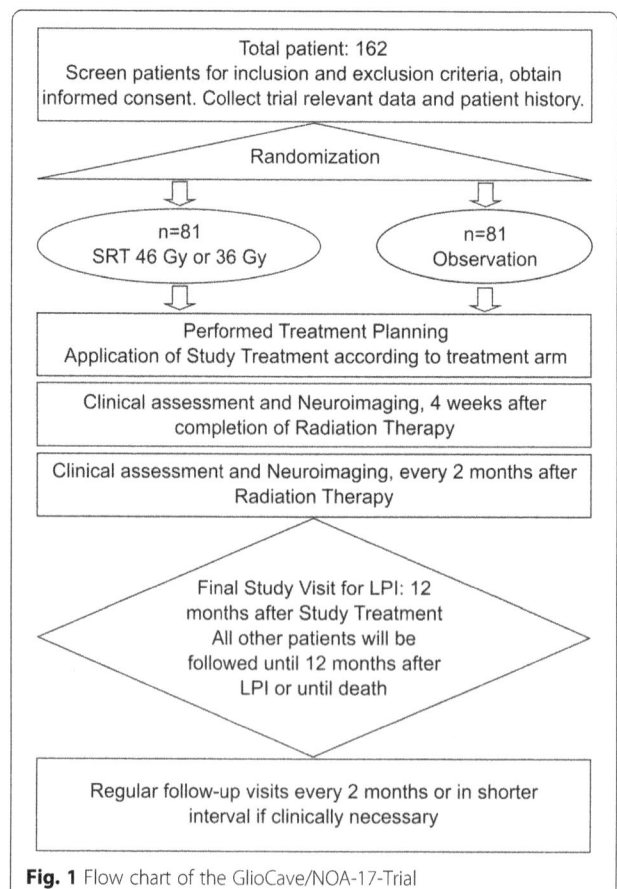

Fig. 1 Flow chart of the GlioCave/NOA-17-Trial

Study objectives and endpoints

The trial is designed to allow the comparison of observation as a standard treatment to adjuvant radiotherapy after GTR of recurrent GBM.

The primary objective of the study is progression-free survival during the follow up phase of at least 12 months. Progression will be defined according to the RANO-HGG as well as to the MacDonald-Criteria [29, 30]. Progression free survival should be preferred as primary endpoint for trials on recurrent glioblastoma as the general aggressiveness of offered treatments influences overall survival in glioblastoma [31]. PFS is thus deemed to be less biased by further therapeutic approaches.

The secondary objectives are overall survival during the follow-up phase of at least 12 months (starting with diagnosis of recurrent disease). Toxicity will be assessed by type, incidence and severity according to the CTCAE v4.02. The EORTC QLQ-C30 version 3.0 questionnaire will be used to monitor for quality of life. Neurocognitive function will be tested at selected centers every 6 months, beginning after randomization. Patients will be followed until death. All study related data will be stored at the MiRO-Database of the Department of Radiation Oncology of the Technical University of Munich.

Patients

Patients with the diagnosis of recurrent GBM presented will be evaluated and screened for the protocol. All patients fulfilling the inclusion and exclusion criteria will be informed about the study.

Inclusion criteria

- Unifocal, supratentorial recurrent glioblastoma
- Prior course of standard treatment
- Complete resection of all contrast enhancing areas
- age ≥ 18 years of age
- Karnofsky Performance Score ≥ 60%
- For women with childbearing potential, (and men) adequate contraception.
- Ability of subject to understand character and individual consequences of the clinical trial
- Written informed consent (must be available before enrolment in the trial)

Exclusion criteria

- Multifocal glioblastoma or gliomatosis cerebri
- Time interval of less than 6 months after primary radiotherapy
- Previous re-irradiation or prior radiosurgery of prior treatment with interstitial radioactive seeds
- refusal of the patients to take part in the study

- Patients who have not yet recovered from acute toxicities of prior therapies
- Known carcinoma < 5 years ago (excluding Carcinoma in situ of the cervix, basal cell carcinoma, squamous cell carcinoma of the skin) requiring immediate treatment interfering with study therapy
- Pregnant or lactating women
- Participation in another clinical study or observation period of competing trials, respectively.

Radiotherapy

Treatment planning will be based on preoperative imaging studies as well as on postoperative MRI and planning MRI.

The clinical target volume (CTV) will contain the margins of the resection cavity of the recurrent tumor, including all contrast enhancing areas +5 mm.

A 1–3 mm expansion will be added to CTV to receive the planning target volume (PTV) depending on individual setup.

Radiotherapy will be prescribed to 95% of the PTV receiving the prescribed dose of either 46 Gy in 2 Gy per fraction or 36 Gy in 3 Gy per fraction.

Systemic therapy

Chemotherapy is not part of this protocol. However, systemic treatments can be offered to the patients at best investigators choice.

Statistics

The study is designed to demonstrate that addition of stereotactic fractionated radiotherapy to the resection cavity can significantly improve the progression free survival compared to a maximum safe resectionwithout a further adjuvant radiotherapy (standard treatment).

The data analytical and the statistical aspects of the study will be in accord with the Guidelines of International Conference on Harmonization (ICH):

- ICH E3: Structure and Contents of Clinical Study Reports
- ICH E6: Good Clinical Practice (GCP). Consolidated Guideline
- ICH E9: Note for Guidance on Statistical Principles in Clinical Trials

In the present context we will use an $\alpha = 0.1$ (one-sided), as a one-sided type I error $\alpha = 0.1$ presents little risk but increases the statistical power of the study. This is supported by a recent communication from the EORTC [32]. The sample size was calculated assuming a progression free survival (PFS) of 7 months after complete resection of a recurrent glioblastoma (control group) and a PFS of 10 months after additive radiotherapy to the resection cavity. With a planned total trial duration of 48 months, containing a recruitment phase of 36 months and a minimum follow up phase of 12 months and a hazard ration of 0.7, a sample of 81 patients per group is necessary to gain a statistical power of 0.8.

The primary endpoint will be analyzed on the per-protocol-group. Calculations will be made within the SAS-LIFETEST-Procedure. This includes non-parametric tests such as Kaplan-Meier-Estimators as well as lifetime-table-based calculations. Statistics for the secondary endpoint Overall Survival (OS) will be calculated similar.

Secondary endpoints will be described descriptively with the use of a Cox-regression model. Age, Karnofsky Performance Score, Recursive Partitioning Analysis, MGMT-status and initial IDH-1-status will be taken into account for the application of an ingression model.

Interim analysis

The interim analysis for safety parameters will be done as soon as 20 patients have been treated and observed for at least 6 months.

Ethical considerations

A positive vote from the local ethical committee of the technical university of Munich, Germany (continuous registration code 525/15 S) was obtained. The study was registered at chlinicaltrials.gov and received the ID NCT02715297.

The protocol received a positive vote from the "Unabhängiges Expertengremium der DEGRO". By that, no further review is necessary.

SPIRIT

The protocol was designed according to the Standard Protokocol Items: Recommendations for Interventional Trials (SPIRIT) criteria and underwent a peer review process.

Discussion

Adjuvant radiotherapy is an established treatment in primary glioblastoma, independent to the extent of resection [3]. For a long time, a second course of radiotherapy was deemed to be unfeasible due to an expected increase in the risk of severe side effects in patients with completely resected recurrences. Adjuvant treatment after GTR of recurrent glioblastoma currently has therefore been limited to chemotherapy. However, during the last decade, re-irradiation-approaches for macroscopic disease have been established successfully with only limited toxicity [11, 15]. With a small margin around the resection cavity, an acceptable amount of brain tissue

will undergo re-irradiation (Manuscript under preparation, Straube et al.). It is therefore worth considering to offer a second course of adjuvant radiotherapy to patients with GTR.

GlioCave is the first phase II trial that will investigate the efficacy as well as the toxicity-profile of this approach.

Abbreviations

CT: Computed tomographie; CTV: Clinical target volume; DEGRO: Deutsche Gesellschaft für Radioonkologie; FSRT: Fractionated stereotactic radiotherapy; GBM: Glioblastoma; GCP: Good clinical practice; GTR: Gross tumor resection; GTV: Gross tumor volume; ICH: International Conference of Harmonization; KPS: Karnofsky performance score; MRI: Magnet resonance imaging; OS: Overall survival; PFS: Progression free survival; PTV: Planning target volume; RS: Radiosurger; TMZ: Temozolomide

Acknowledgments

We are thankful for the support by the German Neurooncological Network (Neuroonkologische Arbeitsgemeinschaft, NOA) and the Working Group Radiation Oncology (Arbeitsgemeinschaft Radiologische Onkologie, ARO) of the German Cancer Society (Deutsche Krebsgesellschaft, DKG). Furthermore, we gratefully acknowledge Prof. Volker Budach and Prof. Wolfgang Wick, members of the DMC, for their advisory opinion.

Funding

The Technical University Munich, Faculty of Medicine, Ismaninger Str. 22, 81,675 Munich, is the sponsor of this trial.
We declare, that we currently do not receive any funding for the trial.

Authors' contributions

CS and SC designed the study protocol obtained ethic's and all other regulatory votes, and wrote the manuscript. HS provided statistical calculations. BM, CZ, JG, JK and FSG will provide patient care. All authors read, edited and approved the final manuscript.

Competing interests

The authors declare that they have no competing interests.

Author details

[1]Klinik für RadioOnkologie und Strahlentherapie, Technische Universität München (TUM), Ismaninger Straße 22, 81675 Munich, Germany. [2]Institute of Computational Biology, Helmholtz Zentrum München, Deutsches Forschungszentrum fuer Gesundheit und Umwelt (GmbH), Ingolstaedter Landstr.1, 85764 Neuherberg, Germany. [3]Neurochirurgische Klinik und Poliklinik, Technische Universität München (TUM), Ismaninger Straße 22, 81675 Munich, Germany. [4]Abteilung für diagnostische und interventionelle Neuroradiologie, Technische Universität München (TUM), Ismaninger Straße 22, 81675 Munich, Germany. [5]Neurologische Klinik und Poliklinik, Technische Universität München (TUM), Ismaninger Straße 22, 81675 Munich, Germany. [6]Institut für Innovative Radiotherapie (iRT), Department of Radiation Sciences (DRS), Helmholtz Zentrum München, Ingolstädter Landstraße 1, 85764 Neuherberg, Germany. [7]Deutsches Konsortium für Translationale Krebsforschung (DKTK) - Partner Site Munich, 81675 Munich, Germany.

References

1. DeAngelis LM. Brain tumors. N Engl J Med. 2001;344:114–23. https://doi.org/10.1056/NEJM200101113440207.

2. Combs S, Schmid T, Vaupel P, Multhoff G. Stress response leading to resistance in Glioblastoma—the need for innovative radiotherapy (iRT) concepts. Cancers. 2016;8:15. https://doi.org/10.3390/cancers8010015.

3. Stupp R, Mason WP, van den Bent MJ, Weller M, Fisher B, Taphoorn MJB, Belanger K, Brandes AA, Marosi C, Bogdahn U, Curschmann J, Janzer RC, Ludwin SK, Gorlia T, Allgeier A, Lacombe D, Cairncross JG, Eisenhauer E, Mirimanoff RO. Radiotherapy plus concomitant and adjuvant temozolomide for glioblastoma. N Engl J Med. 2005;352:987–96. https://doi.org/10.1056/NEJMoa043330.

4. Chinot OL, Wick W, Mason W, Henriksson R, Saran F, Nishikawa R, Carpentier AF, Hoang-Xuan K, Kavan P, Cernea D, Brandes AA, Hilton M, Abrey L, Cloughesy T. Bevacizumab plus radiotherapy-temozolomide for newly diagnosed glioblastoma. N Engl J Med. 2014;370:709–22. https://doi.org/10.1056/NEJMoa1308345.

5. Lai A, Tran A, Nghiemphu PL, Pope WB, Solis OE, Selch M, Filka E, Yong WH, Mischel PS, Liau LM, Phuphanich S, Black K, Peak S, Green RM, Spier CE, Kolevska T, Polikoff J, Fehrenbacher L, Elashoff R, Cloughesy T. Phase II study of bevacizumab plus temozolomide during and after radiation therapy for patients with newly diagnosed glioblastoma multiforme. J Clin Oncol. 2011;29:142–8. https://doi.org/10.1200/JCO.2010.30.2729.

6. Wen PY, Chang SM, Lamborn KR, Kuhn JG, Norden AD, Cloughesy TF, Robins HI, Lieberman FS, Gilbert MR, Mehta MP, Drappatz J, Groves MD, Santagata S, Ligon AH, Yung WKA, Wright JJ, Dancey J, Aldape KD, Prados MD, Ligon KL. Phase I/II study of erlotinib and temsirolimus for patients with recurrent malignant gliomas: north American brain tumor consortium trial 04-02. Neuro-Oncology. 2014;16:567–78. https://doi.org/10.1093/neuonc/not247.

7. Chakravarti A, Wang M, Robins HI, Lautenschlaeger T, Curran WJ, Brachman DG, Schultz CJ, Choucair A, Dolled-Filhart M, Christiansen J, Gustavson M, Molinaro A, Mischel P, Dicker AP, Bredel M, Mehta M. RTOG 0211: a phase 1/2 study of radiation therapy with concurrent gefitinib for newly diagnosed glioblastoma patients. Int. J. Radiat. Oncol. Biol. Phys. 2013;85:1206–11. https://doi.org/10.1016/j.ijrobp.2012.10.008.

8. Friday BB, Anderson SK, Buckner J, Yu C, Giannini C, Geoffroy F, Schwerkoske J, Mazurczak M, Gross H, Pajon E, Jaeckle K, Galanis E. Phase II trial of vorinostat in combination with bortezomib in recurrent glioblastoma: a north central cancer treatment group study. Neuro-Oncology. 2012;14:215–21. https://doi.org/10.1093/neuonc/nor198.

9. Sneed PK, Gutin PH, Larson DA, Malec MK, Phillips TL, Prados MD, Scharfen CO, Weaver KA, Wara WM. Patterns of recurrence of glioblastoma multiforme after external irradiation followed by implant boost. Int J Radiat Oncol Biol Phys. 1994;29:719–27. https://doi.org/10.1016/0360-3016(94)90559-2.

10. Weller M, Cloughesy T, Perry JR, Wick W. Standards of care for treatment of recurrent glioblastoma-are we there yet? Neuro-Oncology. 2013;15:4–27. https://doi.org/10.1093/neuonc/nos273.

11. Niyazi M, Siefert A, Schwarz SB, Ganswindt U, Kreth F-W, Tonn J-C, Belka C. Therapeutic options for recurrent malignant glioma. Radiother Oncol. 2011;98:1–14. https://doi.org/10.1016/j.radonc.2010.11.006.

12. Combs SE, Thilmann C, Edler L, Debus J, Schulz-Ertner D. Efficacy of fractionated stereotactic reirradiation in recurrent gliomas: long-term results in 172 patients treated in a single institution. J Clin Oncol. 2005;23:8863–9. https://doi.org/10.1200/JCO.2005.03.4157.

13. Combs SE, Widmer V, Thilmann C, Hof H, Debus J, Schulz-Ertner D. Stereotactic radiosurgery (SRS): treatment option for recurrent glioblastoma multiforme (GBM). Cancer. 2005;104:2168–73. https://doi.org/10.1002/cncr.21429.

14. Combs SE, Gutwein S, Thilmann C, Debus J, Schulz-Ertner D. Reirradiation of recurrent WHO grade III astrocytomas using fractionated stereotactic radiotherapy (FSRT). Strahlenther Onkol. 2005;181:768–73. https://doi.org/10.1007/s00066-005-1415-6.

15. Amichetti M, Amelio D. A review of the role of re-irradiation in recurrent high-grade Glioma (HGG). Cancers. 2011;3:4061–89. https://doi.org/10.3390/cancers3044061.

16. Kim HR, Kim KH, Kong D-S, Seol HJ, Nam D-H, Lim DH, Lee J-I. Outcome of salvage treatment for recurrent glioblastoma. J Clin Neurosci. 2015;22:468–73. https://doi.org/10.1016/j.jocn.2014.09.018.

17. Park JK, Hodges T, Arko L, Shen M, Dello Iacono D, McNabb A, Olsen Bailey N, Kreisl TN, Iwamoto FM, Sul J, Auh S, Park GE, Fine HA, Black PM. Scale to predict survival after surgery for recurrent Glioblastoma Multiforme. J Clin Oncol. 2010;28:3838–43. https://doi.org/10.1200/JCO.2010.30.0582.

18. Woernle CM, Péus D, Hofer S, Rushing EJ, Held U, Bozinov O, Krayenbühl N, Weller M, Regli L. Efficacy of surgery and further treatment of progressive Glioblastoma. World Neurosurg. 2015;84(2):301–7. https://doi.org/10.1016/j.wneu.2015.03.018.

19. Gobitti C, Borsatti E, Arcicasa M, Roncadin M, Franchin G, Minatel E, Skrap M, Zanotti B, Tuniz F, Cimitan M, Capra E, Drigo A, Trovò MG. Treatment of recurrent high-grade gliomas with GliaSite brachytherapy: a prospective mono-institutional Italian experience. Tumori. 2011;97:614–9. https://doi.org/10.1700/989.10721.

20. Vogelbaum MA. The benefit of surgical resection in recurrent Glioblastoma. 2016;18:1–2. https://doi.org/10.1093/neuonc/now004.

21. Grosu AL, Weber WA, Franz M, Stärk S, Piert M, Thamm R, Gumprecht H, Schwaiger M, Molls M, Nieder C. Reirradiation of recurrent high-grade gliomas using amino acid PET (SPECT)/CT/MRI image fusion to determine gross tumor volume for stereotactic fractionated radiotherapy. Int J Radiat Oncol Biol Phys. 2005;63:511–9. https://doi.org/10.1016/j.ijrobp.2005.01.056.

22. Arcicasa M, Roncadin M, Bidoli E, Dedkov A, Gigante M, Trovò MG. Reirradiation and lomustine in patients with relapsed high-grade gliomas. Int J Radiat Oncol Biol Phys. 1999;43:789–93. https://doi.org/10.1016/S0360-3016(98)00457-X.

23. Combs SE, Bischof M, Welzel T, Hof H, Oertel S, Debus J, Schulz-Ertner D. Radiochemotherapy with temozolomide as re-irradiation using high precision fractionated stereotactic radiotherapy (FSRT) in patients with recurrent gliomas. J Neuro-Oncol. 2008;89:205–10. https://doi.org/10.1007/s11060-008-9607-4.

24. Gutin PH, Iwamoto FM, Beal K, Mohile NA, Karimi S, Hou BL, Lymberis S, Yamada Y, Chang J, Abrey LE. Safety and efficacy of Bevacizumab with Hypofractionated stereotactic irradiation for recurrent malignant Gliomas. Int J Radiat Oncol Biol Phys. 2009;75:156–63. https://doi.org/10.1016/j.ijrobp.2008.10.043.

25. Mandl ES, Dirven CMF, Buis DR, Postma TJ, Vandertop WP. Repeated surgery for glioblastoma multiforme: only in combination with other salvage therapy. Surg Neurol. 2008;69:506–9. https://doi.org/10.1016/j.surneu.2007.03.043.

26. Larson DA, Suplica JM, Chang SM, Lamborn KR, Mcdermott MW, Sneed PK, Prados MD, Wara WM, Nicholas MK, Berger MS. Permanent iodine 125 brachytherapy in patients with progressive or recurrent glioblastoma multiforme. Neuro-Oncology. 2004;6:119–26. https://doi.org/10.1215/S1152851703000425.

27. Halligan JB, Stelzer KJ, Rostomily RC, Spence AM, Griffin TW, Berger MS. Operation and permanent low activity 125I Brachytherapy for recurrent high-grade astrocytomas. Int J Radioation Oncology Biol Phys. 1996;35:541–7.

28. Gabayan AJ, Green SB, Sanan A, Jenrette J, Schultz C, Papagikos M, Tatter SP, Patel A, Amin P, Lustig R, Bastin KT, Watson G, Burri S, Stea B. GliaSite brachytherapy for treatment of recurrent malignant gliomas: a retrospective multi-institutional analysis. Neurosurgery. 2006;58:701–8. https://doi.org/10.1227/01.NEU.0000194836.07848.69.

29. Wen PY, Macdonald DR, Reardon DA, Cloughesy TF, Sorensen AG, Galanis E, DeGroot J, Wick W, Gilbert MR, Lassman AB, Tsien C, Mikkelsen T, Wong ET, Chamberlain MC, Stupp R, Lamborn KR, Vogelbaum MA, Van Den Bent MJ, Chang SM. Updated response assessment criteria for high-grade gliomas: response assessment in neuro-oncology working group. J Clin Oncol. 2010;28:1963–72. https://doi.org/10.1200/JCO.2009.26.3541.

30. Macdonald DR, Cascino TL, Schold SCJ, Cairncross JG. Response criteria for phase II studies of supratentorial malignant glioma. J Clin Oncol. 1990;8:1277–80.

31. Sughrue ME, Sheean T, Bonney PA, Maurer AJ, Teo C. Aggressive repeat surgery for focally recurrent primary glioblastoma: outcomes and theoretical framework. 2015;38:1–7. https://doi.org/10.3171/2014.12.FOCUS14726.DISCLOSURE.

32. Gray R, Manola J, Saxman S, Wright J, Dutcher J, Atkins M, Carducci M, See W, Sweeney C, Liu G, Stein M, Dreicer R, Wilding G, DiPaola RS. Phase II clinical trial design: methods in translational research from the genitourinary Committee at the Eastern Cooperative Oncology Group. Clin Cancer Res. 2006;12:1966–9. https://doi.org/10.1158/1078-0432.CCR-05-1136.

16

In search of druggable targets for GBM amino acid metabolism

Eduard H. Panosyan[1*], Henry J. Lin[1], Jan Koster[2] and Joseph L. Lasky III[1]

Abstract

Background: Amino acid (AA) pathways may contain druggable targets for glioblastoma (GBM). Literature reviews and GBM database (http://r2.amc.nl) analyses were carried out to screen for such targets among 95 AA related enzymes.

Methods: First, we identified the genes that were differentially expressed in GBMs (3 datasets) compared to non-GBM brain tissues (5 datasets), or were associated with survival differences. Further, protein expression for these enzymes was also analyzed in high grade gliomas (HGGs) (*proteinatlas.org*). Finally, AA enzyme and gene expression were compared among the 4 TCGA (The Cancer Genome Atlas) subtypes of GBMs.

Results: We detected differences in enzymes involved in glutamate and urea cycle metabolism in GBM. For example, expression levels of BCAT1 (branched chain amino acid transferase 1) and ASL (argininosuccinate lyase) were high, but ASS1 (argininosuccinate synthase 1) was low in GBM. Proneural and neural TCGA subtypes had low expression of all three. High expression of all three correlated with worse outcome. ASL and ASS1 protein levels were mostly undetected in high grade gliomas, whereas BCAT1 was high. GSS (glutathione synthetase) was not differentially expressed, but higher levels were linked to poor progression free survival. ASPA (aspartoacylase) and GOT1 (glutamic-oxaloacetic transaminase 1) had lower expression in GBM (associated with poor outcomes). All three GABA related genes – glutamate decarboxylase 1 (GAD1) and 2 (GAD2) and 4-aminobutyrate aminotransferase (ABAT) – were lower in mesenchymal tumors, which in contrast showed higher IDO1 (indoleamine 2, 3-dioxygenase 1) and TDO2 (tryptophan 2, 3-diaxygenase). Expression of PRODH (proline dehydrogenase), a putative tumor suppressor, was lower in GBM. Higher levels predicted poor survival.

Conclusions: Several AA-metabolizing enzymes that are higher in GBM, are also linked to poor outcome (such as BCAT1), which makes them potential targets for therapeutic inhibition. Moreover, existing drugs that deplete asparagine and arginine may be effective against brain tumors, and should be studied in conjunction with chemotherapy. Last, AA metabolism is heterogeneous in TCGA subtypes of GBM (as well as medulloblastomas and other pediatric tumors), which may translate to variable responses to AA targeted therapies.

Keywords: Glioblastoma (GBM), Amino-acid (AA) metabolism, BCAT1 (branched chain amino acid transaminase 1), Asparagine (Asn), Glutamine (Gln)

Background

In addition to surgery and radiation, brain tumors are subject to systemic therapies, which circulate in the bloodstream and affect cancer cells all over the body. The systemic therapies for cancer can be grouped into 4 main categories: (1) DNA damaging and/or repair suppressing agents [1] (e.g., cytotoxic chemotherapy); (2) cell signaling inhibition [1–3] (e.g., blocking tumor angiogenesis and tyrosine kinases); (3) immunotherapy [4, 5]; and (4) metabolic strategies [6]. Metabolic approaches are based on assumed differences in metabolism in cancer cells compared to normal tissues [6, 7]. Antimetabolites largely act by diminishing synthesis of molecules essential for cancer cell survival, either by substrate depletion or by interfering with enzyme (s) [6]. Classic examples include asparaginase for acute leukemias [8] and the anti-folate drug, methotrexate, for a variety of tumors [9]. A major advantage of antimetabolites is the absence of direct DNA damage,

* Correspondence: epanosyan@labiomed.org
[1]Los Angeles Biomedical Research Institute and Department of Pediatrics at Harbor-UCLA Medical Center, Box 468, 1000 W. Carson Street, N25, Torrance, CA 90509, USA
Full list of author information is available at the end of the article

which leads to significant bone marrow toxicity [10], and may cause secondary malignancies [11]. Although signaling inhibition and immunotherapy also lack myelosuppression, clinical efficacy of these "targeted" strategies has been limited to only certain types of cancer [3, 5].

The recent discovery of mutations in IDH (isocitrate dehydrogenase, a Krebs cycle enzyme) in some gliomas [12] has renewed interest in antimetabolic approaches in neuro-oncology [13]. In addition to the use of IDH1 and IDH2 inhibitors [12], targeting lipid [14] and carbohydrate (i.e., energy) metabolism has also been an area of research (e.g., use of metformin [15]). Moreover, the augmented amino acid metabolism in brain tumors has led to enhanced neuro-imaging with radiolabeled amino acids as a diagnostic tool [16, 17]. However, manipulation of amino acid metabolism remains an under-studied topic in current neuro-oncology research, and is therefore the topic of this investigation.

Methods

Publically available databases and published literature were used for this study. Our general hypotheses were: (a) differential expression of genes related to amino-acid (AA) metabolism and the corresponding enzymes can help to identify potential drug targets for glioblastoma treatment; (b) correlations among certain genes (or enzymes) and patient survival may indicate clinical relevance; and (c) subtypes of brain tumors may show heterogeneity in AA metabolism.

First, we constructed a list of 95 genes that code for amino-acid metabolizing enzymes, based on known biochemical pathways (Table 1) [18]. Analyses of 22 AA KEGG (Kyoto Encyclopedia of Genes and Genomes) pathways suggested by TCGA data were also used in developing the list. To assess potential differential expression, we used the "R2: Genomic Analysis and Visualization Platform" database (s) at http://r2.amc.nl [19]. R2 contains multiple datasets on various pathological conditions from gene expression microarrays. Datasets generated on 2 Affymetrix chip types, both analyzed by MAS5.0, were used in our study. In addition, certain datasets allowed patient survival analysis in relation to gene expression levels. Selected glioblastoma (GBM) datasets in R2 also allowed analysis based on TCGA subtypes.

Eight datasets, including 3 with GBM and 5 with non-GBM brain tissues, were used to review metabolic differences in GBM (Table 2). In order to minimize ambiguity, we selected 5 non-GBM/control datasets containing information on non-neoplastic brain tissues with or without concomitant conditions (such as mild cognitive impairment, agonal stress or Parkinson's disease). Initially, we screened the entire pool of 95 genes in 3 of the largest GBM datasets, using R2 bar-graphing

tools and Kaplan-Meier curves to identify potentially relevant candidates (representative graphs are shown in Results). Gene probes were selected based on higher expression and availability of the same probe across the datasets and for Kaplan-Meier analysis. About a third of the genes appeared to be either differentially expressed, or have significant association with clinical outcome (i.e., progression free survival and/or overall survival). A few genes were included in our analysis solely based on literature reports on relevance to GBM. For the 34 genes resulting from this initial analysis, we aimed to verify quantitative expression in GBMs and compare these values to expression levels in non-GBM brain tissues.

Statistics for differential gene expression in GBM versus non-GBM

Datasets 1–5 from Table 2 were generated by Affymetrix Human Genome U133 Plus 2.0 arrays (u133p2), and datasets 6–8 by u133pa. To avoid possible misinterpretation of results due to use of the two different arrays, the average gene expression levels were kept in two groups: Mean-A (for datasets 1, 2 and 3); and Mean-B (for datasets 6 and 7). Next, for each gene we calculated 3 ratios of expression, from 3 GBM datasets (using GBM/non-GBM from the same array):

1) Ratio 1 = Gene expression from dataset #4 over Mean-A,
2) Ratio 2 = Gene expression from dataset #5 over Mean-A, and
3) Ratio 3 = Gene expression from dataset #8 over Mean-B.

Last, averages (± standard errors) of ratios 1, 2 and 3 were calculated for each gene (Fig. 1). This procedure allowed us to evaluate differential expression more reliably, and to eliminate a few genes that were proposed in the initial screen.

Protein expression of AA related enzymes in high grade gliomas

Gene expression levels may not always correlate with protein production. Therefore, further verification of our findings at the protein level was considered. An online database (Proteinatlas.org) contains immunohistochemical (IHC) data on most human proteins in a variety of tissues, including gliomas, as part of a cancer atlas project [20]. The database was used to evaluate protein expression for the panel of 34 genes with possible differential expression in high grade gliomas (HGGs). Each tested tumor has a semi-quantitative antibody staining score (i.e., high, medium, low or not detected; representative examples are shown in Fig. 2). The average number of high grade glioma specimens tested for each protein was 8 (range, 5–11).

Table 1 Ninety-five genes for amino acid metabolism related enzymes that were subjected to initial screening

Pathways	Gene/Enzyme
Alanine, asparagine, aspartate, glutamine, & glutamate metabolism:	1. ABAT: 4-aminobutyrate aminotransferase 2. ADSL: adenylosuccinate lyase 3. ADSS: adenylosuccinate synthetase 4. AGXT: alanine-glyoxylate aminotransferase 5. DDO: D-aspartate oxidase 6. ASNS: aspargine synthetase 7. ASPA: aspartoacylase 8. GAD1: glutamate decarboxylase 1 9. GAD2: glutamate decarboxylase 2 10. GOT1: glutamic-oxaloacetic transaminase 1, soluble (i.e., AST: aspartate transaminase or aminotransferase, AspAT/ASAT/AAT or SGOT) 11. GOT2: glutamic-oxaloacetic transaminase 2, mitochondrial 12. GPT: glutamic-pyruvate transaminase (i.e. ALT: alanine aminotransferase) 13. GLUD1: glutamate dehydrogenase 1 14. GLUD2: glutamate dehydrogenase 2 15. ALDH5A1: Aldehyde Dehydrogenase 5 Family, Member A1 16. GLUL: glutamine synthetase (i.e., GS) 17. GFPT2: glutamine-fructose-6-phosphate transaminase 2 18. MECP2: methyl CpG binding protein 2 19. GLS: glutaminase
Histidine metabolism:	20. ALDH1B1: aldehyde dehydrogenase 1 family, member B1 21. CNDP2: CNDP dipeptidase 2 (metallopeptidase M20 family) 22. HDC: Histidine dexarboxylase 23. HAL: histidine ammonia-lyase (i.e., Histidase: HIS or HSTD)
Leucine, isoleucine, & valine metabolism:	24. BCAT1: branched chain amino-acid transaminase 1, cytosolic 25. BCAT2: branched chain amino-acid transaminase 2, mitochondrial 26. LRS: Leucyl-tRNA synthetase 27. BCKDHB: branched chain keto acid dehydrogenase E1, beta polypeptide 28. ILVBL: ilvB (bacterial acetolactate synthase)-like 29. PCCB: propionyl CoA carboxylase, beta polypeptide
Lysine metabolism:	30. AASDHPPT: L-aminoadipate-semialdehyde dehydrogenase-phosphopantetheinyl transferase 31. PIPOX: pipecolic acid oxidase 32. WHSC1L1: Wolf-Hirschhorn syndrome candidate 1-like 1
Phenylalanine metabolism:	33. PAH: phenylalanine hydroxylase 34. FAH: fumarylacetoacetate hydrolase (fumarylacetoacetase)
Serine, glycine, & threonine metabolism:	35. ALAS1: 5'-aminolevulinate synthase 1 36. ALAS2: 5'-aminolevulinate synthase 2 37. GCAT: glycine C-acetyltransferase 38. PHGDH: phosphoglycerate dehydrogenase 39. PSAT1: phosphoserine aminotransferase 1 40. PSPH: phosphoserine phosphatase 41. SDS: serine dehydratase 42. SHMT1: serine hydroxymethyltransferase 1 43. SHMT2: serine hydroxymethyltransferase 2 44. SPTLC1: serine palmitoyltransferase, long chain base subunit 1 45. SPTLC2: serine palmitoyltransferase, long chain base subunit 2 46. SPTLC3: serine palmitoyltransferase, long chain base subunit 3 47. PPP2R4: protein phosphatase 2A activator, regulatory subunit 4 (i.e., PP2A) 48. ALAD: Aminolevulinic dehydrase
Tyrosine metabolism:	49. PNMT: phenylethanolamine N-methyltransferase 50. TH: tyrosine hydroxylase 51. TAT: tyrosine aminotransferase 52. DDC: DOPA decarboxylase (aromatic L-amino acid decarboxylase)
Cysteine, methionine, & glutathione metabolism:	53. CCBL1: cysteine conjugate-beta lyase, cytoplasmic 54. CCBL2: cysteine conjugate-beta lyase 2 55. LDHA: lactate dehydrogenase A 56. AHCY: adenosylhomocysteinase 57. MDH2: malate dehydrogenase 2, NAD (mitochondrial) 58. TYMS: thymidylate synthase 59. CTH: cystathionine gamma-lyase 60. GCLC: glutamate-cysteine ligase, catalytic subunit 61. GCLM: glutamate-cysteine ligase, modifier subunit 62. GSS: Glutathione synthetase 63. MTR: 5-methyltetrahydrofolate-homocysteine methyltransferase

Table 1 Ninety-five genes for amino acid metabolism related enzymes that were subjected to initial screening *(Continued)*

	64. MAT2A: methionine adenosyltransferase II, alpha
Arginine and proline metabolism:	65. OAT: ornithine aminotransferase
	66. CKM: creatine kinase, muscle
	67. LAP3: leucine aminopeptidase 3
	68. ASL: argininosuccinate lyase
	69. ASS1: argininosuccinate synthetase 1
	70. ADC: arginine decarboxylase
	71. DDAH2: dimethylarginine dimethylaminohydrolase 2
	72. GATM: glycine amidinotransferase (L-arginine:glycine amidinotransferase) (i.e., AGAT: arginine:glycine amidinotransferase)
	73. ARG1: arginase 1
	74. PADI2: peptidyl arginine deiminase, type II
	75. PYCR1: pyrroline-5-carboxylate reductase 1
	76. PRODH: proline dehydrogenase (oxidase) 1
Tryptophan metabolism:	77. AANAT: aralkylamine N-acetyltransferase
	78. TDO2: tryptophan 2,3-dioxygenase
	79. TPH1: Tryptophan hydroxylase 1
	80. IDO1: indoleamine 2,3-dioxygenase 1
Selenocompound metabolism:	81. MARS: methionyl-tRNA synthetase
	82. SEPHS1: selenophosphate synthetase 1
Other:	83. AADAT: aminoadipate aminotransferase
	84. UROS: Uroporphyrineogen synthase
	85. UROD: uroporphyrinogen decarboxylase
	86. CPS1: carbamoyl-phosphatesynthase 1, mitochondrial
	87. OTC: ornithine carbamoyltransferase
	88. PDXP: pyridoxal (pyridoxine, vitamin B6) phosphatase
	89. PNPO: pyridoxamine 5′-phosphate oxidase
Amino acid transporters:	90. SLC3A2: solute carrier family 3 (amino acid transporter heavy chain), member 2 (i.e., 4F2hc)
	91. SLC7A11: solute carrier family 7 (anionic amino acid transporter light chain, xc- system), member 11 (i.e., xCT)
	92. SLC7A7 solute carrier family 7 (amino acid transporter light chain, y + L system), member 7 (i.e., LAT3)
	93. SLC7A5: solute carrier family 7 (amino acid transporter light chain, L system), member 5 (i.e., LAT1)
	94. SLC1A5: solute carrier family 1 (neutral amino acid transporter), member 5 (i.e., ASCT2)
	95. SLC6A14: solute carrier family 6 (amino acid transporter), member 14

Figure 2 shows the numbers of tumors with each of the 4 levels of antibody staining, for a given protein. IHC for a few proteins was done with more than one antibody. Selection was based on the most consistent staining pattern, for these proteins.

TCGA database in R2: subtypes and survival analyses

This enriched database contains 540 GBM samples and is the largest among the 3 tested. It allows detailed analysis of patient survival with the Kaplan-Meier method. Comparison of expression of various genes among the

Table 2 Five brain tumor (3 GBM) and five non-brain tumor datasets used

#	Name of dataset	Number of samples	Platform - Chiptype
1	Normal Brain regions - Berchtold	172	u133p2
2	Normal Brain PFC – Harris	44	u133p2
3	Disease[a] Brain - Liang	34	u133p2
4	Tumor Glioblastoma - Loeffler	70	u133p2
5	Tumor Glioblastoma - Hegi	84 (80 tumors)	u133p2
6	Normal Brain agonal stress - Li	1168	u133a
7	Disease Brain Parkinson - Moran	47	u133a
8	Tumor Glioblastoma - TCGA	540	u133a
9	Mixed Pediatric Brain (Normal-Tumor) – Donson	130 (117 tumors)	u133p2
10	Tumor Medulloblastoma – Gilbertson	76 (73 tumors)	u133p2

[a]Brain tissues are from individuals who had been diagnosed with mild cognitive impairment. Detailed description of each dataset is available at http://r2.amc.nl

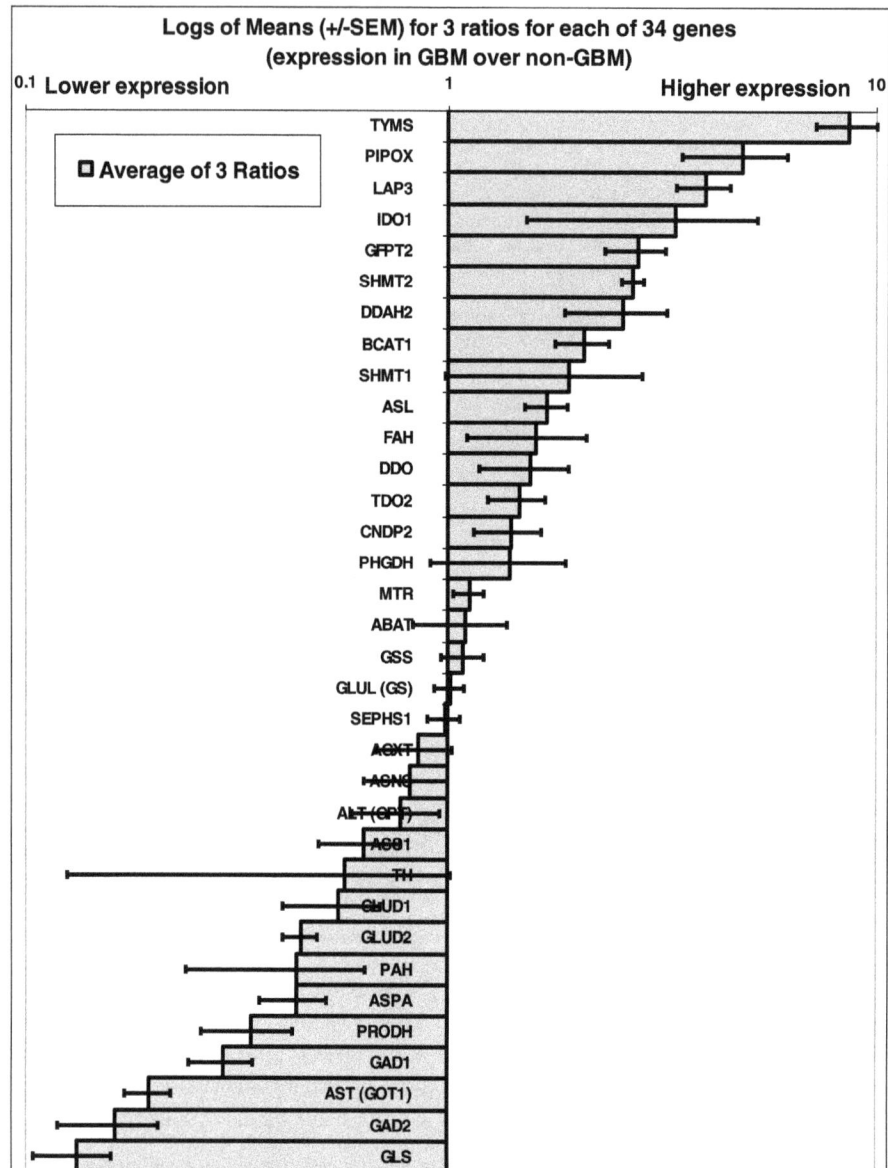

Fig. 1 Differential expression of 34 genes in glioblastoma (GBM). The *x-axis* represents the logarithm of the ratio of gene expression in GBM over expression in normal brain tissue (calculations as described in Methods). Each horizontal bar with errors represents a gene, and ratios are shown as means ± standard errors. Genes listed starting from TDO2 and above are over-expressed genes. Genes listed starting from ASS1 and below are under-expressed genes. Refer to Table 1 for abbreviations. Log of Mean values = 1 indicates equal expression in GBMs and normal brain tissue

4 TCGA subtypes is also possible (proneural, neural, classical and mesenchymal; 85 specimens). For Kaplan-Meier analysis, both progression-free survival (PFS) and overall survival (OS) were assessed for each of the genes with various cut-offs, aiming for *P* values <0.05 (which were considered significant). However, survival analysis in relation to gene expression levels within each subtype was not feasible, due to small sample sizes.

Gene expression "heat maps" for 34 genes

Heat maps were constructed using 3 datasets from R2 (datasets 8, 9 and 10, Table 2). We aimed to display heterogeneity in the form of under- versus over-expression of 34 genes in the 4 GBM and 4 medullo-blastoma subtypes (as defined in TCGA; Fig. 4 and Additional file 1: Figure S1, respectively), as well as in 4 types of pediatric brain tumors versus non-diseased brain (Additional file 2: Figure S2).

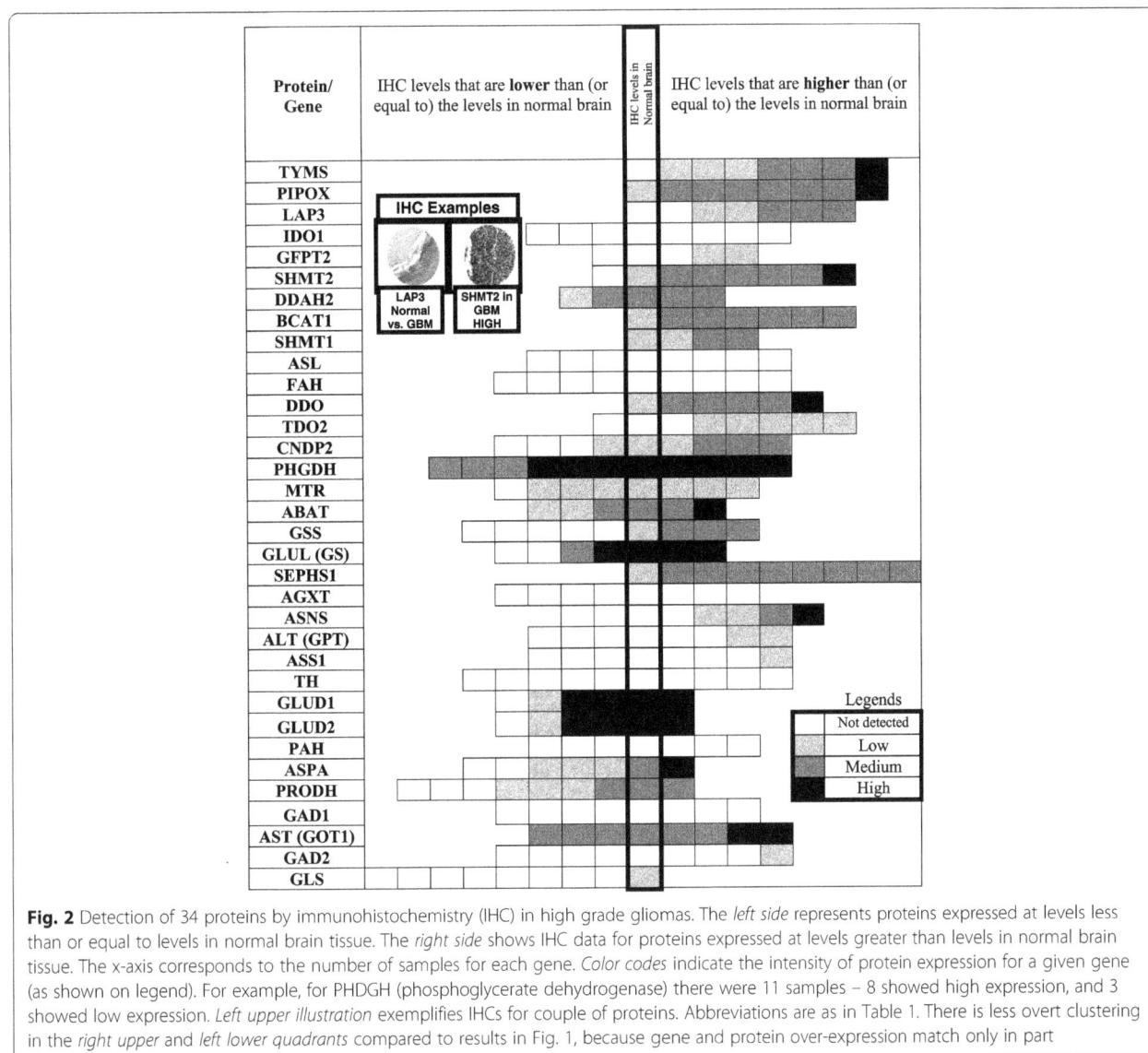

Fig. 2 Detection of 34 proteins by immunohistochemistry (IHC) in high grade gliomas. The *left side* represents proteins expressed at levels less than or equal to levels in normal brain tissue. The *right side* shows IHC data for proteins expressed at levels greater than levels in normal brain tissue. The x-axis corresponds to the number of samples for each gene. *Color codes* indicate the intensity of protein expression for a given gene (as shown on legend). For example, for PHDGH (phosphoglycerate dehydrogenase) there were 11 samples – 8 showed high expression, and 3 showed low expression. *Left upper illustration* exemplifies IHCs for couple of proteins. Abbreviations are as in Table 1. There is less overt clustering in the *right upper* and *left lower quadrants* compared to results in Fig. 1, because gene and protein over-expression match only in part

The heat maps were obtained by hierarchical clustering on samples within every defined subgroup of a dataset separately, followed by clustering over the genes (complete cohort).

Results

Differential expression of enzyme genes in GBM and proteins in HGG

Differential expression was defined as a ≥40% difference (higher or lower) in gene expression for any gene, in GBM compared to non-GBM specimens. Fewer than 30 genes involved in AA metabolism met this criterion (Fig. 1). Protein detection by IHC reflected gene expression levels in roughly two-thirds of the 34 genes (Fig. 2). Specifically, over-expressed genes had a higher proportion of samples with medium to high IHC staining of the expressed protein. In contrast, under-expressed

genes were associated with low or undetected protein staining. This observation was true for most, but not all, genes and enzymes analyzed.

Survival in relation to gene expression

Expression of some of the 34 genes correlated with progression free and/or overall survival (Fig. 3). For example, higher levels of some genes that are upregulated in GBM were associated with poor outcome, or via versa. However, other genes showed the reverse (occasionally following predictions based on protein levels). Some genes did not play a role in patient outcome altogether (Table 3). Interestingly, we also identified a group of genes that may play a role in outcome, but were not differentially expressed. Overall, it appears that dramatic differences in expression are more likely to result in survival differences, especially when gene

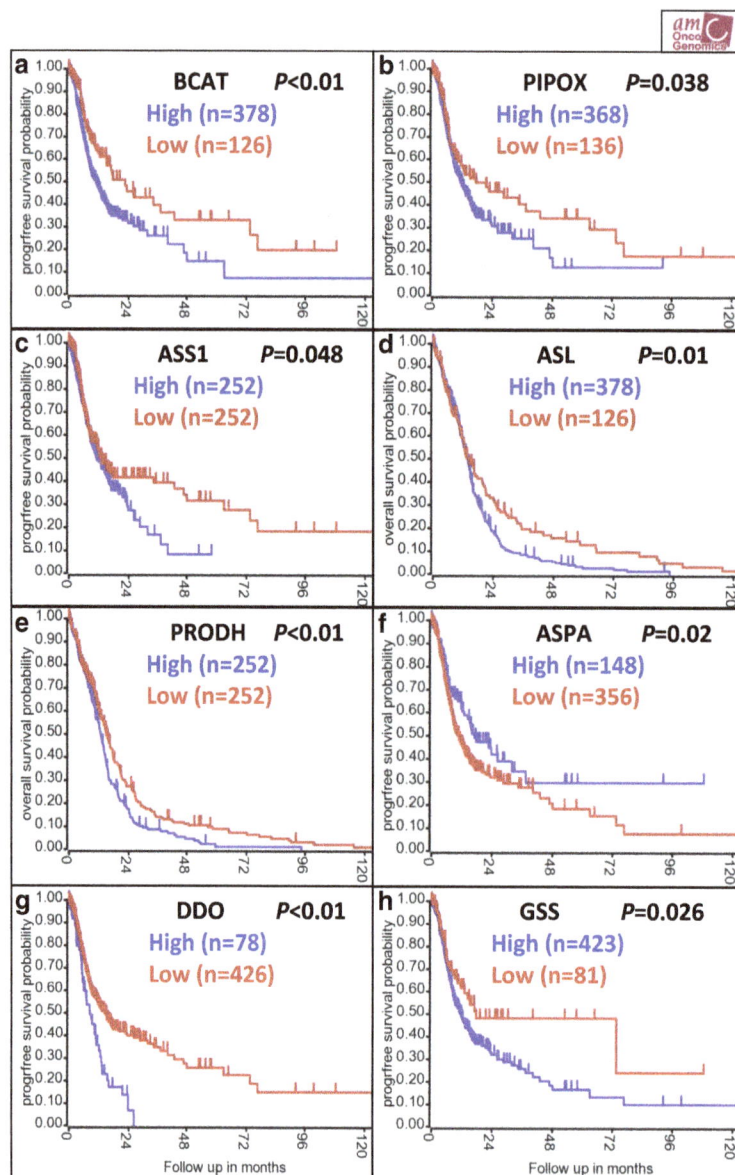

Fig. 3 Representative Kaplan-Meier curves showing associations between expression of selected genes and patient survival. Gene names, numbers of samples with high versus low expression, and *P* values are shown in *boxes*. *X-axes* show follow-up in months, and *Y-axes* show survival probability. Panels **a**, **b**, **c**, **f**, **g**, and **h** show progression-free survival. Panels **d** and **e** show overall survival

expression correlates with protein production (Table 3). Genes that are over-expressed in GBM and also associated with poor survival at high expression levels may be the top candidates for therapeutic inhibition (dark gray shaded box in Table 3).

TCGA subtypes demonstrate heterogeneity for genes involved in AA metabolism
Thirty-four genes were tested in one of the datasets, where TCGA grouping was available for 85 samples (17 neural, 17 classical, 27 mesenchymal and 24 proneural). A complex pattern of heterogeneity was observed (Fig. 4).

Although further confirmation is needed, the results suggest distinct patterns of amino acid metabolism in the 4 TCGA subtypes, as measured by gene expression.

Pediatric brain tumor types and medulloblastoma subtypes also may have distinct signatures of AA metabolism
In addition to GBM, we analyzed the same 34 genes in two other datasets in R2 (#9 and #10 in Table 2). One contains pediatric brain tumor samples (15 pilocytic astrocytomas, 34 glioblastomas, 22 medulloblastomas and 46 ependymomas). The other is a medulloblastoma

Table 3 Relationship between expressions of 34 selected genes and Kaplan-Meier analysis

	Enzymes for which …		
	higher expression is linked to poor survival	lower expression is linked to poor survival	expression is not correlated with survival
Enzymes with higher expression in GBM	**BCAT1**[a] ASL[a] **LAP3** **PIPOX**[a] **GFPT2** **DDO**[a] FAH	DDAH2 **SHMT2** **TYMS** SHMT1	**TDO2** IDO1
Enzymes with expression as in normal brain	CNDP2 **GSS**[a] **GLUL (GS)**	PHGDH SEPHS1 **ABAT** ALT (GPT) **AGXT**	ASNS **MTR**
Enzymes with lower expression in GBM	**PRODH**[a] **ASS1**[a]	AST (GOT1) **ASPA**[a] PAH	**GLUD1/GLUD2** GAD1/GAD2 **GLS** TH

[a]Survival curves for footnoted genes are shown in Fig. 3. Genes in bold have concordant protein (by IHC) and mRNA expression (by microarray)

dataset, grouped into 4 subtypes (10 SHH, 8 WNT, 16 G3, and 39 G4). As for GBM TCGA subtypes above (Fig. 4), we prepared gene expression heat maps reflecting over- and under-expression of genes in medulloblastoma subtypes and pediatric brain tumors (Additional file 1: Figure S1 and Additional file 2: Figure S2, respectively). In both cases, one can appreciate AA gene expression variability among the subtypes. There were no proteins or patient survival data available for analysis. However, these observations provide preliminary findings for further analysis and preclinical therapeutics development.

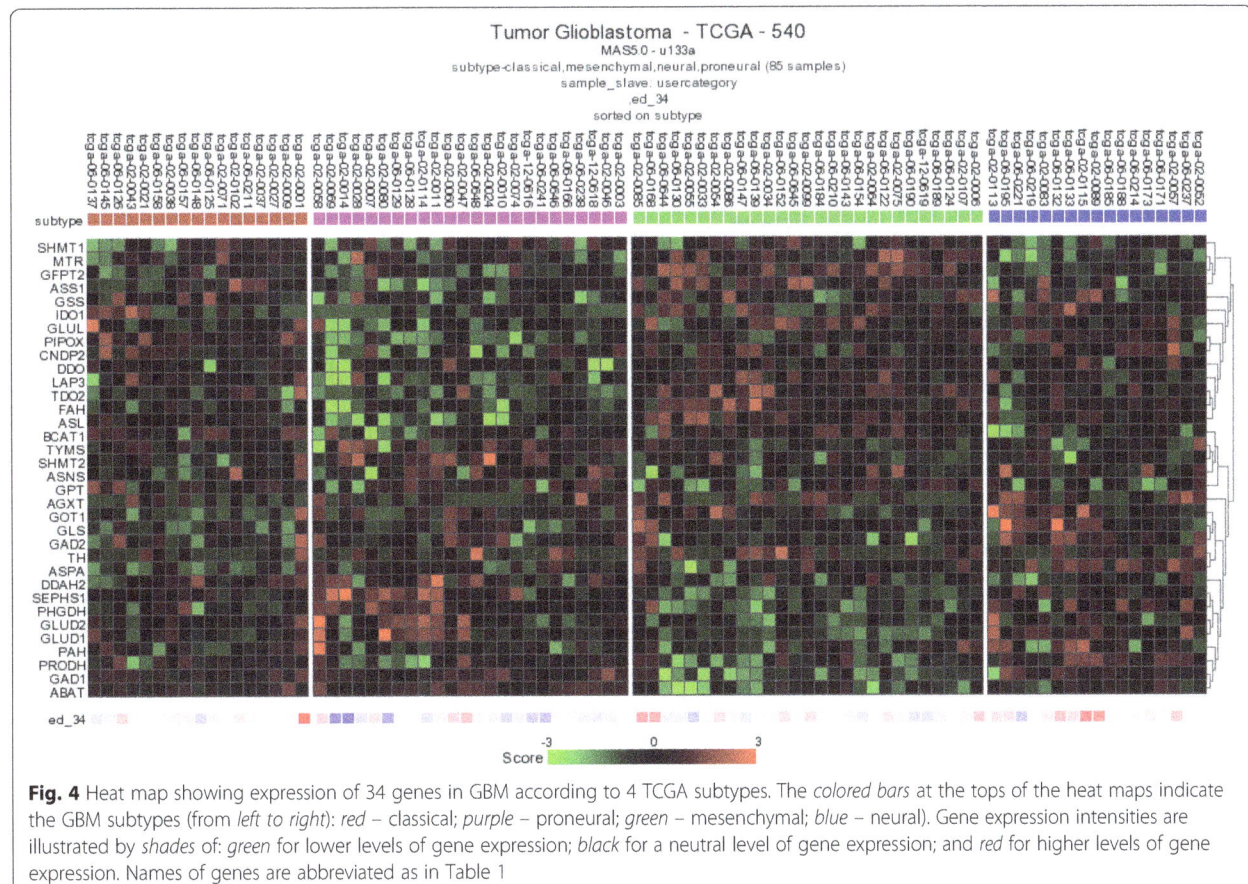

Fig. 4 Heat map showing expression of 34 genes in GBM according to 4 TCGA subtypes. The *colored bars* at the tops of the heat maps indicate the GBM subtypes (from *left to right*): *red* – classical; *purple* – proneural; *green* – mesenchymal; *blue* – neural. Gene expression intensities are illustrated by *shades* of: *green* for lower levels of gene expression; *black* for a neutral level of gene expression; and *red* for higher levels of gene expression. Names of genes are abbreviated as in Table 1

Findings on specific genes and enzymes are addressed in the Discussion section.

Discussion

Glioblastoma therapy continues to remain a major clinical challenge due to poor outcomes, with >90% of patients succumbing from their disease within 3 years of diagnosis [21]. Although immunotherapy and inhibition of cancer cell signaling hold promise, the "cornerstone" of current therapy against GBM remains DNA damaging strategies combined with surgery [22]. Targeting cancer metabolism by starving cancers of essential nutrients should be combinable with DNA damaging chemotherapy, due to lack of myelosuppression. Because lipid and energy metabolism is being investigated more intensively, this pilot study was designed to review brain tumor databases, to identify potentially druggable sites by interrogating amino acid-related metabolic pathways in GBM. Gene and protein expression patterns, in conjunction with survival data in GBM, were used as the main tools for searching for such targets. In addition, known amino acid depleting strategies, based on the available armamentarium and reported efficacy, are also considered in this discussion (Fig. 5). The analysis showed that 7 enzymes, namely, BCAT1, ASL, LAP3,

PIPOX, GFPT2, DDO and FAH were upregulated variably in GBMs and were associated decreased survival. However, ASL and FAH upregulation did not translate into protein overproduction (Table 3 and Fig. 2). While it remains unclear how patient survival is affected by expression of these enzymes, a deeper follow-up metabolic exploration of brain cancers and other malignancies may be useful.

BCAT1 (branched chain amino acid transaminase 1)

The enzyme catalyzes the reversible transamination of branched-chain alpha-keto acids to branched-chain L-amino acids. BCAT1 has a well proven role in IDH^{WT} GBM reported in the literature [23]. In our study, there is higher expression of BCAT1 in GBM compared to non-GBM. Both PFS and OS are affected adversely by higher levels of expression in GBM, as well as by high levels of the protein (detected by IHC in HGGs). Taken together, these results suggest that development of BCAT1 inhibitors may have promising clinical potential. Neural and proneural tumors have lower BCAT1, making them less likely to respond to BCAA metabolism manipulation. The role of BCAT1 in other cancers may also be investigated.

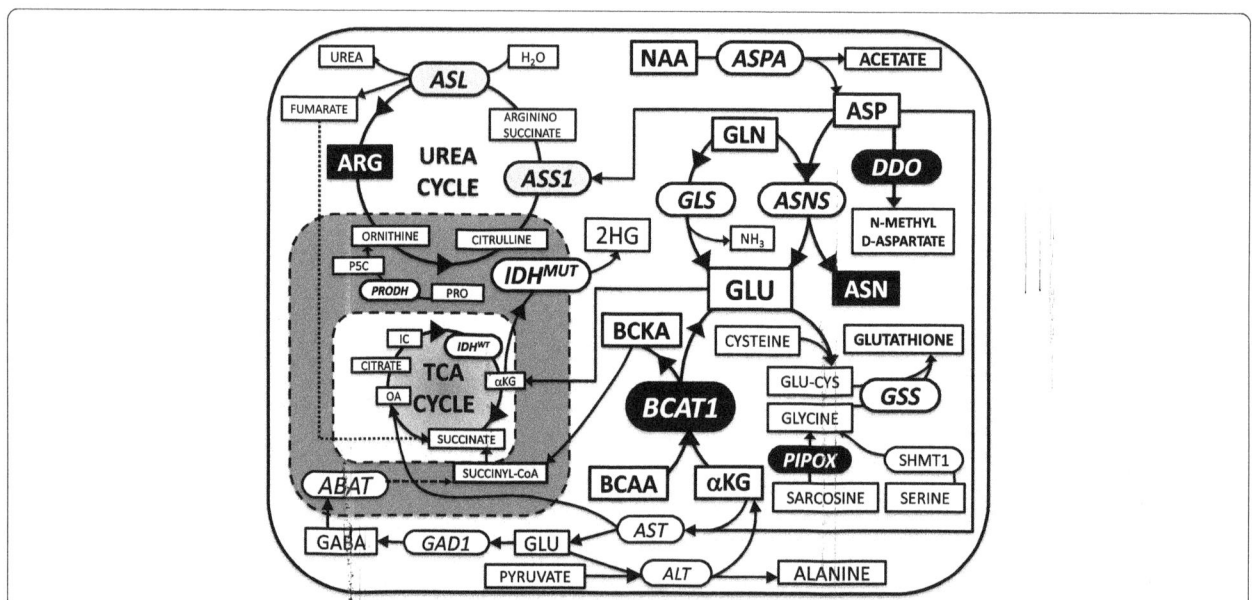

Fig. 5 Summary of metabolic pathways in relation to selected potential targets for GBM therapy. The complex interplay among biochemical reactions in amino-acid metabolism in a metabolic network affects mitochondrial energy production and nitrogen utilization. Enzymes are in *rounded boxes*, and substrates are in *squared boxes*. A *few black boxes* highlight the most relevant targets. Abbreviations: ABAT, 4-aminobutyrate aminotransferase; αKG, alpha-keto-glutarate; ALT, alanine aminotransferase (also known as GPT); ARG, arginine; ASL, argininosuccinate lyase; ASN, asparagine; ASNS, asparagine synthetase; ASP, aspartate; ASPA, aspartoacylase; ASS1, argininosuccinate synthase 1; AST, aspartate aminotransferase (also known as GOT1); BCAAs, branched-chain amino acids; BCAT1, branched chain amino-acid aminotransferase 1; BCKA, branched chain ketoacids; CYS, cysteine; DDO, D-aspartate oxidase; GABA, gamma-amino butyric acid; GAD1, glutamate decarboxylase 1; GLN, glutamine; GLU, glutamate; GLS, glutaminase; GSS, glutathione synthetase; IC, isocitrate; IDH^{MUT} isocitrate dehydrogenase, mutated; 2HG, 2-hydroxyglutarate; NAA, N-acetyl-L-aspartic acid; OA, oxaloacetate; P5C, 1-pyrroline-5-carboxylate; PIPOX, pipecolic acid and sarcosine oxidase; PRO, proline; PRODH, proline dehydrogenase; SHMT1, serine hydroxymethyltransferase 1; TCA, tricarboxylic acid

Arginine metabolism

Higher expression of ASS1 (argininosuccinate synthase 1) and ASL (argininosuccinate lyase) genes are associated with poor PFS and/or OS. However, only the ASL gene is differentially over-expressed in GBMs. And at the protein level, both ASL and ASS1 enzymes are low or undetected in HGGs. In spite of this complex pattern, it has been shown recently that human recombinant arginase-induced arginine depletion is selectively cytotoxic to human glioblastoma cells [24]. Moreover, arginine deiminase is active against GBM in vitro and in vivo [25]. Low ASS1 and ASL proteins in HGGs support further testing of arginine-depletion against GBM. An alternative formulation to be considered is PEG-ADI, which was used in a phase 2 trial for hepatocellular carcinoma [26].

Amino-acid depleting enzymes, such as arginase or asparaginase are large molecules, which may not penetrate an intact blood–brain barrier (BBB). Nevertheless, it is well documented that CSF asparagine, for instance, decreases significantly after asparaginase administration to acute lymphoblastic leukemia patients [27]. Therefore, penetration of these enzymes into parenchyma may not be necessary for an anti-tumor effect, inasmuch as substrate depletion influences the extra-vascular microenvironment of the CNS. In addition, parts of the BBB may not be completely intact [28] – theoretically allowing direct entry of enzymes. Intracranial brain tumor mouse model testing will be the best next step to assess potential synergy of amino-acid depleting strategies with other therapies.

Methionine

MTR (5-methyltetrahydrofolate-homocysteine methyltransferase) was the main methionine related enzyme, whose gene expression levels were slightly elevated in GBM. However, expression levels did not meet our definition of differential expression. MTR was not associated with clinical outcome. Moreover, there was neither differential expression in TCGA subtypes, nor high protein levels. Nevertheless, clinical observations, such as great diagnostic yields from 11C-MET PET uptake testing [29], support recently suggested research on methionine-free diets in combination with temozolomide against GBM (https://clinicaltrials.gov/ct2/show/NCT00508456). This study was terminated due to low accrual. Yet, preclinical research continues to support methionine deprivation as a potential therapy for GBM [30].

Alanine and asparagine-glutamine networks

Some findings in these biochemical pathways can be summarized as differential under-expression of ASPA (aspartoacylase) and GOT1 (glutamic-oxaloacetic transaminase 1; previously known as AST, or aspartate aminotransferase) in GBM. Both are associated with poor outcome at lower gene levels, as is lower GPT (glutamic-pyruvic transaminase; previously known as ALT, or alanine aminotransferase). The neural group had higher GOT1 and ASPA gene expression, but lower GPT. Protein counterparts of GPT and GOT1 are overall more detectable in HGGs, compared to normal tissue, whereas ASPA protein is less detectable. ASPA catalyzes conversion of N-acetyl-L-aspartic acid (NAA) to acetate and is mutated in patients with Canavan disease. Detection of elevated NAA by magnetic resonance spectroscopy (MRS) is indicative of GBM progression. Some investigators have suggested that acetate supplementation (used for Canavan disease) may serve as an adjuvant therapy against GBM [31]. Acetate use against GBM may be supported by our findings of under-expression of the ASPA gene in GBM and the ASPA protein in HGGs. Acetate use is also supported by a strong signal from another over-expressed gene in our study – PIPOX (pipecolic acid and sarcosine oxidase). PIPOX also shows high protein levels in HGGs, and high PIPOX is associated with poor outcome in GBM. PIPOX converts sarcosine to glycine (used by GSS, or glutathione synthetase) and can be inhibited by acetate [32].

The only individual, key-enzyme gene effect observed for glutamine metabolism in our study was for GLUL (glutamate-ammonia ligase; previously known as GS, or glutamine synthetase). Low GLUL levels correlated with better OS (Table 3). Nevertheless, a large body of literature suggests that the asparagine-glutamine node of amino acid metabolism may contain a credible potential target against GBM metabolism [33]. The combined effect of increased ASNS (asparagine synthetase), GLUL, and/or BCAT1 expression was shown in one of our recent studies to have a detrimental effect on patient outcomes [34]. Therefore, we consider and propose asparaginase/glutaminase as another potential adjuvant strategy against GBM. Differential expression of ASNS in ependymomas and certain types of medulloblastomas also supports asparaginase testing against these pediatric brain tumors.

GABA metabolism

Mixed gene expression for GABA related enzymes indicated that decreased production and possibly increased catabolism may be linked to poor outcome. Gabapentin, a GABA analog, inhibits substance P-induced NF-kB activation in rat gliomas and may play role in regulating inflammation-related intracellular signaling [35]. However, the hypothesis of a significant antitumor effect of GABA against GBM remains unexplored, because its analogue, gabapentin (widely used in clinical practice without major anti-GBM effects), has no direct effect on GABA binding, uptake or degradation.

Glutathione synthetase (GSS)

Interestingly, overexpression of the rate-limiting enzyme in glutathione synthesis (GCLM, or glutamate-cysteine ligase modifier subunit) was not detected in these analyses. Likewise, GSS levels were not much altered at baseline. One may predict that a potential role of GSS inhibition by the available agent, buthionine sulfoximine (BSO), may be limited to chemotherapy-induced, GSS-up-regulation cases. This has been a subject of significant research for other cancers, but not GBM [36]. A study to assess GSS upregulation after chemotherapy in GBM may be useful. Analysis of enzymatic and non-enzymatic components of antioxidant pathways – apart from amino-acid metabolism – is another valid topic for study.

Tryptophan

IDO1 (indoleamine 2, 3-dioxygenase 1) catalyzes tryptophan breakdown. Its inhibitors are aimed at suppressing tryptophan catabolism-induced cancer immunotolerance and are in clinical trials (https://www.clinicaltrials.gov/show/NCT02052648). No survival link or differential expression was observed in our analysis for GBM versus non-GBM brain tissues for IDO1 or TDO2 (tryptophan 2, 3-dioxygenase, also involved in tryptophan catabolism). However, our findings showed higher TDO2 and IDO1 in GBM, and particularly in the mesenchymal subtype, which may show better responses to immunotherapy [37]. These reports further support a potential role for manipulating tryptophan metabolism for cancer immunomodulation effects [30, 38].

Other genes

Potential targets can be expanded to a few other important genes based on our results, including: GFPT2 (glutamine-fructose-6-phosphate transaminase 2; previously reported to be high in GBM [39]); LAP3 (leucine aminopeptidase); DDO (D-aspartate oxidase); and PRODH (proline dehydrogenase, a putative tumor suppressor). Retrospective studies and preclinical validations are needed, because gene and protein databases used in this study are not the same. Also, no protein data were available on pediatric tumors and medulloblastoma. Furthermore, changes may occur in response to chemo/radiation treatments, and the tumors may harbor unknown mutations in some of these pathways (a possible subject of future studies).

Conclusions

Brain tumors have distinct gene expression patterns for certain amino acid-metabolizing enzymes. These enzymes may provide valid targets for therapeutics development. Although drugs used clinically, such as asparaginase and arginase, are readily available for preclinical testing,

inhibitors have yet to be developed against other promising targets, such as BCAT1 or PIPOX. Heterogeneity is evident in various types (and subtypes) of brain tumors, which indicates the possible need for tailored manipulation of amino acid metabolism to achieve enhanced therapeutic effects and less toxicity than encountered with conventional chemotherapy.

Abbreviations

2HG: 2-hydroxyglutarate; AA: Amino-acids; ABAT: 4-aminobutyrate aminotransferase; ARG: Arginine; ASL: Argininosuccinate lyase; ASN: Asparagine; ASNS: Asparagine synthetase; ASP: Aspartate; ASPA: Aspartoacylase; ASS1: Argininosuccinate synthase 1; BBB: Blood–brain barrier; BCAAs: Branched-chain amino acids; BCAT1: Branched chain amino acid transaminase 1; BCKA: Branched chain ketoacids; DDO: D-aspartate oxidase; GABA: Gamma-amino butyric acid; GAD1: Glutamate decarboxylase 1; GAD2: Glutamate decarboxylase 2; GBM: Glioblastoma; GFPT2: Glutamine-fructose-6-phosphate transaminase 2; GLN: Glutamine; GLS: Glutaminase; GLU: Glutamate; GLUL: Glutamate-ammonia ligase; GOT1: Glutamic-oxaloacetic transaminase 1; GPT: Glutamic-pyruvic transaminase; GSS: Glutathione synthetase; IC: Isocitrate; IDH^{MUT}: Isocitrate dehydrogenase, mutated; IDH^{WT}: Isocitrate dehydrogenase, wild type; IDO1: Indoleamine 2,3-dioxygenase 1; KEGG: Kyoto Encyclopedia of Genes and Genomes; LAP3: Leucine aminopeptidase; MRS: Magnetic resonance spectroscopy; MTR: 5-methyltetrahydrofolate-homocysteine methyltransferase; NAA: N-acetyl-L-aspartic acid; NFkB: Transcription factor complex nuclear factor-kappa-B; OA: Oxaloacetate; OS: Overall survival; PFS: Progression-free survival; PIPOX: Pipecolic acid and sarcosine oxidase; PRO: Proline; PRODH: Proline dehydrogenase; PRODH: Proline dehydrogenase; TCGA: The Cancer Genome Atlas; TDO2: Tryptophan 2,3-dioxygenase

Acknowledgements

We acknowledge support of the Department of Pediatrics at Harbor UCLA Medical Center and LA BioMed.

Funding

None.

Authors' contributions

All authors have read and approved the manuscript. EP study design, data acquisition and analysis, manuscript drafting and writing. HL contributions to conception and design, analytical discussions, manuscript writing. JK contributions to data acquisition and analysis, manuscript writing. JL contributions to conception and design, analytical discussions, manuscript writing.

Competing interests

The authors declare that they have no competing interests.

Author details

[1]Los Angeles Biomedical Research Institute and Department of Pediatrics at Harbor-UCLA Medical Center, Box 468, 1000 W. Carson Street, N25, Torrance, CA 90509, USA. [2]Department of Oncogenomics, Academic Medical Center of the University of Amsterdam, Amsterdam, The Netherlands.

References

1. Squatrito M, Holland EC. DNA damage response and growth factor signaling pathways in gliomagenesis and therapeutic resistance. Cancer Res. 2011;71(18):5945–9.

2. Scott BJ, Quant EC, McNamara MB, Ryg PA, Batchelor TT, Wen PY. Bevacizumab salvage therapy following progression in high-grade glioma patients treated with VEGF receptor tyrosine kinase inhibitors. Neuro-Oncology. 2010;12(6):603–7.

3. Mellinghoff IK, Lassman AB, Wen PY. Signal transduction inhibitors and antiangiogenic therapies for malignant glioma. Glia. 2011;59(8):1205–12.

4. Reardon DA, Freeman G, Wu C, Chiocca EA, Wucherpfennig KW, Wen PY, Fritsch EF, Curry WT, Sampson JH, Dranoff G. Immunotherapy advances for glioblastoma. Neuro-Oncology. 2014;16(11):1441–58.

5. Weber JS. Current perspectives on immunotherapy. Semin Oncol. 2014; 41(Supplement 5):S14–29.

6. Vander Heiden MG. Targeting cancer metabolism: a therapeutic window opens. Nat Rev Drug Discov. 2011;10(9):671–84.

7. Sciacovelli M, Gaude E, Hilvo M, Frezza C. Chapter One - The Metabolic Alterations of Cancer Cells. In: Lorenzo G, Guido K, editors. Methods in Enzymology. Volume 542, edn. USA: Academic Press; 2014. p. 1–23.

8. Avramis VI, Panosyan EH. Pharmacokinetic/pharmacodynamic relationships of asparaginase formulations: the past, the present and recommendations for the future. Clin Pharmacokinet. 2005;44(4):367–93.

9. Bertino JR. Cancer research: from folate antagonism to molecular targets. Best Pract Res Clin Haematol. 2009;22(4):577–82.

10. Maxwell MB, Maher KE. Chemotherapy-induced myelosuppression. Semin Oncol Nurs. 1992;8(2):113–23.

11. Ezoe S. Secondary leukemia associated with the anti-cancer agent, etoposide, a topoisomerase II inhibitor. Int J Environ Res Public Health. 2012; 9(7):2444–53.

12. Turkalp Z, Karamchandani J, Das S. Idh mutation in glioma: New insights and promises for the future. JAMA Neurol. 2014;71(10):1319–25.

13. Seyfried TN, Flores R, Poff AM, D'Agostino DP, Mukherjee P. Metabolic therapy: A new paradigm for managing malignant brain cancer. Cancer Lett. 2015;356(2, Part A):289–300.

14. Guo D, Bell EH, Chakravarti A. Lipid metabolism emerges as a promising target for malignant glioma therapy. CNS Oncol. 2013;2(3):289–99.

15. Sato A, Sunayama J, Okada M, Watanabe E, Seino S, Shibuya K, Suzuki K, Narita Y, Shibui S, Kayama T, et al. Glioma-initiating cell elimination by metformin activation of FOXO3 via AMPK. Stem Cells Transl Med. 2012;1(11):811–24.

16. Lapa C, Linsenmann T, Monoranu CM, Samnick S, Buck AK, Bluemel C, Czernin J, Kessler AF, Homola GA, Ernestus R-I, et al. Comparison of the amino acid tracers 18 F-FET and 18 F-DOPA in high-grade glioma patients. J Nucl Med. 2014;55(10):1611–6.

17. Langen K-J, Tatsch K, Grosu A-L, Jacobs AH, Weckesser M, Sabri O. Diagnostics of cerebral gliomas with radiolabeled amino acids. Dtsch Arztebl Int. 2008;105(4):55–61.

18. Bender DA. Amino Acids Synthesized from Glutamate: Glutamine, Proline, Ornithine, Citrulline and Arginine. In: Amino Acid Metabolism. Chichester: Wiley; 2012. p. 157–223.

19. R2: Genomics Analysis and Visualization Platform. http://r2.amc.nl. Accessed 5 Jan 2016.

20. The Human Protein Atlas. http://www.proteinatlas.org/cancer. Accessed 5 Jan 2016.

21. Lu J, Cowperthwaite MC, Burnett MG, Shpak M. Molecular predictors of long-term survival in glioblastoma multiforme patients. PLoS ONE. 2016; 11(4):e0154313.

22. Bush NAO, Chang SM, Berger MS. Current and future strategies for treatment of glioma. Neurosurg Rev. 2016;1–14.

23. Tonjes M, Barbus S, Park YJ, Wang W, Schlotter M, Lindroth AM, Pleier SV, Bai AHC, Karra D, Piro RM, et al. BCAT1 promotes cell proliferation through amino acid catabolism in gliomas carrying wild-type IDH1. Nat Med. 2013; 19(7):901–8.

24. Khoury O, Ghazale N, Stone E, El-Sibai M, Frankel A, Abi-Habib R. Human recombinant arginase I (Co)-PEG5000 [HuArgI (Co)-PEG5000]-induced arginine depletion is selectively cytotoxic to human glioblastoma cells. J Neurooncol. 2015;122(1):75–85.

25. Fiedler T, Strauss M, Hering S, Redanz U, William D, Rosche Y, Classen CF, Kreikemeyer B, Linnebacher M, Maletzki C. Arginine deprivation by arginine deiminase of Streptococcus pyogenes controls primary glioblastoma growth in vitro and in vivo. Cancer Biol Ther. 2015;16(7):1047–55.

26. Glazer ES, Piccirillo M, Albino V, Di Giacomo R, Palaia R, Mastro AA, Beneduce G, Castello G, De Rosa V, Petrillo A, et al. Phase II study of Pegylated arginine deiminase for nonresectable and metastatic hepatocellular carcinoma. J Clin Oncol. 2010;28(13):2220–6.

27. Hawkins DS, Park JR, Thomson BG, Felgenhauer JL, Holcenberg JS, Panosyan EH, Avramis VI. Asparaginase pharmacokinetics after intensive polyethylene glycol-conjugated L-asparaginase therapy for children with relapsed acute lymphoblastic leukemia. Clin Cancer Res. 2004;10(16):5335–41.

28. Nduom EK, Yang C, Merrill MJ, Zhuang Z, Lonser RR. Characterization of the blood–brain barrier of metastatic and primary malignant neoplasms. J Neurosurg. 2013;119(2):427–33.

29. D'Souza MM, Sharma R, Jaimini A, Panwar P, Saw S, Kaur P, Mondal A, Mishra A, Tripathi RP. 11C-MET PET/CT and Advanced MRI in the Evaluation of Tumor Recurrence in High-Grade Gliomas. Clin Nucl Med. 2014;39(9):791–8.

30. Palanichamy K, Thirumoorthy K, Kanji S, Gordon N, Singh R, Jacob JR, Sebastian N, Litzenberg KT, Patel D, Bassett E, et al. Methionine and kynurenine activate oncogenic kinases in glioblastoma, and methionine deprivation compromises proliferation. Clin Cancer Res. 2016;22(14):3513–23.

31. Long PM, Tighe SW, Driscoll HE, Fortner KA, Viapiano MS, Jaworski DM. Acetate supplementation as a means of inducing glioblastoma stem-like cell growth arrest. J Cell Physiol. 2015;230(8):1929–43.

32. Frisell WR, Mackenzie CG. The binding sites of sarcosine oxidase. J Biol Chem. 1955;217(1):275–86.

33. Tanaka K, Sasayama T, Irino Y, Takata K, Nagashima H, Satoh N, Kyotani K, Mizowaki T, Imahori T, Ejima Y, et al. Compensatory glutamine metabolism promotes glioblastoma resistance to mTOR inhibitor treatment. J Clin Invest. 2015;125(4):1591–602.

34. Panosyan EH, Lasky JL, Lin HJ, Lai a, Hai Y, Guo X, Quinn M, Nelson SF, Cloughesy TF, Nghiemphu PL. Clinical aggressiveness of malignant gliomas is linked to augmented metabolism of amino acids. J Neurooncol. 2016;128: 57–66.

35. Park S, Ahn ES, Han DW, Lee JH, Min KT, Kim H, Hong Y-W. Pregabalin and gabapentin inhibit substance P-induced NF-κB activation in neuroblastoma and glioma cells. J Cell Biochem. 2008;105(2):414–23.

36. Anderson CP, Matthay KK, Perentesis JP, Neglia JP, Bailey HH, Villablanca JG, Groshen S, Hasenauer B, Maris JM, Seeger RC, et al. Pilot study of intravenous melphalan combined with continuous infusion L-S, R-buthionine sulfoximine for children with recurrent neuroblastoma. Pediatr Blood Cancer. 2015;62(10):1739–46.

37. Prins RM, Soto H, Konkankit V, Odesa SK, Eskin A, Yong WH, Nelson SF, Liau LM. Gene expression profile correlates with T-cell infiltration and relative survival in glioblastoma patients vaccinated with dendritic cell immunotherapy. Clin Cancer Res. 2011;17(6):1603–15.

38. Platten M, von Knebel DN, Oezen I, Wick W, Ochs K. Cancer immunotherapy by targeting IDO1/TDO and their downstream effectors. Front Immunol. 2015;5:673.

39. Wolf A, Agnihotri S, Guha A. Targeting metabolic remodeling in glioblastoma multiforme. Oncotarget. 2010;1:552–62.

17

A 35-gene signature discriminates between rapidly- and slowly-progressing glioblastoma multiforme and predicts survival in known subtypes of the cancer

Azeez A. Fatai and Junaid Gamieldien* ⓘ

Abstract

Background: Gene expression can be employed for the discovery of prognostic gene or multigene signatures cancer. In this study, we assessed the prognostic value of a 35-gene expression signature selected by pathway and machine learning based methods in adjuvant therapy-linked glioblastoma multiforme (GBM) patients from the Cancer Genome Atlas.

Methods: Genes with high expression variance was subjected to pathway enrichment analysis and those having roles in chemoradioresistance pathways were used in expression-based feature selection. A modified Support Vector Machine Recursive Feature Elimination algorithm was employed to select a subset of these genes that discriminated between rapidly-progressing and slowly-progressing patients.

Results: Survival analysis on TCGA samples not used in feature selection and samples from four GBM subclasses, as well as from an entirely independent study, showed that the 35-gene signature discriminated between the survival groups in all cases ($p < 0.05$) and could accurately predict survival irrespective of the subtype. In a multivariate analysis, the signature predicted progression-free and overall survival independently of other factors considered.

Conclusion: We propose that the performance of the signature makes it an attractive candidate for further studies to assess its utility as a clinical prognostic and predictive biomarker in GBM patients. Additionally, the signature genes may also be useful therapeutic targets to improve both progression-free and overall survival in GBM patients.

Keywords: Glioblastoma multiforme, Prognostic genes, Risk groups, Chemoradiation resistance pathways

Background

Glioblastoma multiforme (GBM) is the most common and highly aggressive brain tumour. Patients with GBM have very poor prognosis, with the median OS time of 14.5 months [1]. Chemotherapy and radiotherapies are intended to improve patient survival, but are, however, hampered by development of resistance. Methylation of the promoter of the MGMT gene, which encodes O-6-methylguanine-DNA methyl-transferase, a DNA-repair enzyme that removes alkylating groups at the O6 of guanine residues, is a predictor of treatment response in GBM. Most studies that considered progression-free survival assessed only the prognostic value of MGMT promoter methylation [2–4]. Tumours with hypermethylated MGMT promoters are expected to benefit from temozolomide, an alkylating agent used for treating GBM, but reports regarding the prognostic value of this biomarker have been conflicting [5, 6].

Several gene expression prognostic and predictive signatures have been translated into clinical applications for cancer treatment. Oncotype DX is a 21-gene qRT-PCR assay used to predict likelihood of recurrence in women with estrogen receptor positive breast cancer [7, 8]. Mammostrat is prognostic immunohistochemical test that uses antibodies specific for SLC7A5, p53, HTF9C,

*Correspondence: junaid@sanbi.ac.za
South African Bioinformatics Institute and SAMRC Unit for Bioinformatics Capacity Development, University of the Western Cape, Bellville, 7535, 7530 Western Cape, South Africa

NDRG1, and CEACAM5 to classify ER-positive, lymph node negative breast cancer cases into low-, moderate- or high-risk groups [9, 10]. Mammaprint is a 70-gene microarray-based test for predicting risk of metastasis in breast cancer [11].

In light of the lack of standardised prognostic biomarkers for GBM, we aimed to identify a mRNA expression derived prognostic signature using data from the Cancer Genome Atlas (TCGA - http://cancergenome.nih.gov/). As current prognostic feature selection approaches lack reproducibility and do not take chemoradioresistant pathways into consideration, we used a combination of pathway enrichment analysis and Support Vector Machine based Recursive Feature Elimination (SVM-RFE) to ensure that the genes selected as having predictive potential would also be biologically relevant to the phenoptype. We here describe a multigene signature that successfully predicts both progression-free and overall survival in glioblastoma multiforme.

Methods

Gene-centric expression data

Five hundred fifty eight GBM gene expression profiles generated by the Cancer Genome Atlas (TCGA) were downloaded from the NCI Genomic Data Commons Data Portal (https://portal.gdc.cancer.gov/projects/TCGA-GBM). Five hundred forty eight of the these profiles were obtained from GBM patients, and ten were from non-neoplastic patients. One profile was selected for each of the samples profiled two or more times. Five hundred twenty nine profiles left after removing those of non-neoplastic samples were used in this study (Additional file 1). The expression were profiled on Affymetrix HT HG-U133A platform. As gene expression of the TCGA samples was profiled in batches which could introduce bias in classification analysis [12], the statistical significance of batch effect was assessed as a function of the selected genes using guided Principal Component Analysis (gPCA) from the R package *gPCA* [13]. The approach used by TCGA (2008) [14] and Verhaak et al. (2011) [15] was employed to generate gene-centric expression data. The probe sequences of HT HG-U133A downloaded from Affymetrix were mapped against a database composed of RefSeq version 41 and GenBank 178 complete coding sequences using SpliceMiner [16]. Only perfect matches were considered and probes mapping to more than one gene were excluded. The output file from SpliceMiner and the HT HG-U133A chip definition file (cdf) were passed to the alternate cdf-generating function *makealtcdf* of AffyProbeMiner [17]. Probe sets with less than five probes were excluded from the resulting alternative cdf, which was then converted to an R package using *makecdfenv*. The cdf was used to perform Robust Multi-array Average normalization and summarization of the gene expression data, resulting in gene-centric data for 12161 genes.

An independent validation data set (GSE7696) profiled on HG-U133 Plus 2 Affymetrix platform and downloaded from the NCBI Gene Expression Omnibus (https://www.ncbi.nlm.nih.gov/geo/query/acc.cgi?acc=GSE7696) was equivalently treated. This data set contained gene expression data for 80 GBM and four non-neoplastic samples, and was chosen because of the availability of patients' treatment information.

Sample selection

To ensure that treatment did not introduce confounding effects, samples from patients that received adjuvant chemotherapy and radiation and had uncensored days to death or progression were selected. Figure 1 shows sample selection for the identification of genes with prognostic value. Four hundred fifteen patients received the standard GBM treatment. Semantically, tumour progression is a radiologically documented increase in tumour size after a subtotal surgical excision [18]. The time for this to occur is known as time to progression, which is the same as uncensored progression-free survival (PFS) [19]. Two hundred one patients had associated uncensored progression-free survival (PFS) times, and 380 had overall survival OS times (censored or uncensored).

Clinical data for all the patients used in this study were obtained from TCGA. PFS times for patients who experienced tumour progression within the follow-up period were obtained from the TCGA file for new tumour events. The GBM subtypes of samples used in our study were obtained from the supplementary clinical file provided by Brennan et al., (2013) [20].

There is no standard for classifying patients as rapid and slow GBM progressors after standard treatment. While the median PFS after treatment could be used as a separation point, it does not provide a 'buffer zone' to filter out borderline samples close to the median that may fall in the incorrect group due to unknown confounding factors. Rather than defining an arbitrary exclusion range, we used the first (Q1) and third (Q3) quartiles, 120 and 341 days respectively, as boundaries to divide patients into three classes, since they are still dependent on the median and not influenced by extreme outliers. Class 1 contained 48 patients having PFS times between 6 and 120 days (rapidly-progressing) and class 2 contained 35 patients having PFS times between 358 and 720 days (slow progressing). Classes 1 and 2 were used in feature selection and the 118 remaining samples (Class 3) that fell within the inter-quartile range were used in PFS and OS analysis.

Selection of genes discriminating between rapidly and slowly progressing GBM patients

In this present study, genes in the cancer-related pathways were considered in our feature selection because of

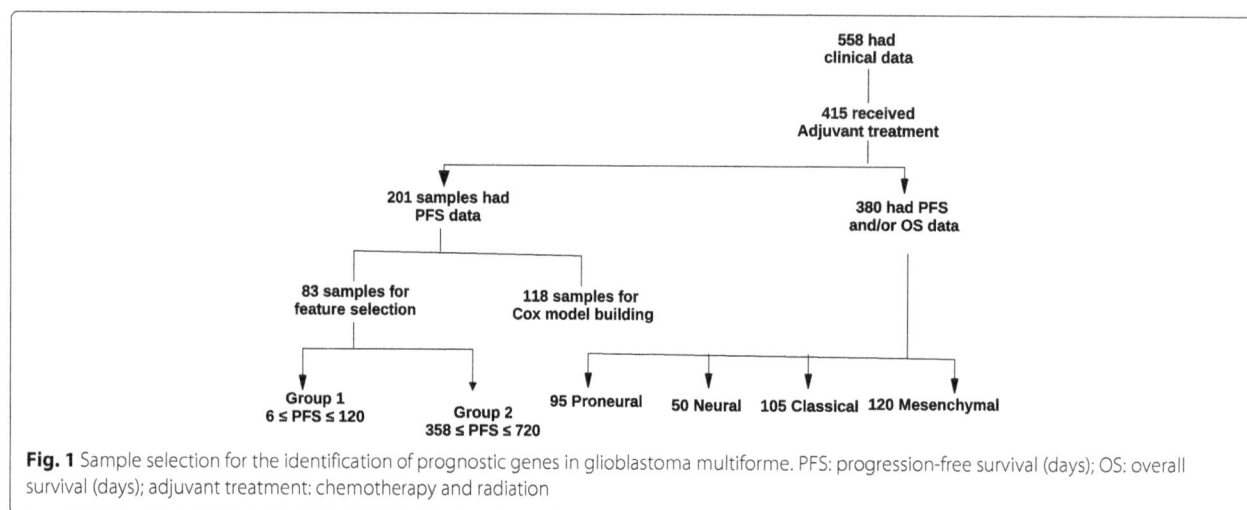

Fig. 1 Sample selection for the identification of prognostic genes in glioblastoma multiforme. PFS: progression-free survival (days); OS: overall survival (days); adjuvant treatment: chemotherapy and radiation

their known roles in chemoradiation resistance, and to reduce the likelihood of selecting genes related to survival by chance. Studies have identified pathways and processes that drive resistance to chemotherapy and radiotherapy in cancer. Several of these genes are found in known cancer pathways [21–28]. Several genes in the NF-κB and PI3K/Akt signaling pathways are associated with chemoresistance development in cancer [29, 30]. Also, genes involved in drug inactivation and efflux, DNA repair, and epithelial-mesenchymal transition have been shown to enhance drug resistance mechanisms [26, 31]. Pathway enrichment analysis was performed on the genes with high expression variance (median absolute deviation ≥ 0.5) across the 529 samples using the *Set Analyser* web service provided by the Comparative Toxicogenomics Database [32] . Genes were selected from the pathway categories related to cancer signaling pathways, reactive oxygen species metabolism, DNA repair, and drug transport and metabolism. A set of genes that discriminated between the rapidly-progressing and slowly-progressing groups were selected using a modified Support Vector Machine-Recursive Feature Elimination (SVM-RFE). SVM-RFE, proposed by [33], was modified by introducing 5-fold cross-validation into the SVM classifier step and capturing the error rate generated at this step (the figure showing the workflow for SVM-RFE is attached as Additional file 2).

Survival analysis
The 118 Class 3 patients not used in the feature selection step were used to calculate regression coefficients (β) for the selected genes using univariate Cox proportional hazards analysis. The β's were computed for the genes using *coxph* from the R survival package. Prognostic index, *PI*, was then calculated for each of the patients who received adjuvant chemotherapy and radiation and had PFS and/or OS data using the equation

$$PI = \beta_1 * gene_1 + \beta_2 * gene_2 + \ldots + \beta * gene_g$$

where β_g and $gene_g$ are the regression coefficient and the gene expression value for gene g, respectively. Patients in Class 3 were classified into low-risk and high-risk groups by choosing a value between the highest and lowest PI that ensured proper patients distribution based on *PI*. Patients with *PI* scores greater or equal than the chosen value were assigned to the high-risk group, whereas those with *PI* scores less than the value were assigned to the low-risk group. 380 patients with OS times were also classified into low-risk and high-risk groups in the same way.

Assessment of signature prognostic value in GBM subtypes
Verhaak et al. (2010) [15] identified four subtypes of GBM, namely proneural, neural, classical and mesenchymal, using gene expression data from 200 GBM samples. Brennan et al. (2013) [20] assigned additional 342 TGCA samples into the four subtypes using single-sample gene set enrichment analysis. A summarised clinical file provided by the authors was used in our study to assign patients to GBM subtypes. 95, 60, 105 and 120 of the 380 patients with available OS times were assigned to proneural, neural, classical and mesenchymal subtypes, respectively. 51, 33, 51 and 66 of the 201 patient group having associated PFS times were assigned to proneural, neural, classical and mesenchymal subtypes, respectively. We further categorised patients in each subtype into low-risk and high-risk groups.

Assessment of signature prognostic value in an independent dataset
The prognostic value of the selected gene signature was validated with the data from patients in the Murat et al. [34] validation dataset who had primary tumours and received adjuvant chemo- and radiotherapy. *PI* was

calculated for the patients using the β's obtained from the TCGA training set and the expression values of the selected genes in the samples from the patients. They were classified into low-risk and high-risk groups in such a manner as to ensure proper patient distribution between the two groups. Survival of the low-risk and high-risk groups were determined for both the TCGA and validation cohorts using the Kaplan-Meier method. Differences in survival between the risk groups were estimated statistically by log rank test. Survival differences between groups was said to be statistically significant if $p < 0.05$. Hazard ratios (HR) between risk groups were determined by Cox proportional hazards regression model.

Mutivariate survival analysis to assess independent prognostic value

A multivariate Cox survival model was built using three variables: our prognostic index, MGMT promoter methylation, and age. Ages of patients at diagnosis were obtained from the clinical file provided by TCGA. MGMT promoter methylation status data were obtained from the clinical file provided by Brennan et al. [20] The univariate Cox analysis was first carried out on each variable followed by multivariate Cox analysis on all the variables. The coxph function in the R *survival* package was used for the analysis. Using the median *PI* value, the patients were assigned into low-risk or high-risk groups. Those with *PI* values lower than the median were assigned to low-risk groups, and those with *PI* to high-risk groups. The low-risk and the MGMT methylated promoter groups were used as references for prognostic index and MGMT promoter methylation status, respectively. Correlation of variables with PFS and OS was considered statistically significant at $p(Wald) < 0.05$.

Identifying functional interactions between signature genes

We used the STRING database of known and predicted protein-protein interactions (https://string-db.org/) [35] to construct an interaction network for the signature genes and to perform KEGG pathway enrichment analysis on the derived subnetwork.

Results and discussion

In this present study, pathway-based and modified SVM-RFE-based methods were used to select a set of genes that discriminated between rapidly- and slowly-progressing GBM patients and combined into a signature. The prognostic value of the signature in predicting PFS and OS was accessed in the risk groups of GBM patients and validated on data set from an independent study. The independence of the signature in predicting PFS and OS was assessed by a multivariate Cox's proportional hazards analysis. Studies on the identification of protein-coding

multigene prognostic signatures in GBM focused on OS [7–9]. Overall survival (OS) is dependent on other factors besides gene expression. Progression-free survival, on the other hand, is expected to be a function of the expression of certain key genes. Genes whose expression across a cohort of patients correlated with OS were selected for survival analysis in these previous studies. This method has be shown to produce inconsistent signature genes in different data sets [36, 37].

35 genes discriminate between rapidly- and slowly-progressing GBM patients

GBM is a highly aggressive brain tumour, and the median survival of patients with GBM is 14.6 months [38]. We hypothesized that the tumour's pre-treatment expression of genes in pathways associated with chemoradioresistance in cancer would be predictive of how rapidly a GBM patient would experience progression after standard treatment. Signaling pathways (MAPK, JAK/STAT, WNT, NOTCH, Hedgehog, PIK3/AKT), cell cycle, drug transporters, reactive oxygen species metabolism and DNA repair system are known to be involved in chemoradioresistance in cancer [29, 39–41]. We also reasoned that PFS times were more appropriate than OS times in grouping patients. PFS times were expected to be more closely related to expression of key genes, while other factors including age and treatment after disease progression are also associated with OS.

Pathway enrichment analysis was performed on 3899 genes (Additional file 2) that had varied expression ($MAD \geq 0.5$) across 529 GBM samples. 18 of the 159 gene sets from the enrichment analysis were annotated for the known chemoradioresistance-associated pathways (Table 1). Assessment of batch effect in TGCA expression data set from 529 GBM samples as a function of the 356 genes extracted from the pathways (Additional file 3) showed that the data set did not have significant batch effect ($p = 0.118$). Inspection of the unguided principal component analysis plot of the first two principal components also showed that no batch effect was present (Additional file 4). The extracted genes were used in gene selection by the modified SVM-RFE. Our modified SVM-RFE was used to identify genes that discriminated between 48 rapidly-progressing patients (between 6 and 120 days PFS) and 35 slowly-progressing patients (between 358 and 720 days PFS). Figure 2 shows the plot of 5-fold cross-validation error rate against number of genes at each recursive step, starting with the 356 genes extracted from the pathways. The CV error rate decreased with decreasing number of genes until it reached 35 genes, which discriminated between rapidly- and slowly-progressing GBM patients at 100% accuracy. Further decreases in the number of genes resulted in increasing error rate.

Table 1 Selected pathway categories associated with chemoradiation resistance by pathway enrichment analysis on genes with high expression variance

Pathway	Number of genes
Cell cycle	62
MAPK signaling	87
p53 signaling	39
WNT signaling	48
Glutathione metabolism	23
TGF-β signaling	30
Insulin signaling	40
ErbB signaling	29
Phosphatidylinositol signaling	25
Mismatch repair	12
Inositol phosphate metabolism	20
JAK-STAT signaling	22
Apoptosis	25
VEGF signaling	22
Nucleotide excision repair	15

The PFS times and expression levels of selected genes in the 118 Class 3 patients were used in multivariate Cox regression analysis to compute β's for the genes. Table 2 shows the β's calculated for the 35 selected genes. *PI* scores were calculated for all patients who received adjuvant chemotherapy and radiation (380) by substituting β's and expression levels of selected genes into the prognostic index formula. The scores were then used to classify samples into low- and high-risk groups in survival analysis.

All the seed pathways in Table 1 except mismatch repair had at least one representative in the signature. Cell cycle had the highest number of genes (eight), followed by WNT pathway, which had five. The expression of four of the selected genes were significantly correlated with PFS ($p < 0.05$): *DKK1, FZD7,* and *PPARGC1A* showed positive correlation ($\beta > 0$), and *CCNE1* displayed negative correlation ($\beta < 0$) (Table 2).

Several signature genes are linked to survival in other cancers

Several genes in the signature have been reported to be associated with progression-free and/or overall survival in other cancers. DKK1, FZD3, FZD7, SFRP1, and SFRP4 are regulators of the Wnt/β pathway. Overexpression of DKK1 is predictive of unfavourable overall survival and time to recurrence in intrahepatic cholangiocarcinoma patients [42]. Overexpression of FZD3 in colorectal patients was correlated with poor survival [43]. Underexpression of SFRP1 is associated with poor survival and may be an independent predictive and prognostic factor for prostate cancer [44]. SFRP4 increased the sensitivity of ovarian cancer cell lines to cisplatin, suggesting it is a predictive marker of chemoresistance in the cancer [45]. CCNA1, CCND1, CCNE1, CDC6, CDK2, CDKN1C and CDKN2A regulate the cell cycle. CCND1 amplication was associated with poor prognosis in estrogen receptor positive breast cancer [46] and [47] found it to be

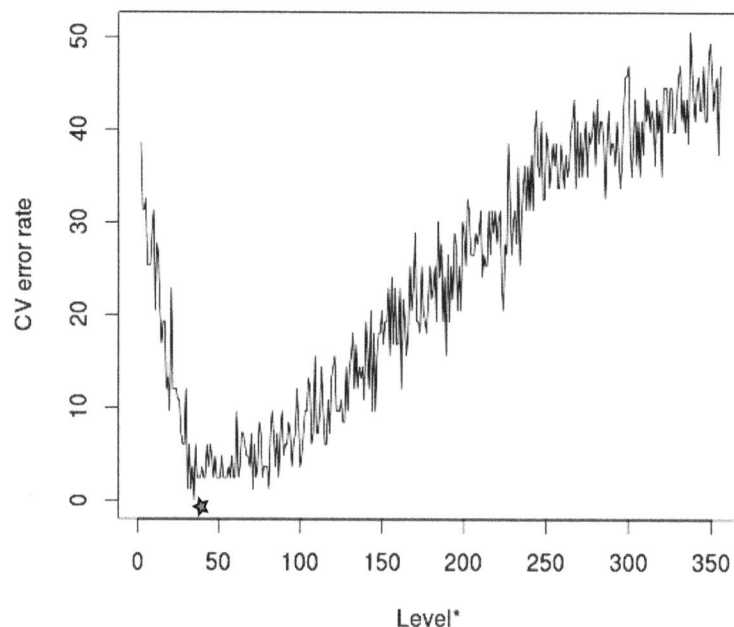

Fig. 2 Cross-validated error rates of R-SVM in each recursive steps. *The number of features used for SVM classification in each step. Parameters for SVM: kernel = linear, cost = 10, and 5% cross-validation. The red star represents the level at which the minimal cross-validation error was achieved

Table 2 Correlation of the expression of the 35 signature genes with progression-free survival using univariate Cox model

Gene	Contained pathway	Coefficient (β)	HR	p
ABL1	Cell cycle	-0.1215	0.886	0.650
	ErbB pathway			
CCNA1	Cell cycle	-0.0899	0.914	0.520
CCND1	Cell cycle	0.0746	1.077	0.620
CCNE1	Cell cycle	-0.4975	0.608	0.032
CDC6	Cell cycle	0.2324	1.262	0.410
CDK2	Cell cycle	-0.5268	0.591	0.150
CDKN1C	Cell cycle	-0.0285	0.972	0.900
CDKN2A	Cell cycle	0.1415	1.152	0.170
	p53 pathway			
DKK1	WNT pathway	0.1759	1.192	0.040
FZD3	WNT pathway	0.2434	1.276	0.230
FZD7	WNT pathway	0.4934	1.638	0.022
GADD45G	MAPK pathway	0.2850	1.330	0.200
GHR	JAK-STAT pathway	-0.2292	0.795	0.180
GSTT1	Glutathione metabolism	0.0485	1.050	0.590
HSPA1B	JAK-STAT pathway	-0.1244	0.883	0.340
ID4	TGF-β pathway	-0.1680	0.845	0.350
IGFBP3	p53 pathway	0.1103	1.117	0.340
INHBB	TGF-β pathway	-0.1187	0.888	0.390
IRS2	Insulin signaling	-0.0665	0.936	0.790
LIFR	ErbB pathway	-0.1009	0.904	0.670
PDGFRA	MAPK pathway	0.0262	1.027	0.760
PIK3CA	Phosphatidylinositol signaling	0.1479	1.159	0.420
PLA2G5	Phosphatidylinositol signaling	-0.0176	0.983	0.900
POLE3	Nucleotide excision repair	0.0615	1.063	0.840
PPARGC1A	MAPK pathway	0.4121	1.510	0.045
PRKAR2B	Insulin signaling	0.0641	1.066	0.660
PYGB	Insulin signaling	-0.4071	0.666	0.160
SFRP1	WNT pathway	-0.1216	0.886	0.270
SFRP4	WNT pathway	0.1461	1.157	0.270
SH2B2	Insulin signaling	-0.0199	0.980	0.950
STAG3L4	JAK-STAT pathway	-0.0001	1.000	1.000
STMN1	MAPK pathway	0.0837	1.087	0.750
THBS2	Focal adhesion	-0.1319	0.876	0.330
THBS3	Focal adhesion	-0.3916	0.767	0.160
VEGFA	VEGFA signaling	-0.0268	0.974	0.810

an independent prognostic factor in primary tumours and metastases as well as an independent prognostic factor in metastasis. CDC6 expression was correlated with overall and recurrence survival in non-small cell lung cancer patients [48]. CDKN2A promoter methylation was correlated with poor prognosis of colorectal cancer

patients [49, 50]. CDK2, regulated by CDKN2A, is a known oncogene and regulator of the cell cycle. Its regression coefficient ($\beta < 0$) in our study, however, showed that it was positively associated with progression-free survival. Its overexpression was associated with shorter survival in oral cancer [51]. GADD45G is implicated in stress signaling responses to physiological or environmental stressors, resulting in cell cycle arrest, DNA repair, cell survival and senescence, or apoptosis [52, 53]. GADD45G methylation and protein expression were independently associated with survival of gastric cardia adenocarcinoma patients [54] and esophageal squamous cell carcinoma patients [55].

The 35-gene signature predicts progression-free and overall survival in both TCGA and independent dataset

The 35 genes that discriminated between rapidly- and slowly-progressing patients were combined into a signature and its prognostic value first assessed in the patients that were not used in the feature selection step (Class 3). The prognostic index (PI) scores of these patients were standardized and used to split the patients into low- and high-risk groups. Figures 3a and 3b show the PFS and OS Kaplan Meier plots, respectively, for the two prognostic groups. The median PFS and OS times for the low-risk group (256 days, 95% CI = 232 - 299 days and 635 days, 95% CI = 502 - 1024 days) were significantly higher than those of the high-risk group (175 days, 95% CI = 158 - 204 days and 393 days, 95% CI = 345 - 454 days) ($p < 0.05$).

Two hundred seventy nine of the 380 patients who received adjuvant chemotherapy and radiotherapy died before the end of the follow-up period. The remaining 101 patients were alive at the end of follow-up or were lost to follow-up. The 380 patients were split into low- and high-risk groups. Figure 3c shows the OS plots for these prognostic groups. There was a statistically significant difference in OS between the groups ($p < 0.05$). The median OS time (548 days, 95% CI = 486 - 646) of the low-risk group was significantly higher than that (442 days, 95% CI = 394 - 476) of the high-risk group ($p < 0.05$).

Thirty nine patients in the validation cohort received adjuvant chemotherapy and radiation. The β's computed with the TCGA cohort and the expression levels of the signature genes in the validation cohort were used to calculate PI scores for the patients in the validation cohort. The patients were then split into low- and high-risk groups. The median OS of the low-risk group was higher than that of the high-risk group, and the difference in OS between the groups was statistically significant ($p < 0.05$) (Fig. 3d).

The results show that the 35-gene signature identified from the TCGA dataset may be a generically applicable predictor of progression-free and overall survival in GBM,

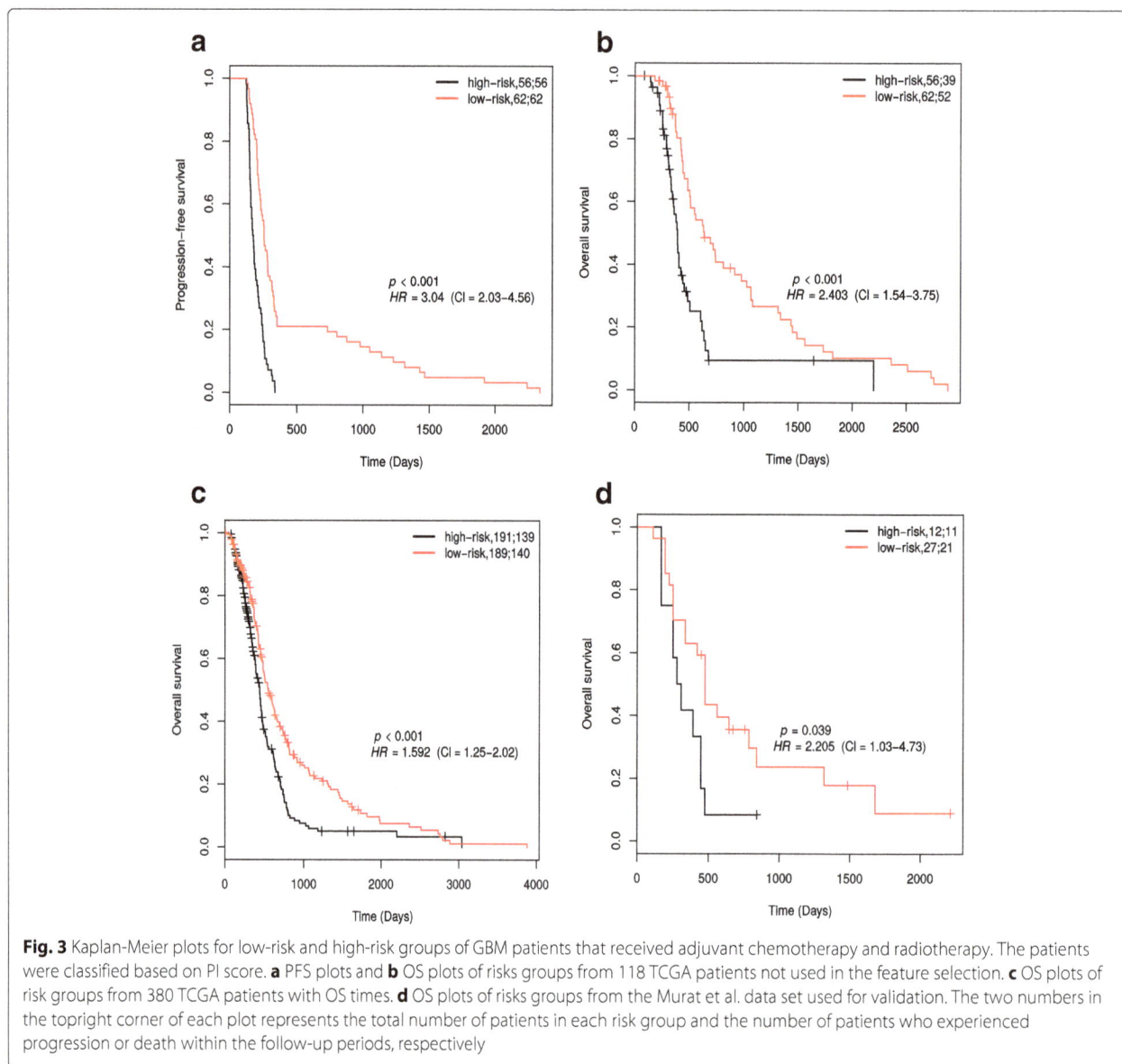

Fig. 3 Kaplan-Meier plots for low-risk and high-risk groups of GBM patients that received adjuvant chemotherapy and radiotherapy. The patients were classified based on PI score. **a** PFS plots and **b** OS plots of risks groups from 118 TCGA patients not used in the feature selection. **c** OS plots of risk groups from 380 TCGA patients with OS times. **d** OS plots of risks groups from the Murat et al. data set used for validation. The two numbers in the topright corner of each plot represents the total number of patients in each risk group and the number of patients who experienced progression or death within the follow-up periods, respectively

since prognostic value in the prediction of overall survival was validated in an independent cohort.

The 35-gene signature predicts progression-free and overall survival in four GBM subtypes

The prognostic value of the signature in predicting PFS and OS in subtypes of GBM was assessed. 51, 51, 3 and 66 patients belonged to the classical, proneural, neural, and mesenchymal subtypes, respectively. Figure 4 shows the results of the PFS survival analysis in the subtypes. There was statistically significant difference in survival between low- and high-risk groups in all the subtypes ($p < 0.05$). In the classical subtype, the median PFS times of low- and high-risk groups were 256 and 186 days respectively. In the mesenchymal subtype, the median PFS times were

269 and 146 days respectively. In the neural subtype, the median PFS times were 358 and 172 days, respectively. In the proneural subtype, the median PFS times were 304 and 172 days, respectively.

One hundred five classical, 95 proneural, 60 neural and 120 mesenchymal subtype patients were used for subtype-specific OS analysis. Figure 5 shows the Kaplan-Meier OS plots for high-risk and low-risk groups in each subtype. The low- and high-risk groups differed significantly in OS in all the subtypes ($p < 0.05$). In the classical subtype, the median OS times of low- and high-risk groups were 544 and 452 days respectively. In the mesenchymal subtype, the median OS times were 485 and 394 days respectively. In the neural subtype, the median OS times were 476 and 435 days, respectively. In the proneural subtype, the

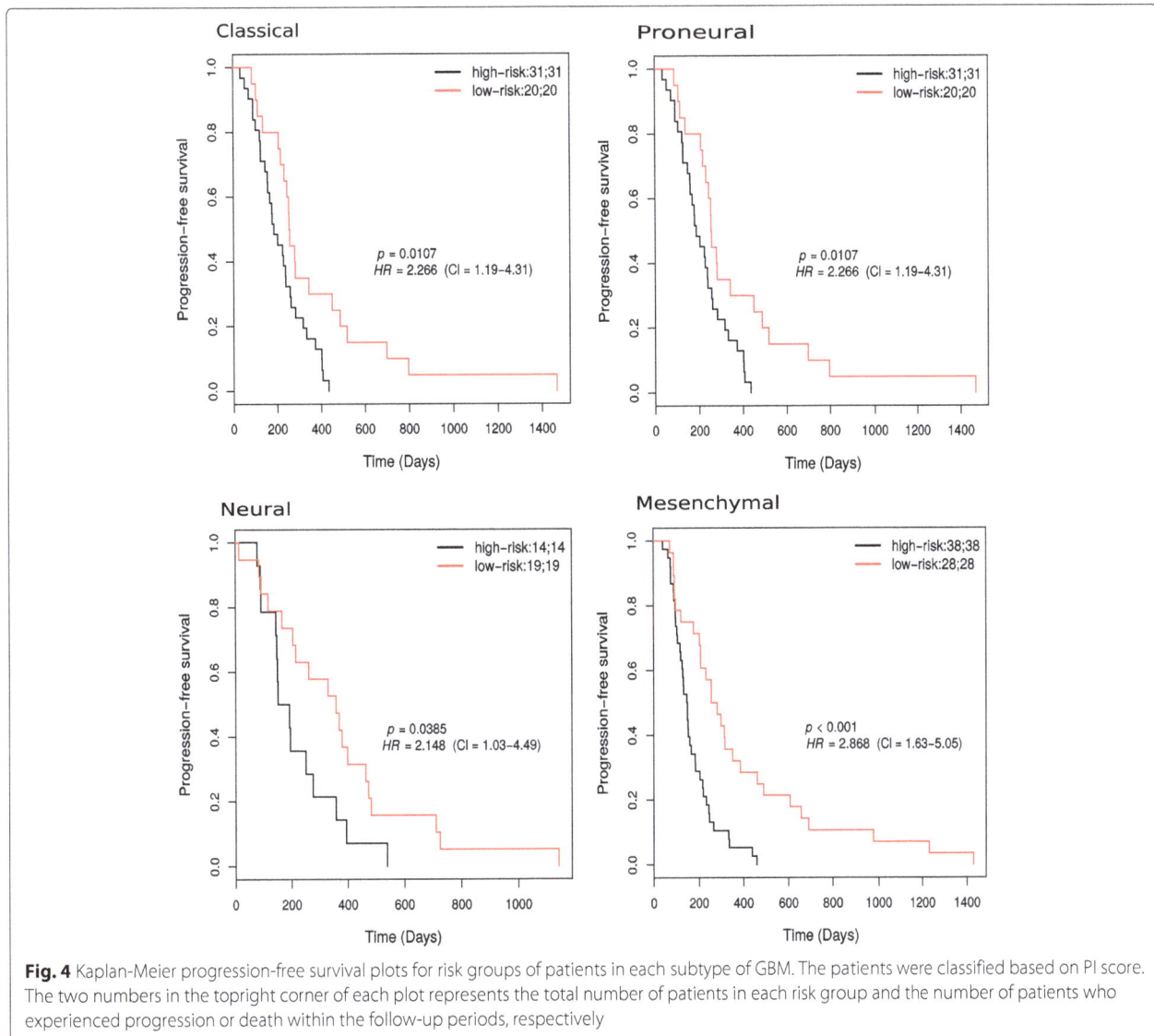

Fig. 4 Kaplan-Meier progression-free survival plots for risk groups of patients in each subtype of GBM. The patients were classified based on PI score. The two numbers in the topright corner of each plot represents the total number of patients in each risk group and the number of patients who experienced progression or death within the follow-up periods, respectively

median OS times were 748 and 395 days, respectively. Reports from previous studies show that the prognostic value of MGMT promoter methylation in GBM patients is controversial. Zhang et al. [56] showed that MGMT promoter methylation was associated with better PFS and OS in patients with GBM regardless of therapeutic intervention, and associated with longer OS in GBM patients treated with alkylating agents. Costa et al. [5] did not find significant association between MGMT promoter methylation and the outcome of Portuguese GBM patients treated with temozolomide. Brennan et al. [20] however reported that MGMT promoter methylation was only correlated with OS in the GBM classical subtypes. The possible explanation for these conflicting reports on the prognostic value of MGMT promoter methylation could thus be due to differences in the GBM subtype

distribution which was not considered in most previous studies. Our 35-gene signature, however, predicted PFS and OS regardless of the subtype, suggesting that it may be a more effective predictor of overall and progression-free survival in GBM.

The 35-gene signature is an independent predictor of PFS and OS in GBM patients

A multivariate Cox regression model analysis involving the prognostic index, age and MGMT promoter methylation was carried to assess the independence of the gene signature to predict PFS and OS. 79 TCGA GBM patients had associated days to progression, and age and MGMT promoter methylation status (38 methylated and 41 unmethylated) data. Two hundred sixty nine patients had days to death and age and MGMT promoter

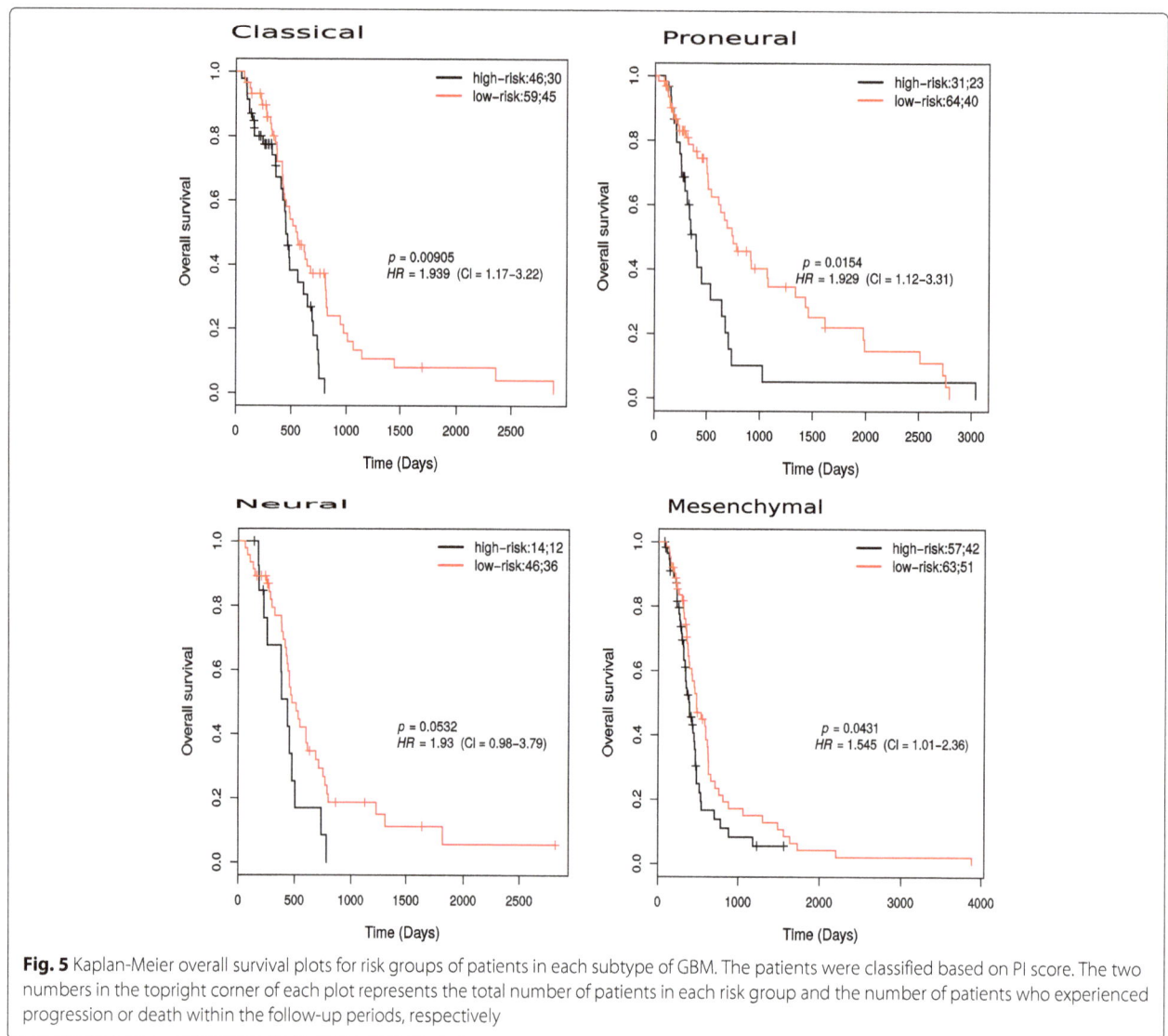

Fig. 5 Kaplan-Meier overall survival plots for risk groups of patients in each subtype of GBM. The patients were classified based on PI score. The two numbers in the topright corner of each plot represents the total number of patients in each risk group and the number of patients who experienced progression or death within the follow-up periods, respectively

methylation (135 methylated and 134 unmethylated) data. The results from the univariate and multivariate analyses on the three variable are shown in Table 3. MGMT promoter methylation was not correlated with PFS in both univariate and multivariate Cox analyses ($p > 0.05$). Prognostic index, age and MGMT promoter methylation were significantly correlated with OS in the univariate and multivariate analyses ($p < 0.05$). The univariate Cox's proportional hazard analysis showed that age and the prognostic index based on the 35-gene signature were both significantly correlated with PFS ($p < 0.05$), but only the prognostic index was significantly correlated with PFS in the multivariate analysis ($p < 0.05$). This showed that the expression signature is an independent predictor of PFS and OS in GBM patients.

Post-treatment tumour progression depends largely on alterations in classical cancer and chemotherapy/radiation resistance-related pathways. This is supported by findings from the multivariate Cox's proportional hazard analysis findings as only the 35-gene prognostic index was significantly associated with PFS and was an independent predictor of PFS. Overall survival, on the other hand, is determined by many factors. Age at diagnosis is one of the most important factors associated with overall survival in cancer and has been demonstrated in GBM [57–59]. While the prognostic value of MGMT promoter methylation in GBM remains controversial, our findings showed that prognostic index, age and MGMT promoter methylation are all independent prognostic factors for overall survival.

Signature genes belong to a functional interaction subnetwork enriched for known cancer pathways

A subnetwork generated from the interactions between the signature genes had significantly more interactions

Table 3 Univariate and multivariate Cox's proportional hazards model analyses of prognostic factors for progression-free and overall survival

Variable	Progression-free survival						Overall survival					
			Univariate		Multivariate				Univariate		Multivariate	
	n	n*	HR	p(Wald)	HR	p(Wald)	n	n*	HR	p(Wald)	HR	p(Wald)
Prognostic groups[1] High-risk[2]	79	79	3.41	3.00E-6	3.13	2.97E-5	269	181	1.63	1.45E-3	1.60	2.46E-3
Age	79	79	1.02	4.30E-2	1.01	3.70E-1	269	181	1.04	3.50E-8	1.03	6.12E-7
MGMT methylation status Unmethylated[3]	79	79	1.33	2.14E-1	1,26	3.20E-1	269	181	1.68	6.59E-4	1.52	7.35E-3

*Number of events; [1]high-risk and low-risk groups; [2]low-risk was used as reference; [3]methylated was used as reference

than would be expected for a random set of proteins of similar size (PPI enrichment $p = 1.11 \times 10^{-16}$) (Fig. 6). The network was also significantly enriched ($p < 0.01$) for KEGG cancer pathways and pathways known to drive tumour initiation and progression, such as the cell cycle and PI3K-Akt, Wnt, p53 and Ras signaling [60, 61].

A subset of the signature genes may be relevant to GBM biology and may have utility in drug discovery

Combinatorial medicine have been proposed for the treatment of tumour recurrence. It involves therapeutically targeting as many genomic alterations responsible for a disease in a patient as possible and has strong implications for overcoming the challenge of tumour progression and drug resistance [62, 63]. One of the ways to overcome this challenge is to prioritise combinations of genes to be targeted based on their unique roles in tumour progression. Of the signature genes, only *ABL1, CCND1,*

CCNE1, PDGFRA, PIK3CA were found to be linked to predisposition to at least one cancer by the Online Mendelian Inheritance in Man (OMIM) database [64]. However, *CCNA1, CDK2, CDKN1C, CDKN2A, FZD3, HSPA1B, IGFBP3, PDGFRA, PIK3CA, PLA2G5, THBS2* and *VEGFA* all have gene ontology annotations related to apoptosis, while *ABL1, FZD7, PDGFRA, PIK3CA, SFRP1, THBS2,* and *VEGFA* are annotated as being involved in angiogenesis (data not shown). Collectively this may indicate differential gene expression explicitly directed towards towards resisting induced cell death by both intrinsic and extrinsic factors and optimising the tumour microenvironment for maximum fitness. This, combined with the knowledge that the signature genes are involved in classical pathways implicated in cancer drug resistance, suggests that the highlighted genes should be further validated and assessed as drug targets in designing novel combinatorial therapies for GBM in future studies.

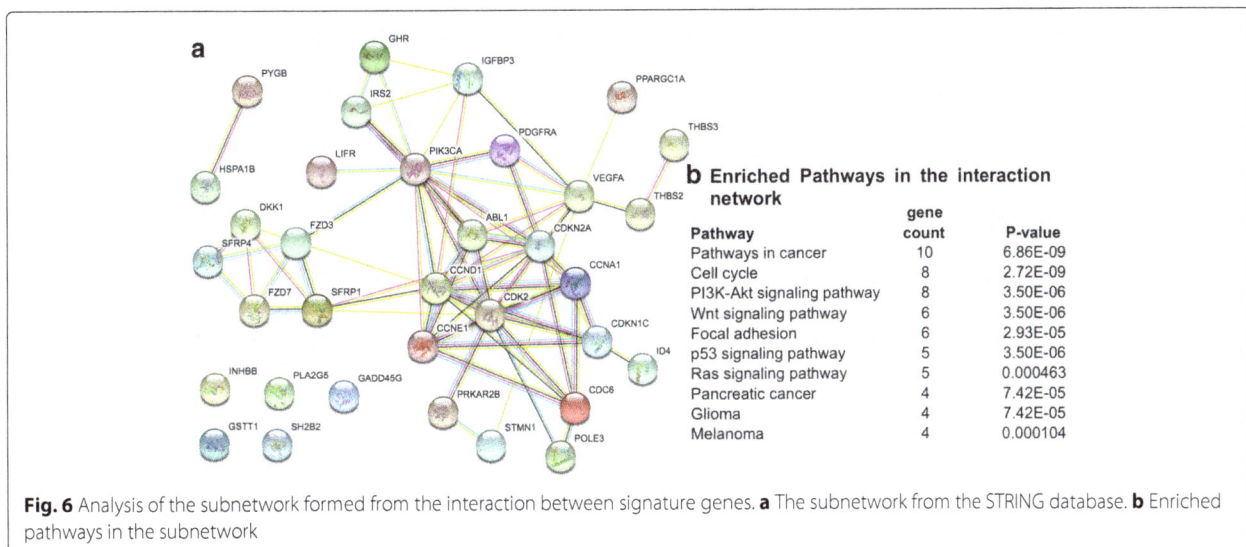

Fig. 6 Analysis of the subnetwork formed from the interaction between signature genes. **a** The subnetwork from the STRING database. **b** Enriched pathways in the subnetwork

Conclusion

We propose that the performance of the signature makes it an attractive candidate for further studies to assess its utility as a clinical prognostic and predictive biomarker in GBM patients, and that its component genes may also have utility as therapeutic targets for improving both progression-free and overall survival.

Additional files

Additional file 1: Workflow of the modified SVM-RFE used for selecting a set of genes that discriminated between rapidly-progressing and slow-progressing GBM patients.

Additional file 2: Genes with high expression variance used in pathway enrichment analysis.

Additional file 3: Unguided principal component analysis to identify batch effect in the TCGA data set as a function of genes from chemoradioresistance-associated pathways. $p = 0.118$, indicating absence of significant batch effect in the data. Samples in each batch are denoted by a different colour and symbol.

Additional file 4: Unguided principal component analysis to assess batch effect.

Acknowledgements
Not applicable.

Authors' contributions
AAF conceived and designed the experiments, and analyzed the data. AAF wrote the paper under JG's guidance. JG supervised all aspects of this work, and read, edited and approved the final manuscript. All authors read and approved the final manuscript.

Authors' information
Not applicable.

Competing interests
The authors declare that they have no competing interests.

References

1. Hegi ME, Diserens AC, Gorlia T, Hamou MF, de Tribolet N, Weller M, Kros JM, Hainfellner JA, Mason W, Mariani L, Bromberg JEC, Hau P, Mirimanoff RO, Cairncross JG, Janzer RC, Stupp R. MGMT Gene Silencing and Benefit from Temozolomide in Glioblastoma. N Engl J Med. 2005;352(10):997–1003. https://doi.org/10.1056/NEJMoa043331.

2. Kim YS, Kim SH, Cho J, Kim JW, Chang JH, Kim DS, Lee KS, Suh CO. MGMT gene promoter methylation as a potent prognostic factor in glioblastoma treated with temozolomide-based chemoradiotherapy: a single-institution study. Int J Radiat Oncol Biol Phys. 2012;84(3):661–7. https://doi.org/10.1016/j.ijrobp.2011.12.086.

3. Shen D, Liu T, Lin Q, Lu X, Wang Q, Lin F, Mao W. MGMT Promoter Methylation Correlates with an Overall Survival Benefit in Chinese High-Grade Glioblastoma Patients Treated with Radiotherapy and Alkylating Agent-Based Chemotherapy: A Single-Institution Study. PLoS ONE. 2014;9(9):107558. https://doi.org/10.1371/journal.pone.0107558.

4. Melguizo C, Prados J, González B, Ortiz R, Concha A, Alvarez PJ, Madeddu R, Perazzoli G, Oliver JA, López R, Rodríguez-Serrano F, Aránega A. MGMT promoter methylation status and MGMT and CD133 immunohistochemical expression as prognostic markers in glioblastoma patients treated with temozolomide plus radiotherapy. J Transl Med. 2012;10(1):250. https://doi.org/10.1186/1479-5876-10-250

5. Costa BM, Caeiro C, Guimarães I, Martinho O, Jaraquemada T, Augusto I, Castro L, Osório L, Linhares P, Honavar M, Resende M, Braga F, Silva A, Pardal F, Amorim J, Nabiço R, Almeida R, Alegria C, Pires M, Pinheiro C, Carvalho E, Lopes JM, Costa P, Damasceno M, Reis RM. Prognostic value of MGMT promoter methylation in glioblastoma patients treated with temozolomide-based chemoradiation: a Portuguese multicentre study. Oncol Rep. 2010;23(6):1655–62.

6. Yin A-a, Zhang L-h, Cheng J-x, Dong Y, Liu B-l, Han N, Zhang X. The Predictive but Not Prognostic Value of MGMT Promoter Methylation Status in Elderly Glioblastoma Patients: A Meta-Analysis. PLoS ONE. 2014;9(1):85102. https://doi.org/10.1371/journal.pone.0085102.

7. Goldstein LJ, Gray R, Badve S, Childs BH, Yoshizawa C, Rowley S, Shak S, Baehner FL, Ravdin PM, Davidson NE, Sledge GW, Perez EA, Shulman LN, Martino S, Sparano JA. Prognostic Utility of the 21-Gene Assay in Hormone Receptor–Positive Operable Breast Cancer Compared With Classical Clinicopathologic Features. J Clin Oncol. 2008;26(25):4063–71. https://doi.org/10.1200/JCO.2007.14.4501.

8. Paik S, Shak S, Tang G, Kim C, Baker J, Cronin M, Baehner FL, Walker MG, Watson D, Park T, Hiller W, Fisher ER, Wickerham DL, Bryant J, Wolmark N. A Multigene Assay to Predict Recurrence of Tamoxifen-Treated, Node-Negative Breast Cancer. N Engl J Med. 2004;351(27):2817–26. https://doi.org/10.1056/NEJMoa041588.

9. Acs G, Kiluk J, Loftus L, Laronga C. Comparison of Oncotype DX and Mammostrat risk estimations and correlations with histologic tumor features in low-grade, estrogen receptor-positive invasive breast carcinomas. Mod Pathol. 2013;26(11):1451–60. https://doi.org/10.1038/modpathol.2013.88.

10. Ring BZ, Seitz RS, Beck R, Shasteen WJ, Tarr SM, Cheang MCU, Yoder BJ, Budd GT, Nielsen TO, Hicks DG, Estopinal NC, Ross DT. Novel prognostic immunohistochemical biomarker panel for estrogen receptor-positive breast cancer. J Clin Oncol Off J Am Soc Clin Oncol. 2006;24(19):3039–47. https://doi.org/10.1200/JCO.2006.05.6564.

11. van 't Veer LJ, Dai H, van de Vijver MJ, He YD, Hart AAM, Mao M, Peterse HL, van der Kooy K, Marton MJ, Witteveen AT, Schreiber GJ, Kerkhoven RM, Roberts C, Linsley PS, Bernards R, Friend SH. Gene expression profiling predicts clinical outcome of breast cancer. Nature. 2002;415(6871):530–6. https://doi.org/10.1038/415530a.

12. Soneson C, Gerster S, Delorenzi M. Batch Effect Confounding Leads to Strong Bias in Performance Estimates Obtained by Cross-Validation. PLoS ONE. 2014;9(6):100335. https://doi.org/10.1371/journal.pone.0100335.

13. Reese SE, Archer KJ, Therneau TM, Atkinson EJ, Vachon CM, de Andrade M, Kocher J-PA, Eckel-Passow JE. A new statistic for identifying batch effects in high-throughput genomic data that uses guided principal component analysis. Bioinformatics. 2013;29(22): 2877–83. https://doi.org/10.1093/bioinformatics/btt480.

14. TCGA: Comprehensive genomic characterization defines human glioblastoma genes and core pathways. Nature. 2008;455(7216):1061–8. https://doi.org/10.1038/nature07385.

15. Verhaak RGW, Hoadley KA, Purdom E, Wang V, Qi Y, Wilkerson MD, Miller CR, Ding L, Golub T, Mesirov JP, Alexe G, Lawrence M, O'Kelly M, Tamayo P, Weir BA, Gabriel S, Winckler W, Gupta S, Jakkula L, Feiler HS, Hodgson JG, James CD, Sarkaria JN, Brennan C, Kahn A, Spellman PT, Wilson RK, Speed TP, Gray JW, Meyerson M, Getz G, Perou CM, Hayes DN. An integrated genomic analysis identifies clinically relevant subtypes of glioblastoma characterized by abnormalities in PDGFRA, IDH1, EGFR and NF1. Cancer Cell. 2010;17(1):98. https://doi.org/10.1016/j.ccr.2009.12.020.

16. Kahn AB, Ryan MC, Liu H, Zeeberg BR, Jamison DC, Weinstein JN. SpliceMiner: a high-throughput database implementation of the NCBI Evidence Viewer for microarray splice variant analysis. BMC Bioinformatics. 2007;8(1):75. https://doi.org/10.1186/1471-2105-8-75.

17. Liu H, Zeeberg BR, Qu G, Koru AG, Ferrucci A, Kahn A, Ryan MC, Nuhanovic A, Munson PJ, Reinhold WC, Kane DW, Weinstein JN. AffyProbeMiner: a web resource for computing or retrieving accurately redefined Affymetrix probe sets. Bioinformatics. 2007;23(18):2385–90. https://doi.org/10.1093/bioinformatics/btm360.

18. Iacob G, Dinca E. Current data and strategy in glioblastoma multiforme. J Med Life. 2009;2(4):386–93.

19. Tang PA, Bentzen SM, Chen EX, Siu LL. Surrogate end points for median overall survival in metastatic colorectal cancer: Literature-based analysis from 39 randomized controlled trials of first-line chemotherapy. J Clin

Oncol. 2007;25(29):4562–8. https://doi.org/10.1200/JCO.2006.08.1935.

20. Brennan CW, Verhaak RGW, McKenna A, Campos B, Noushmehr H, Salama SR, Zheng S, Chakravarty D, Sanborn JZ, Berman SH, Beroukhim R, Bernard B, Wu CJ, Genovese G, Shmulevich I, Barnholtz-Sloan J, Zou L, Vegesna R, Shukla SA, Ciriello G, Yung W, Zhang W, Sougnez C, Mikkelsen T, Aldape K, Bigner DD, Van Meir EG, Prados M, Sloan A, Black KL, Eschbacher J, Finocchiaro G, Friedman W, Andrews DW, Guha A, Iacocca M, O'Neill BP, Foltz G, Myers J, Weisenberger DJ, Penny R, Kucherlapati R, Perou CM, Hayes DN, Gibbs R, Marra M, Mills GB, Lander E, Spellman P, Wilson R, Sander C, Weinstein J, Meyerson M, Gabriel S, Laird PW, Haussler D, Getz G, Chin L. The Somatic Genomic Landscape of Glioblastoma. Cell. 2013;155(2):462–77. https://doi.org/10.1016/j.cell.2013.09.034.

21. Shtivelman E, Hensing T, Simon GR, Dennis PA, Otterson GA, Bueno R, Salgia R, Shtivelman E, Hensing T, Simon GR, Dennis PA, Otterson GA, Bueno R, Salgia R. Molecular pathways and therapeutic targets in lung cancer. Oncotarget. 2014;5(6):1392–433. https://doi.org/10.18632/oncotarget.1891.

22. Bagnyukova TV, Serebriiskii IG, Zhou Y, Hopper-Borge EA, Golemis EA, Astsaturov I. Chemotherapy and signaling: How can targeted therpies supercharge cytotoxic agents? Cancer Biol Ther. 2010;10(9):839–53. https://doi.org/10.4161/cbt.10.9.13738.

23. Riedel RF, Porrello A, Pontzer E, Chenette EJ, Hsu DS, Balakumaran B, Potti A, Nevins J, Febbo PG. A genomic approach to identify molecular pathways associated with chemotherapy resistance. Mol Cancer Ther. 2008;7(10):3141–9. https://doi.org/10.1158/1535-7163.MCT-08-0642.

24. Fojo T. Cancer, DNA repair mechanisms, and resistance to chemotherapy. J Natl Cancer Inst. 2001;93(19):1434–6. https://doi.org/10.1093/jnci/93.19.1434.

25. Sherman-Baust CA, Becker KG, Wood III WH, Zhang Y, Morin PJ. Gene expression and pathway analysis of ovarian cancer cells selected for resistance to cisplatin, paclitaxel, or doxorubicin. J Ovarian Res. 2011;4:21. https://doi.org/10.1186/1757-2215-4-21.

26. Long J, Zhang Y, Yu X, Yang J, LeBrun D, Chen C, Yao Q, Li M. Overcoming Drug Resistance in Pancreatic Cancer. Expert Opin Ther Targets. 2011;15(7):817–28. https://doi.org/10.1517/14728222.2011.566216.

27. Pritchard JR, Lauffenburger DA, Hemann MT. Understanding resistance to combination chemotherapy. Drug Resist Updat. 2012;15(5):249–57. https://doi.org/10.1016/j.drup.2012.10.003.

28. Humphrey RW, Brockway-Lunardi LM, Bonk DT, Dohoney KM, Doroshow JH, Meech SJ, Ratain MJ, Topalian SL, Pardoll DM. Opportunities and challenges in the development of experimental drug combinations for cancer. J Natl Cancer Inst. 2011;103(16):1222–6. https://doi.org/10.1093/jnci/djr246.

29. Reuter S, Gupta SC, Chaturvedi MM, Aggarwal BB. Oxidative stress, inflammation, and cancer: How are they linked? Free Radic Biol Med. 2010;49(11):1603–16. https://doi.org/10.1016/j.freeradbiomed.2010.09.006.

30. West KA, Castillo SS, Dennis PA. Activation of the PI3k/Akt pathway and chemotherapeutic resistance. Drug Resist Updat Rev Commentaries Antimicrob Anticancer Chemother. 2002;5(6):234–48.

31. Housman G, Byler S, Heerboth S, Lapinska K, Longacre M, Snyder N, Sarkar S. Drug Resistance in Cancer: An Overview. Cancers. 2014;6(3):1769–92. https://doi.org/10.3390/cancers6031769.

32. Davis AP, Murphy CG, Johnson R, Lay JM, Lennon-Hopkins K, Saraceni-Richards C, Sciaky D, King BL, Rosenstein MC, Wiegers TC, Mattingly CJ. The Comparative Toxicogenomics Database: update 2013. Nucleic Acids Res. 2013;41(Database issue):1104–14. https://doi.org/10.1093/nar/gks994.

33. Guyon I, Weston J, Barnhill S, Vapnik V. Gene Selection for Cancer Classification using Support Vector Machines. Mach Learn. 2002;46(1-3):389–422. https://doi.org/10.1023/A:1012487302797.

34. Murat A, Migliavacca E, Gorlia T, Lambiv WL, Shay T, Hamou MF, de Tribolet N, Regli L, Wick W, Kouwenhoven MCM, Hainfellner JA, Heppner FL, Dietrich PY, Zimmer Y, Cairncross JG, Janzer RC, Domany E, Delorenzi M, Stupp R, Hegi ME. Stem cell-related "self-renewal" signature and high epidermal growth factor receptor expression associated with resistance to concomitant chemoradiotherapy in glioblastoma. J Clin Oncol Off J Am Soc Clin Oncol. 2008;26(18):3015–24. https://doi.org/10.1200/JCO.2007.15.7164.

35. Szklarczyk D, Morris JH, Cook H, Kuhn M, Wyder S, Simonovic M, Santos A, Doncheva NT, Roth A, Bork P, Jensen LJ, von Mering C. The STRING database in 2017: quality-controlled protein–protein association networks, made broadly accessible. Nucleic Acids Res. 2017;45:362–8. https://doi.org/10.1093/nar/gkw937.

36. Zhao X, Rødland EA, Sørlie T, Naume B, Langerød A, Frigessi A, Kristensen VN, Børresen-Dale AL, Lingjærde OC. Combining gene signatures improves prediction of breast cancer survival. PLoS ONE. 2011;6(3):17845. https://doi.org/10.1371/journal.pone.0017845.

37. Lau SK, Boutros PC, Pintilie M, Blackhall FH, Zhu CQ, Strumpf D, Johnston MR, Darling G, Keshavjee S, Waddell TK, Liu N, Lau D, Penn LZ, Shepherd FA, Jurisica I, Der SD, Tsao MS. Three-gene prognostic classifier for early-stage non small-cell lung cancer. J Clin Oncol Off J Am Soc Clin Oncol. 2007;25(35):5562–9. https://doi.org/10.1200/JCO.2007.12.0352.

38. Stupp R, Mason WP, van den Bent MJ, Weller M, Fisher B, Taphoorn MJB, Belanger K, Brandes AA, Marosi C, Bogdahn U, Curschmann J, Janzer RC, Ludwin SK, Gorlia T, Allgeier A, Lacombe D, Cairncross JG, Eisenhauer E, Mirimanoff RO. European Organisation for Research and Treatment of Cancer Brain Tumor and Radiotherapy Groups, National Cancer Institute of Canada Clinical Trials Group. Radiotherapy plus concomitant and adjuvant temozolomide for glioblastoma. N Engl J Med. 2005;352(10):987–96. https://doi.org/10.1056/NEJMoa043330.

39. Jiang BH, Liu LZ. Role of mTOR in anticancer drug resistance. Drug Resist Updat Rev Commentaries Antimicrob Anticancer Chemother. 2008;11(3):63–76. https://doi.org/10.1016/j.drup.2008.03.001.

40. Niero EL, Rocha-Sales B, Lauand C, Cortez BA, de Souza MM, Rezende-Teixeira P, Urabayashi MS, Martens AA, Neves JH, Machado-Santelli GM. The multiple facets of drug resistance: one history, different approaches. J Exp Clin Cancer Res CR. 2014;33(1):37. https://doi.org/10.1186/1756-9966-33-37.

41. Martin HL, Smith L, Tomlinson DC. Multidrug-resistant breast cancer: current perspectives. Breast Cancer Targets Ther. 2014;6:1–13. https://doi.org/10.2147/BCTT.S37638.

42. Shi RY, Yang XR, Shen QJ, Yang LX, Xu Y, Qiu SJ, Sun YF, Zhang X, Wang Z, Zhu K, Qin WX, Tang ZY, Fan J, Zhou J. High expression of Dickkopf-related protein 1 is related to lymphatic metastasis and indicates poor prognosis in intrahepatic cholangiocarcinoma patients after surgery. Cancer. 2013;119(5):993–1003. https://doi.org/10.1002/cncr.27788.

43. Wong SCC, He CW, Chan CML, Chan AKC, Wong HT, Cheung MT, Luk LLY, Au TCC, Chiu MK, Ma BBY, Chan ATC. Clinical Significance of Frizzled Homolog 3 Protein in Colorectal Cancer Patients. PLoS ONE. 2013;8(11):79481. https://doi.org/10.1371/journal.pone.0079481.

44. Zheng L, Sun D, Fan W, Zhang Z, Li Q, Jiang T. Diagnostic Value of SFRP1 as a Favorable Predictive and Prognostic Biomarker in Patients with Prostate Cancer. PLoS ONE. 2015;10(2):0118276. https://doi.org/10.1371/journal.pone.0118276.

45. Saran U, Arfuso F, Zeps N, Dharmarajan A. Secreted frizzled-related protein 4 expression is positively associated with responsiveness to Cisplatin of ovarian cancer cell lines in vitro and with lower tumour grade in mucinous ovarian cancers. BMC Cell Biol. 2012;13(1):25. https://doi.org/10.1186/1471-2121-13-25.

46. Roy PG, Pratt N, Purdie CA, Baker L, Ashfield A, Quinlan P, Thompson AM. High CCND1 amplification identifies a group of poor prognosis women with estrogen receptor positive breast cancer. Int J Cancer. J Int Du Cancer. 2010;127(2):355–60. https://doi.org/10.1002/ijc.25034.

47. Seiler R, Thalmann GN, Rotzer D, Perren A, Fleischmann A. CCND1/CyclinD1 status in metastasizing bladder cancer: a prognosticator and predictor of chemotherapeutic response. Mod Pathol. 2014;27(1):87–95. https://doi.org/10.1038/modpathol.2013.125.

48. Allera-Moreau C, Rouquette I, Lepage B, Oumouhou N, Walschaerts M, Leconte E, Schilling V, Gordien K, Brouchet L, Delisle MB, Mazieres J, Hoffmann JS, Pasero P, Cazaux C. DNA replication stress response involving PLK1, CDC6, POLQ, RAD51 and CLASPIN upregulation prognoses the outcome of early/mid-stage non-small cell lung cancer patients. Oncogenesis. 2012;1(10):30. https://doi.org/10.1038/oncsis.2012.29.

49. Xing X, Cai W, Shi H, Wang Y, Li M, Jiao J, Chen M. The prognostic value of CDKN2a hypermethylation in colorectal cancer: a meta-analysis. Br J Cancer. 2013;108(12):2542–8. https://doi.org/10.1038/bjc.2013.251.

50. Maeda K, Kawakami K, Ishida Y, Ishiguro K, Omura K, Watanabe G. Hypermethylation of the CDKN2A gene in colorectal cancer is associated

with shorter survival. Oncol Rep. 2003;10(4):935–8. https://doi.org/10.3892/or.10.4.935

51. Mihara M, Shintani S, Nakahara Y, Kiyota A, Ueyama Y, Matsumura T, Wong DT. Overexpression of CDK2 is a prognostic indicator of oral cancer progression. Jpn J Cancer Res Gann. 2001;92(3):352–60.

52. Cretu A, Sha X, Tront J, Hoffman B, Liebermann DA. Stress sensor Gadd45 genes as therapeutic targets in cancer. Cancer Ther. 2009;7(A):268–76.

53. Zerbini LF, Libermann TA. GADD45 Deregulation in Cancer: Frequently Methylated Tumor Suppressors and Potential Therapeutic Targets. Clin Cancer Res. 2005;11(18):6409–13. https://doi.org/10.1158/1078-0432.CCR-05-1475.

54. Guo W, Dong Z, Guo Y, Chen Z, Kuang G, Yang Z. Methylation-mediated repression of GADD45a and GADD45g expression in gastric cardia adenocarcinoma. Int J Cancer J Int Du Cancer. 2013;133(9):2043–53. https://doi.org/10.1002/ijc.28223.

55. Guo W, Zhu T, Dong Z, Cui L, Zhang M, Kuang G. Decreased expression and aberrant methylation of Gadd45g is associated with tumor progression and poor prognosis in esophageal squamous cell carcinoma. Clin Exp Metastasis. 2013;30(8):977–92. https://doi.org/10.1007/s10585-013-9597-2.

56. Zhang K, Wang X-q, Zhou B, Zhang L. The prognostic value of MGMT promoter methylation in Glioblastoma multiforme: a meta-analysis. Familial Cancer. 2013;12(3):449–58. https://doi.org/10.1007/s10689-013-9607-1.

57. Scott JG, Suh JH, Elson P, Barnett GH, Vogelbaum MA, Peereboom DM, Stevens GHJ, Elinzano H, Chao ST. Aggressive treatment is appropriate for glioblastoma multiforme patients 70 years old or older: a retrospective review of 206 cases. Neuro-Oncol. 2011;13(4):428–36. http://dx.doi.org/10.1093/neuonc/nor005.

58. Thumma SR, Fairbanks RK, Lamoreaux WT, Mackay AR, Demakas JJ, Cooke BS, Elaimy AL, Hanson PW, Lee CM. Effect of pretreatment clinical factors on overall survival in glioblastoma multiforme: a Surveillance Epidemiology and End Results (SEER) population analysis. World J Surg Oncol. 2012;10:75. https://doi.org/10.1186/1477-7819-10-75.

59. Bozdag S, Li A, Riddick G, Kotliarov Y, Baysan M, Iwamoto FM, Cam MC, Kotliarova S, Fine HA. Age-Specific Signatures of Glioblastoma at the Genomic. Genetic, and Epigenetic Levels. PLoS ONE. 2013;8(4):62982. https://doi.org/10.1371/journal.pone.0062982.

60. Feitelson MA, Arzumanyan A, Kulathinal RJ, Blain SW, Holcombe RF, Mahajna J, Marino M, Martinez-Chantar ML, Nawroth R, Sanchez-Garcia I, Sharma D, Saxena NK, Singh N, Vlachostergios PJ, Guo S, Honoki K, Fujii H, Georgakilas AG, Amedei A, Niccolai E, Amin A, Ashraf SS, Boosani CS, Guha G, Ciriolo MR, Aquilano K, Chen S, Mohammed SI, Azmi AS, Bhakta D, Halicka D, Nowsheen S. Sustained proliferation in cancer: mechanisms and novel therapeutic targets. Semin Cancer Biol. 2015;35:25–54. https://doi.org/10.1016/j.semcancer.2015.02.006.

61. Zhang J, Chen YH, Lu Q. Pro-oncogenic and anti-oncogenic pathways: opportunities and challenges of cancer therapy. Futur Oncol. 2010;6(4):587–603. https://doi.org/10.2217/fon.10.15.

62. Al-Lazikani B, Banerji U, Workman P. Combinatorial drug therapy for cancer in the post-genomic era. Nat Biotechnol. 2012;30(7):679–92. https://doi.org/10.1038/nbt.2284.

63. Tang J, Karhinen L, Xu T, Szwajda A, Yadav B, Wennerberg K, Aittokallio T. Target inhibition networks: predicting selective combinations of druggable targets to block cancer survival pathways. PLoS Comput Biol. 2013;9(9):1003226. https://doi.org/10.1371/journal.pcbi.1003226.

64. Amberger JS, Bocchini CA, Schiettecatte F, Scott AF, Hamosh A. OMIM.org: Online mendelian inheritance in man (OMIM®), an online catalog of human genes and genetic disorders. 2015;43:789–98. https://doi.org/10.1093/nar/gku1205.

18

Two successful pregnancies following fertility preservation in a patient with anaplastic astrocytoma

Alexandra Peyser[1,2], Sara L. Bristow[1] and Avner Hershlag[1,2*]

Abstract

Background: Astrocytomas are the most common malignant glial tumors. With improved prognosis, it is possible for patients to pursue pregnancy post-treatment. However, with potential gonadotoxicity of oncology treatments, fertility preservation prior to chemotherapy and/or radiation therapy should be considered. This requires close collaboration between the oncologist and reproductive endocrinologist. To our knowledge this is the first report of successful pregnancies following fertility preservation for AA.

Case presentation: 33-year-old nulligravid woman with newly diagnosed anaplastic astrocytoma (AA; WHO grade III, IDH1-negative) sought fertility preservation. Prior to chemotherapy and radiation for AA, the patient underwent in vitro fertilization (IVF) for fertility preservation, resulting in 8 vitrified embryos. Following chemo-radiation, the patient underwent two rounds of frozen embryo transfers (FET), each resulting in a successful singleton pregnancy.

Conclusion: This case illustrates the realistic possibility, in carefully selected patients with brain tumors, of oocyte or embryo cryo-preservation prior to chemo-radiation and subsequent pregnancies.

Keywords: Fertility preservation, Anaplastic astrocytoma, Glioma, Brain cancer

Background

Astrocytomas are the most common malignant glial tumors originating from small star- shaped glial cells (astrocytes) within the central nervous system. Anaplastic astrocytomas (AA) are defined as grade III glial tumors according to the WHO 2000 classification [1]. The incidence of AA is approximately 0.48 per 100,000 person/ years. They occur more often in younger adults ages 30–50 and account for 17% of primary malignant brain tumors [2]. Prognosis in historical studies, which include both IDH (Isocitrate dehydrogenase)-mutant and IDH-wild type AAs, ranges from 3 to 5 five-year-survival. Prognosis is better for a genetically-defined subset of IDH-mutant tumors, with a median survival closer to 10 years [3]. The mainstay of therapy is surgery followed by radiotherapy. Multiple protocols, including various combinations of high dose radiotherapy, chemotherapy, alternative fraction regimens, heavy particle treatment, interstitial brachytherapy and radiosurgery have been proposed to extend survival [3].

Determining the safety of fertility preservation and subsequent pregnancy after treatment of gliomas is difficult due to the lack of data in the literature. Most studies have been done in patients where the glioma was diagnosed during pregnancy; in these cases there have been reports of changes in the growth of the tumors throughout the pregnancy [4–8]. Significantly, it seems that the same hormones and growth factors required for fetal development may also enhance tumor growth [9]. Currently, no guidelines exist for the medical management and treatment of gliomas diagnosed prior to or during pregnancy. Therefore, it is recommended that women with treated gliomas who want to pursue pregnancy should be followed by a high-risk obstetrician as well as a neuro-oncologist and monitored throughout pregnancy.

* Correspondence: zymania1@northwell.edu
[1]Department of Obstetrics and Gynecology, Northwell Health, Division of Reproductive Endocrinology, 300 Community Drive, Manhasset, NY 11030, USA
[2]Hofstra-Northwell School of Medicine, 500 Hofstra Blvd, Hempstead, NY 11549, USA

Case presentation

A 33-year-old nulligravid woman with newly diagnosed AA (WHO grade III, IDH1 negative) presented to our office for fertility preservation. The patient had undergone a craniotomy with complete resection of her right parietal lobe tumor one month prior, and was scheduled to start chemotherapy and radiation in the next month. Her neuro-oncologist recommended that she undergo fertility preservation prior to chemo-radiation. The fertility preservation did not delay the anticipated start of her chemo-radiation treatment.

The patient had no significant medical or gynecological history. On physical exam, the patient was a healthy-appearing woman. She had left lower extremity weakness and instability. Transvaginal ultrasound demonstrated a normal-appearing uterus and ovaries bilaterally. A dominant follicle was noted on her right ovary; therefore, it was decided to administer HCG 10,000 IU at the time of her presentation to trigger ovulation, thus enabling the initiation of gonadotropins two weeks later. The patient had a high antral follicle count (6 on right, 7 on left).

The patient received low dose gonadotropins: 1 ampule of Human Menopausal Gonadotropin (Menopur®, Ferring Pharmaceuticals, Parsippany, NJ, USA), 75–187. 5 IU of FSH (Gonal F®, EMD Serono, Rockland, MA, USA) for 10 days and cetrorelix acetate (Ganirelex®, GnRH antagonist, EMD Serono, Rockland, MA, USA) for the last 6 days. Final oocyte maturation was triggered with Lupron Luprolide Acetate (Lupron®, GnRH agonist, SANDOZ Pharmaceuticals, Princeton, NJ, USA) 40u. Twelve oocytes were retrieved transvaginally under ultrasound guidance. Eight embryos developed and were vitrified in liquid nitrogen (6 on day 3 and 2 on day 5 post-retrieval).

The patient returned to our Center one year later after she was cleared by her neuro-oncologist following the completion of chemotherapy and radiation. The patient had 6 weeks of radiation therapy with Temozolomide (Temodar®, Merck&Co, Inc., Whitehouse Station, NJ, USA) followed by 6 months of maintenance dose. Her last dose of chemotherapy was one month prior to returning to the office. The patient had maintained regular cycles post chemotherapy. The patient underwent a frozen-thaw natural cycle embryo transfer of a single day-3 embryo with vaginal progesterone (Crinone®, Actavis, Parsippany, NJ, USA) luteal phase support. The patient remained on Keppra® 500 TID (levetiracetam, UCB Pharmacueticals, Brussels, Belgium) and Lactulose throughout the pregnancy. A viable singleton pregnancy was seen on ultrasound 1 month later. The patient delivered a healthy female baby weighing 7lbs 5 oz. at term.

The patient returned two years later desirous of another pregnancy. Her neurological status had been stable, was tumor free and was cleared by her oncologist to conceive again. This time the patient was treated with Estrace® (estradiol, Warner Chilcott, Rockaway, NJ, USA) 6 mg a day and underwent a frozen-thaw cycle with a single day-5 blastocyst transferred. The patient conceived with a viable singleton pregnancy and delivered a healthy male at term weighing 6lbs.

Throughout the patient's treatment regimen for fertility preservation and frozen embryo transfers, no adverse or unanticipated events were encountered.

Discussion and conclusions

Women diagnosed with gliomas during child-bearing years may undergo fertility preservation prior to receiving chemotherapy and radiation to harvest oocytes and freeze them or freeze embryos if they have a partner, since their postoperative treatment, especially chemotherapy, is potentially gonadotoxic and may render them sterile. Studies have shown that the risk of ovarian failure as a result of chemotherapy varies based on both the drugs used as well as the patient's age [10, 11]. Temozolomide (Temodar®, Merck&Co, Inc., Whitehouse Station, NJ, USA) is an alkylating agent, and while the effects of other alkylating agents used for chemotherapy on fertility have been studied, little is published about the gonadotoxicity of temozolomide in females. A handful of small studies have shown that fertility potential is affected in males [12, 13], with one case resulting in fathering a healthy child after treatment with temozolomide [13]. A study from France followed fertility outcomes in two groups of glioma survivors who had received temozolomide categorized based on whether the patient pursued fertility preservation [14]. They observed one spontaneous pregnancy in a woman who did not undergo fertility preservation and three pregnancies – one delivery, one spontaneous miscarriage, and one ongoing pregnancy – in women that underwent fertility preservation (four out of 24 women followed for one to five years). In the absence of more data, we recommend to assume high gonadotoxicity level of temozolomide, and pursuing fertility preservation in such patients following clearance by the neuro-oncologist.

A remaining concern for oncologists and oncologic surgeons is whether fertility preservation delays critical treatment. In cases when the patient receives adjuvant therapy, such as the one presented here, there is typically a sufficient interval between surgery and planned adjuvant therapy (chemotherapy and/or radiation) to allow for a short window of opportunity to freeze eggs or embryos without affecting the cancer treatment timeline at all. In addition, if neoadjuvant therapy is recommended in other cases, recent advances in reproductive technologies allows for fertility preservation to be initiated any time during the menstrual cycle ("random start"). This allows patient to start an ovulation induction cycle on the day she presents to the oncofertility specialist, and it is expected that the cycle will be no more than 2 weeks. Thus, fertility preservation should not delay or alter treatment regimens for cancer patients.

The literature is scarce regarding the possible interactions between gliomas and pregnancy. Changes of the biological behavior of some tumor subtypes may occur during pregnancy, such as an accelerated tumor growth and/or malignant transformation. Several reports have discussed interactions between pregnancy and the growth of gliomas. One study analyzed velocity of diametric expansion (VDE) of WHO grade II gliomas in 11 pregnant women and demonstrated an increase in VDE during pregnancy [4]. Multiple case series have demonstrated cases where woman with WHO grade II gliomas developed de-differentiation of the tumor during pregnancy which became apparent either clinically, radiologically or confirmed histologically by post-delivery surgeries [5–7]. A recent case report revealed a malignant transformation from diffuse astrocytoma (WHO grade II) to glioblastoma (WHO grade IV) in a post-partum patient 1 month following the patient's delivery [8].

The mechanism by which tumor growth is enhanced during pregnancy stems from the idea that the large amount of hormones and growth factors excreted during pregnancy simultaneously increase tumor growth. Placental growth factor for example, is an angiogenic element necessary for both fetal development and the growth of gliomas [9]. Due to the relative paucity of cases reported, the majority of cases focus on gliomas diagnosed during pregnancy. There are no guidelines for the management of gliomas diagnosed either during or prior to pregnancy. If a woman with a treated glioma desires a pregnancy it is advised to perform very close neurological follow-up with repeat MRI's in addition to obstetrical monitoring.

The use of antiepileptic drugs (AEDs) during the course of pregnancy may be teratogenic and increase the risk of congenital malformations. Levetiracetam (Keppra®) is considered a safe medication for use during pregnancy. The North American AED pregnancy registry published data collected from pregnant women taking Levetiracetam monotheraphy from 1997 to 2011. The relative risk of major malformations was not increased in comparison to women with epilepsy who did not take AEDs while pregnant [15].

To our knowledge this is the first report of successful pregnancies following fertility preservation for AA. This case illustrates the realistic possibility of oocyte or embryo cryo-preservation prior to chemotherapy and radiation with subsequent embryo transfers. A recent article published in Neuro-Oncology [16], describes a study reviewing primary brain tumor patients age 18–45, referred for fertility preservation. Seventy-three percent

accepted referral to a sperm bank (87% men) or a reproductive endocrinologist (56% women). The study concludes that there is significant interest in fertility preservation among these patients, particularly if they had no children [16]. Patients should be informed at the time of tumor diagnosis about the option of preserving their fertility. Proper referral to a reproductive endocrinologist as well as a mental health professional is recommended to help make informed decisions [17].

It is incumbent upon physicians to engage in discussion of the ethical perspectives of fertility preservation in patients with brain tumors. For childless women, the option of post-treatment pregnancy opens a window of hope that may elevate their mood, helping them cope with a potentially fatal diagnosis and difficult treatment. However, the possibility that pregnancy may negatively affect prognosis remains a major concern.

Abbreviations
AA: Anaplastic Astrocytoma; AED: Antiepileptic Drug; FET: Frozen Embryo Transfer; IDH: Isocitrate Dehydrogenase; IVF: In Vitro Fertilization; VDE: Velocity of Diametric Expansion

Authors' contributions
AP and SLB reviewed the entire case and was a major contributor in writing the manuscript. AH was the primary physician on the case and was a major contributor in writing the manuscript. All authors read and approved the final manuscript.

Competing interests
The authors declare that they have no competing interests.

References
1. Burger PC, Green SB. Patient age, histologic features, and length of survival in patients with glioblastoma multiforme. Cancer [Internet]. 1987 [cited 2017 Feb 14];59:1617–25. Available from: http://www.ncbi.nlm.nih.gov/pubmed/3030531
2. Smoll NR, Hamilton B. Incidence and relative survival of anaplastic astrocytomas. Neuro Oncol. [Internet]. 2014 [cited 2017 Feb 14];16:1400–7. Available from: http://www.ncbi.nlm.nih.gov/pubmed/24723565
3. Reuss DE, Mamatjan Y, Schrimpf D, Capper D, Hovestadt V, Kratz A, et al. IDH mutant diffuse and anaplastic astrocytomas have similar age at presentation and little difference in survival: a grading problem for WHO. Acta Neuropathol. [Internet]. 2015 [cited 2017 Feb 14];129:867–73. Available from: http://link.springer.com/10.1007/s00401-015-1438-8
4. Pallud J, Mandonnet E, Deroulers C, Fontaine D, Badoual M, Capelle L, et al. Pregnancy increases the growth rates of World Health Organization grade II gliomas. Ann Neurol. [Internet]. 2010 [cited 2017 Feb 14];67:398–404. Available from: http://doi.wiley.com/10.1002/ana.21888
5. Lynch JC, Gouvêa F, Emmerich JC, Kokinovrachos G, Pereira C, Welling L, et al. Management strategy for brain tumour diagnosed during pregnancy. Br J Neurosurg. [Internet]. 2011 [cited 2017 Feb 14];25:225–30. Available from: http://www.ncbi.nlm.nih.gov/pubmed/20825287
6. Pallud J, Duffau H, Razak RA, Barbarino-Monnier P, Capelle L, Fontaine D, et al. Influence of pregnancy in the behavior of diffuse gliomas: clinical cases of a French glioma study group. J Neurol. [Internet]. 2009 [cited 2017 Feb 14];256:2014–20. Available from: http://link.springer.com/10.1007/s00415-009-5232-1

7. Daras M, Cone C, Peters KB. Tumor progression and transformation of low-grade glial tumors associated with pregnancy. J Neurooncol. [Internet]. 2014 [cited 2017 Feb 14];116:113–7. Available from: http://link.springer.com/10.1007/s11060-013-1261-9

8. Hanada T, Rahayu TU, Yamahata H, Hirano H, Yoshioka T, Arita K. Rapid malignant transformation of low-grade astrocytoma in a pregnant woman. J Obstet Gynaecol Res. [Internet]. 2016 [cited 2017 Feb 14];42:1385–9. Available from: http://doi.wiley.com/10.1111/jog.13072

9. Yust-Katz S, de Groot JF, Liu D, Wu J, Yuan Y, Anderson MD, et al. Pregnancy and glial brain tumors. Neuro Oncol. [Internet]. 2014 [cited 2017 Feb 14];16:1289–94. Available from: https://academic.oup.com/neuro-oncology/article-lookup/doi/10.1093/neuonc/nou019

10. Meirow D, Lewin A, Or R, Rachmilewitz E, Slavin S, Schenker J, et al. Ovarian failure post-chemotherapy in young cancer patients - risk assessment indicate the need for intervention. Am Soc Reprod Med Annu Meet Cincinatti. 1997;68:S218.

11. Meirow D, Nugent D. The effects of radiotherapy and chemotherapy on female reproduction. Hum Reprod Update [Internet]. 2001 [cited 2017 Feb 14];7:535–43. Available from: http://www.ncbi.nlm.nih.gov/pubmed/11727861

12. Strowd RE, Blackwood R, Brown M, Harmon M, Lovato J, Yalcinkaya T, et al. Impact of temozolomide on gonadal function in patients with primary malignant brain tumors. J Oncol Pharm Pract. [Internet]. 2013 [cited 2017 Feb 14];19:321–7. Available from: http://journals.sagepub.com/doi/10.1177/1078155212469243

13. Palmieri C, Brock C, Newlands ES. Maintenance of fertility following treatment with temozolomide for a high grade astrocytoma. J Neurooncol. [Internet]. 2005 [cited 2017 Feb 14];73:185. Available from: http://link.springer.com/10.1007/s11060-004-3577-y

14. Sitbon Sitruk L, Sanson M, Prades M, Lefebvre G, Schubert B, Poirot C. [Unknown gonadotoxicity chemotherapy and preservation of fertility: example of Temozolomide]. Gynecol Obstet Fertil. [Internet]. 2010 [cited 2017 Feb 14];38:660–2. Available from: https://www.ncbi.nlm.nih.gov/pubmed/21030284

15. Hernandez-Diaz S, Smith CR, Shen A, Mittendorf R, Hauser WA, Yerby M, et al. Comparative safety of antiepileptic drugs during pregnancy. Neurology [Internet]. 2012 [cited 2017 Feb 14];78:1692–9. Available from: http://www.ncbi.nlm.nih.gov/pubmed/22551726

16. Stone JB, Kelvin JF, DeAngelis LM. Fertility preservation in primary brain tumor patients. Neuro-Oncology Pract [Internet]. 2017 [cited 2017 Feb 14]; npw005. Available from: https://academic.oup.com/nop/article-lookup/doi/10.1093/nop/npw005

17. Goossens J, Delbaere I, Van Lancker A, Beeckman D, Verhaeghe S, Van Hecke A. Cancer patients' and professional caregivers' needs, preferences and factors associated with receiving and providing fertility-related information: a mixed-methods systematic review. Int J Nurs Stud [Internet]. 2014 [cited 2017 Feb 14];51:300–19. Available from: http://linkinghub.elsevier.com/retrieve/pii/S0020748913001971

19

Modeling treatment-dependent glioma growth including a dormant tumor cell subpopulation

Marvin A. Böttcher[1][†], Janka Held-Feindt[2][†], Michael Synowitz[2], Ralph Lucius[3], Arne Traulsen[1][†] and Kirsten Hattermann[3][*][†]

Abstract

Background: Tumors comprise a variety of specialized cell phenotypes adapted to different ecological niches that massively influence the tumor growth and its response to treatment.

Methods: In the background of *glioblastoma multiforme*, a highly malignant brain tumor, we consider a rapid *proliferating* phenotype that appears susceptible to treatment, and a *dormant* phenotype which lacks this pronounced proliferative ability and is not affected by standard therapeutic strategies. To gain insight in the dynamically changing proportions of different tumor cell phenotypes under different treatment conditions, we develop a mathematical model and underline our assumptions with experimental data.

Results: We show that both cell phenotypes contribute to the distinct composition of the tumor, especially in cycling low and high dose treatment, and therefore may influence the tumor growth in a phenotype specific way.

Conclusion: Our model of the dynamic proportions of dormant and rapidly growing glioblastoma cells in different therapy settings suggests that phenotypically different cells should be considered to plan dose and duration of treatment schedules.

Keywords: Evolutionary game theory, Glioma, Dormancy

Background

Gliomas are the most common type of primary brain tumors including their highly malignant form, the *glioblastoma multiforme* (GBM), which accounts for about 15% of all brain tumors [1]. Despite current standard treatment of GBM by surgical resection and adjuvant radio- and chemotherapy, the median survival time for GBM patients is still poor, approximating 12–15 months [2], mostly due to unsatisfactory response of the tumor to treatment strategies. Additionally, combined aggressive radio–/chemotherapy is causing severe side effects frequently necessitating interruptions of the therapy due to e.g. blood toxicity [3]. GBMs and also many other tumors are heterogeneous tumors, being composed of cells with different, partly specialized phenotypes [4]. Besides

e.g. rapidly proliferating tumors cells, invading immune cells, endothelial cells and (tumor) stem cells, also a subpopulation of so called *dormant* tumor cells exists in the heterogeneous tumor mass. These cells enter a quiescent state driven by cell-intrinsic or extrinsic factors, including permanent competition for nutrients, oxygen, and space ("cellular dormancy") [5–8]. In several tumors and metastases, dormant cells have been shown to be not proliferative or only very slowly cycling [9–12]. Linking dormancy and effects of chemotherapy, studies on glioma cells showed that cells underwent a prolonged cell cycle arrest upon treatment with temozolomide (TMZ), the most common chemotherapeutic in GBM therapy [13].

Evolutionary forces, such as competition and selection, shape the growth of the tumor and therefore the progression of the cancer. These forces create different ecological niches within the tumor encouraging the adaption of specialized tumor cell phenotypes. Accordingly, the proportional balance between different tumor cellular phenotypes can drastically change with treatment conditions. Indeed,

* Correspondence: k.hattermann@anat.uni-kiel.de

Marvin A. Böttcher and Janka Held-Feindt shared first authorship.
Arne Traulsen and Kirsten Hattermann shared senior authorship.
[†]Equal contributors
[3]Department of Anatomy, University of Kiel, 24098 Kiel, Germany
Full list of author information is available at the end of the article

compared to rapidly proliferating tumor cells, especially dormant cells exhibit a much higher robustness against chemotherapeutic drugs [5]. This dormant state seems to be reversible [13], so that the conversion to dormancy and the exit from dormancy may be a mechanism that facilitates tumor survival and progression even upon adverse or changing conditions. Hence, a better understanding of the proportional dynamics of different cell phenotypes within gliomas under chemotherapeutic treatment may improve further therapeutic approaches.

Mathematical models are beneficial resources to gain insight into key mechanisms of cancer development, growth, and evolution and to help identifying potential therapeutic targets [14]. Among these approaches, evolutionary game theory [15, 16] models the interactions between different individuals as a game between agents playing different strategies and relates the payoff from this game to the reproductive fitness of the corresponding agent [17–21].

Here, we use evolutionary game theory to model the proportions of two different phenotypes of GBM cells in a variety of different treatment conditions, see Basanta and Deutsch [18] for a related approach in GBM. Defining the fitness of the different cell types as growth rate in comparison to cells of the respective other phenotype, we focus especially on the balance between the rapidly proliferating and the cellular dormant phenotype and describe the corresponding payoffs in a payoff matrix which also includes the effect of treatment. Then, we use a special form of the replicator-mutator equation [22, 23], which takes into account that conversion from dormant to rapidly proliferating phenotype and *vice versa* is possible. To strengthen our theoretical assumptions, we analyzed cell numbers and the cellular expression of a dormancy marker under different chemotherapy dosages and the phenotypic conversion modalities in cultured GBM cells in vitro. Taken together, the aim of our study was to develop a simple theoretical model which describes the dynamically changing proportions of two different GBM cell phenotypes, rapidly proliferating and dormant cells, under different treatment conditions. Showing this, we suggest that different properties of cell phenotypes should be taken into account for the development of more efficient, less toxic treatment schedules in order to improve patient's prognosis and quality of life.

Methods
Theoretical model
We analyze the proportions of two different GBM cell phenotypes, dormant (D, please refer to Table 1 for symbols used in the equations) and rapidly proliferating (P) cells, in a mathematical model including the influence of different

Table 1 Overview of all used symbols in the model

n_X	number of cells of type X
x_X	ratio of cells of type X in population
D, P	index for dormant or rapidly proliferating cell type, respectively
ε	Fitness of dormant (D) cells
λ	treatment cost on normally growing cells
σ	probability for spontaneous conversion between types
$\bar{f}$	total average fitness of all cell types in the population

treatment conditions. In the following, we characterize the cells in terms of their fitness, which we define as the growth rate in comparison to cells of the other phenotype. Dormant cells always have a very low or even zero growth rate ε, which we assume to be independent of the exact composition of the population and the treatment condition. Rapidly proliferating P cells, on the other hand, have a very large fitness advantage compared to dormant cells, which means they proliferate much faster, but they also compete with each other for space and resources. Facing another P cell, a focal P cell has an intermediate fitness, which we assume to be still much larger than the growth rate of D cells ε. Their fitness therefore depends on the relative fraction of D vs. P cells. Due to the very slow growth of D cells, P cells will represent the vast majority of glioblastoma cells in the absence of treatment.

Under treatment conditions, however, the population composition changes. Even though D cells still have the same very low (or zero) growth rate ε, P cells experience a fitness cost λ due to treatment. The reduction of the fitness due to treatment only applies to P cells, because cytotoxic drugs mostly affect rapidly dividing cells. The fitness cost parameter λ can be adjusted to account for the strength of the applied treatment. In principle we can continuously vary this parameter. However, for simplicity we focus on two different treatment strategies: In high dosage (HD) chemotherapy the treatment strength parameter λ is large compared to the growth rate of the P type. Since high dosage chemotherapy has strong side effects for the whole organism (for GBM: [3]), in reality this treatment strategy cannot be maintained for extended time periods. Therefore, strong treatment needs to be applied in turns with weaker or no treatment. For low dosage (LD) chemotherapy, λ means only a small reduction of the growth rate of the P cells. As the side-effect stress to the organism should also be lower, this treatment regime could be applied for longer time spans.

Dormant (D) and rapidly proliferating (P) phenotypes in glioblastoma and their aforementioned interactions can be described by the following payoff matrix [18]:

$$
\begin{array}{c}
\begin{array}{cc} & \hspace{-1.2em}\text{D} \hspace{3em} \text{P} \end{array}\\[-0.3em]
\begin{array}{c}\text{D}\\\text{P}\end{array}
\left(
\begin{array}{cc}
\varepsilon & \varepsilon \\
1{-}\varepsilon{-}\lambda & \dfrac{1}{2}{-}\lambda
\end{array}
\right)
\end{array}
$$

This matrix gives the fitness for each type if confronted with any of the two other types. Here, we find for example that the fitness of a focal P cell interacting with a D cell is $1 - \varepsilon - \lambda$, which includes both the small or zero growth rate of D cells ε and the fitness cost for P cells under treatment λ.

As the phenomenon of dormancy is presumably a reversible process that also occurs without any treatment, we assume that conversion between both phenotypes is possible with a small rate σ. Thus, P cells may enter a dormant phenotype, and D cells may exit from their quiescent state, converting into a P phenotype at any time point.

In the following, we include these fitness effects and phenotypic conversion into a set of ordinary differential equations. In general, the growth of a whole cell population can be explained in terms of a differential equation that describes the change in the number of individuals over time

$$
\frac{dn}{dt} = r(n,t)n\,.
$$

Here n is the number of individuals, t is the time and $r(n,t)$ is the growth rate, which can itself depend on the number of cells and the time.

At first, we focus on the number of D cells, n_D, in the population over time, which have a very small but constant growth rate ε

$$
\frac{dn_D}{dt} = \varepsilon\, n_D\,.
$$

For P cells on the other hand, the growth rate of n_P, given by the average fitness from the payoff matrix (weighted to the cell fractions), changes with the composition of the population

$$
\frac{dn_P}{dt} = n_P\left((1{-}\varepsilon{-}\lambda)\frac{n_D}{n_D+n_P} + \left(\frac{1}{2}{-}\lambda\right)\frac{n_P}{n_D+n_P}\right)\,.
$$

Since the system under consideration is constrained, both in terms of nutrients and space, in reality the cell population only grows exponentially as indicated by the growth equations in the very beginning of the process where the constraints regarding space or nutrients are negligible. However, we are mainly interested in the fraction of D cells $x_D = \frac{n_D}{n_D+n_P}$ in the population and vice versa the fraction of P cells $x_P = 1{-}x_D = \frac{n_P}{n_D+n_P}$. To obtain the change in fractions for both types, we subtract the average growth rate $\bar{f}$ of the population from both individual growth rates,

$$
\bar{f} = \varepsilon x_D + \left[(1{-}\varepsilon{-}\lambda)x_D + \left(\frac{1}{2}{-}\lambda\right)x_P\right]x_P
$$

From this we obtain two differential equations for the fractions of D and P cells,

$$
\dot{x}_D = x_D\left(\varepsilon{-}\bar{f}\right)
$$

$$
\dot{x}_P = x_P\left(\left[(1{-}\varepsilon{-}\lambda)x_D + \left(\frac{1}{2}{-}\lambda\right)x_P\right]{-}\bar{f}\right)
$$

Next, we include the spontaneous conversion between phenotypes with a constant rate σ, which is independent of the cellular growth. This leads to an additional term to the differential equation of both phenotypes

$$
\dot{x}_D = \left[\varepsilon{-}\bar{f}\right]x_D + \sigma(x_P{-}x_D)
$$

$$
\dot{x}_P = \left[(1{-}\varepsilon{-}\lambda)x_D + \left(\frac{1}{2}{-}\lambda\right)x_P{-}\bar{f}\right]x_P + \sigma(x_D{-}x_P)
$$

$$\tag{1}$$

These equations have the important difference to the usual replicator-mutator equation [15] that phenotype conversion is a spontaneous process with a constant rate and is independent of the growth in the population. This allows conversion from D to P even if D cells do not grow at all.

Using these equations, we model different therapy schedules combining different treatment strengths in different cycling time plans. Since the equations are non-linear, we use numerical integration with *Odeint* of the Python library Scipy[1] to examine the temporal dynamics of the system under different treatment regimes. Additionally we analytically determine the fixed points of the system and their stability.

Experimental model
Cell culture and cell number determination
The GBM cell line LN229 was purchased from ATCC/LGC Standards (Middlesex, UK, ATCC-CRL 2611) and cultured in Dulbecco's modified eagle medium (DMEM) plus 10% fetal calf serum (FCS, PAN Biotech, Aidenbach, Germany). *Mycoplasma* contaminations were routinely excluded by bisbenzimide staining. The GBM cell line identity was proven routinely by STR (Short Tandem Repeat) profiling at the Department of Forensic Medicine (Kiel, Germany) using the Powerplex HS Genotyping Kit (Promega, Madison, WC). Briefly, DNA was amplified with a STR multiplex PCR, electrophoretic separation was performed with the 3500 Genetic Analyser (Thermo Fisher Scientific, Waltham, MA, USA), and evaluated using the Software GeneMapper ID-X (Thermo Fisher Scientific). For determination of cell numbers after low and high dose chemotherapy treatment, 25,000 cells/well

were seeded in 6 well plates (Greiner Bio-one, Fricken-hausen, Germany). Cells were grown for 24 h, then washed with phosphate buffered saline (PBS), supplemented with fresh DMEM + 10% FCS and temozolomide concentrations (Sigma-Aldrich, St. Louis, MO, USA; dissolved in dimethyl sulfoxide DMSO) as indicated in Fig. 2a (5, 50 or 100 µg/ml for 10 days). Temozolomide (TMZ) is a DNA alkylating drug causing apoptotic cell death and the most commonly used chemotherapeutic in GBM therapy. Control cells were supplemented with 0.5% DMSO, which corresponds to the solvent concentrations of each TMZ stimulated sample. Cells were stimulated for 10 days with TMZ, while media were changed every 2–3 days. After 10 days, cells were detached by trypsination and total cell numbers per well counted using trypan blue exclusion and a Neubauer chamber (Brand, Wertheim, Germany). DMSO stimulated control cells were already detached after 6 days of stimulation, split 1:10 and seeded again to exclude limitations of growth due to space and nutrient limitations. This splitting factor (1:10) was considered when relative cell numbers of TMZ treated samples in comparison to DMSO controls were determined for n = 5–6 independent experiments.

Immunocytochemistry

For immunocytochemistry, 50,000 cells were seeded onto poly-D-lysine coated glass cover slips, grown for 24 h and supplemented with indicated TMZ or DMSO concentrations as described above. From day 6, growth media were additionally supplemented with 10 µM 5-bromo-2´-deoxyuridine (BrdU, Sigma-Aldrich, St. Louis, MO) to allow for incorporation in the DNA in the S phase of the cell cycle. After 10 days, cover slips were fixed with an ice-cold mixture of methanol and acetone (1:1) for 10 min, rinsed with 0.1% Tween / PBS (3 × 5 min), incubated with 1 M HCl for 30 min, neutralized with 0.1 M sodium borate buffer (pH 8.5), and rinsed again with 0.1% Tween/PBS. Afterwards, cells were blocked for unspecific bindings with 0.5% bovine serum albumin (BSA) / 0.5% glycine in PBS (1 h) and incubated over night with the primary antibody against H2BK (1:300, Biorbyt, Cambridge, UK), a marker of glioma dormancy [24, 25] and the primary antibody against BrdU (1:200, Abcam, Cambridge, UK). Then cover slips were incubated with the secondary antibodies (donkey anti-rabbit IgG, labelled with Alexa Fluor 488, and donkey anti-sheep labelled with Alexa Fluor 555, both Invitrogen, Carlsbad, CA, USA) for 1 h at 37°, and 4´, 6-diamidino-2-phenylindole (DAPI; Sigma Aldrich, St. Louis, MO, USA; 1 mg/ml, 1:30,000, 30 min at room temperature) to stain nuclei. Cover slips were embedded using Immu-Mount (Thermo Fisher Scientific, Rockford, IL, USA), and analysed with equal exposure times using an Axiovert

microscope and digital camera (Zeiss, Jena, Germany). H2BK-immunopositive, BrdU-positive and double positive cells were counted and normalized to total cell numbers in 6 (DMSO controls) to 10 (TMZ samples) fields of view for n = 4 independent experiments.

DiO retention and cell countings on phenotype conversion

To monitor the conversion to and from dormancy we used the green fluorescent vital dye DiO (Invitrogen), as rapidly proliferating cells lose the dye due to repeated divisions, while resting, dormant (or very slowly cycling) cells retain the dye and can be detected by fluorescence microscopy. Investigating the conversion to dormancy, 150,000 LN229 cells were seeded into 6-well-plates, stained with Vybrant® DiO Cell-Labeling Solution (Thermo Fisher Scientific, Waltham, MA, USA) following the manufacturer's instructions and stimulated with 100 µg/ml TMZ (or equal volume of the solvent DMSO) for 10–12 days. Cells were photographed combining transmitted-light microscopy and fluorescence microscopy with equal exposure times for TMZ and control treated cells, and green fluorescent cell portions were determined in comparison to total cell counts. To determine the influence of different cell densities on the incidence of conversion, 50,000 and 150,000 cells were seeded, respectively, into 6-well-plates and treated with 100 µg/ml TMZ (or equal volumes of the solvent DMSO) for 10 days. As the DMSO control treated cells rapidly proliferate, cells were detached at day 6 (50,000) or day 3 and 6 (150,000), cell numbers counted using a Neubauer chamber to determine the growth rate over this time period, and seeded again at initial density, to allow for cell growth without limitation of space and nutrients. After 10 days, TMZ and control treated cells were detached and counted. To extrapolate the total cell numbers of control cells, growth rates determined at day 3, 6 and 10 were used, and TMZ surviving cells were calculated as percentage of extrapolated total cells.

Statistical analysis

Statistical analysis and graphical presentation of experimental data were performed with Graph Pad Prism using a two-tailed t-test (*** $p < 0.001$).

Results

Modelling the dynamics of cell frequencies

The temporal dynamics of the proportion of D against P cells in GBM strongly depends on the treatment conditions. Therefore, we first analyze the fixed points of the dynamical system and how they change for different treatment strengths λ, without considering possible conversions of phenotypes. The fixed points mark a stable equilibrium between the portions of P and D cells under certain, predefined conditions and are found by setting Eq. 1 to zero. Of particular interest are *stable* fixed points, as the system returns into this state again after a small perturbation [26].

For our system, there is only one stable fixed point for each treatment condition (Fig. 1a). If we consider the case of no phenotype conversion, $\sigma = 0$, we can give the exact position of this point for each treatment condition λ. The fraction of D cells at the fixed point is then given by

$$
x_D = \begin{cases} 0 & \dfrac{2\lambda}{1-2\varepsilon} \leq 1 \\[2ex] \dfrac{2\lambda}{1-2\varepsilon} - 1 & 1 \leq \dfrac{2\lambda}{1-2\varepsilon} \leq 2 \\[2ex] 1 & 2 \leq \dfrac{2\lambda}{1-2\varepsilon} \end{cases}
$$

For small treatment strengths λ the fraction of D cells in the population at the stable fixed point is zero, but after reaching a threshold, the fraction of dormant cells increases linearly with λ until the whole population consists of dormant cells at very high treatment strengths.

With conversion between the two phenotypes ($\sigma > 0$), the analytical calculation for the stable fixed points is more difficult and the result is not instructive. By contrast to the previous results without phenotype conversion, there is always a small proportion of dormant cells in the population, even at very low treatment strengths. The proportion of dormant cells at the fixed points increases immediately with increasing treatment strength until it approaches a maximum at high treatment strengths. For both D cell growth rates ε ($\varepsilon = 0$, orange lines; and $\varepsilon = 0.1$, blue lines) the population composition is very similar or even the same without phenotype conversion at very small or large treatment strengths λ. In contrast, the largest effect of ε on the population composition is at intermediate values of treatment strength.

The average fitness $\bar{f}$ for the whole tumor cell population including P and D cells decreases linearly from the maximum at treatment strength $\lambda = 0$ until it reaches the minimum of $\bar{f} = \varepsilon$ at the point where the fraction of dormant cells in the population starts to increase (Fig. 1b). Interestingly, with spontaneous conversion $\sigma > 0$, the average fitness at the fixed point can become smaller than ε and even negative for high treatment strengths, potentially leading to a shrinking tumor. This is caused by conversion of D cells into P cells which are then susceptible to treatment.

Comparison to experimental data

To test our mathematical model of phenotype composition upon treatment, we used LN229 cells as an experimental in vitro model. We treated these cells for 10 days with temozolomide (TMZ), the most commonly used cytotoxic drug in glioma therapy. In a first step, we focused on different treatment strength and analysed the portions of surviving cells in comparison to control cultures and the percentage of cells expressing H2BK (histone cluster 1), a marker of glioma dormancy [24, 25], alongside with incorporation of BrdU in the late treatment phase (day 6–10). In general, after 10 days of treatment, samples stimulated with 5, 50 and 100 µg/ml TMZ had significantly less total cell numbers than control treated cells (Fig. 2a). By immunocytochemistry of H2BK, we could detect and quantify the fraction of dormant cells within the cultures, and by adding BrdU to the cells from day 6 of treatment and immunocytochemical staining of BrdU, we could in parallel mark cells that incorporate BrdU in the DNA (examples of microscopic pictures in Fig. 2b). While DMSO-treated control cells showed a low fraction of H2BK-positive cells (mean: 9.7% ± 3.5), TMZ treatment yielded increased numbers of dormant cells reaching a plateau at high concentrations (5 µg/ml: mean 26.8% ± 9.0, 50 µg/ml: mean: 82.8% ± 5.3, 100 µg/ml: 87.7% ± 8.0, compare Fig. 2b, grey graph portions). In parallel, we investigated the incorporation of

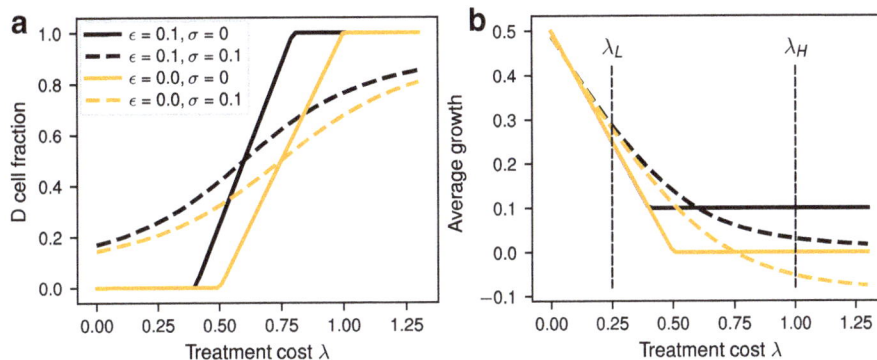

Fig. 1 a Equilibrium fraction of dormant cells depending on treatment cost λ. **b** Average growth rate at the fixed point depending on treatment cost λ. Blue lines indicate a growth rate of D cells of $\varepsilon = 0$ and orange lines a growth rate $\varepsilon = 0.1$. Solid lines are for the absence of phenotype conversion ($\sigma = 0$) and dashed lines with phenotype conversion ($\sigma = 0.1$)

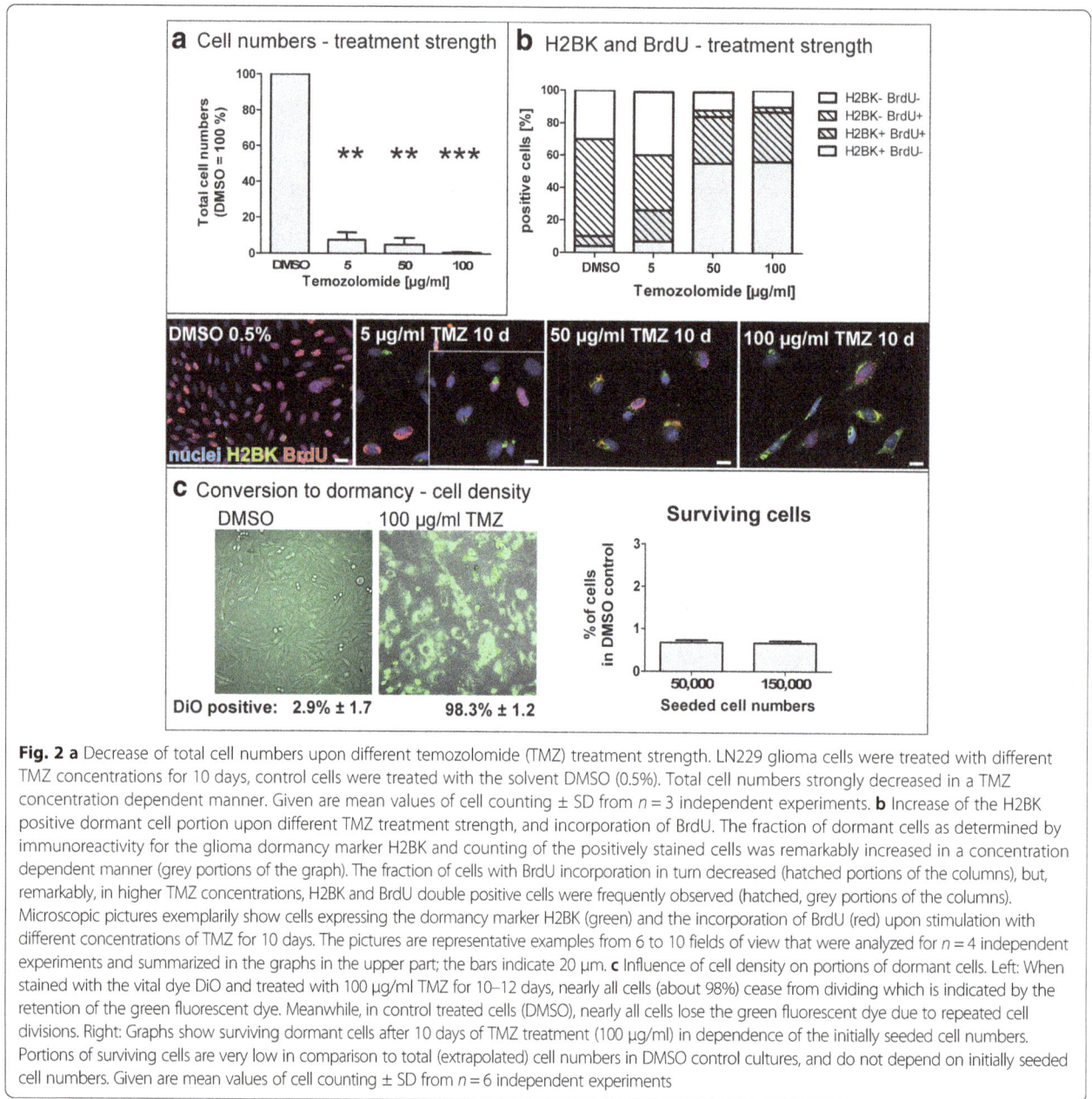

Fig. 2 a Decrease of total cell numbers upon different temozolomide (TMZ) treatment strength. LN229 glioma cells were treated with different TMZ concentrations for 10 days, control cells were treated with the solvent DMSO (0.5%). Total cell numbers strongly decreased in a TMZ concentration dependent manner. Given are mean values of cell counting ± SD from $n = 3$ independent experiments. **b** Increase of the H2BK positive dormant cell portion upon different TMZ treatment strength, and incorporation of BrdU. The fraction of dormant cells as determined by immunoreactivity for the glioma dormancy marker H2BK and counting of the positively stained cells was remarkably increased in a concentration dependent manner (grey portions of the graph). The fraction of cells with BrdU incorporation in turn decreased (hatched portions of the columns), but, remarkably, in higher TMZ concentrations, H2BK and BrdU double positive cells were frequently observed (hatched, grey portions of the columns). Microscopic pictures exemplarily show cells expressing the dormancy marker H2BK (green) and the incorporation of BrdU (red) upon stimulation with different concentrations of TMZ for 10 days. The pictures are representative examples from 6 to 10 fields of view that were analyzed for $n = 4$ independent experiments and summarized in the graphs in the upper part; the bars indicate 20 μm. **c** Influence of cell density on portions of dormant cells. Left: When stained with the vital dye DiO and treated with 100 μg/ml TMZ for 10–12 days, nearly all cells (about 98%) cease from dividing which is indicated by the retention of the green fluorescent dye. Meanwhile, in control treated cells (DMSO), nearly all cells lose the green fluorescent dye due to repeated cell divisions. Right: Graphs show surviving dormant cells after 10 days of TMZ treatment (100 μg/ml) in dependence of the initially seeded cell numbers. Portions of surviving cells are very low in comparison to total (extrapolated) cell numbers in DMSO control cultures, and do not depend on initially seeded cell numbers. Given are mean values of cell counting ± SD from $n = 6$ independent experiments

BrdU in the DNA and determined a high portion (66.0% ± 7.8) of BrdU positive cells in the control cultures and lower portions upon TMZ treatment (5 μg/ml: 53.6% ± 14.5; 50 μg/ml: 33.4% ± 5.3; 100 μg/ml: 33.7% ± 10.1, compare Fig. 2b, hatched graph portions). Interestingly, BrdU incorporation also took place in TMZ treated cultures, so that staining for the dormancy marker H2BK and for BrdU could be observed in the very same cells (compare examples of microscopic photographs in Fig. 2b) indicating that cell cycle arrest may occur after the S phase of the cell cycle. Together with our experiments described in the following section and Fig. 2c, showing that dormant cells hardly divide within our

experimental time frame, these observations suggest that dormant glioma cells are not or only very slowly cycling. Furthermore, taking into account that we use a clonal cell line, the occurrence of dormant cells needs to be a phenotypic adaption to the environmental conditions as all cells are genetically homogenous (as proven by routinely STR profiling, compare Materials and Methods section).

To investigate if the conversion to a dormant phenotype depended on the cell density, initially, we determined in a DiO retention assay that nearly all cells (98.3% ± 1.2) retain the green fluorescent dye when treated with 100 μg/ml ("high dose") TMZ for 10–12 days, while in control cultures (treated with equal volumes of the solvent DMSO) only 2.9% ± 1.7 retained the dye (Fig. 2c, left part). The vital dye is included in every cell at the moment of staining, and is transferred to every daughter cell upon cell division. However, this means the staining is diminishing after several divisions of rapidly proliferating cells, but retained in non-proliferative or very slowly cycling dormant cells. Thus, assuming that nearly all cells that survive treatment with 100 μg/ml TMZ are dormant in our particular setting, we determined the relative incidence of phenotype conversion and the influence of the cell density on this conversion factor by determination of TMZ surviving cells in relation to (extrapolated) total cell numbers of control (DMSO treated) cultures. In our experimental setting, a portion of 0.68% ± 0.13 cells of initially seeded 50,000 LN229 glioblastoma cells survived this high dose treatment, while in cultures of initially seeded 150,000 cells, the portion of surviving cells was nearly similar (0.66% ± 0. 13; Fig. 2c, right part) underlining the assumptions of our theoretical model.

Thus, treatment with TMZ significantly reduced total cell numbers of LN229 cells, while the share of dormant cells within the culture, as detected by the dormancy marker H2BK, was drastically elevated. The incidence of conversion to dormancy did not depend on cell densities in our particular experimental setting.

Treatment schedules

Next, we use our model to analyze the dynamics of the population composition for periodically changing treatment conditions. One example trajectory for a growth rate for D cells $\varepsilon = 0$ and a conversion rate between phenotypes $\sigma = 0.1$ is depicted in Fig. 3. The fraction of D and P cells in the population alternates between the fixed points corresponding to the momentary treatment condition. The trajectory starts with a phase of no treatment, which is characterized by a high average growth rate and a cell population composition of mostly P cells and only very few D cells. After the first phase of unconstrained growth large parts of the tumor are removed (e.g. by surgery), leaving only a small number of cancer cells. Under the following high dosage treatment conditions, the dormant phenotype has the highest fitness and takes over the population. The relative fraction of D cells will increase until the steady state under high treatment conditions is reached. The impact of treatment on P cells leads to a strong initial decline in average growth rate, until the population has a significant proportion of dormant cells and the growth rate starts to recover slightly.

Under the following low dosage treatment conditions, P cells (making up a small fraction of the whole population at the end of the high dosage treatment) are less affected by the treatment and now grow faster. The average growth rate will have a maximum when then

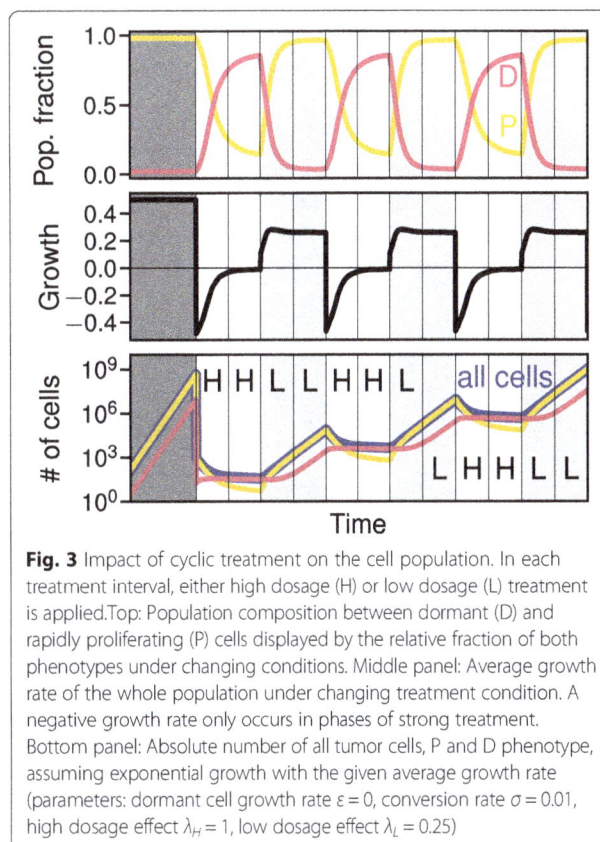

Fig. 3 Impact of cyclic treatment on the cell population. In each treatment interval, either high dosage (H) or low dosage (L) treatment is applied. Top: Population composition between dormant (D) and rapidly proliferating (P) cells displayed by the relative fraction of both phenotypes under changing conditions. Middle panel: Average growth rate of the whole population under changing treatment condition. A negative growth rate only occurs in phases of strong treatment. Bottom panel: Absolute number of all tumor cells, P and D phenotype, assuming exponential growth with the given average growth rate (parameters: dormant cell growth rate $\varepsilon = 0$, conversion rate $\sigma = 0.01$, high dosage effect $\lambda_H = 1$, low dosage effect $\lambda_L = 0.25$)

relative fraction of P cells in the population is still low, since they have a competitive advantage over D cells, and then declines afterwards towards an equilibrium well above the high dosage growth rate. Accordingly, the total number of cells increases strongly again in this regime.

Switching the order of high dosage and low dosage treatment only has a small effect on total number of cells: If treatment starts with low dosage, the system will go into a state with a slightly higher fraction of dormant cells, which makes it less susceptible to the following high dosage treatment. Starting with low dosage therefore does not help to reduce the tumor size.

In Fig. 4 we compare three different treatment schedules: just one switch from initial high (H) dose to low (L) dose treatment (HHHHHHLLLLLL, Fig. 4a, each instance of the letter H or L corresponds to the same time interval), slow cyclic switching (HHHLLL, Fig. 4b), and fast cyclic switching (HLHL, Fig. 4c) for two different growth rates of D cells (left panels $\varepsilon = 0$ and right panels $\varepsilon = 0.1$). In case of only switching once, the fixed points for each treatment are quickly reached. At high dosage treatment the number of cells increases very slowly or even decreases. In the following low treatment phase, however, P cells take over growing particularly fast and jeopardizing any positive effect from the previous strong

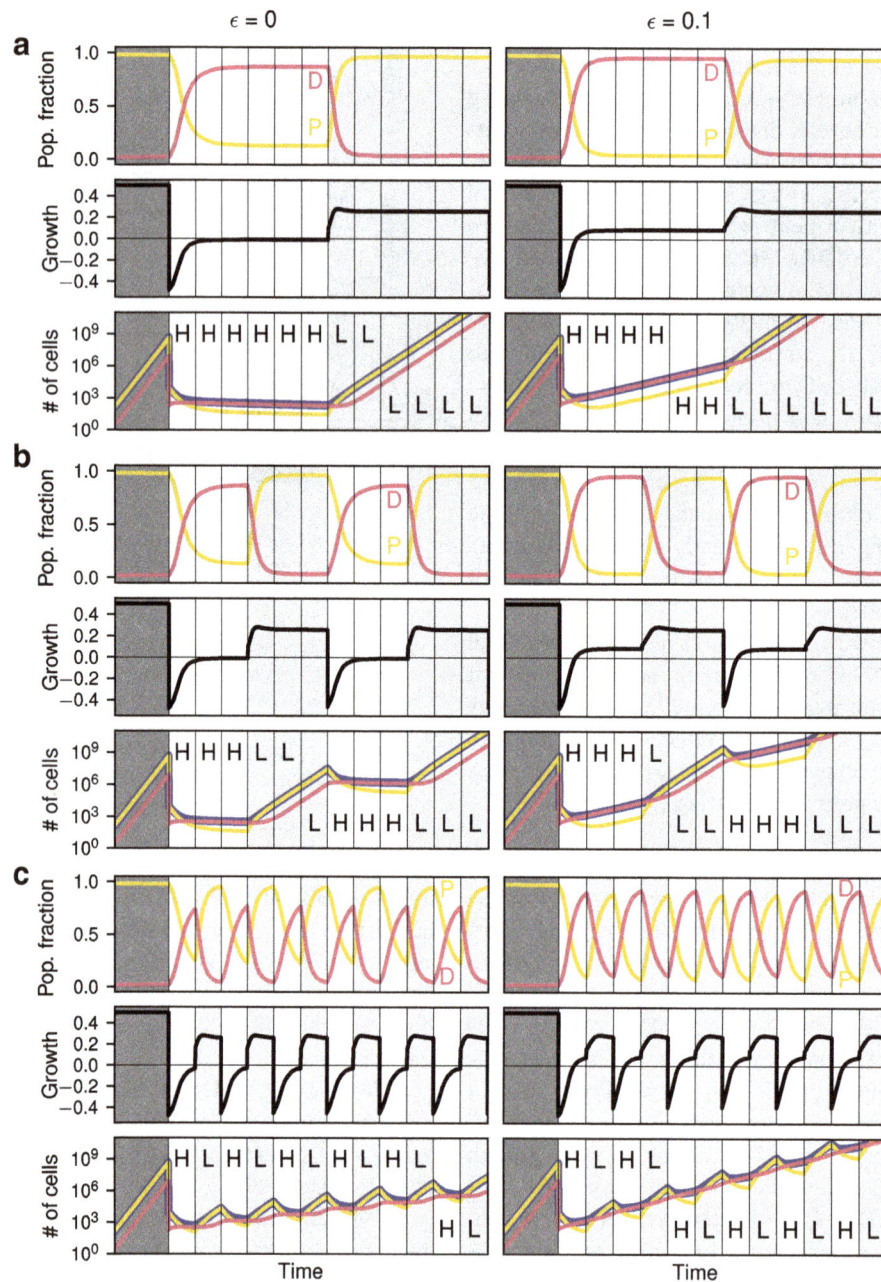

Fig. 4 Comparison of the effect of different treatment cycle lengths on population composition, average growth rate and number of cells, similarly to Fig. 3. All panels on the left have a D cell growth rate of $\varepsilon = 0$, whereas all panels on the right have $\varepsilon = 0.1$. **a** The top row shows the case of high dosage treatment followed by a sustained low dosage treatment. **b** The middle panels use a relatively slow switching between high dosage and low dosage treatment, whereas the bottom panel **c** shows very fast switching. All other parameters as in Fig. 3

treatment. This is true for both treatment strengths of the high dosage phase.

For the fast switching treatment schedule (HLHL, Fig. 4c), the fixed point of the population proportion is not reached before the treatment changes again. Therefore the population dynamics stays between the two stable fixed points for the two treatment regimes, but does not reach them. By contrast, in the slow treatment switching

regime (HHHLLL, Fig. 4b) the fixed points for both high and low dosage treatment are reached such that the composition of the cell population essentially resembles the case of just one switching event (Fig. 4a). However the time spent at these fixed points is still significantly reduced compared to only a single switch.

The bottom panels of Fig. 4a, b and c show the total number of cells based on the average fitness of the population under the assumption of exponential growth. When the growth rate is positive the cell population grows, otherwise it shrinks. Interestingly, the average growth rate of the population is well below zero only for a short period during the high dosage treatment and only if the share of P cells is still very high and the fraction of D cells in the population is small. However, in this regime the fitness recovers fast and approaches equilibrium with an average fitness close to zero, such that the total number of cells does not change anymore. The strongly negative growth rate directly after switching to the high dosage treatment is therefore the reason why the number of cells for quickly changing treatment regimes is significantly smaller than for slowly changing treatment cases.

Population growth

To systematically examine the effect of switching treatment cycles on the growth rate of the population, we analyze the temporal dynamics of the population size for varying treatment cycle durations and two different growth rates of D cells ε (Fig. 5). Unsurprisingly, a lower growth rate of D cells has a diminishing effect on the overall growth of the cells. For increasing treatment cycle length cancer cells have an increasing overall growth, while maintaining the same total high and low dosage treatment durations. The overall growth rate approaches a maximum with increasing treatment cycle length when the dynamics reaches equilibrium in each cycle.

Taken together, our mathematical model allows us to theoretically predict the fitness and proportions of rapidly proliferating and dormant tumor cells under different treatment conditions. Strengthening our theoretical assumptions we could exemplarily show the effect of high and low chemotherapy doses on the cell numbers and the proportion of a dormant cell phenotype in cultured GBM cells in vitro. Simulating different therapy

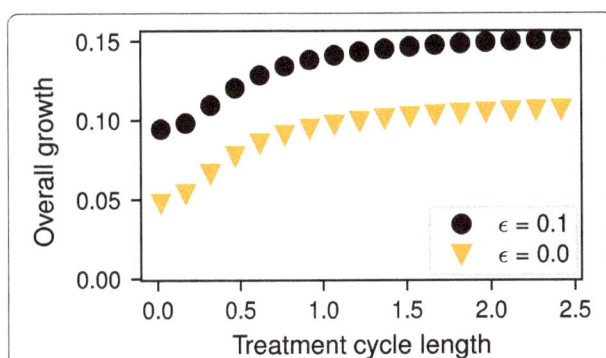

Fig. 5 Overall growth rate for different treatment cycle length and for two different growth rates of dormant cells $\varepsilon = 0$ and $\varepsilon = 0.1$. High and low dosage phases are alternating with the given treatment cycle length for in total 30 cycles. The overall growth rate is then calculated from a linear fit to the log-plot. Other parameters as in Figs. 3 and 4

schedules, we observed that fast switching of low and high treatment doses yields a lower total tumor cell number at equal total drug dose in comparison to low switching schedules.

Discussion

In this study, we established a mathematical model and analyzed the proportions of two different cell phenotypes occurring in GBM, rapidly proliferating and dormant cells. Corroborated by experimental data obtained from in vitro experiments with cultured GBM cells, we observed that treatment strength influences the balance between both phenotypes which in turn influences the growth of the whole tumor population. Sequential switching of treatment strength may thus drastically influence the proportion of dormant and rapidly proliferating cells, especially if switching to the next condition takes place before the population dynamics reaches a steady state.

Dormancy in GBM has been shown by the existence of distinct fraction of temporarily non-proliferative cells in murine models [27], as well as by the identification of clones which were able to generate indolent dormant tumors both in subcutaneous and orthotropic intracranial sites [28]. Additionally, dormancy seems to be characterized by specific features in GBM, such as a non-angiogenic phenotype [24, 28, 29], and is influenced by the (micro-)environment e.g. hypoxia [30] and coagulation [31–33]. However, cellular dormancy in tumors is not only regarded as a state to overcome times of adverse conditions but has also been assigned to DNA repair mechanisms [34]. Interestingly, dormant GBM cells are hallmarked by the upregulation of specific genes like angiomotin, ephrin type-A receptor 5 (EphA5), insulin-like growth factor-binding protein 5 (IGFBP5), and histone cluster 1 (H2BK) [24, 25]. We used the latter as a marker to detect dormant cells in our in vitro experiments and show that the proportion of dormant cells increases with increasing chemotherapy concentrations.

As the fitness in the competition for space and resources depends on the proportions of phenotypically different cell subpopulations, we used evolutionary game theory as a framework for our mathematical model. Previous studies discussed game theoretic interactions with more phenotypes for many different types of cancer, including glioma [35], prostate cancer [36], and multiple myeloma [19, 37] or general tumors [38]. Also, evolutionary game theory is often used in spatially structured populations to answer questions about the effect of environmental constraints on tumor composition and invasiveness of cancer cells [20, 39, 40]. However, including spatial structure in order to increase the realism of the model leads to a large number of additional assumptions and potential pitfalls [41, 42]. Other modeling approaches for dormancy in cancer focus on the interaction between the immune system and the tumor [43–45], the effect of angiogenesis [46], or spatial competition between cells [47]. However, these approaches do not explicitly model the conversion between phenotypes and its consequences under therapy with varying strength.

Thus, we decided to simplify our model on several levels: (i) We do not take spatial structure into account. (ii) We abstract from the interaction with the immune system. (iii) We concentrate on two tumor cell phenotypes – rapidly proliferating and dormant cells – although other cell phenotypes, such as fast migrating cells, cells mimicking vasculature, (cancer) stem cells and invading immune cells (e.g. [48–50]), also contribute to the whole tumor mass. (iv) We focus on the fitness of the respective phenotypes rather than the potentially underlying reasons for phenotypical changes (e.g. genetic or epigenetic changes).

An important aspect of our model is the conversion between the different cell phenotypes. Recent studies suggest that dormant cells may originate from "normal" tumor cells by currently intensively investigated mechanisms (e.g. [51–53]). As a fundamental criterion for tumor dormancy, dormant cells need to be able to reawake and start growing again, so that they then phenotypically resemble the rapidly growing cell phenotype. Thus, we introduced a conversion factor σ into our model capturing these phenotypical transformation processes. Whether such conversions occur spontaneously or can be induced specifically or randomly by extrinsic or intrinsic mechanisms is poorly understood. We thus assumed a spontaneous event which can be modeled by a constant rate.

Using our theoretical approach we showed that dependent on the applied treatment strength an equilibrium balance between rapidly proliferating cells and dormant cells is eventually reached. At this fixed point and with low dosage or no treatment, mostly rapidly proliferating cells dominate the population, similar to the findings of Basanta and colleagues [35]. At stronger treatment, the fraction of dormant cells becomes successively larger, yielding a lower growth rate of the whole tumor. However, high dosage treatment cannot be applied for longer time periods, as it causes severe side effects (for GBM: [3]). Hence, we focused on alternative treatment schedules.

Several previous models discuss the effect different treatment schedules on various aspects of the cancer growth like angiogenesis [44, 54] or evolution of resistance [55]. Here, either the dosage and timing or the type of the chemotherapeutic drug is varied, which can have a massive effect on the growth of the tumor. Accordingly, we combine sequential cycles of low and high dose treatment with different durations. Thereby, we observed that the total growth of the tumor is considerably lower for fast switching compared to a slow switching scheme.

Conclusion

In this study, we have developed a theoretical model to predict the tumor growth kinetics under different treatment strengths including a dormant cell phenotype and underlined our theoretical approach with experimental data. Using our model which allows for phenotypic conversion, we could simulate how different tumor cell phenotypes proportionally contribute to the growing tumor mass in cycling treatment schedules. Additionally, we could observe that switching between high and low dosage treatment (with equal total treatment amounts) remarkably affects tumor growth in a frequency dependent way.

Thus, the dynamic proportions between cell phenotypes should be taken into account in the optimization of treatment schedules in order to control tumor growth.

Abbreviations

D: Dormant cells; DMSO: Dimethyl sulfoxide; FCS: Fetal calf serum; GBM: Glioblastoma *multiforme*; P: Rapidly proliferating cells; SD: Standard deviation; TMZ: Temozolomide

Acknowledgements

We thank Judith Becker, Martina Burmester, Fereshteh Ebrahim and Brigitte Rehmke for expert technical assistance.

Funding

This work was supported by a sponsorship of the Medical Faculty of the University Kiel ("Forschungsförderung 2016" to JHF and KH) and the Deutsche Forschungsgemeinschaft RTG2154 [project 7 (KH) and project 8 (JHF)]. The funding body did not have any influence in the design of the study, collection, analysis and interpretation of data and in writing of the manuscript.

Authors' contributions

MB, JHF, AT and KH designed experimental and theoretical models and prepared the manuscript; MB and AT calculated and visualized the theoretical model; JHF, MS, RL and KH contributed to the experimental model; all authors read and approved the final manuscript.

Competing interests

The authors declare that they have no competing interests.

Author details

[1]Department Evolutionary Theory, Max Planck Institute for Evolutionary Biology, 24306 Plön, Germany. [2]Department of Neurosurgery, University Medical Center Schleswig-Holstein UKSH, Campus Kiel, 24105 Kiel, Germany. [3]Department of Anatomy, University of Kiel, 24098 Kiel, Germany.

References

1. Ohgaki H, Kleihues P. Epidemiology and etiology of gliomas. Acta Neuropathol. 2005;109:93–108.

2. Stupp R, Mason WP, van den Bent MJ, Weller M, Fisher B, Taphoorn MJ, Belanger K, Brandes AA, Marosi C, Bogdahn U, Curschmann J, Janzer RC, Ludwin SK, Allgeier A, Lacombe D, Cairncross JG, Eisenhauer E, Mirimanoff RO. Radiotherapy plus concomitant and adjuvant temozolomide for glioblastomas. N Engl J Med. 2005;35:987–96.

3. Niewald M, Berdel C, Fleckenstein J, Licht N, Ketter R, Ruebe C. Toxicity after radiochemotherapy for glioblastoma using temozolomide - a retrospective evaluation. Rad Oncol. 2011;6:141.

4. Gatenby RA, Gillies RJ, Brown JS. Of cancer and cave fish. Nat Rev Cancer. 2011;11:237–8.

5. Almog N. Molecular mechanisms underlying tumor dormancy. Cancer Lett. 2010;294:139–46.

6. Wikman H, Vessella R, Pantel K. Cancer micrometastasis and tumour dormancy. APMIS. 2008;116:754–70.

7. Bragado P, Sosa MS, Keely P, Condeelis J, Aguirre-Ghiso JA. Microenvironments dictating tumor cell dormancy. Recent Results Cancer Res. 2012;195:25–39.

8. Yeh AC, Ramaswamy S. Mechanisms of Cancer cell dormancy–another Hallmark of Cancer? Cancer Res. 2015;75:5014–22.

9. Zhang XH, Giuliano M, Trivedi MV, Schiff R, Osborne CK. Metastasis dormancy in estrogen receptor-positive breast cancer. Clin Cancer Res. 2013;19:6389–97.

10. Sosnoski DM, Norgard RJ, Grove CD, Foster SJ, Mastro AM. Dormancy and growth of metastatic breast cancer cells in a bone-like microenvironment. Clin Exp Metastasis. 2015;32:335–44.

11. Linde N, Fluegen G, Aguirre-Ghiso JA. The relationship between dormant Cancer cells and their microenvironment. Adv Cancer Res. 2016;132:45–71.

12. Sertil AR. Hypoxia regulation in cellular dormancy. In: Hayat MA, editor. Tumor dormancy, quiescence and senescence, Vol. 3. Dordrecht: Springer Netherlands; 2014. p. 13–24.

13. Hirose Y, Berger MS, Pieper RO. p53 effects both the duration of G2/M arrest and the fate of temozolomide-treated human glioblastoma cells. Cancer Res. 2001;61:1957–63.

14. Altrock PM, Lin LL, Michor F. The mathematics of cancer: integrating quantitative models. Nat Rev Cancer. 2015;15:730–45.

15. Nowak MA. Evolutionary dynamics. Cambridge: Harvard University Press; 2006.

16. Hofbauer J, Sigmund K. Evolutionary games and population dynamics. Cambridge: Cambridge University Press; 1998.

17. Basanta D, Anderson ARA. Exploiting ecological principles to better understand cancer progression and treatment. Interface Focus. 2013;3: 20130020.

18. Basanta D, Deutsch A. A game theoretical perspective on the somatic evolution of Cancer. In: Bellomo N, Angelis E, editors. Selected topics in Cancer modeling. Basel: Springer/ Birkhäuser; 2008. p. 97–112.

19. Dingli D, Chalub FACC, Santos FC, Van Segbroeck S, Pacheco JM. Cancer phenotype as the outcome of an evolutionary game between normal and malignant cells. Brit J Cancer. 2009;101:1130–6.

20. Kaznatcheev A, Scott JG, Basanta D. Edge effects in game-theoretic dynamics of spatially structured tumours. J R Soc Interface. 2015;12: 20150154.

21. Orlando PA, Gatenby RA, Brown JS. Cancer treatment as a game: integrating evolutionary game theory into the optimal control of chemotherapy. Physical Biol. 2012;9:065007.

22. Bomze I, Bürger R. Stability by mutation in evolutionary games. Games Econ Behav. 1995;11:146–72.

23. Page KM, Nowak MA. Unifying evolutionary dynamics. J Theor Biol. 2002; 219:93–8.

24. Almog N, Ma L, Raychowdhury R, Schwager C, Erber R, Short S, Hlatky L, Vajkoczy P, Huber PE, Folkman J, Abdollahi A. Transcriptional switch of dormant tumors to fast-growing angiogenic phenotype. Cancer Res. 2009;69:836–44.

25. Adamski V, Hempelmann A, Flüh C, Lucius R, Synowitz M, Hattermann K, Held-Feindt J. Dormant human glioblastoma cells acquire stem cell characteristics and are differentially affected by Temozolomide and AT101 treatment strategies. Onctarget. 2017;8(64):108064–78.

26. Strogatz S. Nonlinear dynamics and Chaos: with applications to physics, biology, chemistry, and engineering (studies in nonlinearity). New York: Westview Press; 2000.

27. Endaya BB, Lam PY, Meedeniya AC, Neuzil J. Transcriptional profiling of dividing tumor cells detects intratumor heterogeneity linked to cell proliferation in a brain tumor model. Mol Oncol. 2016;10:126–37.

28. Satchi-Fainaro R, Ferber S, Segal E, Ma L, Dixit N, Ijaz A, Hlatky L, Abdollahi A, Almog N. Prospective identification of glioblastoma cells generating dormant tumors. PLoS One. 2012;7:e44395.

29. Naumov GN, Bender E, Zurakowski D, Kang SY, Sampson D, Flynn E, Watnick RS, Straume O, Akslen LA, Folkman J, Almog N. A model of human tumor dormancy: an angiogenic switch from the nonangiogenic phenotype. J Natl Cancer Inst. 2006;98:316–25.

30. Hofstetter CP, Burkhardt JK, Shin BJ, Gürsel DB, Mubita L, Gorrepati R, Brennan C, Holland EC, Boockvar JA. Protein phosphatase 2A mediates dormancy of glioblastoma multiforme-derived tumor stem-like cells during hypoxia. PLoS One. 2012;7:e30059.

31. Magnus N, Gerges N, Jabado N, Rak J. Coagulation-related gene expression profile in glioblastoma is defined by molecular disease subtype. J Thromb Haemost. 2013;11:1197–200.

32. Magnus N, Garnier D, Meehan B, McGraw S, Lee TH, Caron M, Bourque G, Milsom C, Jabado N, Trasler J, Pawlinski R, Mackman N, Rak J. Tissue factor expression provokes escape from tumor dormancy and leads to genomic alterations. Proc Natl Acad Sci U S A. 2014;111:3544–9.

33. Magnus N, D'Asti E, Meehan B, Garnier D, Rak J. Oncogenes and the coagulation system–forces that modulate dormant and aggressive states in cancer. Thromb Res. 2014;133(Suppl 2):S1–9.

34. Evans EB, Lin SY. New insights into tumor dormancy: targeting DNA repair pathways. World J Clin Oncol. 2015;6:80–8.

35. Basanta D, Simon M, Hatzikirou H, Deutsch A. Evolutionary game theory elucidates the role of glycolysis in glioma progression and invasion. Cell Prolif. 2008;41:980–7.

36. Basanta D, Scott JG, Fishman MN, Ayala G, Hayward SW, Anderson ARA. Investigating prostate cancer tumour–stroma interactions: clinical and biological insights from an evolutionary game. Brit J Cancer. 2012;106:174–81.

37. Pacheco JM, Santos FC, Dingli D. The ecology of cancer from an evolutionary game theory perspective. Interface Focus. 2014;4:20140019.

38. Kaznatcheev A, Vander Velde R, Scott JG, Basanta D. Cancer treatment scheduling and dynamic heterogeneity in social dilemmas of tumour acidity and vasculature. Brit J Cancer. 2017;9:1–24.

39. Gerlee P, Anderson ARA. An evolutionary hybrid cellular automaton model of solid tumour growth. J Theoretical Biol. 2007;246:583–603.

40. Anderson ARA, Hassanein M, Branch KM, Lu J, Lobdell NA, Maier J, Basanta D, Weidow B, Narasanna A, Arteaga CL, Reynolds AB, Quaranta V, Estrada L, Weaver AM. Microenvironmental independence associated with tumor progression. Cancer Res. 2009;69:8797–806.

41. Zukewich J, Kurella V, Doebeli M, Hauert C. Consolidating birth-death and death-birth processes in structured populations. PLoS One. 2013;8:e54639.

42. Hindersin L, Traulsen A. Most undirected random graphs are amplifiers of selection for birth-death dynamics, but suppressors of selection for death-birth dynamics. PLoS Comput Biol. 2015;11:e1004437.

43. Wilkie KP, Hahnfeldt P. Tumor-immune dynamics regulated in the microenvironment inform the transient nature of immune-induced tumor dormancy. Cancer Res. 2013;73:3534–44.

44. Hahnfeldt P, Folkman J, Hlatky L. Minimizing long-term tumor burden: the logic for metronomic chemotherapeutic dosing and its antiangiogenic basis. J Theoretical Biol. 2003;220:545–54.

45. Page K, Uhr J. Mathematical models of cancer dormancy. Leuk Lymphoma. 2005;46:313–27.

46. Kareva I. Escape from tumor dormancy and time to angiogenic switch as mitigated by tumor-induced stimulation of stroma. J Theor Biol. 2016;395:11–22.

47. Enderling H, Anderson ARA, Chaplain MAJ, Beheshti A, Hlatky L, Hahnfeldt P. Paradoxical dependencies of tumor dormancy and progression on basic cell kinetics. Cancer Res. 2009;69:8814–21.

48. Adamski V, Schmitt AD, Flüh C, Synowitz M, Hattermann K, Held-Feindt J. Isolation and characterization of fast migrating human glioma cells in the progression of malignant gliomas. Oncol Res. 2017;25:341–53.

49. Hattermann K, Flüh C, Engel D, Mehdorn HM, Synowitz M, Mentlein R, Held-Feindt J. Stem cell markers in glioma progression and recurrence. Int J Oncol. 2016;49:1899–910.

50. Held-Feindt J, Hattermann K, Müerköster SS, Wedderkopp H, Knerlich-Lukoschus F, Ungefroren H, Mehdorn HM, Mentlein R. CX3CR1 promotes recruitment of human glioma-infiltrating microglia/macrophages (GIMs). Exp Cell Res. 2010;316:1553–66.

51. Hoppe-Seyler K, Bossler F, Lohrey C, Bulkescher J, Rösl F, Jansen L, Mayer A, Vaupel P, Dürst M, Hoppe-Seyler F. Induction of dormancy in hypoxic human papillomavirus-positive cancer cells. Proc Natl Acad Sci U S A. 2017; 114:E990–8.

52. Sosa MS, Parikh F, Maia AG, Estrada Y, Bosch A, Bragado P, Ekpin E, George A, Zheng Y, Lam HM, Morrissey C, Chung CY, Farias EF, Bernstein E, Aguirre-Ghiso JA. NR2F1 controls tumour cell dormancy via SOX9- and RARβ-driven quiescence programmes. Nat Commun. 2015;6:6170.

53. Ranganathan AC, Adam AP, Aguirre-Ghiso JA. Opposing roles of mitogenic and stress signaling pathways in the induction of cancer dormancy. Cell Cycle. 2006;5:1799–807.

54. Schättler H, Ledzewicz U, Amini B. Dynamical properties of a minimally parameterized mathematical model for metronomic chemotherapy. J Math Biol. 2016;72:1255–80.

55. Dhawan A, Nichol D, Kinose F, Abazeed ME, Marusyk A, Haura EB, Scott JG. Collateral sensitivity networks reveal evolutionary instability and novel treatment strategies in ALK mutated non-small cell lung cancer. Sci Rep. 2017;7:1232.

20

Survival and clinical outcomes of patients with melanoma brain metastasis in the era of checkpoint inhibitors and targeted therapies

Elham Vosoughi, Jee Min Lee, James R. Miller, Mehdi Nosrati, David R. Minor, Roy Abendroth, John W. Lee, Brian T. Andrews, Lewis Z. Leng, Max Wu, Stanley P. Leong, Mohammed Kashani-Sabet and Kevin B. Kim[*] ⓘ

Abstract

Background: Melanoma brain metastasis is associated with an extremely poor prognosis, with a median overall survival of 4–5 months. Since 2011, the overall survival of patients with stage IV melanoma has been significantly improved with the advent of new targeted therapies and checkpoint inhibitors. We analyze the survival outcomes of patients diagnosed with brain metastasis after the introduction of these novel drugs.

Methods: We performed a retrospective analysis of our melanoma center database and identified 79 patients with brain metastasis between 2011 and 2015.

Results: The median time from primary melanoma diagnosis to brain metastasis was 3.2 years. The median overall survival duration from the time of initial brain metastasis was 12.8 months. Following a diagnosis of brain metastasis, 39 (49.4%), 28 (35.4%), and 24 (30.4%) patients were treated with anti-CTLA-4 antibody, anti-PD-1 antibody, or BRAF inhibitors (with or without a MEK inhibitor), with a median overall survival of 19.2 months, 37.9 months and 12.7 months, respectively. Factors associated with significantly reduced overall survival included male sex, cerebellar metastasis, higher number of brain lesions, and treatment with whole-brain radiation therapy. Factors associated with significantly longer overall survival included treatment with craniotomy, stereotactic radiosurgery, or with anti-PD-1 antibody after initial diagnosis of brain metastasis.

Conclusions: These results show a significant improvement in the overall survival of patients with melanoma brain metastasis in the era of novel therapies. In addition, they suggest the activity of anti-PD-1 therapy specifically in the setting of brain metastasis.

Keywords: Melanoma, Brain, Metastasis, Checkpoint inhibitors, BRAF

Background

Brain metastases are common in patients with advanced melanoma and are a frequent cause of death in patients with this disease [1]. Nearly 20% of patients are found to have brain metastasis at the time of diagnosis of metastatic melanoma, and more than 50% develop brain metastasis during the course of the disease [2–5]. Brain metastasis is associated with a poor prognosis, with

median overall survival from diagnosis of brain metastasis in the range of 17–22 weeks [2, 4, 6, 7]. Until recently, the management of melanoma brain metastasis has included surgical resection, stereotactic radiosurgery, whole-brain radiation therapy, and/or cytotoxic chemotherapy [8, 9], without a clear change in the natural history of melanoma brain metastasis.

Since 2011, a number of targeted therapies, including BRAF inhibitors and MEK inhibitors, and checkpoint inhibitors, such as anti-CTLA4 antibody and anti-PD-1 antibodies, have been approved by the Food and Drug Administration (FDA) in the United States because of

* Correspondence: KimKB@sutterhealth.org
Center for Melanoma Research and Treatment, California Pacific Medical Center Research Institute, 2100 Webster Street, Suite 326, San Francisco, CA 94115, USA

their significant survival benefit, and have emerged as new standard therapies. As of 2016, the median survival duration of patients with unresectable or metastatic melanoma approaches nearly 2 years with these novel drug therapies [10–12], compared to 6–9 months with traditional cytotoxic chemotherapy [13–15]. However, the impact of these new drugs on the clinical outcome and survival of patients with brain metastasis is not well known, although a number of prospective clinical trials have shown promising clinical activity of these agents in the setting of brain metastasis [1, 3]. However, these studies do not address the survival outcomes of patients who are not candidates for systemic therapies or clinical trials. Therefore, there is a lack of current survival data in patients with melanoma brain metastasis in a real world situation in the modern era.

Here, we report the findings of our retrospective analysis of outcomes of patients diagnosed with melanoma brain metastasis in the era of the novel targeted therapies and immunotherapies.

Methods

We searched the Institutional Tumor Registry Database and Melanoma Database at California Pacific Medical Center and San Francisco Oncology Associates for patients with diagnosis of metastatic melanoma to the brain. Under an institutional review board-approved protocol, we performed a retrospective medical record review of all melanoma patients with brain metastases. Because checkpoint inhibitors and BRAF inhibitors have been approved by the FDA beginning in 2011, we limited our search to those who were diagnosed with brain metastasis between January of 2011 and June of 2015. Patients were eligible for inclusion in the study if they had at least 6 months of adequate follow up evaluation since the time of initial brain metastasis, unless they had died within 6 months after the initial date of initial brain metastasis. The final analysis was performed in December of 2016. We utilized Cox regression for univariate and multivariate analyses of the potential association between various clinical or histological factors with overall survival. Kaplan-Meier analysis was used to determine the overall survival of patients, including differences between specific subgroups of patients.

Results

Clinical characteristics of the patients with brain metastasis

A total of 79 patients were identified for this analysis. The demographic and baseline characteristics of the patients are described in Table 1. The median time from primary melanoma diagnosis to brain metastasis was 3. 2 years (range, 0–29.8 years), and the median time from stage IV diagnosis to brain metastasis was 2 months (range, 0–103 months). Forty (50.6%) patients had prior

extracranial metastasis at the time of initial brain metastasis; 28 (35.4%) had concurrent extracranial metastasis at the time of brain metastasis; and 5 (6.3%) patients developed extracranial metastasis subsequently, defined as at least 1 month after initial diagnosis of brain metastasis. Six (7.6%) patients had brain metastasis as the only site of distant metastasis until death or at the time of the analysis.

The cerebrum was the most common site of brain metastasis (72 patients [91.1%]), and 21.5% and 8.9% patients had metastasis to the cerebellum and pons, respectively. Thirty-nine (49.4%) had a solitary brain metastasis at the initial brain metastasis diagnosis, and the largest size of the initial brain metastasis was 10 mm or less in 31.7%. Thirty-six patients (45.6%) had neurological symptoms associated with brain metastasis. Forty-nine (62.0%) of the 79 patients had received systemic therapy prior to or at the time of brain metastasis, including checkpoint inhibitors, targeted drugs, cytotoxic chemotherapy and/or cytokine therapy.

Treatment modalities

Thirty-four patients (43.0%) underwent craniotomy for the management of brain metastasis, and 54 (68.4%) were treated with stereotactic radiosurgery. After diagnosis of brain metastasis, 39 (49.4%), 28 (35.4%), and 24 (30.4%) patients were treated with anti-CTLA-4 antibody, anti-PD-1 antibody, or BRAF inhibitors (with or without a MEK inhibitor), respectively. Thirty-five (44.3%) and ten (12.7%) patients were treated with cytotoxic chemotherapy and interleukin-2 treatment, respectively.

Survival and clinical outcome

Fifty-nine (74.7%) patients had died of melanoma progression at the time of the analysis, among which 32 (40.5%) died with progressing brain metastases. The median overall survival duration from the time of initial brain metastasis was 12.8 months (range, 1.1–71. 9 months) (Fig. 1), and the median overall survival duration from the time of initial melanoma diagnosis was 60.5 months (5.5–367.1 months) for all 79 patients. The median overall survival durations from the time of craniotomy and stereotactic radiosurgery were 17.3 months (2.4–60.7 months) and 15.4 months (1.2–71.8 months), respectively. The median survival durations of patients who received anti-CTLA-4 antibody, anti-PD-1 antibody and BRAF inhibitor (with or without MEK inhibitor) after the diagnosis of brain metastasis were 19.2 months (1.2–65.0 months), 37.9 months (5.3–65.0 months) and 12.7 months (2.7–70.9 months), respectively. Tables 2 and 3 describe the outcomes of the entire cohort as well as specific subsets of patients. Figures 1 and 2 illustrate the Kaplan-Meier curves of overall survival for all patients and for those who were treated with or without anti-PD-1 therapy, respectively.

Table 1 Patient characteristics and treatment ($n = 79$)

Characteristic at the time of initial brain metastasis	No. of patients (%)
Median age (range), years	63 (17–91)
Sex	
Male	53 (67.1%)
Stage prior to initial brain metastasis,	
I/II	13 (16.4%)
III	13 (16.4%)
IV (M1a)	6 (7.6%)
IV (M1b)	8 (10.1%)
IV (M1c)	25 (31.6%)
Unknown primary melanoma/Data not available	14 (17.7%)
Intracranial site of metastasis[a]	
Cerebrum	72 (91.1%)
Cerebellum	17 (21.5%)
Pons	7 (8.9%)
Leptomeninges	2 (2.5%)
Unknown	1 (1.3%)
Number of brain metastasis[a]	
1	39 (49.4%)
2–3	15 (19%)
4–5	6 (7.6%)
6–9	3 (3.8%)
≥ 10	12 (15.2%)
Unknown	4 (5.0%)
Size of the largest brain metastasis[a]	
≤ 10 mm	25 (31.7%)
> 10–30 mm	32 (40.5%)
> 30–50 mm	15 (19.0%)
> 50 mm	3 (3.8%)
Unknown	4 (5.0%)
Symptomatic from brain metastasis	
Yes	36 (45.6%)
Sites of extracranial metastatic organs[a]	
Lung	22 (27.9%)
LN/Soft tissue	21 (26.6%)
Skin/SQ	15 (19.0%)
Bone	12 (15.2%)
Liver	8 (10.1%)
Adrenal gland	3 (3.8%)
V600 BRAF mutation	
Mutated	29 (36.7%)
Wild type	38 (48.1%)
Unknown	12 (15.2%)

Table 1 Patient characteristics and treatment ($n = 79$) (Continued)

Characteristic at the time of initial brain metastasis	No. of patients (%)
Number of systemic therapy given after a diagnosis of brain metastasis	
1	28 (35.4%)
2	22 (27.8%)
3+	20 (25.3%)
Info not available	9 (11.4%)
Type of systemic therapy given after a diagnosis of brain metastasis	
Ipilimumab	39 (49.4%)
Anti PD-1 antibody	28 (35.4%)
Concurrent Nivolumab/Ipilimumab	8 (10.1%)
BRAF inhibitor (+/− MEK inhibitor) only	24 (30.4%)
Cytotoxic chemotherapy	35 (44.3%)
Interleukin-2-based biochemotherapy	10 (12.7%)
Sequence of novel drug therapy after a diagnosis of brain metastasis[b]	
Checkpoint inhibitor followed by BRAF inhibitor (+/− MEK inhibitor)	11 (13.9%)[b]
BRAF inhibitor (+/− MEK inhibitor) followed by checkpoint inhibitor	3 (3.8%)[b]

[a] at the time of initial brain metastasis diagnosis
[b] A total of 14 patients were treated with both checkpoint inhibitor and BRAF inhibitor (+/− MEK inhibitor) after a diagnosis of brain metastasis

Predictive factors for overall survival

We analyzed the potential association between several factors and survival using univariate Cox regression of overall survival (Table 4). Intriguingly, of factors in the primary tumor, increased levels of tumor-infiltrating lymphocytes showed a trend toward improved survival in patients with brain metastasis. Several clinical factors

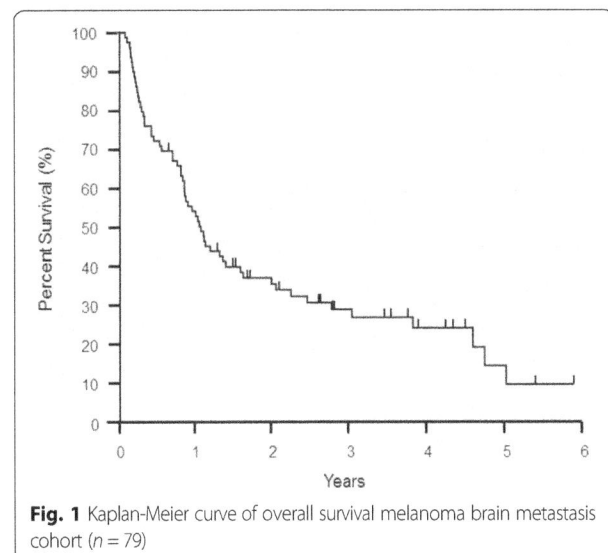

Fig. 1 Kaplan-Meier curve of overall survival melanoma brain metastasis cohort ($n = 79$)

Table 2 Overall survival outcome data

From the time of	Median OS (range), months
initial brain metastasis (*n* = 79)	12.8 (1.1–71.9)
initial melanoma diagnosis (*n* = 79)	60.5 (5.5–367.1)
the first craniotomy (*n* = 34)	17.3 (2.4–60.7)
the first stereotactic radiosurgery (*n* = 54)	15.4 (1.2–71.8)
the first whole brain radiation therapy (*n* = 16)	6.8 (2.2–12.5)

OS, overall survival

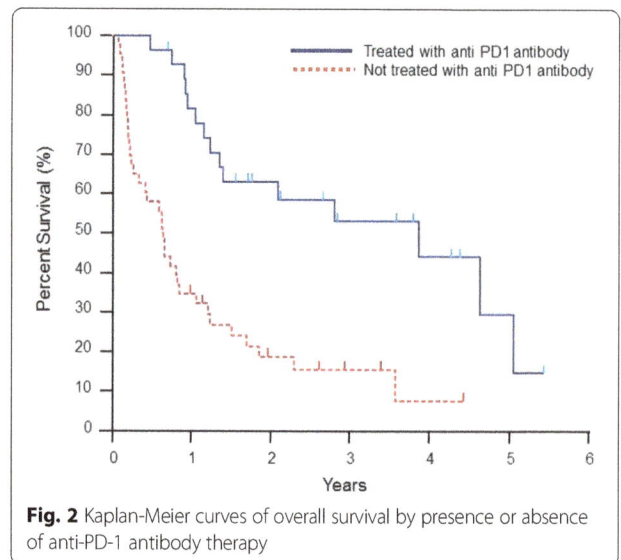

Fig. 2 Kaplan-Meier curves of overall survival by presence or absence of anti-PD-1 antibody therapy

were found to be significantly associated with overall survival in patients with brain metastasis by univariate analysis (Table 4). Factors associated with shorter overall survival included male sex, cerebellar involvement, higher number of metastatic brain tumors, concurrent presence of adrenal metastasis, or treatment with whole-brain radiation therapy. Factors associated with longer overall survival were treatment with craniotomy, stereotactic radiosurgery, or anti-PD-1 antibody therapy after initial diagnosis of brain metastasis.

Multivariate analysis of all eight factors revealed cerebellar involvement, craniotomy, and adrenal involvement as independently predictive of survival (Table 5). There was trend toward significance for treatment with anti-PD-1 antibody (*P = 0.055*).

Discussion

Patients with metastatic melanoma to the brain have been considered to have an extremely poor prognosis with a short median overall survival, and in a vast majority of cases, deaths observed are due to disease progression in the brain. Sampson et al. showed that brain metastasis was responsible for death in 94.5% of patients in their retrospective analysis of patients with melanoma brain metastasis [16]. Although our database do not have the detailed information regarding neurological symptoms at the time of death, we believe that most of our patients have died of the brain metastasis, similar to the historical

Table 3 Subset analyses of overall survival outcomes

OS from the time of initial brain metastasis in patients who:	Median OS, (range), months
Were treated with anti-CTLA-4 antibody therapy	
Before the initial brain metastasis (*n* = 29)	10.5 (2.0–55.3)
After the initial brain metastasis (*n* = 39)	19.2 (1.2–65.0)
Were treated with anti-PD-1 antibody therapy	
Before the initial brain metastasis (*n* = 1)	8.5
After the initial brain metastasis (*n* = 28)	37.9 (5.3–65.0)
Were treated with BRAF and/or MEK inhibitor therapy	
Before the initial brain metastasis (*n* = 16)	10.9 (2.1–55.3)
After the initial brain metastasis (*n* = 24)	12.7 (2.7–70.9)

data. In our study, we report a longer survival of patients with brain metastasis in the era of novel checkpoint inhibitors and BRAF inhibitor-based targeted therapies. The median overall survival duration among all 79 analyzed patients was longer than 1 year. Specifically, among those who were treated with anti-PD-1 antibody, the median survival was nearly 3 years.

Most of the available literature regarding the survival of melanoma patients with brain metastasis was published prior to 2011, when BRAF inhibitor-based therapies and checkpoint inhibitors became available as standard therapies for advanced melanoma. Prior to 2011, most patients were treated with stereotactic radiosurgery to metastatic lesions, whole brain radiation, and/or cytotoxic chemotherapy with or without cytokines, such as interferon-alpha and interleukin-2. As our data show, a vast majority of patients who were diagnosed with brain metastasis since 2011 were treated with the BRAF (and/or MEK)-targeting kinase inhibitors and/or checkpoint inhibitors. Therefore, the prolonged overall survival of the patients in our analysis is most likely due to the clinical benefit of these novel targeted and/or immunotherapeutic drugs. Specifically, patients who were also treated with anti-PD-1 antibody therapy had significantly longer survival, compared to those who had not. Since most patients diagnosed with brain metastasis on or after 2013, when anti-PD-1 antibodies were approved by the FDA, received either nivolumab or pembrolizumab, the longer survival duration is most likely due to the anticancer activity of anti-PD-1 antibody rather than biased patient selection for the treatment, even in the setting of brain metastasis.

One might wonder whether the change in the pattern of therapeutic modality other than the checkpoint inhibitors and BRAF inhibitor-based targeted therapies

Table 4 Univariate Cox regression analysis of association of various clinical factors with overall survival in melanoma patients with brain metastasis

Variable	Chi-squared	Hazard ratio	P value
Gender (male)	4.03	1.85	0.045*
Age	0.826	1.01	0.36
TIL level	2.23	0.628	0.135
Number of positive regional lymph nodes	3.13	1.05	0.077
Characteristics of brain metastasis			
Cerebellar metastases	6.43	2.19	0.011*
Midbrain/pons metastasis	3.24	2.09	0.072
Leptomeningeal disease	0.04	1.07	0.846
Other site metastasis	0.03	0.92	0.867
Size of largest brain metastases	0.816	1.01	0.367
Number of brain metastases	18.8	1.19	< 0.00005*
Presence of neurological symptoms	1.55	2.51	0.214
Required steroid for brain metastasis	1.55	2.51	0.214
Extracranial Metastasis			
Presence of extracranial metastasis	2.29	1.49	0.13
Presence of liver metastasis	2.25	1.94	0.134
Presence of lung metastasis	0.527	1.30	0.468
Presence of bone metastasis	0.06	1.09	0.813
Presence of adrenal metastasis	5.39	4.50	0.02*
Therapy			
Craniotomy	10.0	0.418	0.0015*
Stereotactic radiosurgery	7.72	0.434	0.0055*
Whole brain radiation therapy	16.2	3.85	0.0001*
Number of prior systemic therapies	0.613	1.09	0.434
Anti-CTLA4 antibody after BM	0.658	0.79	0.417
Anti-PD-1 antibody after BM	10.0	0.376	0.0016*
BRAF inhibitor after BM	0.05	1.07	0.82

BM, initial diagnosis of brain metastasis;
*p-value is < 0.05

Table 5 Multivariate Cox regression analysis of association of various clinical factors with overall survival in melanoma patients with brain metastasis

Variable	Chi-squared	Hazard ratio	P value
Gender	0.89	1.93	0.35
Presence of cerebellar metastasis	6.74	4.61	0.009*
Number of brain metastases	0.60	0.93	0.44
Presence of adrenal Metastasis	4.89	9.94	0.027*
Craniotomy	4.45	0.27	0.035*
Stereotactic radiosurgery	0.92	0.51	0.34
Treated with whole brain radiation therapy	1.08	2.13	0.298
Treatment with anti-PD-1 antibody	3.68	0.34	0.055

*p-value is < 0.05

contributed the longer survival of the patients in the recent years. Davies and colleagues showed that there was no significant difference in the median overall survival duration between melanoma patients with brain metastasis diagnosed prior to 1996 and those diagnosed between 1996 and 2004 [4]. Although a stereotactic radiosurgery was likely used more frequently in the latter time period, there was no significant survival improvement in the overall patients. In their study, the median overall survival duration in patients who were initially treated with a stereotactic radiosurgery was 7. 69 months whereas the median survival was 15.4 months post stereotactic radiosurgery in our study. Therefore, we believe that evolution in the pattern of therapeutic

modality for brain metastasis has a minimal impact in overall survival in this patient population until the availability of the checkpoint inhibitors and the targeted therapy drugs.

Our findings showed an improved outcome in this patient population compared to a recent meta-analysis performed by Spagnolo et al., which analyzed 22 clinical studies (including 8 phase I-II studies and 14 "real world" expanded-access program studies), which included 2153 melanoma patients with brain metastasis in the era of MAP-kinase inhibitors and checkpoint inhibitors [2]. In their analysis, the median overall survival of all analyzed patients was 7.9 months and 7.7 months for the phase I-II studies and "real-world" studies, respectively. Although the authors had an intention to report the survival in a "real-world" situation, their results do not necessarily represent all patients with brain metastasis because their findings are based on patients who were able to enroll in the clinical studies, whether or not they are expanded access program studies. It is most likely that only a subset of patients with brain metastasis would meet the eligibility criteria for each study. In addition, the overall survival duration in their analysis was measured from the time of initiation of the novel systemic therapy, not from the time of initial brain metastasis; therefore, patients with brain metastasis who were treated only with local therapy, such as craniotomy, stereotactic radiosurgery or whole brain radiation, without the novel systemic therapy, were not included in their analysis. Lastly, most patients were treated with the targeted therapies and/or ipilimumab, and only 18 of 2153 patients in their analysis received anti-PD-1 antibody therapy. Since anti-PD-1 antibody therapies have shown to be superior to ipilimumab [17, 18], their findings are not likely to represent the true clinical outcome in the current era, where anti-PD-1 antibody therapy has replaced ipilimumab alone as the first-line standard therapy in patients with advanced melanoma.

Our results suggest that the targeted and checkpoint inhibitor drugs have meaningful clinical benefit in patients with brain metastases. This phenomenon was initially observed in phase II studies of ipilimumab and BRAF inhibitors, in which significant regression of active metastatic brain lesions occurred following with treatment with these drugs [1, 3]. More recently, a number of prospective phase II clinical studies have demonstrated that these novel drugs have significant clinical activity in melanoma patients with active brain metastasis [19–21]. The response rates of a combination of nivolumab and ipilimumab were 42%–55% in two of the studies [19, 20] and a combination of dabrafenib and trametininb had an objective response rate of 58% [21]. Unfortunately, a clinical response to a specific therapy could not be appropriately evaluated in our study because most patients were treated with a multimodality therapy, such as a local brain therapy (craniotomy, stereotactic radiosurgery and/or whole brain radiation) administered either concurrently with or shortly followed by a systemic therapy. We believe that our pattern of treatment in patients with active brain metastasis is typical of most community oncology practices, including patients treated outside of a clinical trial.

Our results suggest that the overall survival is especially poor in patients with cerebellar metastasis or in those with concurrent adrenal metastasis. The shorter survival duration for patients with cerebellar involvement in our analysis is consistent with previously reported data [22–24]. Our finding of poor prognosis in those with concurrent brain and adrenal metastasis is interesting and has not been previously been reported. However, due to the small number of patients with this finding, it deserves confirmation in a separate cohort of patients. Similarly, our findings of no significant prognostic impact of the presence of leptomeningeal involvement may be due to the inclusion of a small number of such patients in our analysis.

Our study is the first to show the impact of novel targeted drugs and immunotherapies on the overall survival of patients with brain metastasis. Specifically, our study is the first to show a significantly improved survival of patients receiving anti-PD-1 therapy following the development of brain metastasis. It is particularly interesting that the median survival duration was nearly 3 years in those patients who were treated with anti-PD-1 antibody therapy. Although our study included a relatively small number of patients at a tertiary referral center, our results are very encouraging and show an altered natural history of melanoma brain metastasis, which deserves confirmation in additional, larger cohorts of melanoma patients.

Conclusions

We show significantly improved survival of melanoma patients with brain metastasis in the era of novel targeted and immunotherapeutic drugs. The median overall survival of those with melanoma brain metastasis is longer than 1 year, and nearly 3 years for those who were treated with anti-PD-1 antibody. These results strongly suggest the impact of novel immunotherapies on prolonging the survival of these patients.

Authors' contributions

EV: Design of the study, collection and assembly of data, data analysis and interpretation, writing of the report, critical revision of the report for important intellectual content, and approval of the final manuscript. JRM: Data analysis and interpretation, critical revision of the report for important intellectual content, and approval of the final manuscript. MN: Collection and assembly of data, critical revision of the report for important intellectual content, and approval of the final manuscript. JML DRM, RA, JWL, BTA, LZL, MW, SPL, Collection and assembly of data, and approval of the final manuscript. MKS: Design of the study, data analysis and interpretation, writing of the report, critical revision of the report for important intellectual content, and approval of the final manuscript. KBK: Conception and design of the study, collection and assembly of data, data analysis and interpretation, writing of the report, critical revision of the report for important intellectual content, and approval of the final manuscript.

Competing interests

David R. minor received honoraria from Bristol-Myer Squibb and Merck; Mohammed Kashani-Sabet received research funding from Merck.; Kevin B. Kim received honoraria from Bristol-Myer Squibb, Merck, Novartis and Genentech. Institution received research grant from Bristol-Myer Squibb, Merck and Novartis.

References

1. Margolin K, Ernstoff MS, Hamid O, Lawrence D, McDermott D, Puzanov I, Wolchok JD, Clark JI, Sznol M, Logan TF, et al. Ipilimumab in patients with melanoma and brain metastases: an open-label, phase 2 trial. Lancet Oncol. 2012;13(5):459–65.
2. Spagnolo F, Picasso V, Lambertini M, Ottaviano V, Dozin B, Queirolo P. Survival of patients with metastatic melanoma and brain metastases in the era of MAP-kinase inhibitors and immunologic checkpoint blockade antibodies: a systematic review. Cancer Treat Rev. 2016;45:38–45.
3. Long GV, Trefzer U, Davies MA, Kefford RF, Ascierto PA, Chapman PB, Puzanov I, Hauschild A, Robert C, Algazi A, et al. Dabrafenib in patients with Val600Glu or Val600Lys BRAF-mutant melanoma metastatic to the brain (BREAK-MB): a multicentre, open-label, phase 2 trial. Lancet Oncol. 2012;13(11):1087–95.
4. Davies MA, Liu P, McIntyre S, Kim KB, Papadopoulos N, Hwu WJ, Hwu P, Bedikian A. Prognostic factors for survival in melanoma patients with brain metastases. Cancer. 2011;117(8):1687–96.
5. Bafaloukos D, Gogas H. The treatment of brain metastases in melanoma patients. Cancer Treat Rev. 2004;30(6):515–20.
6. Fife KM, Colman MH, Stevens GN, Firth IC, Moon D, Shannon KF, Harman R, Petersen-Schaefer K, Zacest AC, Besser M, et al. Determinants of outcome in melanoma patients with cerebral metastases. J Clin Oncol. 2004;22(7):1293–300.
7. Eigentler TK, Figl A, Krex D, Mohr P, Mauch C, Rass K, Bostroem A, Heese O, Koelbl O, Garbe C, et al. Number of metastases, serum lactate dehydrogenase level, and type of treatment are prognostic factors in patients with brain metastasis of malignant melanoma. Cancer. 2011;117(8):1697–703.
8. Knisely JP, Yu JB, Flanigan J, Sznol M, Kluger HM, Chiang VL. Radiosurgery for melanoma brain metastases in the ipilimumab era and the possibility of longer survival. J Neurosurg. 2012;117(2):227–33.

9. Chowdhury IH, Ojerholm E, McMillan MT, Miller D, Kolker JD, Kurtz G, Dorsey JF, Nagda SN, Geiger GA, Brem S, et al. Novel risk scores for survival and intracranial failure in patients treated with radiosurgery alone to melanoma brain metastases. Radiat Oncol. 2015;10:248.

10. Robert C, Karaszewska B, Schachter J, Rutkowski P, Mackiewicz A, Stroiakovski D, Lichinitser M, Dummer R, Grange F, Mortier L, et al. Improved overall survival in melanoma with combined dabrafenib and trametinib. N Engl J Med. 2015;372(1):30–9.

11. Larkin J, Ascierto PA, Dreno B, Atkinson V, Liszkay G, Maio M, Mandala M, Demidov L, Stroyakovskiy D, Thomas L, et al. Combined vemurafenib and cobimetinib in BRAF-mutated melanoma. N Engl J Med. 2014;371(20):1867–76.

12. Long GV, Stroyakovskiy D, Gogas H, Levchenko E, de Braud F, Larkin J, Garbe C, Jouary T, Hauschild A, Grob JJ, et al. Dabrafenib and trametinib versus dabrafenib and placebo for Val600 BRAF-mutant melanoma: a multicentre, double-blind, phase 3 randomised controlled trial. Lancet. 2015;386(9992):444–51.

13. Middleton MR, Grob JJ, Aaronson N, Fierlbeck G, Tilgen W, Seiter S, Gore M, Aamdal S, Cebon J, Coates A, et al. Randomized phase III study of temozolomide versus dacarbazine in the treatment of patients with advanced metastatic malignant melanoma. J Clin Oncol. 2000;18(1):158–66.

14. Bedikian AY, Millward M, Pehamberger H, Conry R, Gore M, Trefzer U, Pavlick AC, DeConti R, Hersh EM, Hersey P, et al. Bcl-2 antisense (oblimersen sodium) plus dacarbazine in patients with advanced melanoma: the Oblimersen melanoma study group. J Clin Oncol. 2006;24(29):4738–45.

15. Atkins MB, Hsu J, Lee S, Cohen GI, Flaherty LE, Sosman JA, Sondak VK, Kirkwood JM, Eastern Cooperative Oncology G. Phase III trial comparing concurrent biochemotherapy with cisplatin, vinblastine, dacarbazine, interleukin-2, and interferon alfa-2b with cisplatin, vinblastine, and dacarbazine alone in patients with metastatic malignant melanoma (E3695): a trial coordinated by the eastern cooperative oncology group. J Clin Oncol. 2008;26(35):5748–54.

16. Sampson JH, Carter JH Jr, Friedman AH, Seigler HF. Demographics, prognosis, and therapy in 702 patients with brain metastases from malignant melanoma. J Neurosurg. 1998;88(1):11–20.

17. Robert C, Schachter J, Long GV, Arance A, Grob JJ, Mortier L, Daud A, Carlino MS, McNeil C, Lotem M, et al. Pembrolizumab versus Ipilimumab in advanced melanoma. N Engl J Med. 2015;372(26):2521–32.

18. Larkin J, Chiarion-Sileni V, Gonzalez R, Grob JJ, Cowey CL, Lao CD, Schadendorf D, Dummer R, Smylie M, Rutkowski P, et al. Combined Nivolumab and Ipilimumab or monotherapy in untreated melanoma. N Engl J Med. 2015;373(1):23–34.

19. Tawbi HA, Forsyth PAJ, Algazi AP, Hamid O, Hodi FS, Moschos SJ, Khushalani NI, Gonzalez R, Lao CD, Postow MA, et al. Efficacy and safety of nivolumab (NIVO) plus ipilimumab (IPI) in patients with melanoma (MEL) metastatic to the brain: Results of the phase II study CheckMate 204. J Clin Oncol. 2017;35(15_suppl):9507. (May 20 2017)

20. Long GV, Atkinson V, Menzies AM, Lo S, Guminski AD, Brown MP, Gonzalez MM, Diamante K, Sandhu SK, Scolyer RA, et al. A randomized phase II study of nivolumab or nivolumab combined with ipilimumab in patients (pts) with melanoma brain metastases (mets): The Anti-PD1 Brain Collaboration (ABC). J Clin Oncol. 2017;35(15_supple):9508. (May 20 2017).

21. Davies MA, Saiag P, Robert C, Grob JJ, Flaherty KT, Arance A, Chiarion-Sileni V, Thomas L, Lesimple T, Mortier L, et al. Dabrafenib plus trametinib in patients with BRAF(V600)-mutant melanoma brain metastases (COMBI-MB): a multicentre, multicohort, open-label, phase 2 trial. Lancet Oncol. 2017;18(7):863–73.

22. Chaichana KL, Rao K, Gadkaree S, Dangelmajer S, Bettegowda C, Rigamonti D, Weingart J, Olivi A, Gallia GL, Brem H, et al. Factors associated with survival and recurrence for patients undergoing surgery of cerebellar metastases. Neurol Res. 2014;36(1):13–25.

23. Wronski M, Arbit E. Surgical treatment of brain metastases from melanoma: a retrospective study of 91 patients. J Neurosurg. 2000;93(1):9–18.

24. Liew DN, Kano H, Kondziolka D, Mathieu D, Niranjan A, Flickinger JC, Kirkwood JM, Tarhini A, Moschos S, Lunsford LD. Outcome predictors of gamma knife surgery for melanoma brain metastases. Clinical article J Neurosurg. 2011;114(3):769–79.

21

M1 macrophage recruitment correlates with worse outcome in SHH Medulloblastomas

Chanhee Lee[1], Joongyub Lee[2], Seung Ah Choi[1], Seung-Ki Kim[1], Kyu-Chang Wang[1], Sung-Hye Park[3], Se Hoon Kim[4], Ji Yeoun Lee[1,5] and Ji Hoon Phi[1*] (iD)

Abstract

Background: Recent progress in molecular analysis has advanced the understanding of medulloblastoma (MB) and is anticipated to facilitate management of the disease. MB is composed of 4 molecular subgroups: WNT, SHH, Group 3, and Group 4. Macrophages play a crucial role in the tumor microenvironment; however, the functional role of their activated phenotype (M1/M2) remains controversial. Herein, we investigate the correlation between tumor-associated macrophage (TAM) recruitment within the MB subgroups and prognosis.

Methods: Molecular subgrouping was performed by a nanoString-based RNA assay on retrieved snap-frozen tissue samples. Immunohistochemistry (IHC) and immunofluorescence (IF) assays were performed on subgroup identified samples, and the number of polarized macrophages was quantified from IHC. Survival analyses were conducted on collected clinical data and quantified macrophage data.

Results: TAM (M1/M2) recruitment in SHH MB was significantly higher compared to that in other subgroups. A Kaplan-Meier survival curve and multivariate Cox regression demonstrated that high M1 expressers showed worse overall survival (OS) and progression-free survival (PFS) than low M1 expressers in SHH MB, with relative risk (RR) values of 11.918 and 6.022, respectively.

Conclusion: M1 rather than M2 correlates more strongly with worse outcome in SHH medulloblastoma.

Keywords: Medulloblastoma, Sonic hedgehog, Macrophage, Recruitment, Prognosis

Background

Medulloblastoma (MB) is the most common pediatric brain malignancy that frequently arises below 10 years of age [1, 2]. Approximately 20–30% of patients remain incurable, and high dose radiation and chemotherapy frequently lead to significant long-term sequelae [3]. Progress in molecular diagnostics has revealed that MB is classified into 4 subgroups: WNT, SHH, Group 3 (G3) and Group 4 (G4) [1, 2, 4]. The prognosis of each subgroup ranges from being excellent in WNT MB to intermediate in SHH and G4, to poor in G3 MB [1, 4]. As subgroup-specific prognostication and personalized medicine are in demand, clinically applicable

subgrouping has become essential [3, 5–7]. Practical molecular subgrouping has been developed by multiple researchers via screening subgroup-specific signature genes using various tools, such as nanoString nCounter [3, 4, 6].

The significance of lymphocytes and tumor-associated macrophages (TAMs) in the tumor microenvironment has been perpetually examined for more than a decade; however, their comprehensive role is rather elusive [8–12]. TAMs release growth factors, cytokines, and inflammatory mediators into the environment and are classified according to their functional phenotype [13–16]. The current paradigm of macrophage polarization is undergoing reassessment. It has been commonly accepted that classically activated M1 macrophages suppress tumor growth and progression by production of reactive oxygen species (e.g., nitric oxide), whereas alternatively activated M2

* Correspondence: phi.jihoon@gmail.com
[1]Division of Pediatric Neurosurgery, Seoul National University Children's Hospital, 101 Daehakro, Jongno-gu, 110-744 Seoul, Republic of Korea
Full list of author information is available at the end of the article

macrophages promote tumor growth and progression by releasing growth factors (e.g., epidermal growth factor, fibroblast growth factor 1, vascular endothelial growth factor A) [9, 13–16]. The literature has often described conflicting roles of TAMs in various cancers due to the complexity of the tumor microenvironment and diverse contributing factors, such as immune responses, tumor stages, and types of tumors [11, 13, 17–20].

Despite the molecular insights provided by MB subgroups, relatively little is known about the role of tumor microenvironment with respect to MB and its subgroups [8]. A previous report on the characterization of immunophenotype in pediatric brain tumors suggests that MB is less infiltrated with T lymphocytes and displays an immunosuppressive M2 phenotype compared to other pediatric brain tumors [8]. A recent study demonstrated that TAM recruitment is subgroup-specific in MB, suggesting that the expression of TAM-associated genes was significantly higher in the SHH subgroup [3]. This finding indicates that SHH MB has a distinct tumor microenvironment, which may have important pathophysiological and therapeutic implications. However, the roles of TAMs and their activation phenotypes are inconclusive because the previous study did not present the prognostic connotations of TAMs in SHH MB [3].

In the present study, we investigate the correlation between TAM recruitment in SHH MB with prognosis. We identified that M1 macrophage recruitment rather than total TAM recruitment correlates more strongly with a reduced overall survival outcome within the SHH subgroup. Considering the commonly accepted role of macrophage polarization in various human cancers (M1 tumor-suppressing and M2 tumor-promoting roles), the negative prognostic implication of M1 macrophages in SHH MB is intriguing and requires further investigation.

Methods
Patients and samples
The Institutional Review Board (IRB) of the Seoul National University Hospital (SNUH) approved the study protocol (IRB approval No. 1610–027-797). To identify SHH MB, 48 snap-frozen MB tissues were retrieved from the Brain Bank of the Department of Neurosurgery, Seoul National University Hospital. Tissue samples were collected from 141 MB patients who underwent surgery at Seoul National University Children's Hospital (SNUCH) from 1999 to 2015. The molecular subgroups of the samples were partially verified via immunohistochemistry (IHC) using representative markers [4]. To solidify the molecular subgroup, a nanoString-based RNA assay was performed on these samples. Previously, we provided MB tissues to Dr. M. Taylor from the Hospital for Sick Children (Toronto, Canada) for analysis, and the molecular subgroups were provided for these cases through nanoString [10].

We collected 32 SHH MBs from two sources: cases newly tested for subgrouping ($n = 16$) and cases with subgroup information from Toronto ($n = 16$). Among the 32 known SHH MB patients, 25 patients had available formalin-fixed paraffin-embedded (FFPE) tissues. Two FFPE tissue samples were removed from selection due to small tissue size or the inability to undergo a complete experiment; 23 SHH MB samples were finally recruited from our institution. An additional 7 SHH MB FFPE tissue samples were received from Yonsei University. In total, 30 SHH MB were analyzed in the present study. Subgroups other than SHH were randomly selected with respect to FFPE tissue availability as control groups to validate the correlation between TAM infiltration and the prognosis of the subgroups (WNT = 3, Group 3 = 2, Group 4 = 17).

Subgrouping
Molecular subgroups were identified through gene profiling using nanoString nCounter [6]. Total RNA was extracted from snap-frozen patient tissue samples ($n = 48$) using the miRNeasy kit according to the manufacturer's protocol (Life Technologies, Carlsbad, CA, USA). Procedures related to hybridization, detection and scanning were performed as recommended by nanoString Technologies (Seattle, WA, USA). The collected data were normalized in R, and an algorithm for class prediction analysis was provided by Dr. M. Taylor (Toronto, Canada) [6]. The subgroup of additionally received FFPE tissue samples from Yonsei University, which were identified via immunohistochemistry (IHC), was provided by Dr. SH Kim (Seoul, Korea). For the SHH subgroup, IHC generally yields stable and concordant results with nanoString.

Immunohistochemistry
Macrophage recruitment was investigated using immunohistochemistry (IHC) on FFPE tissue samples ($n = 45$). Human tonsil tissue was used as a positive control (Additional file 1: Figure S1).The recruitment of activated macrophages was identified using the following antibodies: CD68 for total macrophages, CD86 for M1-activation, and CD163 for M2-activation (Additional file 2: Table S1). Five hot spots were randomly selected in each paraffin section, and positive cells among the 300 counterstained cells were counted using the ImageJ Cell Counter plugin [21]. The mean value of the five hot-spots count was used in the following statistical analyses. Researchers engaged in the present experiment were blinded from all clinical data, including subgroup, through data collection.

Immunofluorescence
To confirm the independent localization of M1 and M2 macrophages, an immunofluorescence (IF) assay was performed on FFPE tissue samples. The retrieved blocks

were sectioned at 4 μm using a microtome and transferred to silane-coated slides by the SNUH pathology lab. The slides were deparaffinized in xylene and rehydrated through a graded ethanol series. To retrieve antigen, the slides were microwaved in 10 mM sodium citrate buffer (pH 6.0) for 3 min, with a 15 s cooling interval after 2 min. The slides were washed three times in phosphate-buffered saline (PBS) with 0.1% bovine serum albumin (BSA) for 5 min each and then permeabilized (1× PBS/ Timerasol: 95 mg/L, saponin: 0.6 g/L, normal goat serum: 1%) for 15 min. The slides were subsequently blocked in blocking solution (1 × PBS/ Timerasol: 95 mg/L, saponin: 0.35 g/L, normal goat serum: 3.5%) for 30 min at room temperature [22]. The primary antibody was prepared in a modified blocking solution (1 × PBS/ Timerasol: 95 mg/L, saponin: 0.1 g/L, normal goat serum: 1%), with adequate dilution and incubated overnight at 4 °C. The secondary antibody was similarly diluted accordingly and applied for 1 h at room temperature.

Clinical data

Clinical data, including sex, age at diagnosis, pathology, degree of surgical resection, presence of leptomeningeal seeding at presentation, applied treatment modalities, progression, and survival, were collected independently of the researchers conducting the experiments. Progression-free survival (PFS) refers to the time interval from the day of initial surgery to the date when tumor progression was radiologically identified or the date of the last follow-up [10]. Overall survival (OS) refers to the time interval from the day of initial surgery to the date of patient death or the date of the last follow-up [10].

All 32 patients with SHH MB received chemotherapy. The chemotherapy regimens changed from 1999 to 2015. Prior to 2006, the Children's Cancer Group (CCG) 9921 regimen (3 patients) or the 8 in 1 (6 patients) regimen were applied, and from 2006, the KSPNO (Korean Society for Pediatric Neuro-Oncology) protocols for infant or child MB were applied (14 patients). Eleven patients were aged < 3 yrs. at diagnosis, and radiation therapy (RT) was delayed for these patients. Overall, 20 patients received RT. The RT doses were adapted to the risk status of each patient: the standard risk group: craniospinal axis 19.8–23.4 Gy, tumor bed boost up to 54 Gy; the high risk group: craniospinal axis 28.8–36 Gy, tumor bed boost up to 54 Gy. The three patients for whom RT was delayed did not receive RT. One patient was lost to follow-up prior to initiating RT, while another patient died at 11 months with rapid disease progression, and another patient was cured with chemotherapy alone.

Statistical analysis

Subgroup prediction analysis was conducted in R. IBM SPSS Statistics version 23 was used to perform common statistical analyses, including χ^2, bivariate Pearson's correlation, Cox regression analysis, survival analysis, and the log-rank test as previously described [10]. Appropriate indications are provided in the text and supplementary data.

Results

Identification of molecular subgroupsusing nanoString nCounter

To identify SHH MB, we performed gene profiling on 22 subgroup-specific signature genes on selected samples ($n = 48$) using nanoString nCounter [6]. We identified 5 WNT, 16 SHH, 5 Group3, and 26 Group4 MBs through class prediction analysis (Additional file 1: Figure S2); 7 of the 16 patients identified as SHH subgroup had adequate FFPE tissue samples available. Additionally, 16 SHH samples previously identified by the same method in Toronto were incorporated in the present study, yielding a total number of 23 SHH samples. Moreover, 22 randomly selected non-SHH subgroup samples were analyzed as control groups for the reliability and validity of IHC/IF techniques and counting. The subgroup of the validation cohort was pre-identified by immunohistochemistry only.

Activated macrophage recruitment in the medulloblastoma subgroups

First, we investigated the unique recruitment pattern of tumor-associated macrophages (TAM) in the different MB subgroups. Immunohistochemistry (IHC) analysis was conducted to identify macrophage recruitment (Fig. 1a), and the recruited proportion of CD68-, CD86-, and CD163-positive macrophages were quantified in each subgroup (Fig. 2a & b). The comparison was largely SHH to G4 since the numbers of other subgroups was limited. Notably, CD163-positive M2 macrophages were significantly higher in the SHH subgroup ($n = 23$) compared to that in another subgroup ($n = 22$) ($P < .001$). M1 macrophage recruitment was also significantly higher in the SHH subgroup than that in non-SHH subgroups ($P = .048$). Through immunofluorescence (IF) analysis, we confirmed that M1 and M2 macrophages, identified by CD86 and CD163, respectively, were located in different areas and were independently distinguishable (Fig. 1b).

TAM recruitment and patient characteristics

The M2 macrophage proportion also correlated with patients < 3 years of age ($P = .015$) and the lateral location of the tumor ($P = .008$), which are known indicators of the SHH subgroup (Fig. 2c). We verified that the present quantification method and results were consistent with the findings of a previous study that used a different quantification method [3].

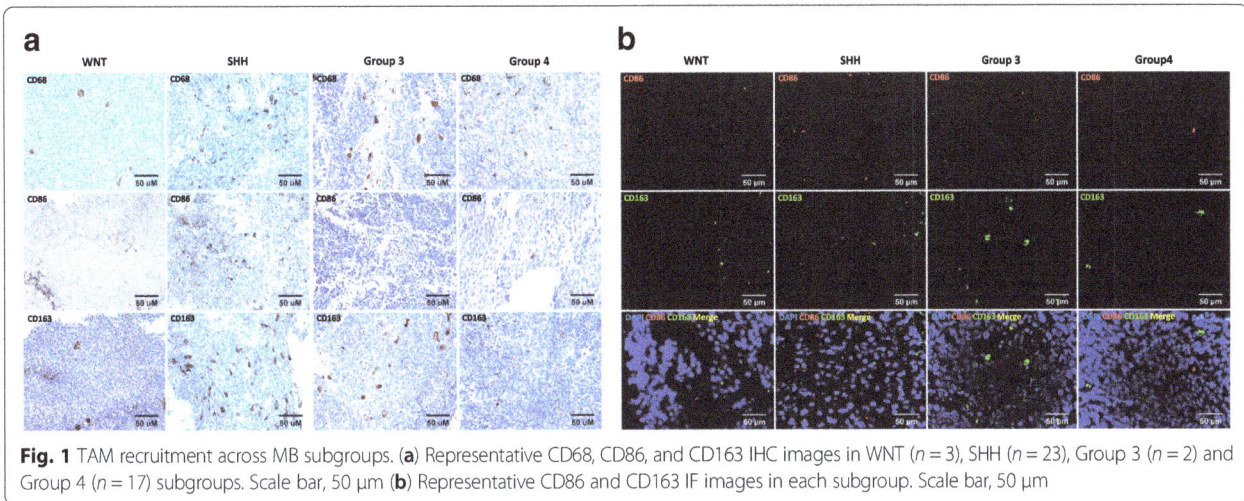

Fig. 1 TAM recruitment across MB subgroups. (**a**) Representative CD68, CD86, and CD163 IHC images in WNT ($n = 3$), SHH ($n = 23$), Group 3 ($n = 2$) and Group 4 ($n = 17$) subgroups. Scale bar, 50 μm (**b**) Representative CD86 and CD163 IF images in each subgroup. Scale bar, 50 μm

TAM recruitment and survival outcomes in MB

Statistical analysis was conducted on the collected data to demonstrate the correlation between TAM in MB and prognosis. We dichotomously defined patient groups of high and low macrophage expressers based on the median-value of the macrophage counts. OS and PFS analyses on counted M1 and M2 activation markers were performed using the Kaplan-Meier plot and log-rank test (Additional file 1: Figure S3). MB patients with high M1 counts showed a considerable trend with shorter OS ($P = .064$). However, patients with high M2 counts showed shorter PFS ($P = .037$), which did not affect the OS of these patients. Considering that

approximately half of all included cases were of the SHH subgroup and TAM is overrepresented only in this subgroup, the prognostic implications may be more clear in the SHH subgroup.

TAM recruitment and survival outcomes in SHH MB

We investigated whether SHH-specific macrophage recruitment showed a correlation with the survival outcomes in SHH MB (Fig. 3). High M1 expressers had shorter OS ($P = .013$) and a trend with shorter PFS ($P = .065$). Prognostic factors those are known to affect the outcomes, such as sex, age, and leptomeningeal seeding, were incorporated in multivariate Cox regression analysis (Tables 1 & 2).

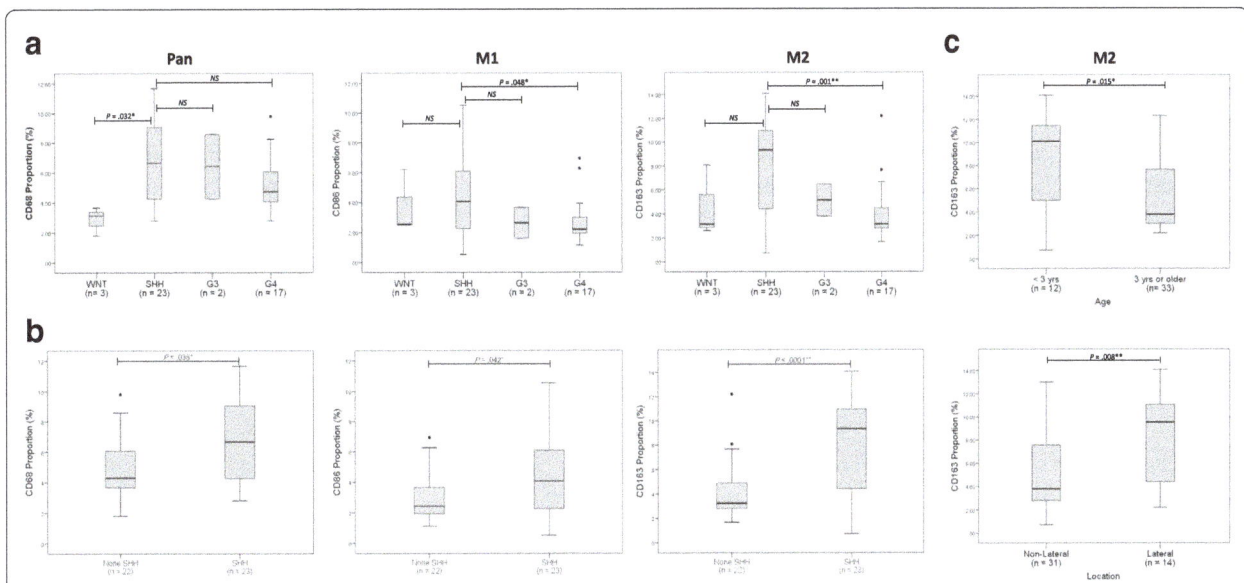

Fig. 2 Proportion of TAM recruitment in MB. (**a**) Comparison of macrophage recruitment between the 4 subgroups. The one-way ANOVA results are presented; however, due to the small number of WNT and Group 3 subgroup samples, statistical significance is neglected. (**b**) Comparison between SHH and non-SHH subgroups; CD68 ($P = .035$), CD86 ($P = .042$), and CD163 ($P < .0001$) were significantly higher in the SHH subgroup than those in the non-SHH subgroups. (**c**) CD163-positive macrophages were significantly higher in patients younger than 3 years-of-age ($P = .015$) as well as the lateral location of the tumor ($P = .008$)

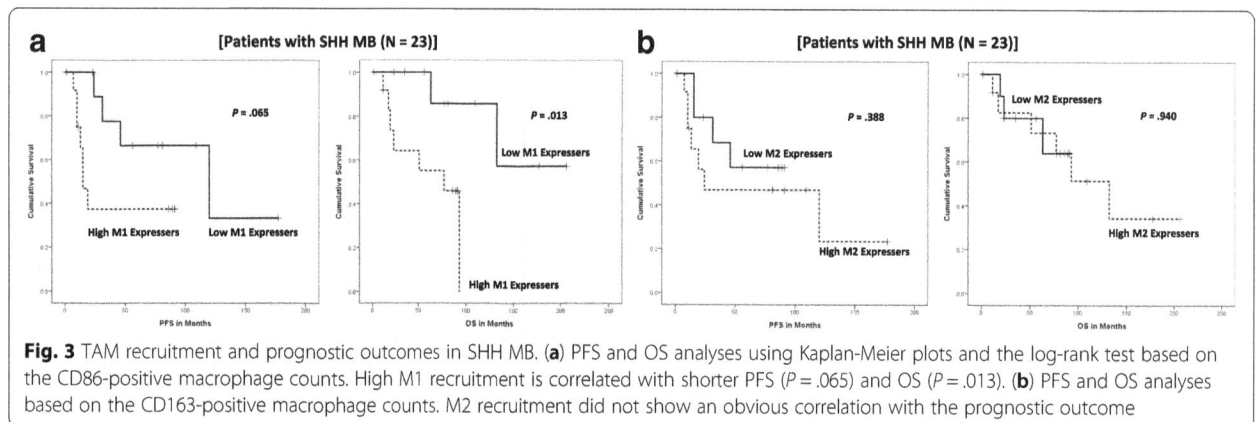

Fig. 3 TAM recruitment and prognostic outcomes in SHH MB. (**a**) PFS and OS analyses using Kaplan-Meier plots and the log-rank test based on the CD86-positive macrophage counts. High M1 recruitment is correlated with shorter PFS (P = .065) and OS (P = .013). (**b**) PFS and OS analyses based on the CD163-positive macrophage counts. M2 recruitment did not show an obvious correlation with the prognostic outcome

Interestingly, high M1 macrophages were significantly correlated with shorter OS (P = .030, RR = 11.918, 95% CI = 1.265–112.282) and PFS (P = .027, RR = 6.022, 95% CI = 1.232–29.433) in the SHH subgroup (Fig. 4). M2 macrophage recruitment did not show an obvious correlation with the outcome of SHH subgroup patients (Fig. 3b, Table 2).

TAM recruitment and other prognostic factors in SHH MB
With respect to the TAM infiltration within MB, other prognostic factors were investigated to identify potential correlations (Table 3). A multivariate analysis using binary logistic regression revealed that age, lateral tumor location, and large residual tumor ($> 1.5 cm^2$) were not significantly related to the M1 and M2 macrophage recruitment patterns in SHH MB (Additional file 2: Table. S2).

TAM and survival outcome correlation in other cohort
To further confirm the correlation between TAM recruitment and survival outcome, 7 additional SHH MB from other cohorts were separately investigated (Additional file 1: Figure S4). Due to the short follow-up (FU) period and small population, the correlation between TAM recruitment and survival outcome was not significant, but the survival graphs showed a considerable trend with the current study cohort.

Discussion
We demonstrate an unconventional correlation between subgroup-specific recruitment of TAM in SHH MB and prognosis. We confirmed subgroup-specific augmentation of M1 and M2 macrophages in SHH MB and compared this result with relevant prognostic factors. Survival analyses and Cox-regression analysis showed that M1 rather than M2 infiltration correlates better with worse OS and PFS in SHH MB, with relative risk values of 11.918 and 6.022, respectively.

The SHH MB subgroup, as suggested by its name, is thought to be driven by alterations in the Sonic-hedgehog signaling pathway [4]. The SHH pathway plays a crucial role in cerebellar development, inducing the proliferation of neuronal precursors [1, 4]. Individuals with germline or somatic mutations in the SHH pathway, such as *PTCH*, *SMO*, *SUFU*, *GLI1*, and *GLI2*, are predisposed to MB [1, 4]. Moreover, SHH MB has an intermediate prognosis among the 4 subgroups but, interestingly, is saturated with the highest number of TAMs, as demonstrated in the present and the previous one [1, 3]. A dichotomous age distribution (< 4 years and > 16 years) is another hallmark of SHH subgroup; the present study showed that the age distribution within SHH MB did not significantly correlate with activated macrophage recruitment [1].

Table 1 Relative risks for shorter PFS in SHH MB estimated with a Cox proportional hazards model

Clinical Factor	Univariate analysis			Multivariate analysis		
	P value	RR	95% CI	P value	RR	95% CI
M1 Count	.085	3.331	.848–13.091	.027	6.022	1.232–29.433
M2 Count	.399	1.727	.485–6.151	.246	2.361	.553–10.076
Age	.700	1.029	.890–1.190	.687	1.031	.890–1.194
Sex (Male)[a]	.098	.316	.081–1.237	.117	.256	.046–1.408
Leptomeningeal Seeding	.319	1.994	.514–7.736	.521	1.721	.328–9.037

RR Relative risk, *CI* Confidence interval

[a]Sex was included in the multivariate analysis model as a basic variable

Table 2 Relative risks for shorter OS in SHH MB estimated with a Cox proportional hazards model

Clinical Factor	Univariate analysis			Multivariate analysis		
	P value	RR	95% CI	P value	RR	95% CI
M1 Count	.038	9.558	1.128–81.002	.030	11.918	1.265–112.282
M2 Count	.940	1.060	.234–4.801	.601	.620	.104–3.710
Age	.111	1.146	.969–1.354	.180	1.118	.950–1.316
Sex (Male)[a]	.044	.117	.014–0.948	.080	.110	.009–1.298
Leptomeningeal Seeding	.064	4.693	.917–24.026	.422	2.097	.344–12.786

RR, Relative risk; *CI*, Confidence interval
[a]Sex was included in the multivariate analysis model as a basic variable

The recognition of microenvironment in tumor biology has escalated over the past few decades, and this emphasis has led researchers to characterize contributing factors, including immunophenotypes, in various cancers [8]. However, these studies are often limited to phenotypic characterization and lacked prognostic connotation. A previous study investigated TAM recruitment in MB and proposed subgroup-specific recruitment in SHH MB [3]. We sought to verify this phenomenal recruitment in MB by a different method. Indeed, we found corroborating results showing augmented TAM recruitment in SHH MB and confirmed its unique microenvironment. Aside from M2 macrophages, we further characterized M1 macrophages in SHH MB and investigated the prognostic connotation of their recruitment.

In the present study, high M1 macrophages correlated with poor prognosis in SHH MB patients. This result apparently contradicts the common view of tumoricidal M1 macrophages. In many cancer types, M1 macrophage infiltration is associated with better prognosis [23–25]. However, recent studies suggest that the dichotomous M1/M2 classification is oversimplified, and the role of TAM in tumors is still controversial [14, 26]. We cannot provide a conclusive role for M1 macrophages in SHH MB because the causality of the worse prognosis

associated with M1 macrophages has not been investigated. However, few plausible hypotheses can be made from the present results: 1) high M1 macrophage recruitment assists growth and progression of SHH MB contrary to its role in other cancers, 2) M1 macrophages are highly recruited to enhance the tumoricidal effect in aggressive group of SHH MB, but this mechanism alone was insufficient to fight the particular malignancy, or 3) high M1 recruitment is an epiphenomenon, and these cells are simply recruited by other SHH MB initiators and do not directly affect prognosis. Interestingly, the literature suggests multiple perspectives. The loss of nitric oxide synthase2 (NOS2) in the Ptch1[+/-]SHH MB mouse model was reported to promote development of medulloblastoma [27]. NOS2 is a key enzyme that produces nitric oxide in M1 macrophages in response to pathogens [26]. This suggests good prognostic role of M1 macrophages, which supports the second hypothesis. However, direct production of interferon-γ, a known stimulatory cytokine of M1 macrophages, in the developing brain was reported to activate the SHH pathway and cerebellar dysplasia. [28]. This activation may suggest that M1 macrophages are coincidentally recruited in response to the abnormal source of IFN-γ in the developing brain, not in recognition of MB or to

Table 3 Patient characteristics according to activated macrophage recruitment in SHH

Macrophage Polarization	CD86 (M1 macrophages)		CD163 (M2 macrophages)	
	High Expressers[a]	Low Expressers[b]	High Expressers[a]	Low Expressers[b]
Number	12	11	12	11
Mean	6.4 ± .6	2.1 ± .3	11.2 ± .4	4.6 ± .7
Age	5.0 ± 1.1	4.6 ± 1.5	5.7 ± 1.4	4.0 ± 1.2
M:F	7:5	5:6	7:5	5:6
Lateral tumor location	7 (30%)	7 (30%)	8 (35%)	6 (26%)
Gross total resection	10 (43%)	6 (26%)	9 (39%)	7 (30%)
Large residual tumor (> 1.5cm^2)	1 (4%)	3 (13%)	2 (9%)	2 (9%)
Leptomeningeal Seeding	3 (13%)	2 (9%)	3 (13%)	2 (9%)

[a]High expressers indicates patients with greater than or equal to median count.
[b]Low expressers indicates patients with lower than median count

destroy it. Such conflicting perspectives may also suggest a context-dependent role for TAM.

The small number of patients is a major limitation of the present study. The heterogeneity of the treatment administered to the patients may also confound the results, although all patients followed modernized treatment protocols in terms of risk stratification, chemotherapy regimen, and RT doses. Further validation in a comparable MB cohort is required to consolidate the role of TAM in SHH MB.

Conclusion

High M1 macrophage recruitment correlated with a worse prognostic outcome in SHH MB. The present results are unconventional, yet intriguing, as the commonly accepted role of M1 macrophages should demonstrate the opposite effect. However, additional follow-up studies are required; the present study is limited because of its small sample size and strong dependence on the IHC results. Further in vitro and in vivo studies should be performed to determine the mechanism and causality of the worse prognostic outcome associated with M1 macrophages in SHH MB.

Additional files

Additional file 1: Figure S1. Macrophage recruitment in human tonsil FFPE tissue. **Figure S2.** Expression heatmap of 22 subgroup-specific signature genes in 48 study patients by the nanoString nCounter System. **Figure S3.** TAM recruitment and prognostic outcomes in the whole patient cohort. **Figure S4.** TAM recruitment and prognostic outcomes in SHH MB from Yonsei University.

Additional file 2: Table S1. List of antibodies used for immunohistochemistry and immunofluorescence assay **Table S2.** Correlation between TAM and other prognostic factors estimated with a logistic regression in SHH MB.

Abbreviations

CD163: Cluster of differentiation 163; CD68: Cluster of differentiation 86; CD86: Cluster of differentiation 86; FFPE: Formalin-fixed paraffin-embedded; G3: Group 3; G4: Group4; IF: Immunofluorescence; IHC: Immunohistochemistry; IRB: Institutional review board; MB: Medulloblastoma; NOS2: Nitric oxide synthase2; OS: Overall survival; PBS: Phosphate-buffered saline; PFS: Progression-free survival; RR: Relative risk; SHH: Sonic hedgehog; TAM: Tumor-associated macrophages; WNT: Wingless/Integrated

Acknowledgments

The authors would like to thank the reviewers and editors for detailed analysis of the present manuscript and constructive comments and suggestions.

Funding

The present study was financially supported by a grant from the National R&D Program for Cancer Control, Ministry for Health and Welfare, Republic of Korea (1420020).

Author's contributions

JHP supervised the development of the study, produced the study, and approved the final manuscript. CL performed the experiments, interpreted the data and drafted the manuscript. JL gave advice on statistical analysis. KCW, SKK, JYL, and SAC critically reviewed the manuscript. SHP reviewed the pathology slides and IHC control verification. SHK reviewed the pathology slides for the validation cohort and the clinical information. All of the authors read and approved the final manuscript.

Competing interests

The authors disclose no potential conflicts of interest.

Author details

¹Division of Pediatric Neurosurgery, Seoul National University Children's Hospital, 101 Daehakro, Jongno-gu, 110-744 Seoul, Republic of Korea. ²Medical Research Collaborating Center, Seoul National University Hospital, Seoul, South Korea. ³Department of Pathology, Seoul National University College of Medicine, Seoul, Republic of Korea. ⁴Department of Pathology, Yonsei University, College of Medicine, Severance Hospital, Seoul, Republic of Korea. ⁵Department of Anatomy, Seoul National University College of Medicine, Seoul, South Korea.

References

1. RM DS, Jones BR, Lowis SP, Kurian KM. Pediatric medulloblastoma - update on molecular classification driving targeted therapies. Front Oncol. 2014;176(4).
2. Louis DN, Perry A, Reifenberger G, von Deimling A, Figarella-Branger D, Cavenee WK, Ohgaki H, Wiestler OD, Kleihues P, Ellison DW. The 2016 World Health Organization classification of tumors of the central nervous system: a summary. Acta Neuropathol. 2016;131(6):803–20.
3. Margol AS, Robison NJ, Gnanachandran J, Hung LT, Kennedy RJ, Vali M, Dhall G, Finlay JL, Erdreich-Epstein A, Krieger MD, et al. Tumor-associated macrophages in SHH subgroup of medulloblastomas. Clinical cancer research : an official journal of the American Association for Cancer Research. 2015;21(6):1457–65.
4. Taylor MD, Northcott PA, Korshunov A, Remke M, Cho YJ, Clifford SC, Eberhart CG, Parsons DW, Rutkowski S, Gajjar A, et al. Molecular subgroups of medulloblastoma: the current consensus. Acta Neuropathol. 2012;123(4):465–72.
5. Kool M, Korshunov A, Remke M, Jones DT, Schlanstein M, Northcott PA, Cho YJ, Koster J, Schouten-van Meeteren A, van Vuurden D, et al. Molecular subgroups of medulloblastoma: an international meta-analysis of transcriptome, genetic aberrations, and clinical data of WNT, SHH, group 3, and group 4 medulloblastomas. Acta Neuropathol. 2012;123(4):473–84.
6. Northcott PA, Shih DJ, Remke M, Cho YJ, Kool M, Hawkins C, Eberhart CG, Dubuc A, Guettouche T, Cardentey Y, et al. Rapid, reliable, and reproducible molecular sub-grouping of clinical medulloblastoma samples. Acta Neuropathol. 2012;123(4):615–26.
7. Triscott J, Lee C, Foster C, Manoranjan B, Pambid MR, Berns R, Fotovati A, Venugopal C, O'Halloran K, Narendran A, et al. Personalizing the treatment of pediatric medulloblastoma: polo-like kinase 1 as a molecular target in high-risk children. Cancer Res. 2013;73(22):6734–44.
8. Griesinger AM, Birks DK, Donson AM, Amani V, Hoffman LM, Waziri A, Wang M, Handler MH, Foreman NK. Characterization of distinct immunophenotypes across pediatric brain tumor types. J Immunol. 2013; 191(9):4880–8.
9. Kennedy BC, Showers CR, Anderson DE, Anderson L, Canoll P, Bruce JN, Anderson RC. Tumor-associated macrophages in glioma: friend or foe? J. Oncol. 2013;2013:486912.
10. Komohara Y, Ohnishi K, Kuratsu J, Takeya M. Possible involvement of the M2 anti-inflammatory macrophage phenotype in growth of human gliomas. J Pathol. 2008;216(1):15–24.
11. Herrera M, Herrera A, Dominguez G, Silva J, Garcia V, Garcia JM, Gomez I, Soldevilla B, Munoz C, Provencio M, et al. Cancer-associated fibroblast and M2 macrophage markers together predict outcome in colorectal cancer patients. Cancer Sci. 2013;104(4):437–44.

12. Sica A, Larghi P, Mancino A, Rubino L, Porta C, Totaro MG, Rimoldi M, Biswas SK, Allavena P, Mantovani A. Macrophage polarization in tumour progression. Semin Cancer Biol. 2008;18(5):349–55.

13. Almatroodi SA, McDonald CF, Darby IA, Pouniotis DS. Characterization of M1/M2 tumour-associated macrophages (TAMs) and Th1/Th2 cytokine profiles in patients with NSCLC. Cancer Microenviron. 2016;9(1):1–11.

14. Martinez FO, Gordon S. The M1 and M2 paradigm of macrophage activation: time for reassessment. F1000prime reports. 2014;6:13.

15. Mills CD. Anatomy of a discovery: m1 and m2 macrophages. Front Immunol. 2015;6:212.

16. Italiani P, Boraschi D. From monocytes to M1/M2 macrophages: phenotypical vs functional differentiation. Front Immunol. 2014;5:514.

17. Zhang M, He Y, Sun X, Li Q, Wang W, Zhao A, Di W. A high M1/M2 ratio of tumor-associated macrophages is associated with extended survival in ovarian cancer patients. Journal of ovarian research. 2014;7:19.

18. Squadrito ML, De Palma M. A niche role for periostin and macrophages in glioblastoma. Nat Cell Biol. 2015;17(2):107–9.

19. Barros MH, Hassan R, Niedobitek G. Tumor-associated macrophages in pediatric classical Hodgkin lymphoma: association with Epstein-Barr virus, lymphocyte subsets, and prognostic impact. Clinical cancer research : an official journal of the American Association for Cancer Research. 2012;18(14):3762–71.

20. Williams CB, Yeh ES, Soloff AC. Tumor-associated macrophages: unwitting accomplices in breast cancer malignancy. NPJ breast cancer. 2016;2

21. Schneider CA, Rasband WS, Eliceiri KW. NIH image to ImageJ: 25 years of image analysis. Nat Methods. 2012;9(7):671–5.

22. Lee JY, Moon YJ, Lee HO, Park AK, Choi SA, Wang KC, Han JW, Joung JG, Kang HS, Kim JE, et al. Deregulation of Retinaldehyde dehydrogenase 2 leads to defective Angiogenic function of endothelial Colony-forming cells in pediatric Moyamoya disease. Arterioscler Thromb Vasc Biol. 2015;35(7):1670–7.

23. Wang XL, Jiang JT, Wu CP. Prognostic significance of tumor-associated macrophage infiltration in gastric cancer: a meta-analysis. Genetics and molecular research : GMR. 2016;15(4)

24. Mei J, Xiao Z, Guo C, Pu Q, Ma L, Liu C, Lin F, Liao H, You Z, Liu L. Prognostic impact of tumor-associated macrophage infiltration in non-small cell lung cancer: a systemic review and meta-analysis. Oncotarget. 2016; 7(23):34217–28.

25. Edin S, Wikberg ML, Dahlin AM, Rutegard J, Oberg A, Oldenborg PA, Palmqvist R. The distribution of macrophages with a M1 or M2 phenotype in relation to prognosis and the molecular characteristics of colorectal cancer. PLoS One. 2012;7(10):e47045.

26. Van Overmeire E, Laoui D, Keirsse J, Van Ginderachter JA, Sarukhan A. Mechanisms driving macrophage diversity and specialization in distinct tumor microenvironments and parallelisms with other tissues. Front Immunol. 2014;5:127.

27. Haag D, Zipper P, Westrich V, Karra D, Pfleger K, Toedt G, Blond F, Delhomme N, Hahn M, Reifenberger J, et al. Nos2 inactivation promotes the development of medulloblastoma in Ptch1(+/−) mice by deregulation of Gap43-dependent granule cell precursor migration. PLoS Genet. 2012;8(3):e1002572.

28. Wang J, Lin W, Popko B, Campbell IL. Inducible production of interferon-gamma in the developing brain causes cerebellar dysplasia with activation of the sonic hedgehog pathway. Mol Cell Neurosci. 2004;27(4):489–96.

22

A randomised trial to compare cognitive outcome after gamma knife radiosurgery versus whole brain radiation therapy in patients with multiple brain metastases: research protocol CAR-study B

Wietske C. M. Schimmel[1,3*], Eline Verhaak[1,3], Patrick E. J. Hanssens[1,2], Karin Gehring[1,2,3] and Margriet M. Sitskoorn[2,3]

Abstract

Background: Gamma Knife radiosurgery (GKRS) is increasingly applied in patients with multiple brain metastases and is expected to have less adverse effects in cognitive functioning than whole brain radiation therapy (WBRT). Effective treatment with the least negative cognitive side effects is increasingly becoming important, as more patients with brain metastases live longer due to more and better systemic treatment options. There are no published randomized trials yet directly comparing GKRS to WBRT in patients with multiple brain metastases that include objective neuropsychological testing.

Methods: CAR-Study B is a prospective randomised trial comparing cognitive outcome after GKRS or WBRT in adult patients with 11–20 newly diagnosed brain metastases on a contrast-enhanced MRI-scan, KPS ≥70 and life expectancy of at least 3 months. Randomisation by the method of minimization, is stratified by the cumulative tumour volume in the brain, systemic treatment, KPS, histology, baseline cognitive functioning and age. The primary endpoint is the between-group difference in the percentage of patients with significant memory decline at 3 months.

Secondary endpoints include overall survival, local control, development of new brain metastases, cognitive functioning over time, quality of life, depression, anxiety and fatigue. Cognitive functioning is assessed by a standardised neuropsychological test battery.

Assessments (cognitive testing, questionnaires and MRI-scans) are scheduled at baseline and at 3, 6, 9, 12 and 15 months after treatment.

Discussion: Knowledge gained from this trial may be used to inform individual patients with BM more precisely about the cognitive effects they can expect from treatment, and to assist both doctors and patients in making (shared) individual treatment decisions. This trial is currently recruiting. Target accrual: 23 patients at 3-months follow-up in both groups.

Keywords: Brain metastases, Gamma knife radiosurgery, Stereotactic radiosurgery, Whole brain radiation therapy, Cognitive functioning, Hopkins verbal learning test, Quality of life, Neuropsychological assessment

* Correspondence: w.c.m.schimmel@tilburguniversity.edu
[1]Gamma Knife Centre Tilburg, Elisabeth TweeSteden Hospital,
Hilvarenbeekseweg 60, 5022, GC, Tilburg, The Netherlands
[3]Department of Cognitive Neuropsychology, Tilburg University, Warandelaan
2, 5037, AB, Tilburg, The Netherlands
Full list of author information is available at the end of the article

Background

Brain metastases (BM) are the most common tumours in the central nervous system, and account for 20% of cancer deaths each year [1]. Twenty to 40% of all cancer patients develop one or multiple BM during the course of their illness [2]. If left untreated, these patients display a median survival of only one or two months [3, 4]. Most BM originate from lung, breast, skin, kidney, gastrointestinal tract, lymphoma, and prostate [1, 5, 6]. The incidence of BM is thought to be rising as a result of the growing elderly population and advances in cancer treatments which prolong life, allowing for BM to develop [2, 7–10].

Most patients with BM already have cognitive deficits prior to BM treatment due to the BM itself, epilepsy or medication use (i.e., corticosteroids, anti-epileptic drugs, chemotherapy, other systemic therapies) [11–13]. Whole brain radiation therapy (WBRT) has long been the mainstay of treatment for patients with BM [14, 15]. However, its use has decreased in recent years due to advances in radiation technology and growing concerns regarding the often persistent adverse effects after 6–24 months on cognitive function (e.g., memory, attention and concentration impairments as measured with objective neuropsychological tests) [9, 16–18]. Meanwhile, treatment has diversified and stereotactic radiosurgery (SRS) is increasingly employed in the management of (multiple) BM to spare healthy tissue and thereby aiming to prevent cognitive side effects [16, 19, 20].

Due to increased efficacy of systemic cancer treatments there is a growing number of patients with BM that live long enough (i.e., > 6 months) to experience radiation-induced brain injury, including cognitive decline [21, 22]. Because cognitive functions are essential for our daily social, occupational and personal life, and are related to therapy compliance and quality of life in general, a full understanding of the cognitive side effects of radiotherapy is essential.

Traditionally, radiation-induced brain injury is divided into three categories: acute, early delayed, and late delayed [23–25]. Acute and early delayed injury (after 1–6 months) are thought to be of a transient nature. Late delayed injury (after 6–24 months) on the other hand is usually more severe and irreversible. Patients with late delayed effects most often exhibit progressive impairments in memory, visual motor processing, problem solving ability, and attention, all of which can be very debilitating in daily life. It has been demonstrated that the extent of delayed cognitive impairment correlates positively with the total dose received and with the time-dose-fractionation scheme [12, 16].

Radiation-induced brain injury can result from direct neurotoxic effects or indirectly through metabolic abnormalities, microvascular changes, enhanced cytokine gene expression, persistent oxidative stress and inflammatory processes [24, 26, 27]. In addition, radiation therapy may, disrupt hippocampal neurogenesis, which may, in turn, negatively affect memory and learning functions [28, 29].

Among patients with 1–4 BM, the use of SRS has received widespread acceptance and is supported by prospective data [19, 30]. In addition, SRS has been proven effective as the initial treatment option for patients with multiple BM: Mostly for patients with 5–10 BM, but also for patients with > 10 BM and even for patients with > 20 BM [31–37]. Yamamoto and colleagues conducted a case-matched study comparing treatment results after SRS for patients with 2–9 versus > 10 BM. Approximately 90% of all patients died of extracranial disease, regardless of the number of BM. Survival times did not differ significantly between groups. It was concluded that these carefully selected patients with > 10 BM (controlled primary cancer, no extracerebral BM, better KPS scores, and higher RPA class) might be favourable candidates for SRS alone [33].

Additionally, according to the US guideline on BM there is growing evidence suggesting that cumulative tumour volume in the brain is a better selection criterion for SRS than the number of BM [38]. Accordingly, guidelines no longer specify an upper limit for the number of brain metastases [38, 39].

In comparison to WBRT, SRS has the better ability to spare healthy tissue because of the high level of precision and the quick dose fall-off. Therefore, treatment with SRS is expected to cause fewer cognitive side effects than WBRT. However, there are no published trials yet directly comparing SRS alone versus WBRT alone, that include objective neuropsychological testing. This prospective randomised study (CAR-Study B), will yield information on which treatment modality, Gamma Knife radiosurgery (a form of SRS) or WBRT, best preserves cognitive function in patients with 11–20 BM, as assessed with reliable and valid neuropsychological tests. These tests are recommended by the International Cognition and Cancer Taskforce (ICCTF) [40]. Knowledge gained from this trial may possibly change clinical practice and international guidelines on BM.

This randomised trial is one of the two Cognition and Radiation studies (The CAR-Studies: CAR-Study A and B). CAR-Study A is a longitudinal trial assessing cognitive functions after Gamma Knife radiosurgery (GKRS) alone in patients with 1–10 BM (Clinicaltrials.gov identifier: NCT02953756).

Objectives

CAR-Study B aims to assess, in a randomised design, change in cognitive performance after treatment with either GKRS or WBRT in patients with multiple (11–20) BM.

The primary objective is to determine the between-group difference in the percentages of patients with significant cognitive decline at 3 months after treatment as assessed by the Hopkins Verbal Learning Test-Revised (a memory task). The primary hypothesis is that the percentage of patients with reliable cognitive decline at 3 months will be significantly higher after treatment with WBRT in comparison to GKRS, in patients with 11–20 newly diagnosed BM.

Secondary outcome measures

- Cognitive functioning over time (max 15 months)
- Overall survival
- Local control
- Development of new BM
- Patient Reported Outcomes (PROs)
- Fatigue
- Depression and anxiety
- Quality of life

Methods/design
Trial design

CAR-Study B is a two-arm randomised trial. Adult cancer patients (n = 46), with 11–20 BM, Karnofsky Performance Status (KPS) $\geq$ 70 and a life expectancy of at least 3 months, are screened for inclusion and exclusion criteria (Table 1) by the radiation-oncologist. Eligible patients are invited for study participation at their first visit at the Gamma Knife Centre. During this first consultation, patients receive an information letter about the study and its procedures.

After signing a written informed consent statement, co-signed by the principle investigator or a formally delegated authorized person, a baseline neuropsychological assessment (NPA) is performed. Subsequently, patients are randomised by the method of minimisation 1:1 to either GKRS (n = 23) or WBRT (n = 23). The trial schema and randomisation factors are shown in Fig. 1. The trial has been approved by the local medical ethics review committee (METC Brabant, The Netherlands). Patients from both arms are followed up at 3, 6, 9, 12 and 15 months after treatment. High rates of attrition and noncompliance are very common in trials in patients with metastatic disease [14, 41]. In an attempt to maximize patient comfort and convenience, the administration of the test battery and additional questionnaires is combined with usual care clinical visits on site (3-monthly contrast MRI-scans and consult with the radiation-oncologist).

In both groups, chemotherapy is administered at the discretion of the primary physician and recorded by the research team. Type and duration of systemic therapy, use of steroids and other medication are accurately monitored and registered. Treatment side effects for both arms are recorded according to the National Cancer Institute Common Terminology Criteria for Adverse Events (CTCAE version 4). Patients in both treatment arms may receive additional GKRS or WBRT, or salvage surgery when recurrences occur at any one of successive follow-ups; these additional treatments are recorded.

Participants

Patients who meet the inclusion and exclusion criteria (Table 1) are eligible for the study. It is projected to include 46 patients.

Table 1 Eligibility criteria - inclusions and exclusions

Inclusion criteria	Exclusion criteria
• Histologically proven malignant cancer	• Primary brain tumour
• Gadolinium-enhanced volumetric MRI-scan showing 11–20 newly diagnosed BM	• A second active primary tumour
	• Small Cell Lung Cancer, Lymphoma, Leukaemia, Meningeal disease
• Cumulative tumour volume in the brain $\leq$30 cm^3	• Prior brain treatment (radiation/surgery)
• Lesion > 3 mm from the optic apparatus	• Upfront planned surgery after GKRS
• Patient age $\geq$ 18 years	• History of a significant neurological or psychiatric disorder
• Karnofsky Performance Status $\geq$70	• Participation in a concurrent study in which neuropsychological or quality of life assessments are involved
• Anticipated survival $\geq$3 months	• Underlying medical condition precluding adequate follow-up
• Patient informed consent obtained (verifying that patients are aware of the investigational nature of this study)	• Patients unable to complete test battery due to any of the following reasons:
• Patients can be undergoing concurrent systemic therapy at the discretion of their treating oncologist	○ Lack of basic proficiency in Dutch
	○ IQ < 85
	○ Severe aphasia
	○ Paralysis grade 0–3 (MRC scale)
	○ Severe visual problems

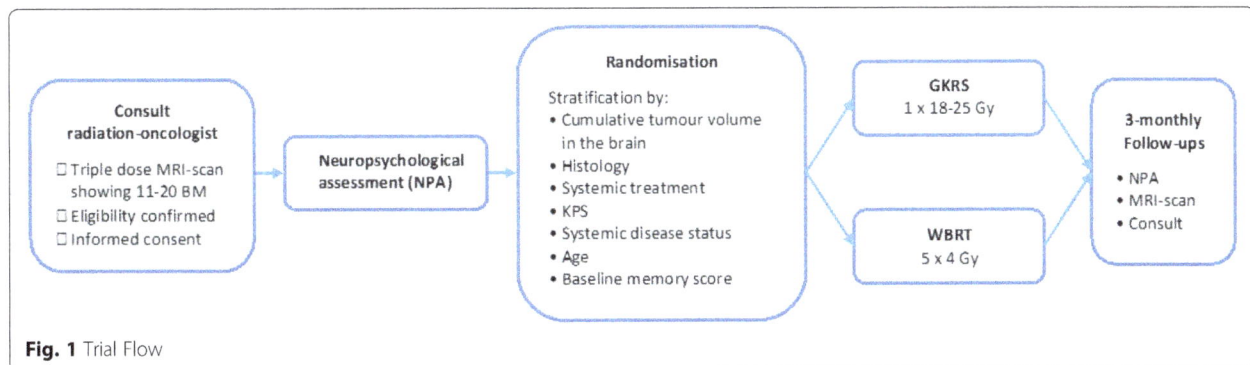

Fig. 1 Trial Flow

Setting
Gamma Knife Centre Tilburg, Department of Neurosurgery, Elisabeth-TweeSteden hospital, The Netherlands.

Interventions
Gamma knife radiosurgery (GKRS)
GKRS is performed with a Leksell Gamma Knife® ICON, Elekta Instruments, AB. Depending upon the volume and location, a dose of 18–25 Gy is prescribed with 99–100% coverage of the target. Dose limits for organs at risk are as follows: brainstem: 18 Gy, optic chiasm or optic nerves: 8–10 Gy.

Whole brain radiation therapy (WBRT)
Dose and fractionation scheme will be at the discretion of the treating radiation oncologist (in a tertiary referral hospital dedicated to radiotherapeutic oncology), though most commonly used dose and fractionation schemes are 20 Gy in 5 fractions of 4 Gy (standard schedule in Europe) and 30 Gy in 10 fractions of 3 Gy (occasionally used schedule).

Neuropsychological assessment (NPA) and patient-reported outcomes (PROs)
A reliable, valid neuropsychological test battery (Table 2) is used to assess cognitive functioning [40, 42, 43] and is administered by a trained neuropsychologist. In addition, measures of patient-reported outcomes (PROs) are used to assess anxiety and depression, quality of life and fatigue (Table 2). The total time for neuropsychological test administration, including assessment of PROs, ranges from approximately 60 to 90 min.

Assessment of outcome
Primary endpoint
The primary endpoint is the between-group difference in the percentages of patients with significant memory decline at 3 months after treatment. Memory decline is defined as a 5-point decrease from baseline in HVLT-R Total Recall score, based on a reliable change index

(RCI) [44]. This definition is based on the result reported by Chang et al. in 2009 [45].

Secondary endpoints

- Differences in percentages of patients with a ≥ 5-point decrease in HVLT-R total recall between treatment arms are evaluated at 6, 9, 12 and 15 months as is done for the primary endpoint at 3 months.
- Group mean scores for all neuropsychological tests and questionnaires are determined for both treatment arms at baseline, 3, 6, 9, 12 and 15 months.
- Percentages of patients with cognitive impairment are determined at baseline, 3, 6, 9, 12 and 15 months.
- Overall survival is calculated as the time from the first day of treatment to date of death.
- The RANO-BM criteria (Response Assessment in Neuro-Oncology Brain Metastases [46]) are used to determine local and distant tumour control.

Randomisation
A software package (ALEA®) is used to support the online patient registration and randomisation, which is based on the minimization method [47]. Groups are balanced on various prognostic factors. This method has been proven to provide more balanced groups in smaller trials when compared with both restricted (stratified) and unrestricted (simple) randomisation, and is able to incorporate more prognostic factors [47–49]. The Dutch Cancer Institute provides access to the online minimization program [50].

Eligible patients are assigned in 1:1 to either GKRS or WBRT. Prognostic factors included in the minimization algorithm are:

- Cumulative tumour volume in the brain (≤10 cm^3 vs. > 10 cm^3).
- Histology (lung vs. other).
- Any systemic treatment (yes vs. no).

Table 2 Neuropsychological test battery and patient-reported outcomes (PROs)

Cognitive Domain	Cognitive Test
Verbal memory	Hopkins Verbal Learning Test-Revised (HVLT-R)
Cognitive flexibility	Trail Making Test B (TMT B)
Word Fluency	Controlled Oral Word Association (COWA)
Working memory	Wechsler Adult Intelligence Scale - Digit Span
Processing speed	Wechsler Adult Intelligence Scale - Digit Symbol
Motor dexterity	Grooved Pegboard (GP)
Patient Reported Outcomes	Questionnaire
Quality of life	Functional Assessment of Cancer Therapy-Brain (FACT-Br)[a]
	• Physical well-being (PWB)
	• Functional well-being (FWB)
	• Social well-being (SWB)
	• Emotional well-being (EWB)
	• Brain Cancer Subscale (BRCS)
Fatigue	Multidimensional Fatigue Inventory (MFI)[a]
	• General fatigue
	• Reduced motivation
	• Physical fatigue
	• Mental fatigue
	• Reduced activity
Anxiety and depression	Hospital Anxiety and Depression Scale (HADS)[b]
	• Anxiety
	• Depression

[a]Published normative data of FACT-Br and MFI are used for the interpretation of quality of life and fatigue scores [55, 56]
[b]A cut-off point ≥8 is used to indicate symptoms of depression or anxiety [57]

- Karnofsky Performance Status (70–80 vs. 90–100).
- Age (18–59 vs. 60 and over).
- Baseline HVLT-R (≤17 vs. 18–27 vs. ≥28, based on the trial by Chang et al., 2009).

Statistical methods

The Bayesian power analysis and interim analyses are based on the randomised trial by Chang and colleagues [45]. An independent statistician will do interim monitoring of this trial using Bayesian statistical methods [51, 52]. Each patient's HVLT-R total recall score recorded at 3 months is assigned a binary outcome: A decline in the total recall score of 5 points or greater compared with baseline will be considered a *failure* (0). A stable or improved score, or a decline of 4 points or less compared with baseline will be considered a *success* (1). The failure rate for treatment k is designated qk. The prior failure rates for both treatment groups will be modelled as Beta(2.09, 2.91)-distributions, with a mean of 0.42 for both groups (for details see Appendix). During the trial, stopping rules specify that in the case of a probability greater than 0.975 for the event that the failure rate of one treatment group is higher than the failure rate of the other

treatment group, we will stop randomising patients to that treatment-arm. In this case, the study is terminated prematurely and the central research question will be answered. If the effect sizes are comparable to earlier accounts in the literature (following Chang et al. an effect size of 0.30 is expected), the early stopping rule will likely come into effect when 46 patients are enrolled (23 patients at 3-months follow-up in both groups; for details see Appendix).

Group analyses are carried out on an intent-to-treat principle. Raw cognitive test scores are compared with published normative values according to age (and, if available, to education) and converted into standardized scores. Cognitive impairment is defined as test performance at or below − 1.5 SD from the normative mean [6, 53]. Reliable change indices (RCI), reflecting change at the individual level in the context of observed changes based on published normative data, correcting for measurement errors are calculated, since group results may mask the variability in individual responses to the intervention [44]. Number of patients, who have improved versus the number of patients who remained stable, or declined, will be counted for all follow-up assessments.

These will be compared over conditions with chi-square tests.

Repeated measures analysis of variance with adjustment for potential confounders will be used, comparing subsequent follow-ups to baseline to assess cognitive change of group means over time and across treatment arms. These analyses are similar to those of the study of Chang et al. in which an identical cognitive endpoint was formulated [45].

Missing data, if not too many, will be explicitly or implicitly (dependent on the statistical technique of choice) imputed to facilitate intention-to-treat analysis. Multiple imputation may be used for explicit imputation of missing values. Alternatively, we may use linear mixed models that implicitly deal with missing data under the assumption of missing at random.

Type and duration of systemic therapy and medication use will be taken into account if necessary.

Operational considerations

In case of new intracranial tumour activity, patients in both treatment arms may receive additional WBRT or GKRS at the discretion of the treating radiation-oncologist.

Discussion

Over the past decade, the management of patients with brain metastases has changed substantially. WBRT has long been the mainstay of treatment, especially in patients with more than 3 or 4 brain metastases. However, increasingly more patients with brain metastases are treated with SRS. SRS is well established in patients with a limited number of brain metastases (1–4) and research on SRS in patients with multiple (> 4) brain metastases is growing steadily. According to the *American Society for Radiation Oncology* (ASTRO) and the *National Comprehensive Cancer Network Clinical Practice Guidelines in Oncology* (NCCN) there now is growing evidence suggesting that the cumulative *volume* of the brain metastases, rather than the *number* of brain metastases, is a better selection criterion for SRS. Accordingly, the NCCN guideline no longer specifies an upper limit for the number of brain metastases [38, 39].

In addition, concerns about the potential late adverse effects of WBRT on cognitive function has led to decreased use of (adjuvant) WBRT. Compared to WBRT, SRS has a better ability to spare healthy tissue because of the high level of precision and quick dose fall-off. Therefore, few(er) negative cognitive side-effects could be expected after treatment with SRS.

Cognitive functions are essential to our daily functioning and quality of life. Since more patients with brain metastases live longer after treatment, reducing or preventing (late) cognitive side effects is of great importance. CAR-Study B will yield information on which treatment modality, GKRS or WBRT, best preserves cognitive functions and quality of life of these patients. In addition to survival and tumour related outcomes, CAR-Study B measures relevant clinical outcomes, such as depression, anxiety and fatigue which are important psychological factors that may influence cognitive functioning [54]. Together with other trials, CAR-Study B may help diminish the controversy about the role of SRS versus WBRT in the management of multiple BM.

We chose the 3-months primary endpoint because *early* effects of radiation on cognition, albeit mostly transient, can negatively affect patients' quality of life. Moreover, at this point in time we will be able to assess cognitive function in as many of the patients enrolled, maintaining the highest possible statistical power.

The more persistent *late delayed* effects of radiation on cognitive functioning become apparent 6–12 months after treatment [22] and may be most disruptive for patients' quality of life. For this reason, we have also included long-term assessments in our design. Information on test performance in long-term survivors is essential for complete comprehension of the course of cognitive functions over time, even though many of the enrolled patients may have deceased at this point in the study.

This study may be highly relevant in clinical decision-making; knowledge gained from this trial may possibly change clinical practice and international guidelines on BM. For example, thus far in the Netherlands, the standard of care for patients with multiple brain metastases (> 4) has remained WBRT. Ultimately, the purpose of CAR-Study B is to inform patients and doctors which treatment modality, GKRS or WBRT, best preserves cognitive functions and quality of life. This will enable patients and doctors to make shared treatment decisions grounded on scientific evidence and consequently maximize the clinical outcome of each individual patient.

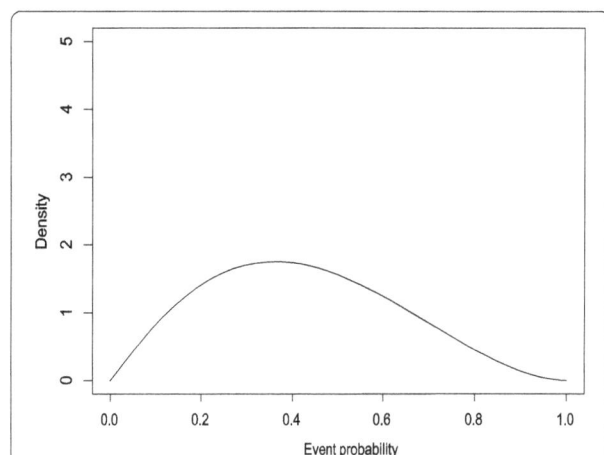

Fig. 2 Prior distributions for failure rates of both groups, with prior mean 0.42

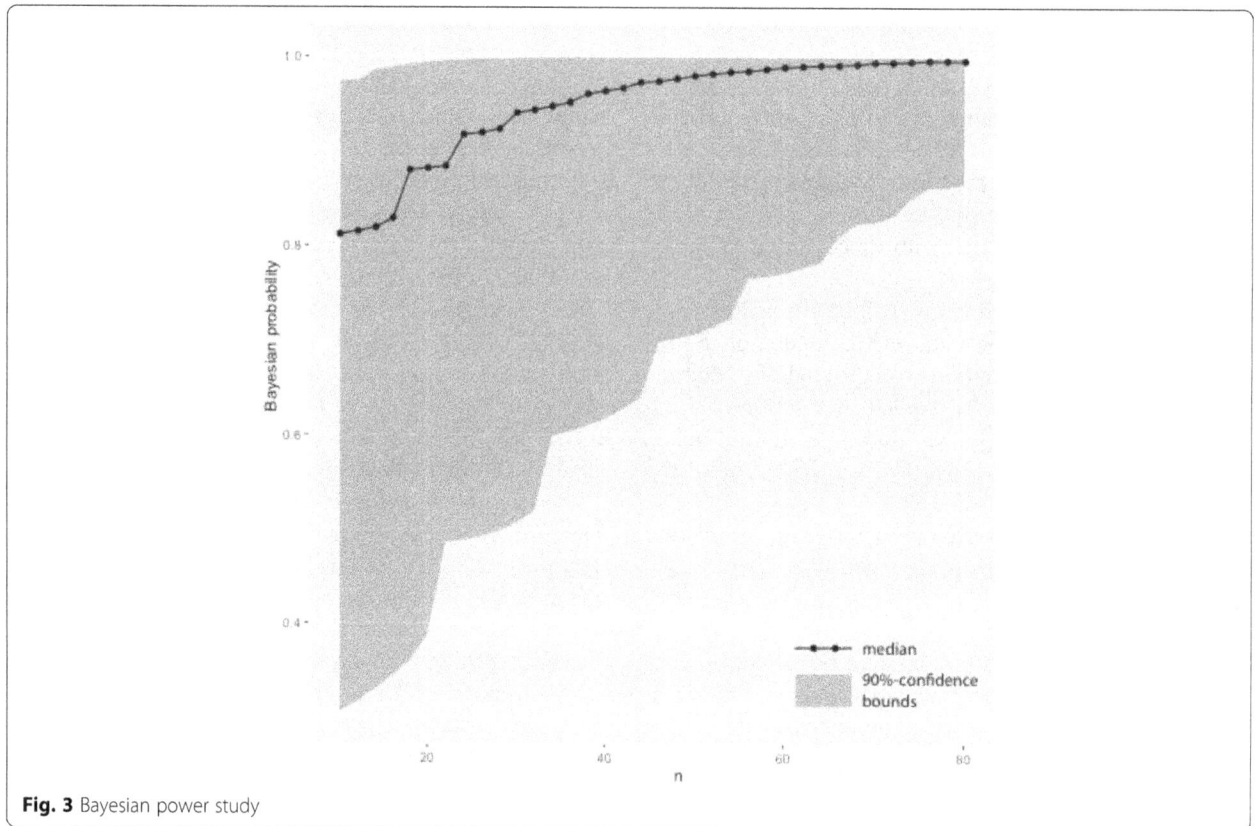

Fig. 3 Bayesian power study

Protocol

A copy of the current study protocol can be requested from Karin Gehring, PhD.

Appendix

For the Bayesian stopping rule, a weakly informative prior is employed with Beta(2.09,2.91)-distributions for both treatment groups. This prior contains the same amount of information as the prior of Chang et al. (2009). Furthermore, the prior mean is equal to 0.42 which is the sample average of the failure rates based on the results of Chang et al. The prior is displayed in Fig. 2.

The trial is terminated prematurely when the probability of the event that the failure rate of one treatment group, as computed under the Bayesian model, is higher than the failure rate of the other treatment group is greater than 0.975. Following Chang et al. an effect size of 0.30 is expected. A power analysis of the Bayesian stopping rule revealed the expected Bayesian probability as a function of the sample size n (Fig. 3). The figure shows that for $n = 46$ (23 patients in each group) and using a 0.3 effect size, it is expected that there is a 0.975 probability that the failure rate of WBRT treatment as found in the study is larger than the failure rate of GKSR treatment. Hence, we deem early stopping relatively likely if the effect sizes are comparable to earlier accounts in the literature.

Abbreviations

BM: Brain metastases; CTCAE: Common Terminology Criteria for Adverse Events; GKRS: Gamma Knife Radiosurgery; Gy: Gray (unit of radiation); KPS: Karnofsky Performance Status; MRI: Magnetic Resonance Imaging; NTR: Netherlands Trial Registry; SRS: Stereotactic Radiosurgery; WBRT: Whole Brain Radiation Therapy

Acknowledgments

The authors would like to thank Dr. Joris Mulder and Dr. Maurits Kaptein from the department of Methodology and Statistics at Tilburg University, the Netherlands, for performing the power analysis based on Bayesian statistical methods.

Funding

CAR-Study B is funded by ZonMw, a Dutch organization for Health Research and Development (Project Number 842003006).

Authors' contributions

WS, EV, PH, KG, MS contributed to the conception and design of the study. All authors critically read and revised the manuscript. All authors approved the final version of the manuscript.

Competing interests

The authors declare that they have no competing interests.

Author details

[1]Gamma Knife Centre Tilburg, Elisabeth TweeSteden Hospital, Hilvarenbeekseweg 60, 5022, GC, Tilburg, The Netherlands. [2]Department Neurosurgery, Elisabeth-TweeSteden Hospital, Hilvarenbeekseweg 60, 5022, GC, Tilburg, The Netherlands. [3]Department of Cognitive Neuropsychology, Tilburg University, Warandelaan 2, 5037, AB, Tilburg, The Netherlands.

References

1. Kaal EC, Niël CG, Vecht CJ. Therapeutic management of brain metastasis. The Lancet Neurology. 2005;4:289–98.

2. Lippitz B, Lindquist C, Paddick I, Peterson D, O'Neill K, Beaney R. Stereotactic radiosurgery in the treatment of brain metastases: the current evidence. Cancer Treatment Reviews Elsevier Ltd. 2014;40:48–59.

3. Khalsa SSS, Chinn M, Krucoff M, Sherman JH. The role of stereotactic radiosurgery for multiple brain metastases in stable systemic disease: a review of the literature. Acta Neurochir. 2013;155:1321–8.

4. Niranjan A, Lunsford LD, Emerick RL. Stereotactic radiosurgery for patients with metastatic brain tumors: development of a consensus radiosurgery guideline recommendation. Basel: Karger. 2012;25:123–38.

5. Rahmathulla G, Toms SA, Weil RJ. The molecular biology of brain metastasis. J Oncol. 2012;2012:1–16.

6. Chang EL, Wefel JS, Maor MH, Hassenbusch SJ, Mahajan A, Lang FF, et al. A pilot study of neurocognitive function in patients with one to three new brain metastases initially treated with stereotactic radiosurgery alone. Neurosurgery. 2007;60:277–83–discussion283–4.

7. Arvold ND, Lee EQ, Mehta MP, Margolin K, Alexander BM, Lin NU, et al. Updates in the management of brain metastases. Neuro-Oncology. 2016;18:1043–65.

8. Elaimy AL, Mackay AR, Lamoreaux WT, Fairbanks RK, Demakas JJ, Cooke BS, et al. Clinical outcomes of stereotactic radiosurgery in the treatment of patients with metastatic brain tumors. World neurosurgery. 2011;75:673–83.

9. Ellis TL, Neal MT, Chan MD. The role of surgery, radiosurgery and whole brain radiation therapy in the Management of Patients with metastatic brain tumors. International Journal of Surgical Oncology. 2012;2012:1–10.

10. Perez-Larraya JG, Hildebrand J. In: Biller J, Ferro JM, editors. Handbook of clinical neurology. Amsterdam: Elsevier; 2014. p. 1143–57.

11. Wefel JS, Parsons MW, Gondi V, Brown PD. Neurocognitive aspects of brain metastasis. Handb Clin Neurol. Amsterdam: Elsevier. 2018;149:155–65.

12. Platta CS, Khuntia D, Mehta MP, Suh JH. Current treatment strategies for brain metastasis and complications from therapeutic techniques. Am J Clin Oncol. 2010;33:398–407.

13. Mehta MP. Survival and neurologic outcomes in a randomized trial of Motexafin gadolinium and whole-brain radiation therapy in brain metastases. J Clin Oncol. 2003;21:2529–36.

14. Barani IJ, Larson DA, Berger MS. Future directions in treatment of brain metastases. Surg Neurol Int. 2013;4:S220–30.

15. McTyre E, Scott J, Chinnaiyan P. Whole brain radiotherapy for brain metastasis. Surg Neurol Int Medknow Publications. 2013;4:S236–44.

16. Abe E, Aoyama H. The role of whole brain radiation therapy for the Management of Brain Metastases in the era of stereotactic radiosurgery. Curr Oncol Rep. 2011;14:79–84.

17. Habets EJJ, Dirven L, Wiggenraad RG, Verbeek-de Kanter A, Lycklama À, Nijeholt GJ, Zwinkels H, et al. Neurocognitive functioning and health-related quality of life in patients treated with stereotactic radiotherapy for brain metastases: a prospective study. Neuro-oncology Oxford University Press. 2016;18:435–44.

18. Brown PD, Jaeckle K, Ballman KV, Farace E, Cerhan JH, Anderson SK, et al. Effect of radiosurgery alone vs radiosurgery with whole brain radiation therapy on cognitive function in patients with 1 to 3 brain metastases. JAMA. 2016;316:401–9.

19. Suh JH. Stereotactic radiosurgery for the management of brain metastases. N Engl J Med. 2010;362:1119–27.

20. Tsao MN. Brain metastases: advances over the decades. Ann Palliat Med. 2015;4:225–32.

21. Cochran DC, Chan MD, Aklilu M, Lovato JF, Alphonse NK, Bourland JD, et al. The effect of targeted agents on outcomes in patients with brain metastases from renal cell carcinoma treated with gamma knife surgery. J Neurosurg. 2012;116:978–83.

22. Greene-Schloesser D, Robbins ME, Peiffer AM, Shaw EG, Wheeler KT, Chan MD. Radiation-induced brain injury: a review. Front Oncol. 2012;2:73.

23. Baschnagel A, Wolters PL, Camphausen K. Neuropsychological testing and biomarkers in the management of brain metastases. Radiat Oncol. BioMed Central Ltd. 2008;3:1–12.

24. Dietrich J, Monje M, Wefel J, Meyers C. Clinical patterns and biological correlates of cognitive dysfunction associated with cancer therapy. Oncologist. 2008;13:1285–95.

25. Soussain C, Ricard D, Fike JR, Mazeron J-J, Psimaras D, Delattre J-Y. CNS complications of radiotherapy and chemotherapy. Lancet. 2009;374:1639–51.

26. Greene-Schloesser D, Moore E, Robbins ME. Molecular pathways: radiation-induced cognitive impairment. Clin Cancer Res American Association for Cancer Research. 2013;19:2294–300.

27. Tofilon PJ, Fike JR. The radioresponse of the central nervous system: a dynamic process. Radiat Res. 2000;153:357–70.

28. Suh JH. Hippocampal-avoidance whole-brain radiation therapy: a new standard for patients with brain metastases? Journal of clinical oncology. Proc Am Soc Clin Oncol. 2014;32:3789–91.

29. Gondi V, Hermann BP, Mehta MP, Tomé WA. Hippocampal dosimetry predicts neurocognitive function impairment after fractionated stereotactic radiotherapy for benign or low-grade adult brain tumors. Radiation Oncology Biology. 2012;83:e487–93.

30. Linskey ME, Andrews DW, Asher AL, Burri SH, Kondziolka D, Robinson PD, et al. The role of stereotactic radiosurgery in the management of patients with newly diagnosed brain metastases: a systematic review and evidence-based clinical practice guideline. J Neuro-Oncol. 2009;96:45–68.

31. Douglas J, Goodkin R. A simple treatment planning strategy for patients with multiple metastases treated with Gamma Knife surgery. J Neurosurg. 2006;105(Suppl):2–4.

32. Park S-H, Hwang S-K, Kang D-H, Lee S-H, Park J, Hwang J-H, et al. Gamma knife radiosurgery for multiple brain metastases from lung cancer. 2008;16:626–9.

33. Yamamoto M, Kawabe T, Sato Y, Higuchi Y, Nariai T, Watanabe S, et al. Stereotactic radiosurgery for patients with multiple brain metastases: a case-matched study comparing treatment results for patients with 2-9 versus 10 or more tumors. J Neurosurg. 2014;121(Suppl):16–25.

34. Ojerholm E, Lee JYK, Kolker J, Lustig R, Dorsey JF, Alonso-Basanta M. Gamma Knife radiosurgery to four or more brain metastases in patients without prior intracranial radiation or surgery. Cancer Med. 2014;3:565–71.

35. Kim C–H, Im Y–S, Nam D–H, Park K, Kim JH, Lee J–I. Gamma knife radiosurgery for ten or more brain metastases. J Korean Neurosurg Soc. 2008;44:358–63.

36. Hunter GK, Suh JH, Reuther AM, Vogelbaum MA, Barnett GH, Angelov L, et al. Treatment of five or more brain metastases with stereotactic radiosurgery. Int J Radiat Oncol Biol Phys Elsevier Inc. 2012;83:1394–8.

37. Suh JH, Chao ST, Angelov L, Vogelbaum MA, Barnett GH. Role of stereotactic radiosurgery for multiple (> 4) brain metastases. J Radiosurg SBRT. 2011;1:31–40.

38. Nabors LB, Portnow J, Ammirati M, Brem H, Brown P, Butowski N, et al. Central nervous system cancers, version 2.2014. Featured updates to the NCCN guidelines. J Natl Compr Cancer Netw. 2014;12:1517–23.

39. Soliman H, Das S, Larson DA, Sahgal A. Stereotactic radiosurgery (SRS) in the modern management of patients with brain metastases. Oncotarget. 2016;7:12318–30.

40. Wefel JS, Vardy J, Ahles T, Schagen SB. International cognition and cancer task force recommendations to harmonise studies of cognitive function in patients with cancer. Lancet Oncol Elsevier. 2011;12:703–8.

41. Rades D, Dziggel L, Segedin B, Oblak I, Nagy V, Marita A, et al. A new survival score for patients with brain metastases from non-small cell lung cancer. Strahlenther Onkol. 2013;189:777–81.

42. Witgert ME, Meyers CA. Neurocognitive and quality of life measures in patients with metastatic brain disease. Neurosurg Clin N Am. 2011;22:79–85.

43. Meyers CA, Brown PD. Role and relevance of neurocognitive assessment in clinical trials of patients with CNS tumors. J Clin Oncol. 2006;24:1305–9.

44. Maassen GH, Bossema E, Brand N. Reliable change and practice effects: outcomes of various indices compared. J Clin Exp Neuropsychol. 3rd ed. Taylor & Francis Group; 2009;31:339–352.

45. Chang EL, Wefel JS, Hess KR, Allen PK, Lang FF, Kornguth DG, et al. Neurocognition in patients with brain metastases treated with radiosurgery or radiosurgery plus whole-brain irradiation: a randomised controlled trial. Lancet Oncol. 2009;10:1037–44.

46. Lin NU, Lee EQ, Aoyama H, Barani IJ, Barboriak DP, Baumert BG, et al. Response assessment criteria for brain metastases: proposal from the RANO group. Lancet Oncol. 2015;16:e270–8.

47. Scott NW, McPherson GC, Ramsay CR, Campbell MK. The method of minimization for allocation to clinical trials: a review. Control Clin Trials. 2002;23:662–74.

48. O'Callaghan CA. OxMaR: open source free software for online minimization and randomization for clinical trials. Añel JA, editor. PLoS One. 2014;9: e110761 e110710.

49. McPherson GC, Campbell MK, Elbourne DR. Use of randomisation in clinical trials: a survey of UK practice. Trials BioMed Central. 2011;13:198–8.

50. ALEA online randomisation software. http://www.aleaclinical.eu. Accessed 14 Feb 2018.

51. Thall PF, Simon R. Practical Bayesian guidelines for phase IIB clinical trials. Biometrics. 1994;50:337–49.

52. Saville BR, Connor JT, Ayers GD, Alvarez J. The utility of Bayesian predictive probabilities for interim monitoring of clinical trials. Clin Trials SAGE Publications. 2014;11:485–93.

53. Lezak MD. Neuropsychological assessment. USA: Oxford University Press; 2004.

54. Dirven L, Armstrong TS, Taphoorn MJB. Health-related quality of life and other clinical outcome assessments in brain tumor patients: challenges in the design, conduct and interpretation of clinical trials. Neurooncol Pract. 2015;2:2–5.

55. Smets EM, Garssen B, Bonke B, De Haes JC. The multidimensional fatigue inventory (MFI) psychometric qualities of an instrument to assess fatigue. J Psychosom Res. 1995;39:315–25.

56. Weitzner MA, Meyers CA, Gelke CK, Byrne KS, Cella DF, Levin VA. The functional assessment of cancer therapy (FACT) scale. Development of a brain subscale and revalidation of the general version (FACT-G) in patients with primary brain tumors. Cancer. 1995;75:1151–61.

57. Bjelland I, Dahl AA, Haug TT, Neckelmann D. The validity of the hospital anxiety and depression scale. An updated literature review J Psychosom Res. 2002;52:69–77.

23

ARL2 overexpression inhibits glioma proliferation and tumorigenicity via down-regulating AXL

Yulin Wang[1†], Gefei Guan[1], Wen Cheng[1], Yang Jiang[1], Fengping Shan[2], Anhua Wu[1], Peng Cheng[1*†] (ID) and Zongze Guo[1*]

Abstract

Background: Glioma is the most common primary brain tumor in adults with a poor prognosis. As a member of ARF subfamily GTPase, ARL2 plays a key role in regulating the dynamics of microtubules and mitochondrial functions. Recently, ARL2 has been identified as a prognostic and therapeutic target in a variety range of malignant tumors. However, the biological functional role of ARL2 in glioma still remains unknown. The aim of this study was to explore the expression and functional role of ARL2 in glioma.

Methods: In this study, we investigated the expression of ARL2 in glioma samples by using RT-PCR, immunohistochemistry and western blot. The correlation between ARL2 expression and the outcomes of glioma patients was evaluated with survival data from TCGA, CGGA and Rembrandt dataset. Lentiviral technique was used for ARL2 overexpression in U87 and U251 cells. CCK8 assay, colony formation assay, wound healing test, transwell invasion assay and in vivo subcutaneous xenograft model were performed to investigated the biological functions of ARL2.

Results: ARL2 expression was down-regulated in glioma, and was inversely associated with poor prognosis in glioma patients. Furthermore, exogenous ARL2 overexpression attenuated the growth and colony-formation abilities of glioma cells, as well as their migration and invasive capabilities. Moreover, elevated expression of ARL2 inhibited in vivo tumorigenicity of glioma cells. Mechanistically, ARL2 regulated AXL expression, which was known as an important functional regulator of proliferation and tumorigenicity in glioma cells.

Conclusion: Our study suggests that ARL2 inhibits the proliferation, migration and tumorigenicity of glioma cells by regulating the expression of AXL and may conduct as a new prognostic and therapeutic target for glioma.

Keywords: ARL2, Glioma, AXL, Tumorgenecity, Brain cancer

Background

Glioma is the most common primary brain tumor in adults [1]. Although a standard treatment including extensive surgical resection followed by radiation and temozolomide chemotherapy has been adopted, the outcomes for glioma patients are still poor [1]. Median survival of glioblastoma multiforme (GBM), the most common and aggressive form of glioma, is 14–15 months and median progression-free survival (FPS) is approximately 6 months [1, 2]. Due to this

dismal situation, great efforts have been made to find out effective approaches to halt the progression of this aggressive cancer. Besides this, recent studies have showed a tremendous understanding of the genetic and molecular mechanisms of glioma, leading to a renewed understanding about potential new therapeutic strategies, including oncogenic signal transduction inhibition/targeted therapy, anti-angiogenesis treatment, therapy targeting glioma stem cells, and immunotherapy [3].

Small G-proteins also known as the Ras superfamily structurally classified into 5 families: Ras, Rho, Rab, Sar/Arf, and Ran, which are involved in multiple cell signaling pathways and various cellular functions, including differentiation, proliferation, vesicle transport, nuclear

* Correspondence: chengpengcmu@sina.com; cmuguozongze@163.com
†Yulin Wang and Peng Cheng contributed equally to this work.
[1]Department of Neurosurgery, The First Hospital of China Medical University, 155 Nanjingbei Street, Heping, Shenyang, Liaoning 110001, People's Republic of China
Full list of author information is available at the end of the article

assembly, and regulation of the cytoskeleton [4, 5]. Recent studies have identified Ras mutations in some human carcinomas [6–8]. It has been reported that activating mutations of KRAS-4B, within the mutated Ras family, occurs in approximately 21% of all human cancers, and accounts for approximately 90% of pancreatic cancers, 45% of colon cancers, and 30% of lung cancers, respectively [6]. The mutated forms of KRAS-4B not only activate their downstream signaling cascades, but also interact with each other and subsequently promote the proliferation of cancer cells and induce resistance to standard cancer therapies [6].

As a member of the ADP-ribosylation factor (ARF) subfamily, ADP ribosylation factor-like GTPase 2 (ARL2) is highly conserved and ubiquitously expressed in eukaryotes [9]. Previous studies show that ARL2 regulates microtubule dynamics through the interaction with tubulin-folding cofactor D (TBC-D), which is required for multiple mitochondrial functions including mitochondrial morphology, motility, asymmetric division, and maintenance of ATP levels [10–12]. Similarly, the trimer consisting of ARL2, tubulin-specific chaperone D and beta-tubulin is required for the maintenance of microtubule network [13–15]. In addition, ARL2 has been proved to be a fundamental regulator of farnesylated cargo and mitochondrial fusion [16, 17]. ARL2 is also involved in regulating nuclear retention of STAT3 with binder of ADP-ribosylation factor-like two (BART) [18–20]. Furthermore, ARL2 inhibition induces the apoptosis of neural progenitor cells derived from human embryonic stem cells [21]. However, the function role of ARL2 in cancer is still controversial. It has been reported that ARL2 expression level modifies cell morphology and influences mitotic and cytokinetic progression in breast cancer [22]. Recent study demonstrates that ARL2 expression is dramatically elevated in hepatocellular carcinoma and might be potentially utilizable as a prognostic marker [23]. Similarly, another study reports that ARL2 functions as an oncogene in cervical cancer [24]. Nevertheless, there is a study showing that breast tumor cells with increased ARL2 content present reduced aggressivity, *both* in vitro *and* in vivo [25]. Decreased ARL2 expression is associated with the regulation of p53 localization and results in a chemoresistant phenotype in breast cancer via a protein phosphatase 2A (PP2A) mediated mechanism [26]. Moreover, the pathophysiologic role of ARL2 in glioma remains unclear.

In this study, we investigated the expression and functional role of ARL2 in glioma. We firstly proved that decreased ARL2 expression level was clinically correlated to the higher grades and poorer outcomes of glioma patients. Secondly, we found that ARL2 overexpression attenuated the proliferation, clone formation, migration, invasive and tumorigenic capabilities of glioma cells by regulating the expression of receptor tyrosine kinase AXL.

Methods

Patients and samples

Twenty-three patient samples were collected at the First Hospital of China Medical University from February to June in 2016, including 20 glioma samples (grade II, 3 cases; grade III, 9 cases; grade IV, 8 cases) and 3 non-tumor brain tissue samples (from partial lobectomy in patients with epilepsy). Nine glioma tissues (grade II-IV, 3 cases for each grade) and 3 non-tumor brain tissue samples were used for qPCR and western blot. To further confirm the data of qPCR and western blot, IHC staining were performed with these 12 samples and other 11 glioma samples (grade III 6 cases and grade IV 5 cases). All glioma patients underwent surgical resection and the histological diagnosis was verified by 2 neuropathologists according to 2016 World Health Organization (WHO) guidelines. All of the samples used for this study were primary tumor samples, except 3 recurrent samples used for IHC staining. This study was approved by the Medical Ethics Committee of the First Hospital of China Medical University, and written informed consent was obtained from each patient. The clinical characteristics of 20 glioma patients were listed in Table 1.

Cell culture

U87-MG (catalogue number TCHu58) and U251 (catalogue number TCHu138) cell lines were obtained from the

Table 1 The clinical characteristics of 20 glioma patients

Characteristics	Number of patients ($n = 20$)
Age(years)	
<50	8 (40%)
≥ 50	12 (60%)
Gender	
Male	12 (60%)
Female	8 (40%)
WHO grade	
II	3 (15%)
III	9 (45%)
IV	8 (40%)
Tumor size	
<4 cm	11 (55%)
≥ 4 cm	9 (45%)
Primary/Recurrent	
Primary	17 (85%)
Recurrent	3 (15%)
IDH1 state	
IDH1(−)	11 (55%)
IDH1(+)	9 (45%)

Chinese Academy of Sciences Cell Bank (Shanghai, China) and maintained in high-glucose Dulbecco's Modified Eagle's Medium (DMEM) (Hyclone, SH30022.01) supplemented with 10% fetal bovine serum (FBS, Hyclone, SV30087), 100 U/ml of penicillin, and 100 U/ml of streptomycin (Hyclone, SV30010) at 37 °C with 5% CO_2.

RNA isolation and quantitative RT-PCR (qPCR)

Total RNA was isolated from U87, U251 cells and 12 clinical samples using TRIzol reagent (Invitrogen), according to the manufacturer's protocol. Total RNA was reversely transcribed into cDNA and used for PCR amplification. Real-time PCR were performed in thermal cycler (Roche LightCycler 480) using TransStart* Top Green qPCR SuperMix Assays (Transgen Biotech, AQ131). PCR conditions were as follows: 1 cycle of 95 °C for 30s, followed by 40 cycles of a two-step cycling program (95 °C for 5 s; 60 °C for 30s). The mRNA expression was normalized to the expression of GAPDH mRNA and calculated by the $2^{-\Delta\Delta Ct}$ method. Specific primers for ARL2, AXL and GAPDH were: ARL2 forward: GGGA GGACATCGACACCA and reverse: AGGACCGCAGGG ACTTCT [27]; AXL forward: 5-GTTTGGAGCTGTGA TGGA AGGC-3 and reverse: 5-CGCTTCACTCAGGA AATCCTCC-3 [28]; GAPDH forward: GAAGGTGAA GGTCGGAGTCA and reverse: TTGAGGTCAATGAAG GGGTC [29], respectively.

Protein extraction and western blot analysis

Total proteins from tissue and cells were extracted by whole cell lysis buffer (Wanleibio) and quantified using the bicinchoninic acid (BCA) method. 30 µg of protein from each sample was electrophoresed by 12% SDS-PAGE and transferred to PVDF membranes (0.45 µm, Millipore). After being blocked with 5% skimmed milk or 5% BSA (used for phosphorylated protein), the PVDF membranes were incubated overnight at 4 °C with the primary antibody. Membranes were then washed three times with TBST (5 min each), and incubated with peroxidase-conjugated affinipure goat anti-rabbit (1:5000; Proteintech) or anti-mouse (1:10000; Proteintech) IgG at 37 °C for 1 h. Protein expression was visualized with a chemiluminescence ECL kit (Tanon, 5500). GAPDH served as a loading control, and band intensity was quantified using Image J software.

Immunohistochemistry and immunocytochemistry

For immunohistochemistry, all samples were fixed in 10% neutral formalin and embedded in paraffin. Sections (4 µm thick) were cut from paraffin blocks and mounted on Poly-L-Lysine-coated glass slides. The sections were deparaffinized in xylene and rehydrated in gradient ethanol. Antigen retrieval was performed in 0.01 mol/L citrate buffer (pH 6.0) by microwave oven for 15 min at

95 °C. Endogenous peroxidase activity was blocked with 3% hydrogen peroxide for 10 min and the sections were incubated with normal goat serum to reduce nonspecific binding for 15 min. Sections were incubated with primary antibody in blocking solution at 4 °C overnight in a humidified chamber. After washing three times with PBS, sections were incubated with biotinylated goat anti-rabbit IgG (SP-9001, ZSGB-BIO) for 15 min at room temperature. After washing in PBS, 3, 3′-diaminobenzidine (DAB) was used for developing. Slides were counterstained with hematoxylin for 3 min. Then the sections were dehydrated and mounted with coverslips. German immunohistochemical score (GIS) was applied to evaluate the expression of ARL2 [30]. Percentage of positive cells was classified as 0 (negative), 1 (up to 10%), 2 (11–50%), 3 (51–80%), or 4 (> 80% positive cells), staining intensity was classified as 0 (no staining), 1 (weak), 2 (moderate), or 3 (strong). The final immunoreactive GIS were defined as the multiplication of both grading results (percentage of positive cells × staining intensity). The IHC expression value of ARL2 and related sample information were listed in Table 2.

For immunocytochemistry, 5×10^3 cells were seeded into confocal dish per well and incubated at 37 °C with 5% CO_2 for 24 h. Then the cells were fixed with 4% paraformaldehyde and permeated with 0.3% Triton X-100 for 20 min. After blocking with 5% BSA for 1 h, primary antibody was added and incubated at 4 °C overnight. Following incubation with rhodamine(TRITC)-conjugated affinipure goat anti-rabbit IgG (Proteintech, SA00007–2) and DAPI (BOSTER, AR1176), the samples were detected using fluorescence microscope (OLYMPUS, BX53).

ARL2 expression data mining in GEO dataset, TCGA and Rembrandt dataset

ARL2 expression data of TCGA and Rembrandt dataset and the patients' survival data of Rembrandt dataset were extracted from Project Betastasis (http://betastasis.com/). The patients' survival data of TCGA were downloaded from GlioVis portal (http://gliovis.bioinfo.cnio.es). In addition, GEO datasets (GSE50161, Griesinger dataset; GSE4290, Sun dataset) were applied to analyze the expression level of ARL2 in glioma and normal brain [31, 32]. Gene Set Enrichment analysis (GSEA, www.broadinstitu te.org/gsea/index.jsp) was applied to obtain the functional information on ARL2 as previously described [33, 34]. Moreover, the data from Chinese Glioma Genome Atlas (CGGA) were used to analyze ARL2 expression and the patients' survival time [35, 36]. The relevant signaling pathways of ARL2 from KEGG and Reactome were analyzed by pathDIP (http://ophid.utoronto.ca/pathdip/).

Table 2 The ARL2 expression value and information of samples used for IHC

Sample tissues (23 cases in total)		Sample NO.	Age range (years)	GIS score	P value (vs. non-tumor)
Non-tumor tissue (3 cases)		N1	38–65	12	
		N2		12	
		N3		12	
Glioma tissues	Grade II (3 cases)	G0201	26–60	4	0.0074
		G0202		9	
		G0203		6	
	Grade III (9 cases)	G0301	32–70	2	0.0001
		G0302		2	
		G0303		1	
		G0304		3	
		G0305		8	
		G0306		2	
		G0307		1	
		G0308		0	
		G0309		0	
	Grade IV (8 cases)	G0401	37–79	4	0.0001
		G0402		2	
		G0403		0	
		G0404		1	
		G0405		2	
		G0406		4	
		G0407		4	
		G0408		1	

Lentivirus mediated ARL2 and AXL over-expression

Lentiviruses carrying overexpressing ARL2, AXL and control vectors were purchased from GeneChem (Shanghai, China). The lentivirus transduction was performed according to the protocol provided by the company. In brief, after the cells (10^5 cells/well in 1 ml high-glucose DMEM medium supplemented with 10% FBS) were seeded in a 6-well plate for 24 h, 20 µl of lentivirus solution (10^7 IU/mL) were added to each well and the cells were incubated at 37 °C with 5% CO_2 for 12 h. The medium was replaced with fresh DMEM medium containing 10% FBS. After 48 h of transduction, the cells were selected with puromycin (10 µg/mL). Medium was changed every 3 days. Real-time PCR and western blot were performed to assess the transfected efficiency.

In vitro cell proliferation assays

5×10^3 cells in 100 µl medium were seeded into 96-well plates per well and incubated at 37 °C with 5% CO_2 for 6 days. The cell proliferation was measured at day 0, 2, 4 and 6 by adding 10 µl CCK8 (DojinDo) into the wells

and following 4 h incubation at 37 °C. Then OD values of each well were measured by microplate reader (BIO-RAD 15033) at the absorbance of 450 nm. Growth curves were plotted according to the OD value of each well.

Colony formation assay

After transduced with ARL2, AXL overexpression or control lentiviruses for 72 h, the cells were collected and resuspended as single cells. Cells were seeded into the wells of a six-well plate and incubated at 37 °C with 5% CO_2. After 2 weeks, the cells were washed with PBS twice and stained with crystal violet staining solution. The number of colonies (more than 50 cells) was counted under a microscope (Leica, 090–135.001).

Wound healing test

The cells (5×10^5 per well) were seeded into six-well plates. After 24 h, the cells overspread the bottom and were scratched by a 200 µl pipette tip. PBS was used to wash out cell debris and suspension cells. Fresh serum-free medium was added, and the cells incubated at 37 °C with 5% CO_2 to allow the wound to heal. Photographs of the wound were taken at 0 and 24 h at the same position. The percentage of wound closure was measured according to previous reports [37, 38]. In brief, the wound areas were evaluated by image J software and the percentage of wound closure were calculated via the formula as follow: (original wound area - actual wound area)/area of the original wound × 100.

Transwell invasion assay

Transwell chambers with a pore size of 8 µm filter membrane (Corning, 3422) were used to perform invasion assay. 100 µl Matrigel (Corning, 356,234) (diluted with serum-free DMEM by 1:8) was plated in transwell chamber, and preserved in an incubator. Four hours later, 200 µl of serum-free medium containing 10^5 cells was added into top chambers of transwell inserts, and 750 µl DMEM containing 10% FBS was added into bottom chambers. The cells were incubated at 37 °C in 5% CO_2 for 16 h. Matrigel and cells in top chambers were removed by cotton swab. After fixation with 4% paraformaldehyde, the cells traversing the membrane were stained with crystal violet staining solution and counted under five different high-power microscope fields per well. The experiment was performed in triplicate.

In vivo subcutaneous tumor transplantation

All animal procedures were conformed to protocols approved by the Animal Care Committee of China Medical University. For xenograft subcutaneous transplantation, 6-week-old male immune-deficient nude mice (BALB/C-Null) were purchased from Beijing Vital River Laboratory Animal Technology Company. Mice were raised in laminar flow cabinets under specific pathogen free (SPF) conditions and were fed ad libitum. U87 cells (transduced with ARL2 overexpression or control vector) were injected into the back flanks of nude mice at a density of 10^7 cells per 0.3 ml as previous described [39, 40]. The tumor size was measured using a Vernier caliper per 4 days, and the tumor volume was calculated using the formula: V = (length x width^2) / 2 [41]. The mice were sacrificed at day 28 after implantation, and the tumors were weighed and photographed.

Statistical analysis

Data are presented as mean ± SD. The number of replicates for each experiment is stated in the figure legend. Statistical differences between and among groups were determined by two tailed *t*-test or one-way analysis of variance (ANOVA) followed by Dunnett's post-test, respectively. Statistical analysis was performed by Microsoft Excel 2013 and Graphpad Prism 6.0, unless mentioned otherwise in the figure legend. $P < 0.05$ was considered as statistically significant.

Results

ARL2 expression is decreased in glioma

The expression of ARL family members in TCGA were studied through GlioVis, and ARL2 was significantly differentially expressed between glioma and non-tumor samples (Additional file 1: Figure S1). To further investigate ARL2 expression in glioma, we assessed mRNA and protein levels in a series of clinical glioma specimens and cell lines. Twelve human clinical specimens were collected including 9 glioma tissues (grade II-IV, 3 cases separately) and 3 non-tumor brain tissue samples. Quantitative PCR was performed on these specimens. The result showed that ARL2 mRNA levels decreased with the increase in grade of tumor tissues (Fig. 1a, $P < 0.01$), as well as U87 and U251 glioma cells (Additional file 2: Figure S2A, $P < 0.0001$). Similarly, ARL2 protein expression levels were down-regulated in grade IV glioma samples (Fig. 1b, $P < 0.05$), as well as U251 and U87 cells than non-tumor samples (Additional file 2: Figure S2B, $P < 0.001$). We then examined ARL2 expression in 20 gliomas tissue samples (grade II, 3 cases; grade III, 9 cases; grade IV, 8 cases) and 3 non-tumor brain tissue samples by immunohistochemistry. The data showed that ARL2 protein expression was reduced in high grade glioma samples (Fig. 1c, grade III, $P < 0.01$; grade IV, $P < 0.0001$). We also collected ARL2 expression data from CGGA, Rembrandt database and TCGA. The results confirmed that ARL2 expression level significantly decreased in GBM (grade IV) (CGGA, Fig. 1d, $P < 0.0001$; Rembrandt database, Fig. 1e, $P < 0.0001$). In TCGA, a decreased ARL2 expression could be observed in all subtypes (Proneural, Mesenchymal, Neural and Classical) of GBM, compared to non-tumor samples (Fig. 1f, $P < 0.05$). Data from Sun (Additional file 2: Figure S2C, $P < 0.001$) and Griesinger dataset (Additional file 2: Figure S2D, $P < 0.05$) also demonstrated the consistent results. Taken together, these results demonstrated that ARL2 expression significantly decreased in glioma.

ARL2 expression is clinical relevant with the poor prognosis of glioma patients

Recently, ARL2 has been identified as a potential prognosis marker for hepatocellular carcinoma [23]. To examine whether ARL2 expression is associated with glioma patient outcomes, we analyzed the data from CGGA, Rembrandt database, and TCGA to investigate the clinical relevance of ARL2. The data from CGGA showed decreased ARL2 expression was clinical relevant to the poor prognosis of glioma patients (Fig. 1g, $P = 0.0003$). Similar results were obtained from Rembrandt, and the patients with a higher ARL2 expression had a favorable survival (Fig. 1h, $P = 0.011$). Finally, we verified the result in TCGA. The consistent elevated expression of ARL2 was also associated with prolonged survival (Fig. 1i, $P = 0.048$).

ARL2 attenuated the growth and colony-formation abilities of glioma cells

To investigate the physiological role of ARL2 in glioma, we first overexpressed ARL2 through transducing lentiviral ARL2 vector in glioma cell lines (U87 and U251), and then examined the effects on cell growth. qPCR and Western blotting assay showed that both of ARL2 mRNA and protein expression level were significantly elevated at 48 h after transduction (Fig. 2a, $P = 0.0099$, and b, $P = 0.0316$; Additional file 3: Figure S3A $P < 0.0001$, and S3B, $P = 0.0075$). As a result, ARL2 overexpression significantly suppressed the proliferation of U251 and U87 cells, compared with cells transduced with the control vector (Fig. 2c and d). Moreover, the colony formation assay was performed to examine the foci formation ability of these cells. As expected, foci formation abilities of U251 or U87 cells infected with lentiviral ARL2 overexpression vector were dramatically decreased in comparison with control cells (Fig. 2e and f). In addition, we measured the cell cycles in U251 cells transfected with or without ARL2 overexpression vector. The percentage of cells at G0/G1 phase in U251 cells with ARL2 overexpression was increased and the proportion at S and G2/M phase was decreased, oppositely (Additional file 3: Figure S3C, G0/G1 phase $P = 0.0014$, S phase $P = 0.0049$, and G2/M phase $P = 0.0111$). This data indicated ARL2 overexpression induced G0/G1 arrest in glioma cells and inhibited their proliferation. Taken together, these results indicated that ARL2 overexpression inhibited the growth and clonogenicity of glioma cells.

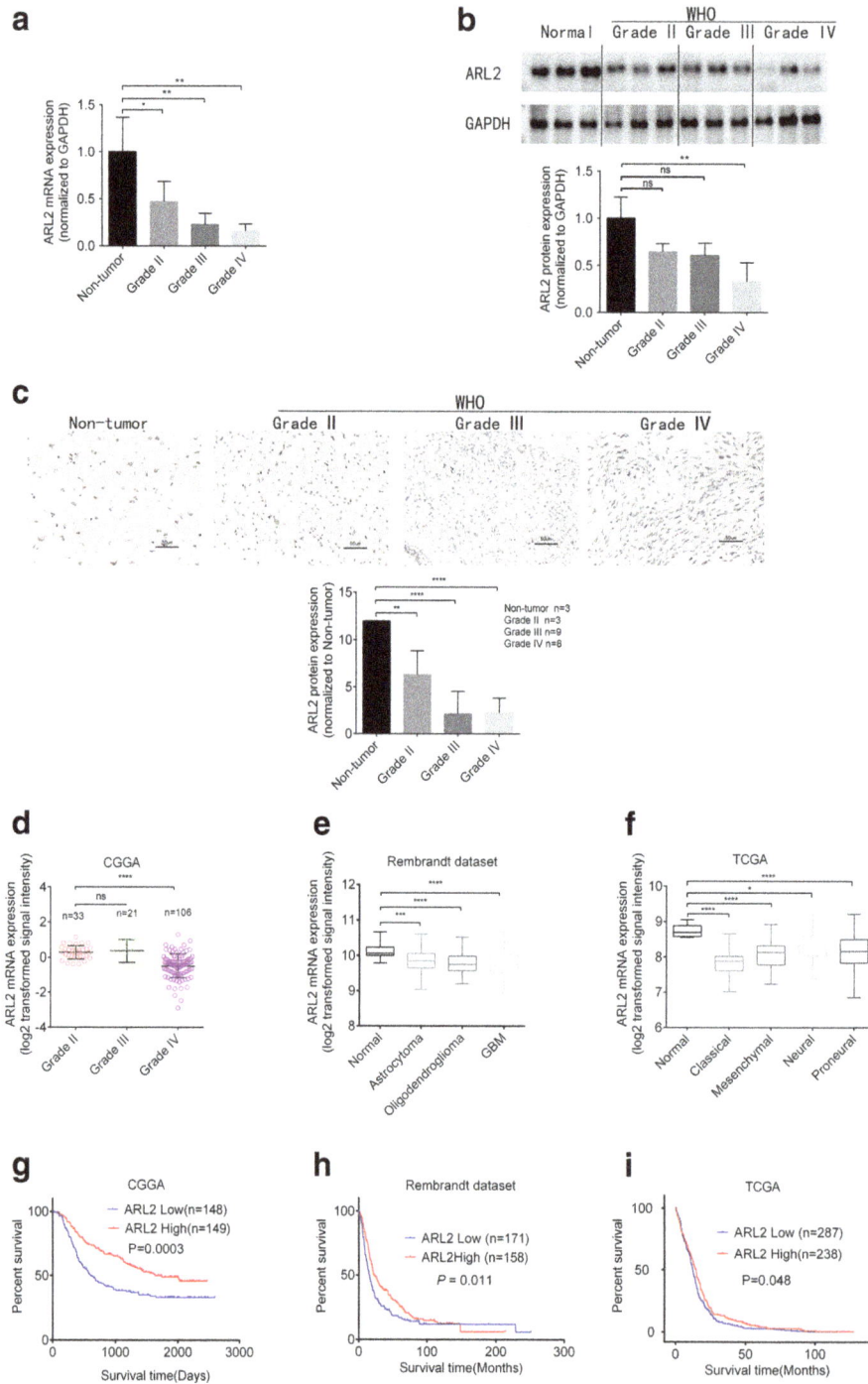

Fig. 1 (See legend on next page.)

Fig. 1 Decreased ARL2 expression is clinically relevant with poor prognosis of glioma patients. **a** qRT-PCR analyses of *ARL2* mRNA in WHO grade II-IV glioma and non-tumor samples (grade II, $n = 3$; grade III, $n = 3$; grade IV, $n = 3$, non-tumor $n = 3$) (non-tumor vs. grade II, $P = 0.0489$; non-tumor vs. grade III, $P = 0.0075$; non-tumor vs. grade IV, $P = 0.0046$; one-way ANOVA). **b** Western blot analyses of ARL2 protein in WHO grade II-IV glioma and non-tumor samples (grade II, $n = 3$; grade III, $n = 3$; grade IV, $n = 3$, non-tumor $n = 3$) (non-tumor vs. grade II, $P = 0.0761$; non-tumor vs. grade III, $P = 0.0512$; non-tumor vs. grade IV, $P = 0.0033$; one-way ANOVA). **c** Representative immunohistochemistry images and analyses of ARL2 protein in WHO grade II-IV glioma and non-tumor brain samples (grade II, $n = 3$; grade III, $n = 9$; grade IV, $n = 8$; non-tumor $n = 3$). Scale bar, 50 μm. (non-tumor vs. grade II, $P = 0.0074$; non-tumor vs. grade III, $P < 0.0001$; non-tumor vs. grade IV, $P < 0.0001$; one-way ANOVA). **d** Data from CGGA showed ARL2 mRNA expression decreased in grade IV compared to grade II (grade II, $n = 33$; grade III, $n = 21$; grade IV, $n = 106$) (grade II vs. grade IV, $P < 0.0001$; grade II vs. grade III, $P = 0.8438$, one way ANOVA). **e, f** Data from Rembrandt database (**e**, non-tumor, $n = 28$; astrocytoma, $n = 148$; oligodendroglioma, $n = 67$; GBM, $n = 228$) (non-tumor vs. Astrocytoma, $P = 0.0007$; non-tumor vs. oligodendroglioma, $P < 0.0001$; non-tumor vs. GBM, $P < 0.0001$; one-way ANOVA) and TCGA (F, normal, $n = 11$; classical, $n = 54$; mesenchymal, $n = 58$; neural, $n = 33$; proneural, $n = 57$) (normal vs. classical, $P < 0.0001$; normal vs. mesenchymal, $P < 0.0001$; normal vs. neural, $P = 0.0188$; normal vs. proneual, $P < 0.0001$ one-way ANOVA) revealed that ARL2 mRNA expression decreased in glioblastoma, compared with non-tumor brain tissues. **g-i** Data from CGGA (G, $P = 0.0003$, low, $n = 148$; high, $n = 147$), Rembrandt database (**h**, low, $n = 171$; high, $n = 158$) and TCGA (**i**, low, $n = 287$; high, $n = 238$) indicated ARL2 was opposite relevant to the poor prognosis of glioma patients

ARL2 inhibited the migration and invasive capabilities of glioma cells.

Since microtubule network plays a crucial role in the regulation of cell migration and invasion, wounding healing test and Transwell invasion assay were performed to examine whether ARL2 overexpression inhibited the migration and invasion of glioma cells. As shown in Fig. 2g and h, glioma cells with ARL2 overexpression migrated significantly more slowly than control cells (Fig. 2g, $P < 0.05$, and H, $P < 0.01$). Similar results were obtained from Transwell assay, ARL2 overexpressed cells exhibited decreased invasive capabilities (Fig. 2i, $P < 0.01$, and j, $P < 0.01$). These data indicated that ARL2 diminished the migration and invasion abilities of glioma cells.

ARL2 suppressed the tumorigenicity of glioma cells in vivo

To determine whether ARL2 is important to the tumorigenicity of glioma cells in vivo, we injected U87 cells infected with ARL2 overexpression vector or control vector into the flank regions of nude mice and measured tumor volumes every 4 days. The results demonstrated that the upregulation of ARL2 expression resulted in a reduction in subcutaneous growth of U87 glioma cells (Fig. 3a). Consistently, after 4 weeks of xenograft transplantation, although ARL2 overexpression didn't alter the tumorigenesis, the mean volume and weight of subcutaneous tumors in ARL2 overexpression group were obviously smaller and lighter than the control group (Fig. 3b-d). Collectively, these results showed that ARL2 could suppress glioma tumorigenicity in vivo.

ARL2 decreased AXL expression in glioma cells

Due to the functional role of ARL2 in glioma, we investigated the downstream target of ARL2 via Gene Set Enrichment Analysis (GSEA). Adhesion dependent cell spreading signaling pathway were enriched, including 33 genes, such as ILK, ITGA8, and AXL (Fig. 4a). Furthermore, another two signaling pathway were enriched

(epidermal growth factor and epidermal growth factor stimulus) (Additional file 4: Figure S4A and S4B). It has been reported that AXL is closely relevant to EGFR signaling pathway and mediates the resistance to EGFR inhibition in lung cancer and GBM [42–44]. We then explored the relationship among AXL and enriched genes in these two datasets separately via STRING (https://string-db.org/). The data also confirmed the close relationship between AXL and these enriched genes (Additional file 4: Figure S4C and S4D). Moreover, pathway analysis through pathDIP (http://ophid.utoronto.ca/pathdip/) was performed to inquire the relevant signaling pathways of ARL2 in KEGG and Reactome (Additional file 4: Figure S4E). It was revealed that ARL2 was relevant to several downstream signaling pathways, including PI3K-Akt, ERK/MAPK and EGFR. These pathways were also downstream targets relevant to AXL [42, 43]. In addition, previous report and our previous study proved that AXL played a critical role in the functional regulation of glioma cells [29, 45]. Based on these observations, we further investigated the effect of ARL2 expression on AXL in glioma cells. Firstly, western blot was applied to examine AXL expression in glioma cells infected with ARL2 overexpression or control vector. The results demonstrated that ARL2 overexpression decreased AXL protein expression (Fig. 4b, $P = 0.038$, and c $P = 0.0053$). Secondly, immunocytochemistry confirmed that ARL2 overexpression attenuated AXL expression in U251 cells (Fig. 4d). Thirdly, IHC staining of ARL2 and AXL in U87 xenograft were consistent with the results of western blot and ICC (Fig. 4e). The upregulated ARL2 expression induced a reduced AXL expression. Finally, phospho-AXL (Tyr702) protein expression in U251 cells was also inhibited after ARL2 overexpression (Fig. 4f, $P = 0.0018$). We also observed that the expression level of phospho-ERK decreased in U251 cells with ARL2 overexpression (Fig. 4g, $P < 0.01$). In contrast, there was no significant change in total ERK, total AKT and phospho-AKT expression (Fig. 4f and Additional file 5: Figure S5).

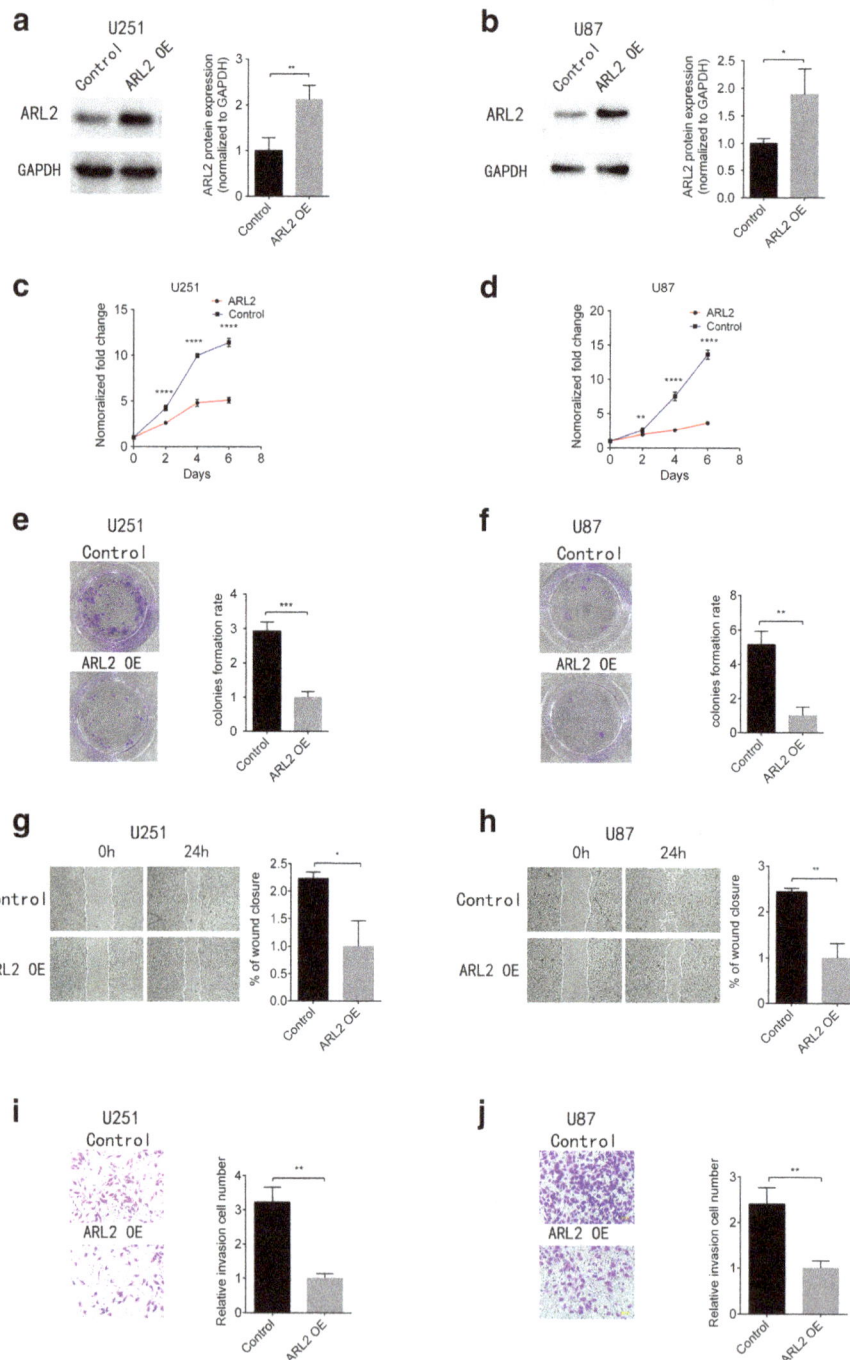

Fig. 2 ARL2 regulated the growth, colony formation, migration and invasion capabilities of glioma cells. **a, b** The representative western blot images and analyses of ARL2 in U251 (**a**) and U87 (**b**) glioma cells transduced with lentiviral ARL2 vector or its control vector (U251, $P = 0.0099$; U87, $P = 0.0316$; $n = 3$; t test). **c, d** In vitro growth assay showed that ARL2 overexpression inhibited the proliferation of U251 (**c**) and U87 (**d**) (** $P < 0.01$; **** $P < 0.0001$; $n = 5$, t test). **e, f** Colony formation assay revealed that ARL2 overexpression reduces clone formation ability of U251 (**e**) and U87 (**f**) cell lines (500 cells/well; U251, $P = 0.0004$; U87, $P = 0.0014$; $n = 3$; t test). **g, h** Wound healing test showed that ARL2 overexpression decreased the migration abilities of U251 (**g**) and U87 (**h**) cells (U251, $P = 0.0111$; U87, $P = 0.0015$; $n = 3$, t test). **i, j** Transwell assay demonstrated that ARL2 overexpression inhibited the invasion capabilities of U251 (**i**) and U87 (**j**) cells. Scale bar, 100 μm. ($P < 0.01$, $n = 3$, with t test)

We further performed qPCR to detect *ARL2* and *AXL* mRNA level in U251 cells transfected with ARL2 overexpression vector or control vector. The data demonstrated that the expression level of ARL2 was increased significantly after transduction (Additional file 6: Figure S6A, $P < 0.0001$). But *ARL2* overexpression didn't lead to significant

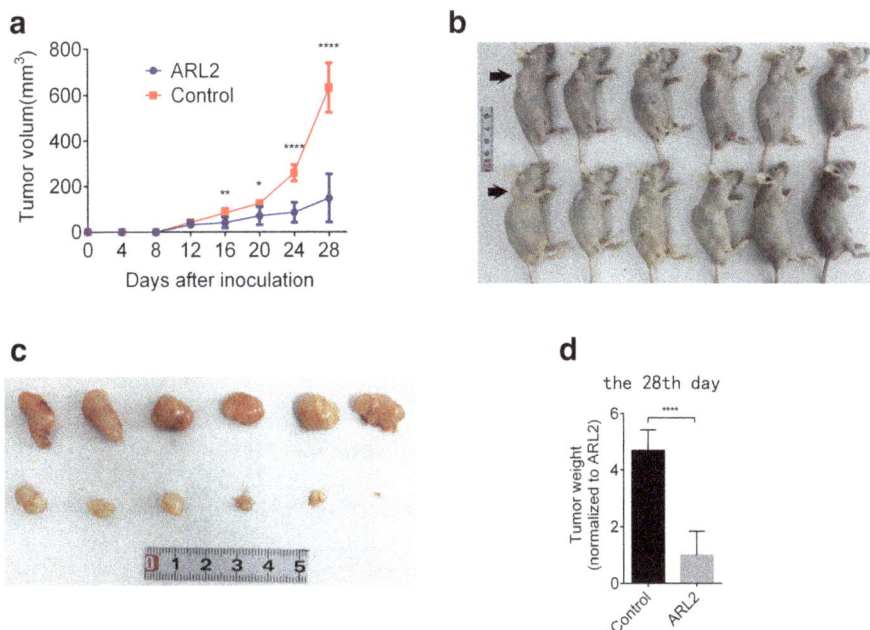

Fig. 3 ARL2 inhibits in vivo tumor formation capability of glioma cells. **a** The size analysis of subcutaneous tumors measured every four days from nude mice transduce with ARL2 overexpression or control vector transduced U87 cells. **b, c** Images of mice (**b**) and subcutaneous (**c**) tumors at 28th day after subcutaneous transplantation of ARL2 overexpression or control vector transduced U87 cells. **d** The weight of tumor from nude mice at 28th day after transplantation of U87 cells transduced with ARL2 overexpression or control vector

decrease in *AXL* mRNA expression (Additional file 6: Figure S6B, $P = 0.7087$). In addition, Ubibrowser (http://ubibrowser.ncpsb.org/) were applied to analyze the high confidence E3 ligases that interacted with AXL. The result showed that STUB1 was one of high confidence E3 ligases that interacted with AXL (Additional file 6: Figure S6C). Finally, TCGA data were used to investigate whether these genes were coexpressed with ARL2. The result showed that STUB1 was positively correlated to ARL2 expression (Additional file 6: Figure S6D). Altogether, these results indicated that ARL2 overexpression suppressed the expression of AXL and the activation of ERK in glioma cells.

AXL overexpression partially rescued the phenotype induced by ARL2 overexpression in U251 cells

To explore the physiological role of ARL2-AXL axis in glioma cells, we evaluated whether AXL overexpression rescue the phenotype induce by ARL2 overexpression in glioma cells. Therefore, we transduced ARL2 overexpression U251 cells with lentiviral AXL overexpression vector (Fig. 5a and b). As a result, the reduced in vitro cell growth and clone formation capabilities of U251 cells by ARL2 overexpression were partially restored by AXL overexpression (Fig. 5c and d). Consistently, we found that their inhibited migration and invasive abilities by ARL2 overexpression were also partially rescued by AXL overexpression, yet not completely (Fig. 5e and f).

Discussion

Microtubule network dynamics is crucial to the regulation of physiological processes like cell mitosis and migration. As a key regulator of microtubule, ARL2 has been implicated in several malignant tumors, such as breast cancer, cervical cancer, and pancreatic cancer [24, 26, 46]. But the pathophysiologic role and expression pattern of ARL2 in cancer is still controversial [23, 24], and the function of ARL2 in glioma remains unknown. In this study, we identified ARL2 expression pattern and its clinical significance in glioma. The downregulation of ARL2 implies the poor prognosis in glioma patients. Furthermore, our results confirmed that ARL2 reduced the growth, clone formation, migration and invasive abilities of glioma cells, as well as in vivo tumorigenicity. These data indicate a promising potential role of ARL2 in malignant glioma treatment.

Another novel finding in this study is that AXL expression is regulated by ARL2. AXL is a member of the TAM (TYRO3, AXL, MER) subfamily of receptor tyrosine kinases [47]. Earlier report and our previous works have described the function of AXL in regulating cell growth, migration and tumorigenesis of glioma [29, 45]. Our study provides the first evidence for the role of ARL2 upregulation in modifying AXL expression. To clarify the mechanism that ARL2 reduced the expression of AXL, qPCR was performed to detect *ARL2* and *AXL*

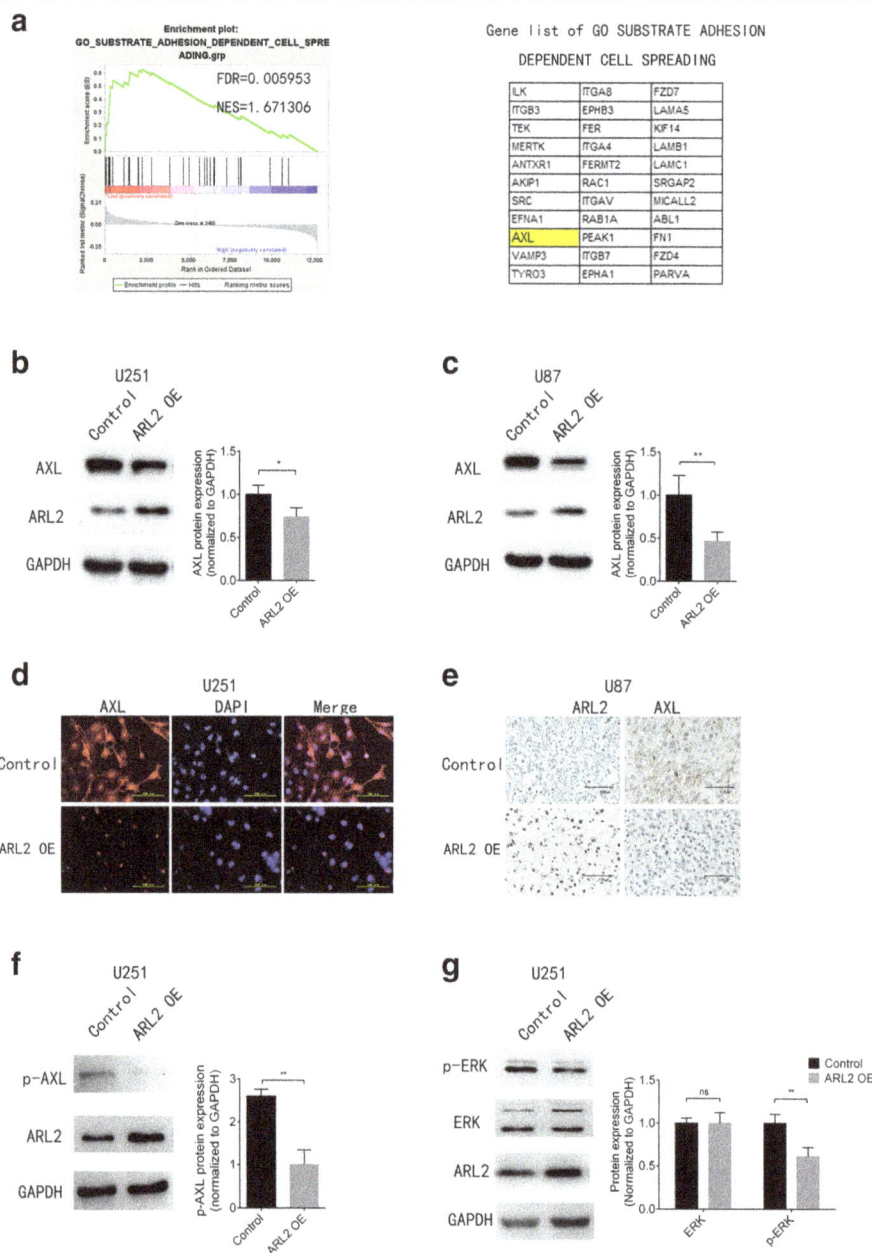

Fig. 4 ARL2 decreases AXL expression in glioma cells. **a** GSEA analysis showed that the expression of ARL2 is associated with substrate adhesion dependent cell spreading signaling pathway (33 genes were enriched and AXL was involved, http://www.broadinstitute.org/gsea/index.jsp). The normalized enrichment scores (NES) and the p values are shown in the plot. **b, c** Representative images and analysis of western blot demonstrated that ARL2 overexpression decreased AXL protein expression in U251 (**b**) and U87 (**c**) cells. (U251, $P = 0.038$, $n = 3$; U87, $P = 0.0053$; $n = 4$, t test). **d** Representative images of immunocytochemistry showed that ARL2 overexpression decreased AXL expression. **e** The IHC staining of U87 xenograft confirmed that AXL expression decreased after ARL2 overexpression. Scale bar = 100 μm. **f** ARL2 overexpression decreased phospho-AXL protein expression in U251 cells ($P = 0.0018$, $n = 3$, t test). **g** ARL2 overexpression inhibited phospho-ERK expression (total ERK, $P = 0.9975$; phospho-ERK, $P = 0.0019$, $n = 4$, t test)

mRNA level in U251 cells after ARL2 overexpression. The result showed that *ARL2* overexpression didn't lead to significant decrease in *AXL* mRNA expression. Therefore, we concluded that ARL2 might regulate AXL expression through post-transcriptional mechanism. Previous studies showed that Ras family members like

Rab35, Rac1, Cdc42 and Rnd3 mediate ubiquitin modification [48–50]. Based on these observations, we used Ubibrowser to analyze the high confidence E3 ligases that interacted with AXL. We also applied TCGA data to explore whether these genes were coexpressed with ARL2. The result showed that STUB1 was not only one

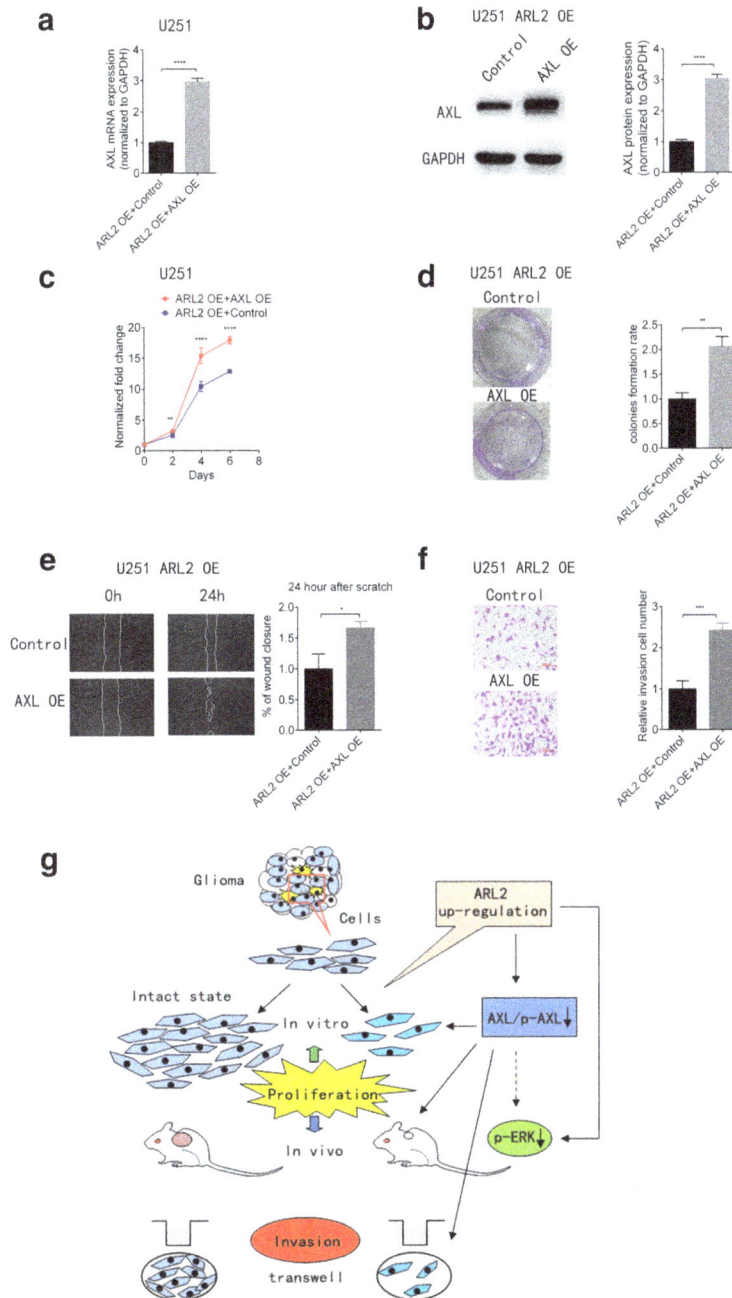

Fig. 5 AXL overexpression partially restores the phenotype change induced by ARL2 overexpression. **a** qPCR analyses of AXL in U251 cells transduced with lentiviral ARL2 overexpression vector together with AXL overexpression or control vector. ($P < 0.0001$, $n = 3$, t test). **b** Western blot images and analyses of AXL in U251 glioma cells transduced with lentiviral ARL2 overexpression vector together with AXL overexpression or control vector. ($P < 0.0001$, $n = 3$, t test). **c** In vitro growth assay showed that the inhibition of U251 proliferation induced by ARL overexpression could be partly rescued by AXL overexpression. (Day 2,$P = 0.0055$;Day 4,$P < 0.0001$; Day 6, $P < 0.0001$; $n = 6$, t test). **d** Colony formation assay revealed that the inhibition of clone formation capabilities in U251 cells induced by ARL2 overexpression could be partially rescued by AXL overexpression. (1000 cells/well, $P < 0.001$, $n = 3$, t test). **e** Wound healing test showed that the inhibition of migration capabilities in U251 cells induced by ARL2 overexpression could be partially rescued by AXL overexpression. ($P < 0.01$, $n = 3$, t test). **f** Transwell assay confirmed that AXL overexpression can partially rescued the invasion capability inhibition in U251 cells induced by ARL2 overexpression. Scale bar, 100 μm. ($P < 0.01$, $n = 3$, t test). **g** The diagram illustrated that ARL2 up-regulation decreased the capabilities of proliferation, invasion and tumorigenesis via inhibiting the expression of AXL in glioma cells

of high confidence E3 ligases that interacted with AXL, but also positively correlated to ARL2 expression. Taken together, these results indicate that ubiquitination and degradation may be a possible mechanism how ARL2 regulate AXL expression. Further studies are needed to fully elucidate the detail mechanism of ARL2-AXL axis. In addition, the restoration of AXL by exogenous expression did not fully rescue the defects in U251 glioma cells caused by ARL2 overexpression, which suggested that there might be additional molecular downstream targets associated with ARL2 overexpression.

Conclusion

In conclusion, this study described the downregulation of ARL2 in clinical glioma samples and its clinical relevance to poor prognosis in glioma patients. Secondly, this study provided the evidence that elevated ARL2 expression in glioma cell lines inhibits the abilities of proliferation, clone formation, migration and invasion. Thirdly, we demonstrated that ARL2 was associated with the regulation of tumorigenicity of glioma cells in vivo. Finally, it was proved in this study that ARL2 regulated AXL expression and activated phospho-ERK in glioma. Altogether, our data suggest that ARL2 serves as an important suppressor for the proliferation, migration and tumorigenicity of glioma cells by regulating the expression of AXL. Therefore, it may conduct as a new prognostic and therapeutic target for glioma. Supplementary methods are available in Additional file 7.

Additional files

Additional file 1: Figure S1. The mRNA expression level of ARL family members in GBM and non-tumor samples from TCGA.

Additional file 2: Figure S2. ARL2 expression decreased in GBM.

Additional file 3: Figure S3. ARL2 overexpression increased the proportion of cells at G0/G1 phase and decreased the proportion of cells at S and G2/M phase.

Additional file 4: Figure S4. The relevant signaling pathway analysis showed that ARL2 expression was correlated with EGFR and AXL signaling.

Additional file 5: Figure S5. Western blot showed that ARL2 overexpression in U251 cells didn't affect the expression of total and phospho-form AKT.

Additional file 6: Figure S6. ARL2 overexpression didn't increase the expression of AXL mRNA.

Additional file 7: Supplementary Methods.

Abbreviations

ARF: ADP-ribosylation factor; ARL2: ADP ribosylation factor-like GTPase 2; BART: Binder of ADP-ribosylation factor-like two; CGGA: Chinese Glioma Genome Atlas; FPS: median progression-free survival; GSEA: Gene Set Enrichment Analysis; PP2A: Protein phosphatase 2A; STUB1: E3 ubiquitin-protein ligase CHIP; TCGA: The Cancer Genome Atlas

Acknowledgements

We thank all the members in Dr. Wu AH's lab for helpful discussion to our study.

Funding

This study was supported by Natural Science Foundation of China (grant no. 30901781, P. C.) and Liaoning Science and Technology Plan Projects (grant no. 2012225014, P. C., and no. 2012225070, Z. Z. G.). None of the funding bodies had a role in the design of this study and the collection, analysis, and interpretation of data and in the preparation of the manuscript.

Authors' contributions

YW and PC conceived and designed the study; YW, GG, WC, FS, and YJ performed the experiments and collected data; PC, ZG, and AW were responsible for the analysis and interpretation of data; PC, ZG, and AW drafted the manuscript; ZG and AW supervised the study and revised the manuscript. All authors read and approved the final manuscript.

Competing interests

The authors declare that they have no competing interests.

Author details

[1]Department of Neurosurgery, The First Hospital of China Medical University, 155 Nanjingbei Street, Heping, Shenyang, Liaoning 110001, People's Republic of China. [2]Department of Immunology, School of Basic Medical Science, China Medical University, Shenyang 110122, Liaoning, China.

References

1. Wen PY, Kesari S. Malignant gliomas in adults. N Engl J Med. 2008;359(5): 492–507.
2. Prados MD, Yung WK, Wen PY, Junck L, Cloughesy T, Fink K, Chang S, Robins HI, Dancey J, Kuhn J. Phase-1 trial of gefitinib and temozolomide in patients with malignant glioma: a north American brain tumor consortium study. Cancer Chemother Pharmacol. 2008;61(6):1059–67.
3. Fine HA. New strategies in glioblastoma: exploiting the new biology. Clin Cancer Res. 2015;21(9):1984–8.
4. Matozaki T, Nakanishi H, Takai Y. Small G-Protein networks: their crosstalk and signal cascades. Cell Signal. 2000;12(8):515–24.
5. Paduch M, Jelen F, Otlewski J. Structure of small G proteins and their regulators. Acta Biochim Pol. 2001;48(4):829–50.
6. Zhang F, Cheong JK. The renewed battle against RAS-mutant cancers. Cellular and molecular life sciences : CMLS. 2016;73(9):1845–58.
7. Stephen AG, Esposito D, Bagni RK, McCormick F. Dragging ras back in the ring. Cancer Cell. 2014;25(3):272–81.
8. Cox AD, Fesik SW, Kimmelman AC, Luo J, Der CJ. Drugging the undruggable RAS: mission possible? Nat Rev Drug Discov. 2014;13(11):828–51.
9. Clark J, Moore L, Krasinskas A, Way J, Battey J, Tamkun J, Kahn RA. Selective amplification of additional members of the ADP-ribosylation factor (ARF) family: cloning of additional human and Drosophila ARF-like genes. Proc Natl Acad Sci U S A. 1993;90(19):8952–6.
10. Bhamidipati A, Lewis SA, Cowan NJ. ADP ribosylation factor-like protein 2 (Arl2) regulates the interaction of tubulin-folding cofactor D with native tubulin. J Cell Biol. 2000;149(5):1087–96.
11. Newman LE, Zhou CJ, Mudigonda S, Mattheyses AL, Paradies E, Marobbio CM, Kahn RA. The ARL2 GTPase is required for mitochondrial morphology, motility, and maintenance of ATP levels. PLoS One. 2014;9(6):e99270.
12. Chen K, Koe CT, Xing ZB, Tian X, Rossi F, Wang C, Tang Q, Zong W, Hong WJ, Taneja R, et al. Arl2- and Msps-dependent microtubule growth governs asymmetric division. J Cell Biol. 2016;212(6):661–76.
13. Francis JW, Newman LE, Cunningham LA, Kahn RA, Trimer A. Consisting of the tubulin-specific chaperone D (TBCD), regulatory GTPase ARL2, and beta-tubulin is required for maintaining the microtubule network. J Biol Chem. 2017;292(10):4336–49.
14. Nithianantham S, Le S, Seto E, Jia W, Leary J, Corbett KD, Moore JK, Al-Bassam J. Tubulin cofactors and Arl2 are cage-like chaperones that regulate the soluble alphabeta-tubulin pool for microtubule dynamics. eLife. 2015;4: e08811.
15. Zhou C, Cunningham L, Marcus AI, Li Y, Kahn RA. Arl2 and Arl3 regulate different microtubule-dependent processes. Mol Biol Cell. 2006;17(5):2476–87.

16. Newman LE, Schiavon CR, Zhou C, Kahn RA. The abundance of the ARL2 GTPase and its GAP, ELMOD2, at mitochondria are modulated by the fusogenic activity of mitofusins and stressors. PLoS One. 2017;12(4): e0175164.

17. Ismail SA, Chen YX, Rusinova A, Chandra A, Bierbaum M, Gremer L, Triola G, Waldmann H, Bastiaens PI, Wittinghofer A. Arl2-GTP and Arl3-GTP regulate a GDI-like transport system for farnesylated cargo. Nat Chem Biol. 2011;7(12): 942–9.

18. Muromoto R, Sekine Y, Imoto S, Ikeda O, Okayama T, Sato N, Matsuda T. BART is essential for nuclear retention of STAT3. Int Immunol. 2008;20(3): 395–403.

19. Zhang T, Li S, Zhang Y, Zhong C, Lai Z, Ding J. Crystal structure of the ARL2-GTP-BART complex reveals a novel recognition and binding mode of small GTPase with effector. Structure. 2009;17(4):602–10.

20. Bailey LK, Campbell LJ, Evetts KA, Littlefield K, Rajendra E, Nietlispach D, Owen D, Mott HR. The structure of binder of Arl2 (BART) reveals a novel G protein binding domain: implications for function. J Biol Chem. 2009;284(2):992–9.

21. Zhou Y, Jiang H, Gu J, Tang Y, Shen N, Jin Y. MicroRNA-195 targets ADP-ribosylation factor-like protein 2 to induce apoptosis in human embryonic stem cell-derived neural progenitor cells. Cell Death Dis. 2013;4:e695.

22. Beghin A, Honore S, Messana C, Matera EL, Aim J, Burlinchon S, Braguer D, Dumontet C. ADP ribosylation factor like 2 (Arl2) protein influences microtubule dynamics in breast cancer cells. Exp Cell Res. 2007;313(3):473–85.

23. Hass HG, Vogel U, Scheurlen M, Jobst J. Gene-expression analysis identifies specific patterns of dysregulated molecular pathways and genetic subgroups of human hepatocellular carcinoma. Anticancer Res. 2016;36(10):5087–95.

24. Peng R, Men J, Ma R, Wang Q, Wang Y, Sun Y, Ren J. miR-214 down-regulates ARL2 and suppresses growth and invasion of cervical cancer cells. Biochem Biophys Res Commun. 2017;484(3):623–30.

25. Beghin A, Belin S, Hage-Sleiman R, Brunet Manquat S, Goddard S, Tabone E, Jordheim LP, Treilleux I, Poupon MF, Diaz JJ, et al. ADP ribosylation factor like 2 (Arl2) regulates breast tumor aggressivity in immunodeficient mice. PLoS One. 2009;4(10):e7478.

26. Beghin A, Matera EL, Brunet-Manquat S, Dumontet C. Expression of Arl2 is associated with p53 localization and chemosensitivity in a breast cancer cell line. Cell Cycle. 2008;7(19):3074–82.

27. Wang K, Li P, Dong Y, Cai X, Hou D, Guo J, Yin Y, Zhang Y, Li J, Liang H, et al. A microarray-based approach identifies ADP ribosylation factor-like protein 2 as a target of microRNA-16. J Biol Chem. 2011;286(11):9468–76.

28. Gioia R, Leroy C, Drullion C, Lagarde V, Etienne G, Dulucq S, Lippert E, Roche S, Mahon FX, Pasquet JM. Quantitative phosphoproteomics revealed interplay between Syk and Lyn in the resistance to nilotinib in chronic myeloid leukemia cells. Blood. 2011;118(8):2211–21.

29. Cheng P, Phillips E, Kim SH, Taylor D, Hielscher T, Puccio L, Hjelmeland AB, Lichter P, Nakano I, Goidts V. Kinome-wide shRNA screen identifies the receptor tyrosine kinase AXL as a key regulator for mesenchymal glioblastoma stem-like cells. Stem cell reports. 2015;4(5):899–913.

30. Cheng P, Wang J, Waghmare I, Sartini S, Coviello V, Zhang Z, Kim SH, Mohyeldin A, Pavlyukov MS, Minata M, et al. FOXD1-ALDH1A3 signaling is a determinant for the self-renewal and Tumorigenicity of mesenchymal glioma stem cells. Cancer Res. 2016;76(24):7219–30.

31. Sun L, Hui AM, Su Q, Vortmeyer A, Kotliarov Y, Pastorino S, Passaniti A, Menon J, Walling J, Bailey R, et al. Neuronal and glioma-derived stem cell factor induces angiogenesis within the brain. Cancer Cell. 2006;9(4):287–300.

32. Griesinger AM, Birks DK, Donson AM, Amani V, Hoffman LM, Waziri A, Wang M, Handler MH, Foreman NK. Characterization of distinct immunophenotypes across pediatric brain tumor types. J Immunol. 2013;191(9):4880–8.

33. Cheng W, Zhang C, Ren X, Jiang Y, Han S, Liu Y, Cai J, Li M, Wang K, Liu Y, et al. Bioinformatic analyses reveal a distinct notch activation induced by STAT3 phosphorylation in the mesenchymal subtype of glioblastoma. J Neurosurg. 2017;126(1):249–59.

34. Subramanian A, Tamayo P, Mootha VK, Mukherjee S, Ebert BL, Gillette MA, Paulovich A, Pomeroy SL, Golub TR, Lander ES, et al. Gene set enrichment analysis: a knowledge-based approach for interpreting genome-wide expression profiles. Proc Natl Acad Sci U S A. 2005;102(43):15545–50.

35. Cheng W, Li M, Jiang Y, Zhang C, Cai J, Wang K, Wu A. Association between small heat shock protein B11 and the prognostic value of MGMT promoter methylation in patients with high-grade glioma. J Neurosurg. 2016;125(1):7–16.

36. Jiang T, Mao Y, Ma W, Mao Q, You Y, Yang X, Jiang C, Kang C, Li X, Chen L, et al. CGCG clinical practice guidelines for the management of adult diffuse gliomas. Cancer Lett. 2016;375(2):263–73.

37. Cormier N, Yeo A, Fiorentino E, Paxson J. Optimization of the wound scratch assay to detect changes in murine mesenchymal stromal cell migration after damage by soluble cigarette smoke extract. J Vis Exp. 2015;106:e53414.

38. Chen J, Tang J, Chen W, Gao Y, He Y, Zhang Q, Ran Q, Cao F, Yao S. Effects of syndecan-1 on the expression of syntenin and the migration of U251 glioma cells. Oncol Lett. 2017;14(6):7217–24.

39. Wu WS, Chien CC, Liu KH, Chen YC, Chiu WT. Evodiamine prevents glioma growth, induces glioblastoma cell apoptosis and cell cycle arrest through JNK activation. Am J Chin Med. 2017;45(4):879–99.

40. Xu X, Cai N, Zhi T, Bao Z, Wang D, Liu Y, Jiang K, Fan L, Ji J, Liu N. MicroRNA-1179 inhibits glioblastoma cell proliferation and cell cycle progression via directly targeting E2F transcription factor 5. Am J Cancer Res. 2017;7(8):1680–92.

41. Naito S, von Eschenbach AC, Giavazzi R, Fidler IJ. Growth and metastasis of tumor cells isolated from a human renal cell carcinoma implanted into different organs of nude mice. Cancer Res. 1986;46(8):4109–15.

42. Guo G, Gong K, Ali S, Ali N, Shallwani S, Hatanpaa KJ, Pan E, Mickey B, Burma S, Wang DH, et al. A TNF-JNK-Axl-ERK signaling axis mediates primary resistance to EGFR inhibition in glioblastoma. Nat Neurosci. 2017;20(8):1074–84.

43. Zhang Z, Lee JC, Lin L, Olivas V, Au V, LaFramboise T, Abdel-Rahman M, Wang X, Levine AD, Rho JK, et al. Activation of the AXL kinase causes resistance to EGFR-targeted therapy in lung cancer. Nat Genet. 2012; 44(8):852–60.

44. Brand TM, Iida M, Corrigan KL, Braverman CM, Coan JP, Flanigan BG, Stein AP, Salgia R, Rolff J, Kimple RJ, et al. The receptor tyrosine kinase AXL mediates nuclear translocation of the epidermal growth factor receptor. Sci Signal. 2017;10(460):eaag1064.

45. Vajkoczy P, Knyazev P, Kunkel A, Capelle HH, Behrndt S, von Tengg-Kobligk H, Kiessling F, Eichelsbacher U, Essig M, Read TA, et al. Dominant-negative inhibition of the Axl receptor tyrosine kinase suppresses brain tumor cell growth and invasion and prolongs survival. Proc Natl Acad Sci U S A. 2006; 103(15):5799–804.

46. Taniuchi K, Nishimori I, Hollingsworth MA. Intracellular CD24 inhibits cell invasion by posttranscriptional regulation of BART through interaction with G3BP. Cancer Res. 2011;71(3):895–905.

47. O'Bryan JP, Frye RA, Cogswell PC, Neubauer A, Kitch B, Prokop C, Espinosa R 3rd, Le Beau MM, Earp HS, Liu ET. Axl, a transforming gene isolated from primary human myeloid leukemia cells, encodes a novel receptor tyrosine kinase. Mol Cell Biol. 1991;11(10):5016–31.

48. Minowa-Nozawa A, Nozawa T, Okamoto-Furuta K, Kohda H, Nakagawa I. Rab35 GTPase recruits NPD52 to autophagy targets. EMBO J. 2017;36(18):2790–807.

49. Ma J, Xue Y, Liu W, Yue C, Bi F, Xu J, Zhang J, Li Y, Zhong C, Chen Y. Role of activated Rac1/Cdc42 in mediating endothelial cell proliferation and tumor angiogenesis in breast cancer. PLoS One. 2013;8(6):e66275.

50. Liu B, Dong H, Lin X, Yang X, Yue X, Yang J, Li Y, Wu L, Zhu X, Zhang S, et al. RND3 promotes snail 1 protein degradation and inhibits glioblastoma cell migration and invasion. Oncotarget. 2016;7(50):82411–23.

Permissions

All chapters in this book were first published in CANCER, by BioMed Central; hereby published with permission under the Creative Commons Attribution License or equivalent. Every chapter published in this book has been scrutinized by our experts. Their significance has been extensively debated. The topics covered herein carry significant findings which will fuel the growth of the discipline. They may even be implemented as practical applications or may be referred to as a beginning point for another development.

The contributors of this book come from diverse backgrounds, making this book a truly international effort. This book will bring forth new frontiers with its revolutionizing research information and detailed analysis of the nascent developments around the world.

We would like to thank all the contributing authors for lending their expertise to make the book truly unique. They have played a crucial role in the development of this book. Without their invaluable contributions this book wouldn't have been possible. They have made vital efforts to compile up to date information on the varied aspects of this subject to make this book a valuable addition to the collection of many professionals and students.

This book was conceptualized with the vision of imparting up-to-date information and advanced data in this field. To ensure the same, a matchless editorial board was set up. Every individual on the board went through rigorous rounds of assessment to prove their worth. After which they invested a large part of their time researching and compiling the most relevant data for our readers.

The editorial board has been involved in producing this book since its inception. They have spent rigorous hours researching and exploring the diverse topics which have resulted in the successful publishing of this book. They have passed on their knowledge of decades through this book. To expedite this challenging task, the publisher supported the team at every step. A small team of assistant editors was also appointed to further simplify the editing procedure and attain best results for the readers.

Apart from the editorial board, the designing team has also invested a significant amount of their time in understanding the subject and creating the most relevant covers. They scrutinized every image to scout for the most suitable representation of the subject and create an appropriate cover for the book.

The publishing team has been an ardent support to the editorial, designing and production team. Their endless efforts to recruit the best for this project, has resulted in the accomplishment of this book. They are a veteran in the field of academics and their pool of knowledge is as vast as their experience in printing. Their expertise and guidance has proved useful at every step. Their uncompromising quality standards have made this book an exceptional effort. Their encouragement from time to time has been an inspiration for everyone.

The publisher and the editorial board hope that this book will prove to be a valuable piece of knowledge for researchers, students, practitioners and scholars across the globe.

List of Contributors

Anja Frömberg and Achim Aigner
Rudolf-Boehm-Institute for Pharmacology and Toxicology, Clinical Pharmacology, University of Leipzig, Haertelstrasse 16 – 18, D-04107 Leipzig, Germany

Michael Rabe
Present address: Deptartment of Pediatrics, University Clinic Heidelberg, Heidelberg, Germany

Henry Oppermann and Frank Gaunitz
Department of Neurosurgery, University Hospital Leipzig, Leipzig, Germany

Tanja Eisemann, Barbara Costa and Peter Angel
Division of Signal Transduction and Growth Control, DKFZ/ZMBH Alliance, Heidelberg, Germany

Jens Strelau
Functional Neuroanatomy, University of Heidelberg, Heidelberg, Germany

Michel Mittelbronn
Institute of Neurology (Edinger-Institute), University Hospital Frankfurt, Goethe University, Frankfurt, Germany
Luxembourg Centre of Neuropathology (LCNP), Dudelange, Luxembourg
Laboratoire National de Santé, Dudelange, Luxembourg
Luxembourg Centre for Systems Biomedicine (LCSB), University of Luxembourg, Esch-sur-Alzette, Luxembourg
Department of Oncology, NORLUX Neuro-Oncology Laboratory, Luxembourg Institute of Health (L.I.H.), Strassen, Luxembourg

Heike Peterziel
Division of Signal Transduction and Growth Control, DKFZ/ZMBH Alliance, Heidelberg, Germany
Present address: Translational Program, Hopp Children's Cancer Center at NCT Heidelberg (KiTZ), University Hospital and DKFZ Heidelberg, Heidelberg Germany
Present address: Clinical Cooperation Unit Pediatric Oncology, DKFZ, Heidelberg, Germany
German Consortium for Translational Cancer Research (DKTK), Heidelberg, Germany

Ravi S. Narayan, Carlos A. Fedrigo, Eelke Brands, Rogier Dik, Ben J. Slotman and Peter Sminia
Department of Radiation Oncology, VU University Medical Center/Cancer Center Amsterdam, Amsterdam 1007, MB, The Netherlands

Lukas J.A. Stalpers
Department of Radiation Oncology, Academic Medical Center, Amsterdam, The Netherlands

Brigitta G. Baumert
Clinical Cooperation Unit Neurooncology, MediClin Robert Janker Klinik and University of Bonn Medical Center, Bonn, Germany
Department of Radiation Oncology, Maastro Clinic, Maastricht, The Netherlands

Bart A. Westerman
Department of Neurosurgery, Neuro Oncology Research Group, VU University Medical Center, Amsterdam, The Netherlands

Godefridus J. Peters
Department of Medical Oncology, VU University Medical Center, Amsterdam, The Netherlands

Xiaoyu Ji, Qiong Zhan, Xinli Zhou and Xiaohua Liang
Department of oncology, Huashan Hospital Fudan University, Shanghai 200040, China

Yingjie Zhuang and Xiangye Yin
Company 4, Battalion 1, Cadet Brigade 1, Fourth Military Medical University, Xi'an 710032, China

Chia-Hsin Chang, Wei-Ting Liu, Hui-Chi Hung and Chun-Lin Su
Department of Pharmacology, College of Medicine, National Cheng Kung University, Tainan, Taiwan

Chia-Yu Gean and Hong-Ming Tsai
Department of Diagnostic Radiology, National Cheng Kung University Hospital, Tainan, Taiwan

Po-Wu Gean
Department of Pharmacology, College of Medicine, National Cheng Kung University, Tainan, Taiwan
Department of Biotechnology and Bioindustry Sciences, College of Bioscience and Biotechnology, National Cheng Kung University, Tainan, Taiwan

Stephen Shannon, Dongxuan Jia, Ildiko Entersz, Paul Beelen, Christian Carcione, Jonathan Carcione, Aria Mahtabfar, Connan Vaca, Michael Weaver and Ramsey A. Foty
Department of Surgery-Rutgers Robert Wood Johnson Medical School, Clinical Academic Building, 125 Paterson Street, New Brunswick, NJ 08901, USA

David Shreiber and Jeffrey D. Zahn
Rutgers-Department of Biomedical Engineering, 599 Taylor Road, Piscataway, NJ 08854, USA

Hao Lin and Miao Yu
Rutgers-Department of Mechanical and Aerospace Engineering, 98 Brett Rd, Piscataway Township, NJ 08854, USA

Liping Liu
Rutgers-Department of Mechanical and Aerospace Engineering, 98 Brett Rd, Piscataway Township, NJ 08854, USA
Rutgers-Department of Mathematics, 110 Frelinghuysen Rd, Piscataway, NJ 08854, USA

Suhas Vasaikar, Giorgos Tsipras, Natalia Landázuri and Mingmei Shang
Unit of Computational Medicine, Center for Molecular Medicine, Department of Medicine, Karolinska Institutet, Stockholm, Sweden

Helena Costa, Vanessa Wilhelmi, Patrick Scicluna, Huanhuan L. Cui, Abdul-Aleem Mohammad, Belghis Davoudi, Sharan Ananthaseshan, Afsar Rahbar, Koon-Chu Yaiw and Cecilia Söderberg-Naucler
Cell and Molecular Immunology, Experimental Cardiovascular Unit, Departments of Medicine and Neurology, Center for Molecular Medicine, Karolinska Institutet, SE-171 76 Stockholm, Sweden

Klas Stråål
Department of Cell and Molecular Biology, Karolinska Institutet, Stockholm, Sweden

Giuseppe Stragliotto
Department of Neurosurgery, Karolinska University Hospital, Stockholm, Sweden

Kum Thong Wong
Department of Pathology, University of Malaya, Kuala Lumpur, Malaysia

Jesper Tegner
Unit of Computational Medicine, Center for Molecular Medicine, Department of Medicine, Karolinska Institutet, Stockholm, Sweden
Biological and Environmental Sciences and Engineering Division (BESE), Computer, Electrical and Mathematical Sciences and Engineering Division (CEMSE), King Abdullah University of Science and Technology (KAUST), Thuwal 23955–6900, Kingdom of Saudi Arabia

Min-joo Ahn and Kanghan Lee
Departments of Internal Medicine, Chonnam National University Medical School, Gwangju 501-757, South Korea

Kyung Hwa Lee
Departments of Pathology, Chonnam National University Medical School, Gwangju 501-757, South Korea

Jin Woong Kim
Departments of Radiology, Chonnam National University Medical School, Gwangju 501-757, South Korea

In-Young Kim
Departments of Neurosurgery, Chonnam National University Medical School, Gwangju 501-757, South Korea
Chonnam National University Hwasun Hospital, 160 Ilsim-ri, Hwasun-eup, Hwasun-gun 519-809, South Korea

Woo Kyun Bae
Departments of Internal Medicine, Chonnam National University Medical School, Gwangju 501-757, South Korea
Chonnam National University Hwasun Hospital, 160 Ilsim-ri, Hwasun-eup, Hwasun-gun 519-809, South Korea

Shang-Yu Chou
Departments of Radiation Oncology, Kaohsiung Chang Gung Memorial Hospital, 123 Ta-Pei Road, Niao-Song Dist, Kaohsiung City 83301, Taiwan

Eng-Yen Huang
Departments of Radiation Oncology, Kaohsiung Chang Gung Memorial Hospital, 123 Ta-Pei Road, Niao-Song Dist, Kaohsiung City 83301, Taiwan
Department of Radiation Oncology, Xiamen Chang Gung Hospital, No. 123, Xiafei Rd., Haicang District, Fujian, China
School of Traditional Chinese Medicine, Chang Gung University College of Medicine, No. 259, Wenhua 1st Rd., Guishan Dist., Taoyuan City, Taiwan
Department of Radiation Oncology, Kaohsiung Chang Gung Memorial Hospital, 123 Ta-Pei Road, Niao-Song Dist, Kaohsiung City 83301, Taiwan

Chao-Cheng Huang
Department of Pathology, Kaohsiung Chang Gung Memorial Hospital, Chang Gung University College of Medicine, Hospital, 123 Ta-Pei Road, Niao-Song Dist, Kaohsiung City 83301, Taiwan
School of Traditional Chinese Medicine, Chang Gung University College of Medicine, No. 259, Wenhua 1st Rd., Guishan Dist., Taoyuan City, Taiwan

Shao-Lun Yen
Department of Pathology, An Nan Hospital, China Medical University, No. 66, Sec.2, Changhe Road, Annan Dist, Tainan City 709, Taiwan

Altay Burak Dalan
Department of Biochemistry, Yeditepe University Medical School, Istanbul, Turkey

Sukru Gulluoglu and Emre Can Tuysuz
Department of Medical Genetics, Yeditepe University Medical School, Istanbul, Turkey
Department of Biotechnology, Institute of Science, Yeditepe University, Istanbul, Turkey

Aysegul Kuskucu
Department of Medical Genetics, Yeditepe University Medical School, Istanbul, Turkey

Cumhur Kaan Yaltirik and Ugur Ture
Department of Neurosurgery, Yeditepe University Medical School, Istanbul, Turkey

Oguz Ozturk
Department of Molecular Medicine, Capa School of Medicine, Istanbul University, Istanbul, Turkey

Omer Faruk Bayrak
Department of Medical Genetics, Yeditepe University Medical School, Istanbul, Turkey
Yeditepe Universitesi Hastanesi Genetik Tani Merkezi, Koftuncu Sokak Acıbadem mahallesi Istek Vakfi 3. Kat 34718 No: 57/1, Kadikoy, Istanbul, Turkey

Zachary C. Gersey, Gregor A. Rodriguez, Eric Barbarite, Anthony Sanchez, Winston M. Walters, Kelechi C. Ohaeto and Ricardo J. Komotar
Department of Neurosurgery, University of Miami Miller School of Medicine, Miami, Florida, USA

Regina M. Graham
Department of Neurosurgery, University of Miami Miller School of Medicine, Miami, Florida, USA
Department of Neurological Surgery, University of Miami Brain Tumor Initiative (UMBTI) Research Laboratory, Lois Pope LIFE Center, 2nd Floor, 1095 NW 14th Terrace, Miami, Florida 33136, USA

Lina Mörén and Henrik Antti
Department of Chemistry, Umeå University, SE 901 87 Umeå, Sweden

Richard Perryman, Julia K. Langer, Kevin Oneill and Nelofer Syed
John Fulcher Neuro-Oncology Laboratory, Imperial College London, London, UK

Tim Crook
St Luke's Cancer Centre, Royal Surrey County Hospital, Guildford, Surrey, UK

Myung-Giun Noh, Se-Jeong Oh, Jae-Hyuk Lee and Kyung-Hwa Lee
Department of Pathology, Chonnam National University Hwasun Hospital and Medical School, 322 Seoyang-ro, Hwasun-eup, Hwasun-gun, Jeollanam-do 519-763, South Korea

Eun-Jung Ahn, Yeong-Jin Kim, Tae-Young Jung, Shin Jung and Kyung-Sub Moon
Department of Neurosurgery, Chonnam National University Hwasun Hospital and Medical School, 322 Seoyang-ro, Hwasun-eup, Hwasun-gun, Jeollanam-do 519-763, South Korea

Kyung-Keun Kim
Medical Research Center of Gene Regulation and Center for Creative Biomedical Scientists, Chonnam National University Medical School, Gwangju, South Korea

Yi Li, Jun Li, Yijun Cai, Marie Chia-mi Lin and Wai Sang Poon
Brain Tumor Centre, Department of Surgery, The Chinese University of Hong Kong, Hong Kong, China

Yat Ming Woo
Department of Neurosurgery, Kwong Wah Hospital, Hong Kong, China

Zan Shen
Department of Oncology, Affiliated 6th People's Hospital, Shanghai Jiaotong University, Shanghai, China

Hong Yao
Jiangsu Eng. Lab of Cancer Biotherapy, Xuzhou Medical College, Xuzhou, China

Christoph Straube
Klinik für RadioOnkologie und Strahlentherapie, Technische Universität München (TUM), Ismaninger Straße 22, 81675 Munich, Germany
Deutsches Konsortium für Translationale Krebsforschung (DKTK) - Partner Site Munich, 81675 Munich, Germany

Hagen Scherb
Institute of Computational Biology, Helmholtz Zentrum München, Deutsches Forschungszentrum fuer Gesundheit und Umwelt (GmbH), Ingolstaedter Landstr.1, 85764 Neuherberg, Germany

Jens Gempt and Bernhard Meyer
Neurochirurgische Klinik und Poliklinik, Technische Universität München (TUM), Ismaninger Straße 22, 81675 Munich, Germany

Jan Kirschke and Claus Zimmer
Abteilung für diagnostische und interventionelle Neuroradiologie, Technische Universität München (TUM), Ismaninger Straße 22, 81675 Munich, Germany

Friederike Schmidt-Graf
Neurologische Klinik und Poliklinik, Technische Universität München (TUM), Ismaninger Straße 22, 81675 Munich, Germany

Stephanie E. Combs
Klinik für RadioOnkologie und Strahlentherapie, Technische Universität München (TUM), Ismaninger Straße 22, 81675 Munich, Germany
Institut für Innovative Radiotherapie (iRT), Department of Radiation Sciences (DRS), Helmholtz Zentrum München, Ingolstädter Landstraße 1, 85764 Neuherberg, Germany
Deutsches Konsortium für Translationale Krebsforschung (DKTK) - Partner Site Munich, 81675 Munich, Germany

Eduard H. Panosyan, Henry J. Lin and Joseph L. Lasky III
Los Angeles Biomedical Research Institute and Department of Pediatrics at Harbor-UCLA Medical Center, Box 468, 1000 W. Carson Street, N25, Torrance, CA 90509, USA

Jan Koster
Department of Oncogenomics, Academic Medical Center of the University of Amsterdam, Amsterdam, The Netherlands

Azeez A. Fatai and Junaid Gamieldien
South African Bioinformatics Institute and SAMRC Unit for Bioinformatics Capacity Development, University of the Western Cape, Bellville, 7535, 7530 Western Cape, South Africa

Sara L. Bristow
Department of Obstetrics and Gynecology, Northwell Health, Division of Reproductive Endocrinology, 300 Community Drive, Manhasset, NY 11030, USA

Alexandra Peyser and Avner Hershlag
Department of Obstetrics and Gynecology, Northwell Health, Division of Reproductive Endocrinology, 300 Community Drive, Manhasset, NY 11030, USA
Hofstra-Northwell School of Medicine, 500 Hofstra Blvd, Hempstead, NY 11549, USA

Marvin A. Böttcher and Arne Traulsen
Department Evolutionary Theory, Max Planck Institute for Evolutionary Biology, 24306 Plön, Germany

Janka Held-Feindt and Michael Synowitz
Department of Neurosurgery, University Medical Center Schleswig-Holstein UKSH, Campus Kiel, 24105 Kiel, Germany

Ralph Lucius and Kirsten Hattermann
Department of Anatomy, University of Kiel, 24098 Kiel, Germany

Elham Vosoughi, Jee Min Lee, James R. Miller, Mehdi Nosrati, David R. Minor, Roy Abendroth, John W. Lee, Brian T. Andrews, Lewis Z. Leng, Max Wu, Stanley P. Leong, Mohammed Kashani-Sabet and Kevin B. Kim
Center for Melanoma Research and Treatment, California Pacific Medical Center Research Institute, 2100 Webster Street, Suite 326, San Francisco, CA 94115, USA

Chanhee Lee, Seung Ah Choi, Seung-Ki Kim, Kyu-Chang Wang and Ji Hoon Phi
Division of Pediatric Neurosurgery, Seoul National University Children's Hospital, 101 Daehakro, Jongno-gu, 110-744 Seoul, Republic of Korea

Joongyub Lee
Medical Research Collaborating Center, Seoul National University Hospital, Seoul, South Korea

Sung-Hye Park
Department of Pathology, Seoul National University College of Medicine, Seoul, Republic of Korea

Se Hoon Kim
Department of Pathology, Yonsei University, College of Medicine, Severance Hospital, Seoul, Republic of Korea

Ji Yeoun Lee
Division of Pediatric Neurosurgery, Seoul National University Children's Hospital, 101 Daehakro, Jongno-gu, 110-744 Seoul, Republic of Korea
Department of Anatomy, Seoul National University College of Medicine, Seoul, South Korea

Wietske C. M. Schimmel and Eline Verhaak
Gamma Knife Centre Tilburg, Elisabeth TweeSteden Hospital, Hilvarenbeekseweg 60, 5022, GC, Tilburg, The Netherlands
Department of Cognitive Neuropsychology, Tilburg University, Warandelaan 2, 5037, AB, Tilburg, The Netherlands

Patrick E. J. Hanssens
Gamma Knife Centre Tilburg, Elisabeth TweeSteden Hospital, Hilvarenbeekseweg 60, 5022, GC, Tilburg, The Netherlands

Department Neurosurgery, Elisabeth-TweeSteden Hospital, Hilvarenbeekseweg 60, 5022, GC, Tilburg, The Netherlands

Karin Gehring
Gamma Knife Centre Tilburg, Elisabeth TweeSteden Hospital, Hilvarenbeekseweg 60, 5022, GC, Tilburg, The Netherlands
Department Neurosurgery, Elisabeth-TweeSteden Hospital, Hilvarenbeekseweg 60, 5022, GC, Tilburg, The Netherlands
Department of Cognitive Neuropsychology, Tilburg University, Warandelaan 2, 5037, AB, Tilburg, The Netherlands

Margriet M. Sitskoorn
Department Neurosurgery, Elisabeth-TweeSteden Hospital, Hilvarenbeekseweg 60, 5022, GC, Tilburg, The Netherlands

Department of Cognitive Neuropsychology, Tilburg University, Warandelaan 2, 5037, AB, Tilburg, The Netherlands

Yulin Wang, Gefei Guan, Wen Cheng, Yang Jiang, Anhua Wu, Peng Cheng and Zongze Guo
Department of Neurosurgery, The First Hospital of China Medical University, 155 Nanjingbei Street, Heping, Shenyang, Liaoning 110001, People's Republic of China

Fengping Shan
Department of Immunology, School of Basic Medical Science, China Medical University, Shenyang 110122, Liaoning, China

Index

www.ingramcontent.com/pod-product-compliance
Lightning Source LLC
Chambersburg PA
CBHW080530200326
41458CB00012B/4390